Medical Complications of Kidney Transplantation

Claudio Ponticelli MD FRCP(Ed)
Former Director, Division of Nephrology
IRCCSS Ospedale Maggiore
and
Consultant, Instituto Scientifico Auxologico
Milan
Italy

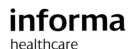
informa
healthcare

© 2007 Informa UK Ltd

First published in the United Kingdom in 2007 by Informa Healthcare, 4 Park Square, Milton Park, Abingdon, Oxon OX14 4RN. Informa Healthcare is a trading division of Informa UK Ltd. Registered Office, 37/41 Mortimer Street, London W1T 3JH. Registered in England and Wales Number 1072954.

Tel: +44 (0)20 7017 6000
Fax: +44 (0)20 7017 6336
E-mail: info.medicine@tandf.co.uk
Website: www.informahealthcare.com

Although every effort has been made to ensure that all owners of copyright material have been acknowledged in this publication, we would be glad to acknowledge in subsequent reprints or editions any omissions brought to our attention.

Although every effort has been made to ensure that drug doses and other information are presented accurately in this publication, the ultimate responsibility rests with the prescribing physician. Neither the publishers nor the authors can be held responsible for errors or for any consequences arising from the use of information contained herein. For detailed prescribing information or instructions on the use of any product or procedure discussed herein, please consult the prescribing information or instructional material issued by the manufacturer.

A CIP record for this book is available from the British Library.

Library of Congress Cataloging-in-Publication Data

Data available on application

ISBN 10 0 415 41715 5
ISBN 13 978 0 415 41715 0

Distributed in North and South America by

Taylor & Francis
6000 Broken Sound Parkway, NW (Suite 300)
Boca Raton, FL 33487, USA

Within Continental USA
Tel: 1(800)272 7737; Fax: 1(800) 374 3401
Outside Continental USA
Tel: (561) 994 0555; Fax: (561)361 6018
E-mail: orders@crcpress.com

Distributed in the rest of the world by
Thomson Publishing Services
Cheriton House
North Way
Andover, Hampshire SP10 5BE, UK
Tel: +44 (0)1264 332424
E-mail: tps.tandfsalesorder@thomson.com

Composition by C&M Digitals (P) Ltd, Chennai, India
Printed and bound by Replika Press Pvt Ltd

CONTENTS

PREFACE

Today kidney transplantation is considered to be the treatment of choice for most patients with end stage renal disease. Yet, in spite of the tremenous advances in immunosuppressive and supportive therapies, the task of transplant clinicians remains very difficult as the morbidity related to kidney transplantation may encompass almost all branches of internal medicine. On the other hand, the recent introduction of newer immunosuppressive drugs and supportive treatments as well as the discovery of new complications that may affect the transplant recipients has considerably modified the results and the clinical scenario of kidney transplantation in the last few years.

This book is designed to acquaint the clinicians with the most frequent problems that may occur after renal transplantation. The typology of the kidney donor and the transplant recipient, which has considerably changed in the recent period, is covered in the first two chapters of the book. Five chapters are focused on the kidney allograft complications and include delayed graft function, acute rejection, chronic allograft nephropathy, recurrent primary diseases and de novo renal diseases. A special chapter is devoted to the toxicity of the currently available immunosuppressive drugs. Three large chapters deal with the most worrying extra-renal complications that may affect the kidney transplant recipient, namely infection, cardiovascular disease and malignancy. The remaining chapters describe the many disorders that may affect the different organs and systems, so impairing the quality of life expectancy of a renal transplant recipient.

It is my hope that the compilation of this material into one volume may be useful to clinicians who are treating renal transplant patients in their daily practice. Appropriate illustrative material and tables have been generously provided. Someone may criticize the fact that this monograph has been written by a single author. This should not be interpreted as a sin of presumption but as an attempt to avoiding discrepancies or conflicting views among different co-authors in a complicated area as renal transplantation is.

I have to acknowledge that the preparation of this monograph would have been impossible without the collaboration of the many doctors, nurses, and patients who lived with me a long fight against renal disease. I wish to deeply thank all of them. A special thought to Antonio Tarantino a skilful clinician who spent most of his professional life in the care of renal transplant patients, and to my other colleagues involved in kidney transplantation Giuseppe Montagnino, Adriana Aroldi, Maria Rosaria Campise, Patrizia Passerini. My gratitude goes to Antonio Vegeto, Luisa Berardinelli and their surgical team for their excellent collaboration. Particular thanks to Giovanni Banfi, a great expert of clinical nephrology and renal histology, who provided most of the figures of the book.

CP

1 SELECTION AND PREPARATION OF THE DONOR

Renal transplantation represents the treatment of choice for many patients with advanced renal failure. When compared with dialysis, a successful renal transplant not only offers improved quality of life (Keown, 2001), better social rehabilitation (Matas et al., 1996), and less economic cost, even in high-risk patients (Whiting et al., 1998, 2000), but also allows a longer life expectancy. By reviewing the mortality of 23 275 first cadaver renal transplant recipients and 46 164 wait-listed dialysis patients, Wolfe et al. (1999) calculated that the relative risk of death during the first 2 weeks after transplantation was 2.84 times as high as that for patients on dialysis who had equal lengths of follow-up since placement on the waiting list, but at 18 months the risk was much lower, the relative risk being 0.32. The long-term mortality rate was 48–82% lower among transplant recipients. Even transplantation of a marginal kidney is associated with a significant survival benefit when compared with maintenance dialysis (Ojo et al., 2001).

As kidney transplantation becomes more and more successful, however, the indications are widening, and the supply of organ donors must be expanded to address the rapidly and continuously growing demand for the large number of patients on the waiting list. In the USA there were over 80 000 patients waiting for an organ at the end of 2004, over 4000 more than at the end of 2003 (Port et al., 2006). Strategies for increasing the number of cadaver donors include better medical organization, educational programs, and the use of marginal and non-heart-beating donors. In the USA this led to an increase in deceased donation of 11% in 2004 (Marks et al., 2006). The utilization of related and unrelated living donors is also increasing. In the past, only parents or siblings of the recipients were considered for living donation. More recently, however, the number of living-unrelated donors has increased. The excellent results obtained using 'unconventional' donors, including spouses, distant relatives, and even friends (Cecka, 1999), has produced a huge increase in the number of living-unrelated donor transplants. In 2001, for the first time, the number of living donors exceeded the number of cadaver donors in the United States (Danovitch and Cecka, 2003).

Cadaver donation

Heart-beating cadaver donors

The large majority of cadaver transplanted kidneys are removed from brain-dead donors with a functional circulation. However, despite the legal and religious acceptance of brain death, many potential donors are not recognized, and many families refuse to donate. Hou (2000) reported that in the USA, 4755 potential donors were lost because of the refusal of families: a number that would close 81% of the gap between the yearly demand and the available kidneys. Thus, there is a considerable need for more education and training in how to inform and support donor relatives. Other problems which make it difficult to convert potential donors into actual donors are the limitations of medical organizations, the societal environment, and different criteria for accepting cadaver donors. The number of cadaver donors per million population varies throughout the world, but no country seems to realize its full potential of cadaver renal donors (Table 1.1). For example, it has been calculated that of 62 500 patients on the waiting list for kidney transplantation in July 2005, only about a quarter of them would receive a transplant within a year, in at least 50% of cases from a living donor (Steinbrook, 2005). Even in Spain, the most active nation in recruiting cadaver donors for organ transplantation, in 2004 the number of cadaver donors utilized for kidney transplantation was 49 per million population (IRODaT, 2005), clearly lower than the expected number of new entries in dialysis, which now ranges around 315 per million population in developed countries (US Renal Data System, 2001).

Table 1.1 Number of cadaver kidneys per million population (pmp) transplanted in 2004. Countries with <1 cadaver transplant per year are not included. Adapted from IRODaT, 2005

Country	Total (pmp)
Argentina	15.3
Australia	18.9
Austria	37.6
Belgium	35.5
Brazil	9.1
Canada	18.8
Chile	15.6
Croatia	21.6
Cyprus	21.4
Czech Republic	39.3
Denmark	25
Estonia	24
Finland	36.8
France	20.9
Greece	10.9
Hong Kong	6.4
Hungary	28.4
Iran	3.0
Israel	10.3
Italy	28.3
Latvia	30.9
Lithuania	16.7
Malta	15
Mexico	4.2
New Zealand	13.8
Poland	27.1
Portugal	39.5
Puerto Rico	14.5
Saudi Arabia	4.2
Slovak Republic	18.3
Slovenia	27.5
Spain	49.2
Sweden	25.5
Switzerland	22.6
Turkey	3.7
UK	24.3
USA	26.5
Uruguay	27.1
Venezuela	3.6

Table 1.2 Contraindications to cadaver kidney procurement

Absolute contraindications	Realtive contraindications (marginal kidneys)
Malignancies other than basal-cell carcinoma	Age over 75 years
Bacteremia due to vancomycin-resistant enterococci, *Streptococcus milleri*, *Salmonella*	Creatinine clearance < 60 ml/min
Fungal or nocardial sepsis	Severe hypertension
Varicella, West Nile virus	Proteinuria > 1 g per day
HIV infection	HBV or HCV positivity
Prolonged hypothermia	Diabetes mellitus

Until a few years ago, the majority of cadaver donors were young patients who had died from brain trauma. However, a decrease in motor vehicle accident deaths and the pressure to enlarge the donor pool have recently prompted the inclusion of increasingly older cadaver donors who have died from cerebrovascular complications. This has led to an increased proportion of cadaver donors older than age 50, from 12% in 1988 to 31% in 2000 in the USA (Rosendale and Dean, 2002). Moreover, there is a growing tendency to accept donors who previously would have been excluded, due to anatomic abnormalities, arterial hypertension, renal dysfunction, proteinuria, diabetes, prolonged cold ischemia time, infections, or poisoning.

Flexibility in accepting kidneys from '*marginal*' donors is increasing. It is possible that, compared with ideal cadaver donors, the acceptance of marginal donors might reduce the 5-year graft survival by 20% (Ojo et al., 2001) and also increase the economic cost (Whiting et al., 1998). On the other hand, even with the use of marginal donors, life expectancy is better (Ojo et al., 2006) and the economic cost is lower (Whiting et al., 2000) than those associated with waiting in dialysis. Moreover, in spite of the older age of the donor and the increased proportion of donors with hypertension, cardiovascular disease, and surgical/radiological interventions before death, the 1-year graft survival and the mean serum creatinine level have improved for cadaver renal transplants performed recently in comparison with transplants performed in the early 1990s, when the age of the donor was younger and most donors died from cerebral trauma (Kyllonen et al., 2005).

Medical evaluation

Once the diagnosis of irreversible brain death has been established for the potential heart-beating cadaver donor, a general clinical evaluation is performed to identify underlying medical conditions that might contraindicate organ procurement, particularly sepsis or malignancies other than basal-cell skin cancers or neoplasms confined to above the tentorium. The evaluation of a cadaver organ donor includes a medical history, physical examination, and laboratory studies. The two main goals of donor evaluation are (1) to exclude donors with severe diseases that can be transmitted to the recipient and (2) to exclude kidneys with severe anatomic or functional changes that could compromise the allograft function. Although today there is a tendency to be more flexible than in the past in accepting suboptimal cadaver donors, whether to accept or reject kidneys from a marginal donor can be a difficult decision in many instances (Table 1.2).

Presence of cancer

Since the ability to transmit cancer from donor to recipient through a transplanted kidney is well documented, donors with cancer should be excluded. Exceptions may be made for donors with *cutaneous basal-cell carcinomas* that do not tend to metastasize. Until recently, also *primary brain tumors* have not been considered as a contraindication to organ donation. However, certain tumors, such as glioblastoma

Table 1.3	Cadaver donor screening for hidden cancer
History	Previous neoplasias?
Radiology	Kidney ultrasonography
	Chest X-ray
Laboratory	Chorionic gonadotropin
	Prostate-specific antigen
Kidney	Careful inspection
	Removal and histologic investigation of any small suspected tumors
Incidental discovery of extra-renal tumors at autopsy	Consider nephrectomy of transplanted kidney

multiforme, medulloblastoma (Kauffman et al., 2002a), and those that have been palliated by means of ventricular shunts, carry a high risk of transmission and should be avoided (Sheil, 2001). Of concern, the possibility of extra-brain spread of the tumor after transplantation has been documented with brain tumor donors even in the absence of the above-reported risk factors (Detry et al., 2000). Reports of donor-to-recipient transmission of choriocarcinoma (Penn, 1991; Doutrelepont et al., 1995) have led to the recommendation that chorionic gonadotropin be measured in all women of childbearing age who have died from a cerebral hemorrhage.

As the number of older donors is increasing, special attention should also be paid to exclude the presence of *prostate cancer*. In the author's experience, kidneys from a patient with prostate cancer revealed only at autopsy were transplanted to two women. The patients both asked to keep the kidney. After 5 years both of them are well, their allografts functioning without any sign of cancer, and with undetectable levels of prostatic antigen. It has been pointed out that transmission of a hidden cancer from an asymptomatic donor is a rare event (Kauffman et al., 2002b). However, fatal cases of the transfer of malignant *melanoma* from a multiorgan donor without a history or clinical evidence of melanoma have been reported (Stephens et al., 2000). Also of concern is the transmission of unrecognized *renal carcinoma*. Because of the relatively high incidence, ultrasound screening and immediate preparation of the kidney surface is recommended, particularly in donors older than 45 years. Microscopic examination of small lesions should be done before transplantation (Wunderlich et al., 2001). Recently, however, Buell et al. (2005) pointed out the possibility of transplanting a kidney with small renal-cell carcinomas. These investigators transplanted 14 kidneys (11 from living donors and three from deceased donors) in which an incidental cancer was found. The median size of the cancer was 4 cm (range 0.5–4.0 cm), and the margins were negative. The patient survival was 100% at 3 years and 93% at 5 years.

To minimize the risks of cancer transmission, a few guidelines should be followed (Table 1.3).

Presence of infection

The presence of *human immunodeficiency virus* (HIV) should preclude use of the organs of the potential donor, as transmission of the virus with the development of fatal infection in the recipient is well documented (Erice et al., 1991). Thus, screening for HIV antibodies in the donor is highly recommended. In children with brain death, it is important to exclude underlying *varicella virus* infection, which may be transmitted to the recipient and thereby introduce a high risk of fatal encephalitis. Serologic assays for latent viruses such as *cytomegalovirus and Epstein–Barr virus* are useful not for deciding whether to accept or refuse the donor, but for allocating the organ to or at least planning preventive strategies in the recipient (Rubin, 1994). *West Nile virus* can also be transmitted by organ transplantation (Iwamoto et al., 2003). Screening with a nucleic acid-based assay for West Nile virus may reduce the risk of this life-threatening infection.

Organs procured from *hepatitis B virus* (HBV)-infected donors may transmit the virus to their recipients. However, kidneys from HBs antigen (HBsAg)-positive donors who are negative for HBeAg carry a minimal risk of transmitting infection if recipients are immune to HBV or are HbsAg-positive (Natov and Pereira, 2002). No case of HBV positivity was seen in seven patients with anti-HBV antibodies treated with post-transplant lamividune after receiving a HBV+ kidney (Berber *et al.*, 2005). Whether or not to use the kidneys of donors who are HB surface-negative and HB core antibody-positive (HBcAb+) has been a matter of controversy until recently. By reviewing the data of cadaver transplants in the UNOS (United Network for Organ Sharing) registry between 1994 and 1999, Fong *et al.* (2002) found that neither donor nor recipient anti-HBcAb status influenced the risk of graft failure or patient death after adjustment for other factors. In an Italian retrospective study, none of 344 recipients of a kidney from anti-HBcAb+ donors developed clinical or biological signs of hepatitis. The patient and graft survival rates were similar to those observed in recipients of HBcAb– donors (De Feo *et al.*, 2006). Therefore, renal allografts from HBcAb+ donors may be considered for transplant. The transmission of *hepatitis C virus* (HCV) by infected donors has also been shown unequivocally (Pereira *et al.*, 1995), although with important differences among centers (Fabrizi *et al.*, 2001). However, since the transplantation of kidneys from HCV-positive donors to HCV-positive recipients is associated with 5-year patient and graft survival rates similar to those observed with HCV-negative donors to HCV-negative recipients (Morales *et al.*, 1995; Ali *et al.*, 1998), the use of HCV-positive donors without active liver disease for HCV-positive recipients with the same virus genotype might be justified. An even better policy could be to offer kidneys of HCV-positive donors only to HCV RNA-positive recipients (Natov, 2003). However, this requires HCV RNA testing of all anti-HCV-positive dialysis patients awaiting renal transplantation (Fabrizi *et al.*, 2003). Instead, transplantation from HCV-positive donors to HCV-negative recipients should be discouraged, as these patients run an increased risk of mortality (Bucci *et al.*, 2002).

Many potential donors acquire *bacterial* or *fungal infections* in the intensive care unit. Transplanting a kidney infected by *Candida* or *Aspergillus* may expose the vascular suture lines, leading to the development of mycotic aneurysms with the consequence of catastrophic rupture. Therefore, the fungal infections of the donor should be treated and the resolution of infection documented prior to procurement (Fishman, 2002). Moreover, the transplant recipient should be given pre-emptive antifungal treatment (Sharma *et al.*, 2005). Kidneys from subjects with severe sepsis and positive blood cultures may be appropriate for donation if the patient is treated with appropriate perioperative antibiotics targeted at an organism with known sensitivities, and with a modified immunosuppressive protocol (Lumbreras *et al.*, 2001; Pauly *et al.*, 2004; Gonzalez-Segura *et al.*, 2005; Cohen *et al.*, 2006). Also, it has been reported that skin contaminants do not pose a risk to the graft (Sharma *et al.*, 2005). In contrast, Rubin and Fishman (1998) propose to exclude donors with septicemia caused by difficult-to-eradicate organisms, such as *vancomycin-resistant enterococci, Streptococcus milleri; Salmonella; or fungal, nocardial, or mycobacterial* etiologies (Table 1.4).

Poisoning

Poisoning as a cause of death does not necessarily represent an absolute contraindication to donation. Organs have been successfully transplanted from donors who died from carbon monoxide (Hebert *et al.*, 1992), cyanide (Barkoukis *et al.*, 1993), anticoagulant rodenticide (Ornstein *et al.*, 1999), the pesticide malathion (Dribben and Kirk, 2001), methanol (Lopez-Navidad *et al.*, 2002), hemlock (Foster *et al.*, 2003), cocaine (Caballero *et al.*, 2003), or paracetamol (Gok *et al.*, 2004) poisoning.

Renal diseases

A history of diabetes mellitus and the presence of more than minimal proteinuria are each usually considered contraindications to donation. However, favorable results have been obtained with kidney transplants harvested from donors with hepatorenal syndrome (Koppel *et al.*, 1969), early diabetic nephropathy (Becker *et al.*, 2002), IgA nephropathy (Cosyns *et al.*, 1998), focal glomerulosclerosis (Rea *et al.*, 2001), lupus nephritis (Schwartzman *et al.*, 2005), or HELLP syndrome, i.e. hemolysis, elevated liver enzymes, and low platelet count (Flynn *et al.*, 2001).

Table 1.4   Contraindications or possible use of donors with infection

Contraindication	Possible use
HIV	Cytomegalovirus: possibly to CMV-positive recipients
Varicella virus	Epstein–Barr virus: possibly to EBV-positive recipients
West Nile virus	Hepatitis B virus: only if donor is negative for HBeAg or recipient has a high titer of anti-HBV antibodies. Little risk if the donor has anti-core antibodies
Fungal infection (unless well-documented resolution)	Hepatitis C virus: only to HCV-positive recipient with the same genotype or to HCV RNA-positive recipients
Vancomycin-resistant staphylococci, *Pseudomonas aeruginosa*, penicillin-resistant streptococci (unless well-documented resolution)	Bacterial endocarditis: only if the isolated micro-organism is sensitive to specific antibiotics
	Bacteremia: if sustained by micro-organisms easy to eradicate

Renal anatomic abnormalities

Most vascular and/or urological abnormalities do not represent a contraindication to donation. Kidneys with multiple vessels, benign cysts, and other urological abnormalities have been transplanted with success (Schulak *et al.*, 1997). The transplantation of a horseshoe kidney either using an *en bloc* technique (Zipitis *et al.*, 2003) or by splitting (Konigsrainer *et al.*, 2006) has also been successfully performed.

Arterial hypertension

Hypertension of the donor is usually considered a variable that may affect the graft outcome. A retrospective analysis of the UNOS database (Cho, 1999) showed that the duration of hypertension in the donor seems to be the most important factor affecting graft survival. Kidneys transplanted from donors with less than a 5-year history of hypertension gave results intermediate between those with kidneys from normotensive donors and those with kidneys from donors with a longer history of hypertension. Di Paolo *et al.* (2002) reported that long-standing donor hypertension was a strong independent risk factor for delayed graft function and 1-year graft function in kidneys with glomerular sclerosis, interstitial fibrosis, and/or vascular damage at time-zero biopsy. Abo-Zenah *et al.* (2002) also reported that, in older donors, hypertension may be a risk factor for delayed graft function and progressive interstitial fibrosis.

Older age

It is well known that *renal reserve* may be reduced after the sixth decade of life: the number of sclerotic glomeruli increases, the tubules may show signs of degeneration, interstitial fibrosis can develop, and the *glomerular filtration rate* may progressively decrease (Rodriguez-Puyol, 1998). However, about one-third of elderly patients show no change in glomerular filtration rate (Lindeman *et al.*, 1985). It has been hypothesized that renal dysfunction of the elderly is due to an accumulation of damage induced by minimal, clinically undetected renal disease rather than by aging itself (Rodriguez-Puyol, 1998). On the other hand, with increasing age, the length of the telomere, which has a finite replicative capacity, shortens, eventually leading to clonal exhaustion (replicative senescence), which is associated with interstitial fibrosis (Halloran *et al.*, 1999; Ferlicot *et al.*, 2003).

Several studies have reported a negative impact of older donor age on graft survival (Hariharan *et al.*, 1997; Cecka 2001; Meier-Kriesche *et al.*, 2002a). However, good results have been reported with the use of elderly donors in single-center experiences (Tarantino *et al.*, 2001; Solá *et al.*, 2002). A retrospective analysis of more than 20 000 renal transplants from adult recipients (Swanson *et al.*, 2002) showed that older donors were not at independently increased risk of graft failure, but rather it was the high donor/recipient age ratio that increased the risk of graft failure. Kasiske and Synder (2002), by reviewing the data of 74 000 renal transplants, found that matching older kidneys with older patients does not improve the overall graft survival.

The clinical impression is that the value of *creatinine clearance* and the *physiological age* of the donor are more important than the chronological age. In this regard it should be remembered that kidneys from cadaver donors with hypertension or diabetes have diminished functional renal reserve that may eventually result in more elevated serum creatinine levels after transplantation (Ojo *et al.*, 2000). Thus, attention should be paid to the history and to the toxic habits of the older patient. A study of the retinal vessels may help to predict the severity of renal lesions caused by hypertension, atherosclerosis, or diabetes. Renal echography may provide useful information about kidney size, parenchymal echogenicity, and corticomedullary ratio, all of which are indirect indices of the degree of renal parenchymal sclerosis. The serum creatinine value on admission is an important index, but in elderly subjects or in patients with small muscle mass, serum creatinine *per se* is not a reliable index of the glomerular filtration rate (GFR). A rapid and reliable estimation of the creatinine clearance is afforded by the formula of Cockroft and Gault (1976):

$$\frac{140 - \text{age (years)} \times \text{body weight (kg)}}{72 \times \text{serum creatinine (mg/dl)}} = \text{creatinine clearance}$$

The result must be multiplied by 0.85 in females.

This formula has been criticized because it may overestimate the GFR. As an alternative, the Modified Diet in Renal Disease (MDRD) formula (Levey *et al.*, 1999) has been proposed:

$$170 \times (\text{plasma creatinine}) - 0.999 \times (\text{age}) - 0.176 \times (\text{urea nitrogen}) - 0.17 \times (\text{serum albumin}) - 0.318$$

The result must be multiplied by 0.762 in women.

A simplified equation (Stevens and Levey 2005) is:

$$186 \times (\text{plasma creatinine}) - 1.154 \times (\text{age}) - 0.203$$

This should be multiplied by 0.742 in women.

It has been recommended that elderly donors with *creatinine clearance lower than 50 ml/min* are not utilized (Lloveras, 1991; Kuo *et al.*, 1996), particularly if the patient is atherosclerotic, hypertensive, and/or diabetic. A final decision must be made in the operating room, particularly in cases of a disparity in renal size.

Macroscopic inspection of the kidneys is a valuable tool for assessing the quality of the organs, particularly when there is evidence of scarring. *Ex vivo* renal *allograft perfusion* provides information about intrarenal vascular resistance. The presence of a benign macroscopic appearance and non-impeded perfusion is considered sufficient by a number of transplant surgeons.

The quality of the kidney may also be assessed by a *renal biopsy*. The degree of glomerular sclerosis is often used to determine whether a kidney can be transplanted (Gaber *et al.*, 1995; Randhawa *et al.*, 2000). However, some studies have reported that wedge biopsies can overestimate the amount of glomerulosclerosis, with the consequent refusal of a kidney that might be available for transplantation (Pokorna *et al.*, 2000; Muruve *et al.*, 2000). In a small number of patients, Remuzzi *et al.* (2006) reported good results using histologic scores for different components of the kidney tissue, namely vessels, glomeruli, tubules, and connective tissue. On the other hand, a poor correlation has been found between the age-associated histologic changes in pre-transplant biopsies and postoperative graft function (Schratzberger and Mayer, 2003; Howie *et al.*, 2004). By reviewing the data of 3444 cadaveric kidneys with reported biopsy, Edwards *et al.* (2004)

Table 1.5 Main criteria used for assessing the availability of cadaver kidneys

Criteria	Comments
History	Caution if previous cancer or history of long-term hypertension (>5 years) or previous renal disease
Age >60 years	Lower GFR may depend on age, or on undetected renal disease. About one-third of elderly subjects may have normal GFR
Creatinine clearance <70 ml/min	Older kidneys with impaired GFR still have functional reserve. Acceptable results may be obtained with donors showing a GFR of 55–60 ml/min
Proteinuria, diabetes	Proteinuria >1 g per day is a sign of underlying renal disease. Only donors with a recent history of diabetes may be considered
Ischemia time, perfusion	A cold ischemia time >36 h may be associated with poor graft survival. Strong resistance may predict delayed graft function and poor outcome, particularly in patients with reduced GFR
Histology	Wedge biopsy may overestimate the percentage of sclerotic glomeruli. Little agreement among pathologists on evaluation of grading of lesions. Histology evaluation should be coupled with data about creatinine clearance, history, hypertension, etc.

found no correlation between the percentage of glomerular sclerosis on donor kidney biopsies and 1-year graft survival, while serum creatinine at 1 year was significantly lower when the donor showed a calculated creatinine clearance >80 ml/min. The reliability of data given by biopsy is made even more complicated by the large variation among pathologists in interpreting the histologic grading, found by an international questionnaire (Furness et al., 2003).

In summary, the decision whether or not to accept the kidneys of an older donor is often subjective and based on a number of factors, including the history, the presence of comorbid conditions, the estimated creatinine clearance at presentation, the quality of kidney perfusion, the macroscopic aspect, and the histologic features in doubtful cases (Table 1.5). Nevertheless, improved survival rates appear to outweigh the increased risk associated with donor age. The relative risk of graft failure was lower for a patient transplanted between 1994 and 1997 with a kidney from a donor aged 75 years than for a patient engrafted between 1983 and 1990 with an organ from a donor aged 30 years (Roodnat et al., 1999).

Pediatric age

In the USA there has been a steady decline in the number of pediatric donors (Seikaly et al., 2001). Some groups are reluctant to transplant the kidney of a pediatric donor to an adult recipient, fearing that the a reduced renal mass might have a detrimental impact on the renal outcome. A study comparing renal function in adults who received pediatric kidneys with that in the recipients of adult kidneys showed no significant differences in either creatinine clearance or the level of proteinuria at 3 years (Al-Bader et al., 1996). In another study, a very wide range of renal mass dosing did not cause differences in medium-term graft evolution (de Petris et al., 2002). On the other hand, the transplantation of single kidneys harvested from children aged younger than 5 years is often associated with poor graft survival. Vascular thrombosis

(Sing et al., 1997) and insufficient recovery of renal function (Johnson et al., 2002) often lead to short-term graft failure. To overcome these problems, en bloc transplantation of both kidneys (EBK) in an adult recipient has been recommended when the kidney has a length of less than 6 cm (Satterthwaite et al., 1997) or when the donor weighs less than 15 kg (Bretan et al., 1997). Good results with EBK transplants to adults have been reported even in the long-term without evidence of glomerular hyperfiltration (Smyth et al., 2005). An analysis of UNOS data from 1987 to 2003 reported that 77% of EBK transplants were from donors <5 years of age. EBK transplants had superior 5-year graft survival compared with single kidney transplants (71% vs. 63%). EBK transplants from very young donors were associated with a significantly lower rate of delayed graft function than were single transplants (Dharnidharka et al., 2005). Good results have been obtained even with donors younger than 2 years by using en bloc kidneys stabilized with a Vicryl® mesh envelope technique (Chinnakotla et al., 2001).

Cold ischemia time

Cold ischemia times longer than 24 hours are usually considered a major risk factor for delayed graft function, and thereby complications that are associated with reduced graft survival (Cecka, 2001; Humar et al., 2002). On the other hand, by reviewing the data of the Collaborative Transplant Study, Opelz (1998) did not find a deleterious effect of cold ischemia times not exceeding 36 hours. This discrepancy may be partly accounted for by the fact that ischemia is only a component of the complex ischemia–reperfusion syndrome, characterized by the increased generation of oxygen free radicals with consequent disturbances in microcirculation, tubular injury, monocyte infiltration, and a T-cell-dominant milieu with overexpression of T cell-associated cytokines (Hoffman et al., 2002; Land, 2005). There is increasing evidence that ischemia–reperfusion injury could be responsible for delayed graft function and may contribute to the development of chronic graft nephropathy by triggering a vicious circle of ischemia–inflammation–rejection.

Renal hemodynamic instability

Many transplant units reject donors who display renal dysfunction immediately before operation. However, a retrospective analysis of French data showed no difference between patients whose last plasma creatinine level was higher than 2.3 mg/dl and patients with lower levels (Alexandre et al., 1996). A review of 1157 renal transplant patients suggested that neither oliguria nor hypotensive episodes in the donor influenced the risk of delayed graft function (Groenewoud and De Boer, 1995). It is not unusual to observe an immediate graft function with excellent serum creatinine level in the long term in kidneys harvested from oligoanuric donors.

Gender

A detrimental influence of female donor gender on the outcome of cadaver kidney grafts has been observed in both primary and retransplant situations (Neugarten and Silbiger, 1994). The donor gender-associated risk ratio for graft loss has been estimated to be 1.15 in female recipients and 1.22 in male recipients (Zeier et al., 2002). Nephron overload, induced by the smaller size of female donor kidneys, might be responsible for the poor outcome of the use of female organs in male recipients (Meier-Kriesche et al., 2002b). However, the possibility of an increased risk of acute rejection or technical failure may also contribute to the poor outcome of female-to-male transplants (Vereerstraeten et al., 1999).

The marginal donor

Donor-related factors, including age, functional status, and anatomic structure of the kidneys, and premorbid conditions, are important conditions that may influence the allograft outcome. Donor age >60 years, the presence of significant glomerulosclerosis at histology, elevated serum creatinine, pre-existing renal diseases, or renal anatomic abnormalities are generally used to define a donor as marginal. In the USA, marginal kidneys account for 20% of all deceased donor kidneys, and the percentage is probably higher in Europe. However, more than 40% of marginal kidneys are discarded, in spite of the evidence that patients receiving a marginal kidney have better survival than those maintained on the waiting list (Ojo et al., 2006).

Single or dual transplant with marginal donors?

A number of investigators have explored the option of grafting two kidneys from a marginal donor into a single recipient in an effort to increase the nephron mass (Johnson et al., 1996; Alfrey et al., 1997, 2003; Stratta and Bennett, 1997). Except for further attenuation of the disparity between the numbers of cadaver donors and recipients, the technique imposes some minor disadvantages for the recipient, including prolonged anesthesia time, a larger field of dissection, and a surgical complication rate that might, in theory, be twice that of conventional, single-kidney grafting.

A major issue concerns the criteria for choosing between two single or one dual transplant from marginal donors. Creatinine clearance (Alfrey et al., 1997), age (Andres et al., 2000), and histologic score (Remuzzi et al., 2006) have been proposed as discriminant criteria. However, none of them is completely satisfactory. Using the criterion of creatinine clearance lower than 90 ml/min, Alfrey et al. (1997) found a greater risk of delayed graft function in single-kidney recipients, compared with dual-transplant recipients. On the other hand, for single-kidney transplants, a number of investigators have used donors with creatinine clearance values of 50–60 ml/min, with good results (Kuo et al., 1996; Berardinelli 2001). Even age alone may be misleading. Although renal function tends to deteriorate with age, less than half of subjects aged more than 70 years have a creatinine clearance lower than 60 ml/min (Maaravi et al., 2006). The role of renal biopsy in selecting the donor has been supported by some investigators who have found a correlation of histologic findings with graft dysfunction (Gaber et al., 1995; Randhawa et al., 2000; Remuzzi et al., 2006), but others have found that the extent of anatomic lesions does not predict the future outcome of a kidney transplant (Lu et al., 2000; Schratzberger and Mayer, 2003).

The main concern with a policy of dual-kidney transplantation is that it may halve, rather than increase, the number of available kidneys. The use of two kidneys from a marginal donor presumes that overload of the reduced nephron mass of a single marginal kidney inexorably leads to progressive allograft dysfunction. However, if chronic graft nephropathy is primarily due to a problem of replicative senescence (Halloran et al., 1999), the benefit of dual-renal transplantation would be less than expected. On the other hand, there is no evidence that basal values of the glomerular filtration rate of the donor represent an independent variable influencing graft outcome. A review of the UNOS data showed that dual transplantation resulted in a 15% lower graft survival at 3 years, and in a higher primary non-function, when compared with single transplants from donors older than 55 years (Bunnapradist et al., 2003). In a French study (Dahmane et al., 2006), the outcomes of 170 kidney transplants from marginal donors refused by at least two centers were compared with those of 170 kidney transplants from optimal cadaver donors. Delayed graft function occurred more frequently and creatinine clearance was significantly lower in marginal kidneys, but the 5-year patient survival (88.2% vs. 88.9%) and graft survival (70.4% vs. 76.7%) rates were similar. Finally, there has been no demonstration that the half-life of a dual transplant is superior to the sum of graft half-lives of two marginal kidneys transplanted in two recipients. Thus, the use of dual-kidney transplantation should be limited to exceptional cases, and the indications should be based on a combination of clinical and histologic data.

Non-heart-beating cadaveric donors

A promising way to increase the actual number of kidneys for transplantation is to expand the donor pool to include non-heart-beating donors (NHBD). Those centers involved with NHBD have reported an increase in kidney transplantation of the order of 16–40% (Brook et al., 2003). In a retrospective review of inpatient hospital deaths, Daemen et al. (1997) found that the utilization of this resource would increase transplant activity 4.5-fold. The possibility of obtaining organs from NHBD who died in the street has also been demonstrated (Alvarez et al., 2000).

Similar long-term graft survival between recipients of kidneys from NHBD and recipients of those from HBD has been found by several investigators (Wijnen et al., 1995; Nicholson et al., 2001; Alonso et al., 2005). A main issue with NHBD is the significantly higher rate of delayed graft function, compared with that associated with heart-beating donors (Keizer *et al.*, 2005). Theoretically, this problem may be at least partially solved by the use of mechanical perfusion and rapid cooling through an intra-aortic catheter inserted via a femoral artery, At any rate, after 3 months, graft function improves to the level seen in grafts from heart-beating donors (Gok *et al.*, 2002), and there is no increased expression of fibrosis-associated genes after the first week (Jain *et al.*, 1999). In a series, graft survival after delayed graft function was better even up to 6 years in kidney recipients from NHBD rather than in recipients from HBD (Brook *et al.*, 2003).

Living donation

Living donation is accepted by law, religion, and bioethics, provided that the donor is aware of the consequences of his/her act and makes the decision without outside pressure or commercialism (Spital 1998). The European Best Practice Guidelines for Renal Transplantation (2000) stated that 'the use of kidney from living donor is recommended whenever possible'. However, living-donor kidney transplant activity varies widely among countries (Table 1.6). In addition, the selection of living donors has caused controversy among members of the transplant community. Some nephrologists do not encourage living-related donation, and some transplant centers rarely or never perform these procedures.

The main arguments against living donation are that cadaver donation represents a valid alternative, that donation is not risk-free, and that living-donor transplantation may represent an excuse not to harvest every possible cadaver donor. On the other hand, the point remains that not a single country in the world can offer cadaver kidneys to all potential recipients. In many countries the shortage of organs is significant, and in countries without the facilities for full renal replacement therapy the shortage of kidneys for transplantation simply means death for uremic patients. Moreover, the results of living kidney transplantation are superior to those of cadaveric renal transplantation, especially in the long term for both related and non-related donors (Table 1.7).

Living versus cadaver donors

There is evidence that delayed graft function (Ojo *et al.*, 1997; Halloran and Hunsicker 2001; Ponticelli *et al.*, 2002) and acute rejection (Cosio *et al.*, 1997; Hariharan *et al.*, 2000) can adversely influence not only the short-term but also the long-term graft survival. Obviously, the risk of *delayed graft function* is considerably lower in living-donor transplants than in cadaver transplants. Also, the incidence of *acute rejection* is lower, not only in living-related transplants with a good HLA match but even in living-unrelated transplants. This is probably because the ischemia–reperfusion injury that may trigger rejection through the activation of innate immunity (Land, 2005) is less frequent and severe with living donation. Moreover, brain death triggers a series of non-specific inflammatory events that increase the intensity of the acute immunologic host response after transplantation (Takada *et al.*, 1998). Studies in rats confirmed that the long-term survival of brain-dead donor transplants was significantly less than that of living-donor transplants. Proteinuria and renal histologic lesions were more severe in rats receiving the transplant from brain-dead donors (Pratschke *et al.*, 2001). There are other potential drawbacks with the use of cadaver transplants. Most donors who die from cerebrovascular complications have diffuse atherosclerosis, which may affect their kidneys. Some donors may be carriers of a hidden viral infection, or have tumors, which can be transmitted to the recipients. Moreover, it can be difficult to assess actual kidney function in many donors under intensive care.

The low risk of delayed graft function and early rejection coupled with the excellent function of kidneys from living donors and the absence of major comorbidity confer a great advantage over cadaver renal transplantation in the long term. By reviewing the UNOS registry, Cecka (2001) showed that the 10-year graft survival rates for transplants between 1988 and 2000 were clustered between 53 and 57% for HLA-mismatched living donors versus 38% for cadaveric transplants. In the experience of our group in Milan, the graft half-life was 31.9 years for living transplants versus 18.7 years for cadaver transplants (Ponticelli *et al.*, 2002). Thus, when compared with cadaver renal transplantation, living-donor transplantation reduces the incidence of delayed graft function and acute rejection, allows longer graft survival, and minimizes the risk of transmitting infections and cancer (Table 1.8).

Table 1.6   Number of living-donor kidneys per million population (pmp) transplanted in 2004. Countries with < 1 living transplant per year are not included. Adapted from IRODaT, 2005

Country	Total (pmp)
Argentina	6.4
Australia	12.2
Austria	5.3
Belgium	3.8
Brazil	9.4
Brunei	8.3
Canada	14.7
Croatia	1.6
Cyprus	41
Czech Republic	3.8
Denmark	9.8
Estonia	3.6
Finland	1.0
France	3.4
Georgia	1.6
Greece	7.1
Hong Kong	3.9
Hungary	1.1
Iceland	10.3
Iran	22.9
Israel	10.9
Italy	2.3
Jordan	34.2
Kuwait	33.2
Lebanon	17.5
Lithuania	1.2
Malaysia	1.4
Malta	10.0
Mexico	11.6
New Zealand	11.8
Norway	20.7
Pakistan	15.1
Poland	1.0
Portugal	3.4
Puerto Rico	6.0
Romania	8.0
Saudi Arabia	11.5
Slovak Republic	3.9

Table 1.6 Continued	
Country	Total (pmp)
Spain	1.8
Sweden	16.8
The Netherlands	15.3
UK	8.0
USA	19.9
Uruguay	2.9
Venezuela	4.2

Table 1.7   Reasons in favor of Living kidney donation

The number of cadaver donors is insufficient to meet the need of candidates for kidney transplantation
The results of transplants from living donors are far better than those of transplants from cadaver donors, particularly in the long term
Living donation permits pre-emptive transplantation
Minimal risk for donors both in the short term and in the long term
Advantages for the recipient, the donor, and society

Table 1.8   Advantages of kidney transplantation from a living donor in comparison with a cadaveric kidney

Better 'quality' of kidney (GFR, renal blood flow, renal functional reserve)
No comorbidity (diabetes, atherosclerosis, hidden tumors, infection, etc.)
No hypotension and renal vasonstriction (less delayed graft function (DGF))
Less ischemia-reperfusion injury (lower risk of DGF, acute rejection)
No over-regulation of cytokines and growth factors caused by intracranial hypertension.
No overexpression of MHC antigens (lower risk of DGF, acute rejection)

What is the best time for transplantation?

A number of reports have pointed out that the longer is the waiting time on dialysis the worse are the results of renal transplantation. Montagnino et al. (1997) found that in patients who received dialysis for more than 5 years, the 10-year graft survival was 45%, while it was 70% in patients with dialysis shorter than 5 years. Cosio et al. (1998) found that the post-transplant mortality rate was 7% in patients transplanted without previous dialysis, 23% in patients dialyzed for less than 3 years, and 44% in patients

Table 1.9 Requirements in considering a subject for potential living kidney donation

Voluntary, altruistic offer
No coercion
Aware of alternative therapies for the recipient
Aware of the benefit/risk for the donor and the recipient
Psychologically suitable
Psychological evaluation in doubtful cases
Fully informed consent

with more than 3 years of dialysis. Mange *et al.* (2001) reported that the relative risk of graft failure was 0.48 at 1 year and 0.18 at 2 years for patients who received a pre-emptive transplantation, 1 being the relative risk for patients who were submitted to regular dialysis before transplantation. Meier-Kriesche *et al.* (2000) reported that in comparison with pre-emptive transplantation, a waiting time on dialysis of 6–12 months conferred an increase in mortality of 37%, and a waiting time of over 24 months increased the mortality by 68%. Kasiske *et al.* (2002) found that the relative risk of graft failure was 0.73 and that of death was 0.69 for patients who received a pre-emptive kidney transplant from living donors, when compared with those transplanted after starting dialysis.

These data underline that increased time on dialysis prior to renal transplantation is associated with decreased graft and patient survival after transplantation. *Pre-emptive* transplantation without dialysis offers the best results. Thus, every effort should be made to perform renal transplantation as soon as possible. This program can be easily realized if a living donor is available. However, it is difficult to give an early transplant to a candidate without penalizing those already on dialysis with a transplant program based on cadaveric donation.

Informed consent

The fully informed consent of the potential living donor and the exclusion of coercion and/or commercial practices are not only ethically necessary, but also mandated by most nations. Thus, even before considering clinical evaluation, it is important to verify that the potential donor is acting voluntarily and altruistically, and is not under pressure (Table 1.9). It is the physician's responsibility to assess the motivation of the donor and to confirm the voluntary nature of the decision to donate an organ. Individuals who cannot be regarded as voluntary for reasons of age (children), mental retardation, or incarceration (prisoners) cannot serve as organ donors unless judicial consent is granted. According to Consensus Conferences (Abecassis *et al.*, 2001; Delmonico, 2005), the living donor should be competent, willing to donate, free from coercion, medically and psychosocially suitable, and fully informed of the risks, benefits, and alternative treatment available to the recipient. The benefits to both donor and recipient must outweigh risks associated with the donation and transplantation of the living donor organ. Donors should be made aware of the maximum level of risk they may incur, as well as the fact that they can change their mind at any point before the operation. A number of transplant centers require a routine psychological evaluation of the potential donor, both to uncover psychiatric disorders that would preclude donation and to ensure that the donor has been informed of the potential risks and benefits of donating a kidney.

Risks to donors

The use of living donors requires nephrectomy not to have severe consequences. The most dreaded complication is *donor death*. Two studies in the United States estimated perioperative mortality at about

0.03–0.02% (Najarian *et al.*, 1992; Matas *et al.*, 2003). A similar rate of mortality was reported in Iran, with three deaths among more than 15 000 living donors (Ghods, 2002). In the long term, donor survival is even better than that of the general population. In a Swedish experience, 85% of donors were alive after 20 years of follow-up, whereas the expected survival rate was 66%. This discrepancy is probably due to the fact that only healthy persons are accepted for living donation (Fehrman-Ekholm *et al.*, 1997), but it is also possible that regular follow-up visits after donation may contribute to longer survival. Ramcharan and Matas (2002) reviewed the outcome of living donor kidney transplants 20–37 years after nephrectomy. Of 464 donors, 84 had died, three of them having had renal failure caused, respectively, by the development of diabetes 10 years after nephrectomy, hemolytic uremic syndrome at 76 years, and pre-renal failure due to cardiac disease.

Apart from the risk of mortality, *major complications* of nephrectomy are rare. The postoperative morbidity depends on the technique and the operator. The classic flank incision is safe and has the advantage of a short operating time. However, hospitalization is longer than with other techniques, the patient may suffer from pain, and bulging and neuralgia may occur. Recently, the anterior subcostal incision has become more popular. It also needs a short operating time, is safe, and does not cause scar discomfort. However, access is limited, and time of hospitalization is medium or even long. The *laparoscopic technique* is now preferred by a number of surgeons. It requires very short hospitalization, allows early mobilization, and is associated with minimal scar discomfort. Disadvantages are a long operating time, and longer cold ischemia time. Some investigators prefer to use the technique for the left side (Mandal *et al.*, 2001), but others have not found differences in results between right and left nephrectomies (Abreu *et al.*, 2004). In the hands of technique-trained surgeons, laparoscopy gave similar results to those with minimal open nephrectomy, but donors had quicker and more complete recovery with laparoscopy (Velidedeoglu *et al.*, 2002; Rajab *et al.*, 2005).

There has been concern about the possibility that patients with a single kidney may develop glomerular hyperfiltration, hypertension, proteinuria, and *renal insufficiency* in the long term. However, the available studies do not support this concern. Najarian *et al.* (1992) found similar mean creatinine clearance, blood pressure, and proteinuria values between 57 donors (mean age 61 years) and 65 healthy siblings (mean age 58 years) evaluated 20 years or more after donation. Narkun-Burgess *et al.* (1993) examined 62 men, 45 years after unilateral nephrectomy following traumatic injuries during World War II. The mortality rates were similar to those of World War II servicemen of the same age, and the prevalence of hypertension was not increased. Five of 28 surviving subjects had levels of proteinuria between 377 and 535 mg/day, and three had increased serum creatinine values (1.7–1.9 mg/dl). The authors asserted that conditions other than nephrectomy could have contributed to the impaired renal function in these patients. Glomerular sclerosis was not increased in ten subjects who had autopsy examinations. Kasiske *et al.* (1995) conducted a meta-analysis of 48 studies reporting the outcome of 1703 normal persons and of 3124 patients who had been unilaterally nephrectomized for a variety of reasons. After nephrectomy, there was a mean decrement of glomerular filtration rate by 17.1 ml/min. However, this decline was not progressive, but tended to improve with each 10 years of follow-up (1.4 ml/min per decade). Although proteinuria increased progressively (76 mg/day per decade) among patients nephrectomized for other reasons, it was negligible after nephrectomy for kidney donation. The prevalence of hypertension did not change after nephrectomy, but systolic blood pressure increased slightly (1.1 mmHg/decade). No evidence of accelerated loss of kidney function in living kidney donors was observed in a cross-sectional follow-up (Fehrman-Ekholm *et al.*, 2001). Ramcharan and Matas (2002) reported five patients with serum creatinine more than 1.7 mg/dl out of 256 donors followed for 20–37 years. According to UNOS data, 56 of more than 50 000 previous kidney donors entered end-stage renal failure and eventually needed a transplant for themselves (Delmonico, 2005). However, in many cases, renal failure was unrelated to glomerular hyperfiltration. Thus, most nephrologists agree that unilateral nephrectomy in healthy subjects does not cause progressive renal dysfunction, but at most may be associated with microalbuminuria and a slight increase in blood pressure. Although these abnormalities are mild and not alarming, it may be prudent to perform a systemic follow-up of kidney donors to detect possible early renal complications.

Benefits to donors

In addition to benefiting recipients and society, living donation may also benefit donors. The immediate postoperative period is commonly marked by minor feelings of depression, especially if the donated kidney has failed. However, after the first days or weeks, most donors have feelings of increased self-esteem and lower scores of depression than in normal controls. These feelings often persist for many years (De Graaf et al., 2001). A review of 11 studies in eight countries reported that the quality of life of donors was usually superior and never inferior to that reported by controls in the general population (Ku, 2005). Furthermore, the vast majority of donors would again donate their kidney if they could, even in cases in which the transplant had failed (Fehrman-Ekholm et al., 2000; Ingelfinger, 2005).

Living-donor evaluation

The evaluation of a candidate to donate a kidney requires an extensive work-up (Table 1.10).

Blood compatibility

Until recently, donors who were ABO-incompatible with recipients were discarded because of the high risk of hyperacute rejection sustained by preformed humoral antibodies. However, in Japan, good results have been obtained with pre-transplant plasmapheresis, splenectomy at the time of transplantation, and a triple therapy based on tacrolimus, mycophenolate mofetil (MMF), and steroids. A 5-year graft survival rate of around 80% has been reported in two large series of ABO-incompatible kidney transplants (Shimmura et al., 2005; Takahashi et al., 2005). No correlation between ABO type and titer of antibodies and long-term results was observed (Shimmura et al., 2005). Good results have been reported in Europe and in the USA without splenectomy, either using immunoadsorption and anti-CD20 monoclonal antibodies (Tyden et al., 2003) or with plasmapheresis and low-dose anti-CMV immunoglobulins (Segev et al., 2005). As an alternative approach, living paired exchanges for cases of ABO incompatibility has also been proposed (Delmonico, 2004) and used successfully (Park et al., 2004; Montgomery et al., 2005).

Tissue compatibility

HLA-A, B, and DR testing of the donor and the recipient should be performed. Generally, one-quarter of siblings will be HLA-identical to the potential recipient, half of siblings will share one haplotype, and the remaining one-quarter will not share any HLA antigen. All parents will share one haplotype with their children.

The ideal transplantation is that between *identical twins*, as it does not require any immunosuppression. The only risks are those related to surgery and to recurrence of the original disease in the graft (Tilney, 1986).

Excellent results are usually obtained with transplants between *HLA-identical siblings*. The UNOS data reported a 5-year graft survival of 85% and a 32-year estimated graft half-life (Cecka, 2001).

Nevertheless, the UNOS and Collaborative Transplant Study registries (Gjertson and Cecka, 2000; Opelz, 2005) showed similar short-term and long-term results for *parent* donor grafts, those from *haploidentical siblings*, and *spouse* donor grafts. These results were better than those obtained with cadaver transplants performed in the same period. Of interest, some authors even found a lower risk of chronic allograft nephropathy in living-unrelated than in non-HLA-identical living-related donors (Humar et al., 2002). The current opinion is that there should be no restriction on live kidney donation based upon HLA match (Delmonico, 2005). This has opened up the possibility of donation also for unrelated individuals, such as spouses, other family members, friends, and anonymous donors (Steinbrook, 2005).

A *T cell crossmatch* between the serum of the recipient and the lymphocytes of the donor should be performed in an attempt to discover preformed antibodies against donor HLA antigens. More debatable is the significance of the *B cell crossmatch*, which may reduce by 4–6% the graft survival at 5 years (Cho and Cecka, 2002).

Table 1.10   Main investigations for a potential living donor

Laboratory tests	Instrumental investigations	Special consultations
ABO-HLA	Electrocardiogram, echocardiogram, non-invasive cardiac stress (over 40 years)	Gynecologist (over 40 years) Cardiologist Psychologist
Hematology	Chest X-ray	
Creatinine clearance (double check)	Abdominal ultrasonography (aorta, kidneys, bladder, prostate, liver, spleen)	
BUN–serum uric acid	Mammography (women over 30 years)	
Serum electrolytes	Sequential renal scintigraphy	
Serum electrophoresis, cholesterol, transaminases, bilirubin, glucose, glycosylated HbA1c (optional), amylases, lipases	Renal angiography with pyelographic images (alternative MRI or spiral CT)	
PSA (men over 40 years), Pap (cervical smear) (women over 30 years)		
Occult blood in the stool		
HIV, HBAg, HCV, CMV, EBV		
Urinalysis, urine culture		

Medical evaluation

Several considerations affect the identification of a living donor and/or the selection of an operative approach. Living-donor evaluation, including a medical history and physical examination, laboratory tests, serologic screening for infectious diseases, renal scintigraphy, and radiologic imaging, seeks to exclude donors with evidence of ongoing illness, as well as individuals at significant risk for subsequent development of hypertension or renal disease. In the *medical history*, attention should be paid to diseases that can preclude transplantation, such as cancer, severe hypertension, renal disease, diabetes, or systemic diseases with potential renal involvement. *Physical examination* should uncover any condition that may contraindicate donation, such as uncontrolled hypertension, chronic cardiovascular disease, chronic pulmonary disease, chronic infection, or malignancy. In addition to taking a careful history and performing a meticulous physical examination, a number of *virological* and *laboratory tests* should be performed routinely. In younger donors without apparent risk factors, an electrocardiogram and chest X-radiography may be sufficient to evaluate the *cardiac status*. For older donors with cardiovascular risk factors, and/or for those with cardiac symptoms or an abnormal electrocardiogram, non-invasive cardiac stress testing and an echocardiogram should be obtained. *Glucose tolerance tests* are usually limited to donors with elevated fasting glucose or with a strong family history of diabetes; glycosylated hemoglobin A1c values may also be useful. To exclude the presence of *neoplasia* in donors above 50 years, we also recommend echography of the abdomen and a search for occult blood in the stool, as well as a mammogram and Pap (cervical smear) test in women or prostate-specific antigen determination in men.

Table 1.11   History of cancer that precludes kidney donation

Melanoma
Testicular cancer
Cell carcinoma of kidney
Choriocarcinoma
Hematological malignancy
Bronchial carcinoma
Breast cancer

Medical contraindications

Generally, patients being considered for donation should be healthy or have only mild diseases that do not cause functional limitations. Patients with jugular venous distension, recent infarction, premature atrial or ventricular contractions, important aortic valvular stenosis, or poor general condition should be excluded due to the increased risk for *cardiac complications*. *Diabetics* are generally excluded because of the increased risk of postoperative complications in the short term and because of the potential risk of developing diabetic nephropathy in the long term (Kasiske *et al.*, 1996).

Patients with *HIV infection* should be excluded from living donation, since the virus is transmittable with the transplanted kidney. For the same reason, carriers of *hepatitis viruses* should also be excluded, with the possible exception of desperate cases in which both donor and recipient give informed consent. Evidence of an *active infection* should delay the transplantation until the infection is completely cured.

Not only patients who are carriers of cancer but also patients with a previous history of some types of tumors should be excluded (Table 1.11).

Renal evaluation

Most centers use serum creatinine and creatinine clearance to estimate the glomerular filtration rate (GFR). In evaluating whether the values of creatinine clearance are normal, one should consider the impact of multiple factors, including diet, muscle mass, and the ability to perform a urine collection accurately. In particular, values of glomerular filtration are strongly influenced by age, with a progressive decline after age 30–40 years. It should also be pointed out that inadequate urine collection may underestimate the actual value of creatinine clearance. Some centers prefer to calculate the clearance from serum creatinine by using the Cockroft–Gault formula (1996). It has been suggested that to index the results by height rather than by body surface area is more correct (Bertolatus and Goddard, 2001). Other investigators prefer to use the MDRD formula, which probably gives better results (Poggio *et al.*, 2006a). The present recommendation is that a GFR below 80 ml/min or two standard deviations below normal should preclude living donation (Delmonico, 2005). Blood urea and electrolytes, urinalysis, and urine culture should also be obtained prior to the acceptance of a living donor for kidney transplantation.

Renal echography and sequential scintigraphy are useful for assessing the morphological and functional characteristics of the two kidneys. The greatest hurdle for the potential donor in the evaluation process has been the *aortogram*, which seeks to define the renal artery anatomy and carries a 1.4% complication rate from puncture-site bleeding, groin hematoma, arterial dissection, thrombosis, contrast reactions, contrast-induced renal failure, and, rarely, angina and neurotropic injuries (Egglin *et al.*, 1995). Advances in spiral *computerized tomography* (CT) methods and *magnetic resonance* (MR) have simplified the procedure of defining donor vascular anatomy. These techniques permit intravenous rather than intra-arterial delivery of modest amounts of contrast and overcome all the complications of angiography except for allergic reactions. In addition, these methods identify with a greater degree of accuracy the presence of multiple renal arteries, ureteral duplication, vascular plaques and calcifications, and/or aberrant or anomalous retro- or

Table 1.12 Types of stones that represent a contraindication to kidney donation

Cystine stones
Struvite stones, or stones with infection difficult to eradicate
Stones associated with hereditary disorders or systemic diseases
Stones associated with chronic intestinal diseases (Crohn's disease, ulcerative colitis, etc.)
Frequently recurring stones

circumaortic renal veins. Lerner et al. (1999) found that CT is as accurate as renal angiography for artery anatomy and more sensitive in evaluating venous and parenchymal anomalies. El Diasty et al. (2005) reported 96% accuracy in identifying the arterial supply with MR angiography and an overall accuracy of 98% with MR venography. Only in patients with screening studies suggesting vascular abnormalities is it useful to perform an angiogram with selective renal artery injections.

Hypertension

There are no precise guidelines regarding donation from patients with arterial hypertension. It is now accepted that systolic blood pressure greater than 140 mmHg is a much more important cardiovascular risk factor than raised diastolic blood pressure, but whether patients with mildly increased systolic blood pressure should be excluded from donation may be challenged. In fact, there is little evidence that well-controlled hypertension may lead to kidney damage in an otherwise healthy subject. According to a Consensus Conference held in Amsterdam (Delmonico, 2005), there is no reason to reject as a kidney donor a subject more than 50 years of age who has a normal blood pressure on therapy with a GFR >80 ml/min and proteinuria <300 mg per day. Ambulatory blood pressure monitoring is more sensitive than office blood pressure measurements in identifying hypertension in living donors (Ozdemir et al., 2000).

Renal diseases

Adult relatives of patients with polycystic kidney disease can be accepted for donation if they have a normal CT or renal ultrasound scan. Opinions differ about the acceptance of potential donors with nephrolithiasis. After nephrectomy, the donor could develop recurrent stones, obstruction, and/or infection, which might injure the remaining kidney. It seems reasonable to accept as donors only those subjects without stones at the time of evaluation and with normal values within a 24-hour urine collection of calcium, urate, and oxalate. According to a Consensus Conference (Delmonico, 2005), patients with stones caused by inherited disorders, inflammatory bowel disease, or systemic disease are at high risk of recurrence and should not be considered for donation (Table 1.12).

In families with inherited Alport's syndrome, inheritance may be X-linked; however, in up to 15% of cases, the syndrome develops due to a new mutation. Male relatives without hematuria do not carry the abnormality and can be considered to be suitable donors. Female relatives with isolated hematuria rarely progress to renal failure. The decision whether to accept a mother for kidney donation depends on the age of the woman and on the presence of other mild renal abnormalities. Female relatives without hematuria may donate, although the absence of hematuria does not completely exclude the possibility that the woman is a carrier of Alport's syndrome (Kasiske et al., 1996).

Whether individuals with thin basement membrane nephropathy (TBMN) may be accepted for kidney donation is still controversial. Most persons with TBMN have a benign prognosis, but some may develop end-stage renal failure. Unfortunately, it is difficult to predict the long-term outcome for the single case. Therefore, the long-term risks for the donor remain unknown. Moreover, any effects of the thinned membranes themselves on allograft function are unclear (Ierino and Kanellis, 2005).

Older age

In the USA the proportion of living donors older than 50 years increased from 10 to 35% between 1988 and 2000, while kidneys from donors older than 60 years accounted for only 3% of first living donor transplants (Cecka, 2001). The limited use of living donors older than 60 years may be due to the fact that a review reported reduced graft survival rates and higher baseline creatinine values among recipients of kidneys from donors over the age of 60 years (Kasiske and Bia, 1995). However, better results have recently been reported by large registries. The Collaborative Transplant Study found the same 78% 5-year graft survival in transplants from living donors aged 16–40 years and from those aged more than 65 years (Collaborative Transplant Study, 2005). The UNOS data reported an 84% graft survival at 5 years with living donors aged more than 60 years (Cecka, 2001). A major problem with older living donors may be represented by the progressive decline of renal function with age, associated with comorbidity. Subjects with hypertension of duration greater than 10 years and creatinine clearance lower than 70 ml/min are bad candidates for living donation.

Pediatric age

Most laws do not allow minors to donate organs. In some countries, the law permits a minor to donate if he or she possesses the mental capacity to make such a decision, or if he or she does not object. However, a questionnaire among centers in the United States showed that only 11% of these centers would exclude a younger donor due to age alone (Bia et al., 1995).

Obesity

There is a potential concern with obese donors due both to technical considerations to retrieve a well-functioning kidney and to the increased risk of postoperative complications. To minimize these risks, obese donors are encouraged to lose weight. A retrospective analysis of a large series of obese donors showed that they had more frequent wound-related complications and a longer operation time than did non-obese donors. Nevertheless, major complications were not observed in the short term (Pesavento et al., 1999; Heimbach et al., 2005), and graft survival was not influenced by the high body mass index (BMI) of the donor (Gore et al., 2006). However, there is little information on the long-term follow-up of obese donors. Of some concern, in patients submitted to unilateral nephrectomy for various reasons, those with a BMI >30 had a significantly higher risk of developing proteinuria or renal dysfunction in the long term than did those with a BMI <30 (Praga et al., 2000). The Consensus Conference held in Amsterdam discouraged donation from persons with a BMI higher than 35 (Delmonico, 2005).

Renal anatomic abnormalities

The vascular anatomy constitutes another important consideration. Because renal veins collateralize, only the largest vein must usually be anastomosed to drain the kidney. However, a particularly short right renal vein or a retroaortic left renal vein may present an operative challenge. In contrast, renal arteries are end-arteries and must all be anastomosed. Atherosclerosis of the renal artery, a not-infrequently encountered finding, generally tends to involve only the aortic origin and not to present a problem for organ retrieval. In contrast, a tortuous, bead-like appearance of the artery suggests the presence of fibromuscular hyperplasia. While severe hyperplasia (irregularity with greater than 50% stenosis or with aneurysms) represents a formal contraindication to donation, selected subjects with mild anatomic abnormalities have been used as renal donors with satisfactory transplant outcomes (Kolettis et al., 2004).

Isolated microhematuria

Microscopic hematuria may be seen in about 8–21% of the general population (Kouschik et al., 2005). The detection of microscopic hematuria in an adult donor necessitates careful evaluation (Fogazzi and Ponticelli, 1996; Figure 1.1). In young adults, particularly women, the risk of an underlying cancer is small if the ultrasound scan is normal. There is a much higher risk of hematuria, reflecting an underlying

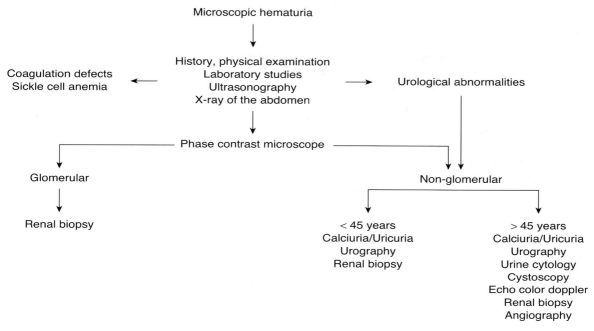

Microscopic hematuria

↓

History, physical examination
Laboratory studies
Ultrasonography
X-ray of the abdomen

Coagulation defects
Sickle cell anemia ←

→ Urological abnormalities

↓

——— Phase contrast microscope ———

Glomerular

Non-glomerular

↓

Renal biopsy

< 45 years
Calciuria/Uricuria
Urography
Renal biopsy

> 45 years
Calciuria/Uricuria
Urography
Urine cytology
Cystoscopy
Echo color doppler
Renal biopsy
Angiography

Figure 1.1 Algorithm for screening potential kidney donors having microscopic hematuria

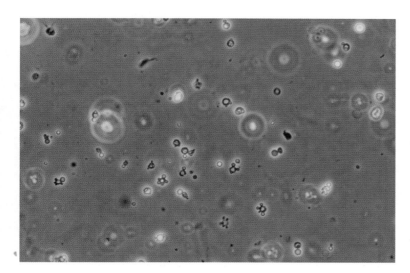

Figure 1.2 Dysmorphic erthyrocyclic. Most erythrocytes appear to be distorted; many show characteristics protrusions of different size and shapte (acanthocytes). This image is typical of glomerular diseases

cancer, among men aged more than 45–50 years; such donors require careful investigation. As ultrasonography may be limited in detecting solid tumors less than 3 cm in diameter, helical computed tomography is recommended as a screening procedure (Cohen and Brown, 2003).

An accurate study of the urine sediment using a phase-contrast microscope may also be helpful. The finding of more than 75–80% distorted red blood cells is strongly suggestive of glomerular disease, particularly when more than 4–5% of cells are acanthocytes (Figure 1.2). The finding of monomorphic

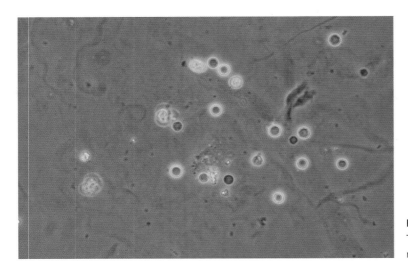

Figure 1.3 Monomorphic erythrocyturia. The erythrocytes are isomorphic and round, with different hemoglobin content

erythrocytes suggests a possible lower urinary tract abnormality as the cause of the hematuria (Figure 1.3), although exceptions may occur, particularly in patients afflicted with IgA nephropathy.

Proteinuria

If a patient is polyuric, the evaluation of spot urine tests for protein can produce a negative result despite the presence of proteinuria. Thus, the assessment of proteinuria should be performed on a 24-hour urine collection. A well accepted option is the ratio of urinary protein/urinary creatinine (Up/Ucr) in a random specimen, which correlates well with the 24-hour urinary protein (K/DOQI Guidelines 2002). Urinary protein excretion in healthy subjects is less than 150 mg/day (or 0.15 Up/Ucr). An amount of proteinuria below 300 mg/day is not considered a contraindication to donation in the absence of microhematuria, hypertension, or pyuria (Karpinski *et al.*, 2006). Postural proteinuria is now recognized as a benign condition and does not represent a contraindication to donating a kidney.

Leukocyturia

Leukocyturia and bacteriuria may be caused by contamination from vaginal discharge or by a trivial urinary tract infection, but may also be associated with chronic pyelonephritis, tubulointerstitial disorders, or renal parenchymal diseases. The persistence of significant leukocyturia in a potential donor necessitates a thorough investigation to determine possible nephrologic or urologic abnormalities.

Nephron mass disparity

A drawback with kidneys of small donors is represented by the low nephron mass. The higher is the size mismatch, the higher is the risk of graft dysfunction in the long term (Sanchez-Fructuoso *et al.*, 2001; Nicholson *et al.*, 2000; El-Agroudy *et al.*, 2003). Poggio *et al.* (2006b) reported that a transplanted kidney volume greater than 120 cm³/1.73 m² was independently associated with a better estimated glomerular filtration rate at 2 years post-transplant when compared with recipients of lower transplanted kidney volumes. Body size and male gender were independent correlates of larger kidney volume. Thus, it would be prudent to avoid extreme mismatching between allograft and recipient size.

Postoperative care

Three major management problems arise during the early postoperative period. *First*, pain control is critical, and may be treated by the use of an epidural catheter for instillation of and/or preferably by patient-controlled intravenous delivery of a narcotic infusion. *Second*, due to the sedation for pain control, the medical team must provide aggressive pulmonary toilet to prevent significant atelectasis and consequent development of pneumonia, as well as perform active and passive motion of the patient's extremities to avert deep venous thrombosis due to extended periods of bed-rest. *Third*, urine output during the early postoperative period should be maintained, with fluid and diuretics, at levels greater than 1 ml/kg per hour. The Foley catheter is removed the morning after surgery, and virtually all patients void without difficulty within 6 hours.

In patients with a previous history of deep vein thrombosis or coagulation abnormality, heparin prophylaxis is recommended. The patient is discharged from the hospital when intestinal function returns, usually on the fourth or fifth postoperative day. The major postoperative complications, which in aggregate occur in 0.23% of donors, include pneumonia, atelectasis, urinary tract infection, wound infection, and pneumothorax.

References

Abecassis M, Adams M, Adams P, et al. Consensus statement on the live organ donor. JAMA 2001; 285:1440–1.

Abo-Zenah H, Katsoudas S, de Takats D, et al. Early progressive interstitial fibrosis in human renal allografts. Clin Nephrol 2002; 57: 9–18.

Abreu SC, Goldfarb DA, Derweesh I, et al. Factors related to delayed graft function after laparoscopic live donor nephrectomy. J Urol 2004; 171: 52–7.

Al-Bader W el-R, Landsberg D, Manson AD, Levin A. Renal function changes over time in adult recipients of small pediatric kidneys. Transplantation 1996; 62: 611–15.

Alexandre L, Eschwege P, Blanchet P, et al. Effect of last donor creatininemia >200 μmol/L on kidney graft function. Transplant Proc 1996; 28: 188.

Alfrey EJ, Lee CM, Scandling JD, et al. When should expanded criteria donor kidneys be used for single versus dual kidney transplants? Transplantation 1997; 64: 1142–6.

Alfrey EJ, Boissy AR, Lerner SM. Dual Kidney Registry. Dual kidney transplants: long-term results. Transplantation 2003; 75: 1232–6.

Ali MK, Light JA, Barhyte DY, et al. Donor hepatitis C virus status does not adversely affect short-term outcomes in HCV+ recipients in renal transplantation. Transplantation 1998; 66: 1694–7.

Alonso A, Fernandez-Rivera C, Villaverde P, et al. Renal transplantation from non-heart-beating donors: a single-center 10-year experience. Transplant Proc 2005; 37: 3658–60.

Alvarez J, Barrio R, Javier A, et al. Non-heart beating donors from the streets. An increasing donor pool source. Transplantation 2000; 70: 314–17.

Andres A, Morales JM, Herrero JC, et al. Double versus single renal allografts from aged donors. Transplantation 2000; 69: 2060–6.

Barkoukis TJ, Sarbak CA, Lewis D, Whitter FC. Multiorgan procurement from a victim of cyanide poisoning: a case report and review of the literature. Transplantation 1993; 55: 1434–6.

Becker YT, Leverson GE, D'Alessandro AM, et al. Diabetic kidneys can safely expand the donor pool. Transplantation 2002; 74: 141–5.

Berardinelli L, Beretta C, Raiteri M, et al. Long-term results of 211 single necrokidney transplantations from extreme-age donors: why dual allograft? Transplant Proc 2001; 33: 3774–6.

Berber L, Aydin C, Turkmen F, et al. The effect of HBsAg-positivity of kidney donors on long-term patient and graft outcome. Transplant Proc 2005; 37: 4173–5.

Bertolatus JA, Goddard L. Evaluation of renal function in potential living donors. Transplantation 2001; 71: 256–60.

Bia MJ, Ramos EL, Danovitch GM, et al. Evaluation of living donors. The current practice of US transplant centers. Transplantation 1995; 60: 322–7.

Bretan PN, Friese C, Goldstein RB, et al. Immunologic and patient selection strategies for successful utilization of less than 15 kg pediatric donor kidneys—long-term experience with 40 transplants. Transplantation 1997; 63: 233–7.

Brook NR, Waller JR, Nicholson ML. Nonheart-beating kidney donation: current practice and future developments. Kidney Int 2003; 63: 1516–29.

Bucci JR, Matsumoto CS, Swanson SJ, et al. Donor hepatitis C seropositivity: clinical correlates and effect on early graft and patient survival in adult cadaveric kidney transplantation. J Am Soc Nephrol 2002; 13: 2974–82.

Buell JF, Hanaway MJ, Thomas M, et al. Donor kidney with small renal cell cancers: can they be transplanted? Transplant Proc 2005; 37: 581–2.

Bunnapradist S, Gritsch HA, Peng A, et al. Dual kidney from marginal adult donors as a source for cadaveric renal transplantation in the United States. J Am Soc Nephrol 2003; 14: 1031–6.

Caballero F, Lopez-Navidad A, Gomez M, Sola R. Successful transplantation of organs from a donor who died from acute cocaine intoxication. Clin Transplant 2003; 17: 89–92.

Cecka JM. Results of more than 1000 recent living-unrelated donor transplants in the United States. Transplant Proc 1999; 31: 234.

Cecka JM. The UNOS renal transplant registry. In Cecka JM, Terasaki PI, eds. Clinical Transplants 2000. Los Angeles: UCLA Tissue Typing Laboratory, 2001: 1–18.

Chinnakotla S, Leone JP, Taylor RJ. Long-term results of en bloc transplantation of pediatric kidneys into adults using a vicryl mesh envelope technique. Clin Transplant 2001; 15: 388–92.

Cho YW. Expanded criteria for donors. In Cecka JM, Terasaki PI, eds. Clinical Transplants 1998. Los Angeles: UCLA Tissue Typing Laboratory, 1999: 421–36.

Cho YW, Cecka JM. Cross-match tests. An analysis of UNOS data from 1991–2000. In Cecka JM, Terasaki PI, eds. Clincial Transplants 2001. Los Angeles: UCLA Tissue Typing Laboratory, 2002: 237–46.

Cockroft D, Gault MH. Prediction of creatinine clearance from serum creatinine. Nephron 1976; 16: 31–41.

Cohen J, Michowiz R, Ashkenazi T, et al. Successful organ transplantation from donors with *Acinetobacter baumannii* septic shock. Transplantation 2006; 81: 853–5.

Cohen RA, Brown RS. Microscopic hematuria. N Engl J Med 2003; 348: 2330–8.

Collaborative Transplant Study. CTS Newsletter 2005; 1.

Cosio FG, Pelletier RP, Falkenhain ME, et al. Impact of acute rejection and early allograft function on renal allograft survival. Transplantation 1997; 63: 1611–15.

Cosio FG, Alamir A, Yim S, et al. Patient survival after renal transplantation: I. The impact of dialysis pre-transplant. Kidney Int 1998; 53: 767–72.

Cosyns JP, Malaise J, Hanique G, et al. Lesions in donor kidneys: nature, incidence, and influence on graft function. Transpl Int 1998; 11: 22–7.

Daemen JW, Oomen AP, Kelders WP, Kootstra G. The potential pool of non-heart-beating kidney donors. Clin Transplant 1997; 11: 149–54.

Dahmane D, Audrad V, Hiesse C, et al. Retrospective follow-up of transplantation of kidneys from marginal donors. Kidney Int 2006; 69: 546–52.

Danovitch GM, Cecka JM. Allocation of deceased donor kidneys: past, present, and future. Am J Kidney Dis 2003; 42: 882–90.

De Feo TM, Grossi P, Poli F, et al. Kidney transplantation from anti-HBc+ donors: results from a retrospective Italian study. Transplantation 2006; 81: 76–80.

De Graaf OW, Bogetti-Dumlao A. Living donors' perception of their quality of health after donation. Prog Transplant 2001; 11: 108–15.

Delmonico F. Exchanging kidneys. Advances in living-kidney transplantation. N Engl J Med 2004; 350: 1812–14.

Delmonico F, Council of the Transplantation Society. A report of the Amsterdam forum on the care of the live kidney donor: data and medical guidelines. Transplantation 2005; 79 (Suppl 6): S53–66.

De Petris L, Faraggiana T, Rizzoni G. Renal mass dosing and graft function in children transplanted from pediatric donors. Pediatr Nephrol 2002; 17: 433–7.

Detry O, Honore P, Hans MF, et al. Organ donors with primary central nervous system tumor. Transplantation 2000; 70: 249–50.

Dharnidharka VR, Stevens G, Howard RJ. En-bloc kidney transplantation in the United States: an analysis of United Network of Organ Sharing (UNOS) data from 1987 to 2003. Am J Transplant 2005; 5: 1513–17.

Di Paolo S, Stallone G, Schena A, et al. Hypertension is an independent predictor of developed graft function and worse renal function only in kidneys with chronic pathologic lesions. Transplantation 2002; 73: 623–7.

Doutrelepont JM, Mat O, Abramowicz D, et al. Inadvertent transfer of choriocarcinoma with renal transplantation: characteristics of the donor-recipient pairs. Transplant Proc 1995; 27: 1789–90.

Dribben WH, Kirk MA. Organ procurement and successful transplantation after malathion poisoning. J Toxicol Clin Toxicol 2001; 39: 633–6.

EBPG; European Renal Association; European Society for Organ Transplantation. European Best Practice Guidelines for Renal Transplantation. Nephrol Dial Transplant 2000; 15(Suppl 7): 1–85.

Edwards E, Posner MP, Maluf DG, Kauffman HM. Reasons for non-use of recovered kidneys: the effect of donor glomerulosclerosis and creatinine clearance on graft survival. Transplantation 2004; 77: 1411–15.

Egglin TK, O'Moore PV, Feinstein AR, Waltman AC. Complications of peripheral arteriography: a new system to identify patients at increased risk. J Vasc Surg 1995; 22: 787–94.

El-Agroudy AE, Hassan NA, Bakr MA, et al. Effect of donor/recipient body weight mismatch on patient and graft outcome in living-donor kidney transplantation. Am J Nephrol 2003; 23: 294–9.

El Diasty TA, El Ghar ME, Shocker AA, et al. Magnetic resonance imaging as a sole method for the morphological and functional evaluation of live kidney donors. BJU Int 2005; 96: 111–16.

Erice A, Rhame FS, Heussner RC, et al. Human immunodeficiency virus infection in patients with solid organ transplants: report of five cases and review. Rev Infect Dis 1991; 13: 537–42.

Fabrizi F, Martin P, Ponticelli C. Hepatitis C virus infection and renal transplantation. Am J Kidney Dis 2001; 38: 919–34.

Fabrizi F, Bunnapradist S, Lunghi G, Martin P. Transplantation of kidneys from HCV-positive donors: a safe strategy? J Nephrol 2003; 16: 617–25.

Fehrman-Ekholm I, Elinder CG, Stenbeck M, et al. Kidney donors live longer. Transplantation 1997; 64: 976–8.

Fehrman-Ekholm I, Brink B, Ericsson C, et al. Kidney donors don't regret: follow-up of 370 donors in Stockholm since 1964. Transplantation 2000; 69: 2067–71.

Fehrman-Ekholm I, Duner F, Brink B, et al. No evidence of accelerated loss of kidney function in living kidney donors: results from a cross-sectional follow-up. Transplantation 2001; 72: 444–9.

Ferlicot S, Durrbach A, Ba N, et al. The role of replicative senescence in chronic allograft nephropathy. Hum Pathol 2003; 34: 924–8.

Fishman JA. Overview: fungal infections in the transplant patient. Transpl Infect Dis 2002; 4(Suppl 3): 3–11.

Flynn MF, Power RE, Murphy DM, et al. Successful transplantation of kidneys from a donor with HELLP syndrome-related death. Transpl Int 2001; 14: 108–10.

Fogazzi GB, Ponticelli C. Microscopic hematuria. Diagnosis and management. Nephron 1996; 72: 125–34.

Fong TL, Bunnapradist S, Jordan SC, Cho YW. Impact of hepatitis B core antibody status on outcomes of cadaveric renal transplantation: analysis of United Network of Organ Sharing database between 1994 and 1999. Transplantation 2002; 73: 85–9.

Foster PF, McFadden R, Trevino R, et al. Successful transplantation of donor organs from a hemlock poisoning victim. Transplantation 2003; 76: 874–6.

Furness P, Taub N, Assmann KJ, et al. International variation in histologic grading is large, and persistent feedback does not improve reproducibility. Am J Surg Pathol 2003; 27: 805–10.

Gaber LW, Moore LW, Alloway RR, et al. Glomerulosclerosis as a determinant of posttransplant function of older donor renal allografts. Transplantation 1995; 60: 334–9.

Ghods A. Renal transplantation in Iran. Nephrol Dial Transplant 2002; 17: 222–8.

Gjertson DW, Cecka JM. Living unrelated kidney transplantation. Kidney Int 2000; 58: 491–9.

Gok MA, Buckley PE, Shenton BK, et al. Long-term renal function in kidneys from non-heart beating donors: a single-center experience. Transplantation 2002; 74: 664–9.

Gok MA, Gupta A, Olschewski P, et al. Renal transplants from non-heart beating paracetamol overdose donors. Clin Transplant 2004; 18: 541–6.

Gonzalez-Segura C, Pascual M, Garcia Huete L, et al. Donors with positive blood culture: could they transmit infections to the recipients? Transplant Proc 2005; 37: 3664–6.

Gore JL, Pham PT, Danovitch GM, et al. Obesity and outcome following renal transplantation. Am J Transplant 2006; 6: 357–63.

Groenewoud A, De Boer J. Potential risk factors affecting delayed graft function after kidney transplantation. Transplant Proc 1995; 27: 3527.

Halloran PF, Melk A, Barth C. Rethinking chronic allograft nephropathy: the concept of accelerated senescence. J Am Soc Nephrol 1999; 10: 167–81.

Halloran PF, Hunsicker LG. Delayed graft function. Am J Transplant 2001; 1: 115–20.

Hariharan S, McBride MA, Bennett LE, Cohen EP. Risk factors for renal allograft survival from older cadaver donors. Transplantation 1997; 64: 1748–54.

Hariharan S, Johnson CP, Bresnahan BA. Improved graft survival after renal transplantation in the United States, 1988 to 1996. N Engl J Med 2000; 342: 605–12.

Hebert MJ, Boucher A, Beaucage G. Transplantation of kidneys from a donor with carbon monoxide poisoning. N Engl J Med 1992; 326: 1571.

Heimbach JK, Taler SJ, Prieto, et al. Obesity in living kidney donors: clinical characteristics and outcomes in the era of laparoscopic donor nephrectomy. Am J Transplant 2005; 5: 1057–64.

Hoffmann SC, Kampen RL, Amur S, et al. Molecular and immunohistochemical characterization of the onset and resolution of human renal allograft ischemia/reperfusion injury. Transplantation 2002; 74: 916–23.

Hou S. Expanding the kidney donor pool: ethical and medical considerations. Kidney Int 2000; 58: 1820–36.

Howie AJ, Ferreira MA, Lipkin GW, Adu D. Measurement of chronic damage in the donor kidney and graft survival. Transplantation 2004; 77: 1058–65.

Humar A, Ramcharan T, Kandaswamy RJ, et al. Risk factors for slow graft function after kidney transplants: a multivariate analysis. Clin Transplant 2002; 16: 425–9.

Ierino FL, Kanellis J. Thin basement membrane nephropathy and renal transplantation. Semin Nephrol 2005; 25: 184–7.

Ingelfinger JR. Risks and benefits to the living donor. N Engl J Med 2005; 353: 447–9.

IRODaT. 2004 Donation and transplantation international values. Organ Tissues 2005; 8: 79–82.

Iwamoto M, Jernigan DB, Guasch A, et al. Transmission of West Nile virus from an organ donor to four transplant recipients. N Engl J Med 2003; 348: 2196–203.

Jain S, Bicknell GR, White SA, et al. Comparison of the expression of fibrosis-associated genes in glomeruli after renal transplantation between conventional cadaveric and non-heart beating donors. Br J Surg 1999; 86: 1264–8.

Johnson LB, Kuo PC, Dafoe DC, et al. Double adult renal allografts: a technique for expansion of the cadaveric kidney donor pool. Surgery 1996; 230: 580–4.

Johnson RJ, Armstrong S, Belger MA, et al. The outcome of pediatric renal transplantation in the UK and Eire. Pediatr Transplant 2002; 6: 367–77.

Karpinski M, Knoll G, Cohn A, et al. The impact of accepting living kidney donors with mild hypertension or protein-uria on transplantation rates. Am J Kidney Dis 2006; 47: 317–23.

Kasiske BL, Bia MJ. The evaluation and selection of living kidney donors. Am J Kidney Dis 1995; 26: 387–98.

Kasiske BL, Ma JZ, Louis TA, Swan K. Long-term effects of reduced renal mass in humans. Kidney Int 1995; 48: 814–19.

Kasiske BL, Ravenscraft M, Ramos EL, et al. The evaluation of living renal transplant donors: clinical practice guidelines. Ad Hoc Clinical Subcommittee of the Patient Care and Education Committee of the American Society of Transplant Physicians. J Am Soc Nephrol 1996; 17: 2288–313.

Kasiske BL, Snyder I. Matching older kidneys with older patients does not improve allograft survival. J Am Soc Nephrol 2002; 13: 1067–72.

Kasiske BL, Snyder JJ, Matas AJ, et al. Preemptive kidney transplantation: the advantage and the advantaged. J Am Soc Nephrol 2002; 13: 1358–64.

Kauffman HM, McBride MA, Cherikh WS, et al. Transplant tumor registry: donors with central nervous system tumors. Transplantation 2002a; 73: 579–82.

Kauffman HM, McBride MA, Cherikh WS, et al. Transplant tumor registry: donor related malignancy. Transplantation 2002b; 4: 358–62.

Keizer KM, de Fijter JW, Haase-Kromwijk BJ, Weimar W. Non-heart-beating donor kidneys in the Netherlands: allocation and outcome of transplantation. Transplantation 2005; 79: 1195–9.

Keown P. Improving quality of life. The new target for transplantation. Transplantation 2001; 72 (Suppl 12): S67–74.

Kolettis PN, Bugg CE, Lockhart ME, et al. Outcomes for live donor renal transplantation using kidneys with medial fibroplasia. Urology 2004; 63: 656–9.

Konigsrainer I, Knubben K, Thiel C, Steurer W, Konigsrainer A. Successful transplantation to two recipients after splitting a large horseshoe kidney with complicated anatomy. Transpl Int 2006; 19: 521–2.

Koppel MH, Coburn JW, Mims MM, et al. Transplantation of cadaveric kidneys from patients with hepatorenal syndrome. Evidence for the functional nature of renal failure in advanced liver disease. N Engl J Med 1969; 280: 1367–71.

Kouschick R, Garvey C, Manivel JC, et al. Persistent asymptomatic microscopic hematuria in prospective kidney donors. Transplantation 2005; 80: 1425–9.

Ku JH. Health-related quality of life of living kidney donors: review of the short form 36-health questionnaire survey. Transpl Int 2005; 12: 1309–17.

Kuo PC, Johnson LB, Schweitzer EJ, et al. Utilization of the older donor for renal transplantation. Am J Surg 1996; 172: 551–7.

Kyllonen L, Kahu J, Kyllonen L, Salmela K. Kidney transplantation from 1119 deceased donors in Finland, 1991 to 2003: impact of donor factors. Transplant Proc 2005; 37: 3248–52.

Land W. The role of postischemic reperfusion injury and other nonantigen-dependent inflammatory pathways in transplantation. Transplantation 2005; 79: 505–14.

Lerner LB, Henriques HF, Harris RD. Interactive 3-dimensional computerized tomography reconstruction in evaluation of the living renal donor. J Urol 1999; 161: 403–7.

Levey AS, Bosch JP, Lewis JB, et al. A more accurate method to estimate glomerular filtration rate from serum creatinine: a new prediction equation. Modification of Diet in Renal Disease Study Group. Ann Intern Med 1999; 130: 461–70.

Lindeman RD, Tobin J, Shock NW. Longitudinal studies on the rate of decline in renal function with age. J Am Geriatr Soc 1985; 33: 278–85.

Lloveras J. The elderly donor. Transplant Proc 1991; 23: 2592–5.

López-Navidad A, Caballero F, Gonzalez-Segura C, et al. Short- and long-term success of organs transplanted from acute methanol poisoned donors. Clin Transplant 2002; 16: 151–2.

Lu AD, Desai D, Myers BD, et al. Severe glomerular sclerosis is not associated with poor outcome after kidney transplantation. Am J Surg 2000; 180: 470–4.

Lumbreras C, Sanz F, Gonzales A, et al. Clinical significance of donor-unrecognized bacteremia in the outcome of solid-organ transplant recipients. Clin Infect Dis 2001; 33: 722–6.

Maaravi Y, Bursztyn M, Hammerman-Rozenberg R, et al. Moderate renal insufficiency at 70 years predicts mortality. QJM 2006; 99: 97–102.

Mandal AK, Cohen C, Montgomery RA, et al. Should the indications for laparascopic live donor nephrectomy of the right kidney be the same as for the open procedure? Anomalous left renal vasculature is not a contraindication to laparoscopic left donor nephrectomy. Transplantation 2001; 71: 660–4.

Mange KC, Joffe MM, Feldman HI. Effect of the use or non use of long-term dialysis on the subsequent survival of renal transplantation from living donors. N Engl J Med 2001; 344: 726–31.

Marks WH, Wagner D, Pearson TC, et al. Organ donation and utilization, 1995–2004: entering the collaborative era. Am J Transplant 2006; 6: 1101–10.

Matas AJ, Lawson W, McHugh L, et al. Employment patterns after successful kidney transplantation. Transplantation 1996; 61: 729–33.

Matas AJ, Bartlett ST, Leichtman AB, Delmonico FL. Morbidity and mortality after living kidney donation, 1999–2001: survey of United States transplant centers. Am J Transplant 2003; 3: 830–4.

Meier-Kriesche HU, Port FK, Ojo AO, et al. Effect of waiting time on renal transplant outcome. Kidney Int 2000; 58: 1311–17.

Meier-Kriesche HU, Cibrik DM, Ojo AO, et al. Interaction between donor and recipient age in determining the risk of chronic renal failure. J Am Geriatr Soc 2002a; 50: 195–7.

Meier-Kriesche HU, Amdorfer JA, Kaplan B. The impact of body mass index on renal transplant outcomes: a significant independent risk factor for graft failure and patient death. Transplantation 2002b; 73: 70–4.

Montagnino G, Tarantino A, Cesana B, et al. Prognostic factors of long-term allograft survival in 632 CyA-treated recipients of a primary renal transplant. Transpl Int 1997; 10: 268–75.

Montgomery RA, Zachary AA, Ratner LE, et al. Clinical results from transplanting incompatible live kidney donor/recipient pairs using kidney paired donation. JAMA 2005; 294: 1655–63.

Morales JM, Campistol JM, Bruguera M, et al. Hepatitis C virus and organ transplantation. Lancet 1995; 345: 1174–5.

Muruve NA, Steinbecker KM, Luger AM. Are wedge biopsies of cadaver kidneys obtained at procurement reliable? Transplantation 2000; 69: 2384–8.

Najarian JS, Chavers BM, McHugh LE, Matas AJ. 20 years or more of follow-up of living kidney donors. Lancet 1992; 340: 807–10.

Narkun-Burgess DM, Nolan CR, Norman JE, et al. Forty-five year follow-up after uninephrectomy. Kidney Int 1993; 43: 1110–15.

Natov SN. Transmission of viral hepatitis by kidney transplantation: donor evaluation and transplant policies (Part 1: hepatitis B virus). Transpl Infect Dis 2003; 4: 124–31.

Natov SN, Pereira BJ. Transmission of viral hepatitis by kidney transplantation: donor evaluation and transplant policies. Transpl Infect Dis 2002; 43: 117–23.

Neugarten J, Silbiger S. The impact of gender on renal transplantation. Transplantation 1994; 58: 1145–52.

Nicholson ML, Metcalfe MS, White SA, et al. A comparison of the results of renal transplantation from non-heart beating donors, conventional cadaveric and living donors. Kidney Int 2001; 58: 2585–91.

Nicholson ML, Windmill DC, Horsburgh T, Harris KP. Influence of allograft size to recipient body-weight ratio on the long-term outcome of renal transplantation. Br J Surg 2000; 87: 314–19.

Ojo AO, Wolfe RA, Held PJ, et al. Delayed graft function: risk factors and implications for renal allograft survival. Transplantation 1997; 63: 968–72.

Ojo AO, Leichtman AB, Punch JD, et al. Impact of preexisting donor hypertension and diabetes mellitus on cadaveric renal transplant outcomes. Am J Kidney Dis 2000; 36: 153–9.

Ojo AO, Hanson JA, Meier-Kriesche H, et al. Survival in recipients of marginal cadaveric donor kidneys compared with other recipients and wait-listed transplant candidates. J Am Soc Nephrol 2001; 12: 589–97.

Ojo AO, Luan F, Sung RS, Merion RM. The use of expanded criteria donor organs for transplantation. Transplant Rev 2006; 20: 41–8.

Opelz G. Cadaver kidney graft outcome in relation to ischemia time and HLA match. Collaborative Transplant Study. Transplant Proc 1998; 30: 4294–6.

Opelz G; Collaborative Transplant Study. Non-HLA transplantation immunity revealed by lymphocytotoxic antibodies. Lancet 2005; 365: 1570–6.

Ornstein DL, Lord KE, Yanofsky NN, et al. Successful donation and transplantation of multiple organs after fatal poisoning with brodifacoum, a long-acting anticoagulant rodenticide: case report. Transplantation 1999; 67: 475–8.

Ozdemir FN, Guz G, Sezer S, et al. Ambulatory blood pressure monitoring in potential renal transplant donors. Nephrol Dial Transplant 2000; 15: 1038–40.

Park K, Lee JH, Huh KH, et al. Exchange living-donor kidney transplantation: diminution of donor organ shortage. Transplant Proc 2004; 36: 2949–51.

Pauly RP, Rayner D, Murray AG, et al. Transplantation in the face of severe donor sepsis: pushing the boundaries? Am J Kidney Dis 2004; 44: 64–7.

Penn I. Donor transmitted disease: cancer. Transplant Proc 1991; 23: 2629–31.

Pereira B, Wright T, Schmid C, Levy AS. A controlled study of hepatitis C transmission by organ transplantation. The New England Organ Bank Hepatitis C Study Group. Lancet 1995; 345: 484–7.

Pesavento TC, Henry ML, Falkenhain ME, et al. Obese living kidney donors: short-term results and possible complications. Transplantation 1999; 68: 1491–6.

Poggio ED, Wang X, Weinstein DM, et al. Assessing glomerular filtration rate by estimation equations in kidney transplant recipients. Am J Transplant 2006a; 6: 100–8.

Poggio ED, Hila S, Stephany B, et al. Donor kidney volume and outcomes following live donor kidney transplantation. Am J Transplant 2006b; 6: 616–24.

Pokorna E, Vitko S, Chadimova M, et al. Proportion of glomerulosclerosis procurement wedge renal biopsy cannot alone discriminate for acceptance of marginal donors. Transplantation 2000; 69: 36–43.

Ponticelli C, Villa M, Cesana B, et al. Risk factors for late kidney allograft failure. Kidney Int 2002; 62: 1848–52.

Port FK, Merino RM, Goodrich NP, Wolfe RA. Recent trends and results for organ donation and transplantation in the United States, 2005. Am J Transplant 2006; 6: 1095–100.

Praga M, Hernandez E, Herrero JC, et al. Influence of obesity on the appearance of proteinuria and renal insufficiency after unilateral nephrectomy. Kidney Int 2000; 58: 2111–18.

Pratschke J, Wilhelm MJ, Laskowski I, et al. Influence of donor brain on chronic rejection of renal transplants in rats. J Am Soc Nephrol 2001; 12: 2474–81.

Rajab A, Mahoney JE, Henry ML, et al. Hand-assisted laparoscopic versus open nephrectomies in living donors. Can J Surg 2005; 48: 123–30.

Ramcharan T, Matas AJ. Long-term (20–37 years) follow-up of living kidney donors. Am J Transplant 2002; 2: 959–64.

Randhawa PS, Minervini MI, Lombnardero M, et al. Biopsy of marginal donor kidneys: correlation of histologic findings with graft dysfunction. Transplantation 2000; 69: 36–43.

Rea R, Smith C, Sandhu K, et al. Successful transplant of a kidney with focal glomerulosclerosis. Nephrol Dial Transplant 2001; 16: 416–17.

Remuzzi G, Cravedi P, Perna A, et al. Long-term outcome of renal transplantation from older donors. N Engl J Med 2006; 354: 343–52.

Rodriguez-Puyol D. The aging kidney. Kidney Int 1998; 54: 2247–65.

Roodnat JJ, Zietse R, Mulder PGH, et al. The vanishing importance of age in renal transplantation. Transplantation 1999; 67: 576–80.

Rosendale JD, Dean JR. Organ donation in the United States: 1988–2000. Clin Transplant 2002; 93–104.

Rubin RH. Infection in the organ transplant recipient. In Rubin RH, Young LS, eds. Clinical Approach to Infection in the Immunocompromised Host, 3rd edn. New York: Plenum Press, 1994: 629–705.

Rubin RH, Fishman JA. A consideration of potential donors with active infection – is this a way to expand the donor pool? Transpl Int 1998; 11: 333–5.

Sanchez-Fructuoso AI, Prats D, Marques M, et al. Does renal mass exert an independent effect on the determinants of antigen-dependent injury? Transplantation 2001; 71: 381–6.

Satterthwaite R, Aswad S, Sunga V, et al. Outcome of en bloc and single kidney transplantation from very young cadaveric donors. Transplantation 1997; 63: 1405–10.

Schratzberger G, Mayer G. Age and renal transplantation: an interim analysis. Nephrol Dial Transplant 2003; 18: 471–6.

Schulak JA, Matthews LA, Hricik DE. Renal transplantation using a kidney with a large cyst. Transplantation 1997; 63: 783–5.

Schwartzman MS, Zhang PL, Potdar S, et al. Transplantation and 6-month follow-up of renal transplantation from a donor with systemic lupus erythematosus and lupus nephritis. Am J Transplant 2005; 5: 1772–6.

Segev DL, Simpkins RA, Hartman EC, et al. ABO incompatible high-titer transplantation without splenectomy or anti-CD20 treatment. Am J Transplant 2005; 5: 2750–5.

Seikaly M, Ho PL, Emmett L, Tejani A. The 12th Annual Report of the North American Pediatric Renal Transplant Cooperative Study: renal transplantation from 1987 through 1998. Pediatr Transplant 2001; 5: 215–31.

Sharma AK, Smith G, Smith D, et al. Clinical outcome of cadaveric renal allografts contaminated before transplantation. Transpl Int 2005; 18: 824–7.

Sheil AG. Donor-derived malignancy in organ transplant recipients. Transplant Proc 2001; 33: 1827–9.

Shimmura H, Tanabe K, Ishida H, et al. Lack of correlation between results of ABO-incompatible living kidney transplants and anti-ABO blood type titers under current immunosuppression. Transplantation 2005; 80: 985–8.

Sing A, Stablein D, Tejani A. Risk factors for vascular thrombosis in pediatric renal transplantation. A special report of the North American Pediatric Renal Transplant Cooperative Study. Transplantation 1997; 63: 1263–7.

Smyth GP, Eng MP, Power RP, et al. Long-term outcome of cadaveric pediatric en bloc transplantation – a 15-year experience.Transplant Proc 2005; 37: 4228–9.

Solá R, Guirado L, Diaz JM, et al. Elderly donor kidney grafts into young recipients: results at 5 years. Transplantation 2002; 73: 1673–5.

Spital A. Living kidney donors: still a valuable resource. Curr Opin Organ Transplant 1998; 3: 205–11.

Steinbrook R. Public solicitation of organ donors. N Engl J Med 2005; 353: 441–4.

Stephens JK, Everson GT, Elliott CL, et al. Fatal transfers of malignant melanoma from multiorgan donor to four allograft recipients. Transplantation 2000; 70: 232–6.

Stevens LA, Levey AS. Measurement of kidney function. Med Clin North Am 2005; 89: 457–73.

Stratta RJ, Bennett L. Preliminary experience with double kidney transplants from adult cadaveric donors. Analysis of United Network for Organ Sharing data. Transplant Proc 1997; 29: 3375–6.

Swanson SJ, Hypolite IO, Agodoa LY, et al. Effect of donor factors on early graft survival in adult cadaveric renal transplantation. Am J Transplant 2002; 2: 68–75.

Takada M, Nadeau KC, Hancock WW, et al. Effects of explosive brain death on cytokine activation of peripheral organs in the rat. Transplantation 1998; 65: 1533–42.

Takahashi K, Takahara S, Uchila K, et al. Successful results after 5 years of tacrolimus therapy in ABO-incompatible kidney transplantation in Japan. Transplant Proc 2005; 37: 1800–3.

Tarantino A, Montagnino G, Cesana B, et al. Renal transplantation from older donors. Transplant Proc 2001; 33: 3769–70.

Tilney NL. Transplantation between identical twins: a review. World J Surg 1986; 10: 381–5.

Tyden G, Kumlien G, Fehrman I. Successful ABO-incompatible kidney transplantations without splenectomy using antigen-specific immunoadsorption and rituximab. Transplantation 2003; 76: 730–1.

US Renal Data System. USRDS 2001 Annual Data Report. Incidence and prevalence of ESRDS. Am J Kidney Dis 2001; 38 (Suppl 3): S17–36.

Velidedeoglu E, Williams N, Brayman KL, et al. Comparison of open, laparoscopic, and hand-assisted approaches to live-donor nephrectomy. Transplantation 2002; 74: 169–72.

Vereerstraeten P, Wissing M, De Pauw L, et al. Male recipients from female donors are at increased risk of graft loss from both rejection and technical failure. Clin Transplant 1999; 13: 181–6.

Whiting JF, Golconda M, Smith R, et al. Economic cost of expanded criteria donors in renal transplantation. Transplantation 1998; 65: 204–7.

Whiting JF, Woodward RS, Zavala EY, et al. Economic cost of expanded criteria donors in cadaveric renal transplantation: analysis of Medicare payments. Transplantation 2000; 70: 755–60.

Wijnen RM, Booster MH, Stubenitsky BM, et al. Outcome of transplantation of non-heart-beating donor kidneys. Lancet 1995; 345: 1067–70.

Wolfe RA, Ashby VB, Milford EL, et al. Comparison of mortality in all patients on dialysis, patients on dialysis awaiting transplantation and recipients of a first cadaveric transplant. N Engl J Med 1999; 341: 1725–30.

Wunderlich H, Willhelm S, Reichelt O, et al. Renal cell carcinoma in renal graft recipients and donors: incidence and consequences. Urol Int 2001; 67: 24–7.

Zeier M, Dohler B, Opelz G, Ritz E. The effect of donor gender on graft survival. J Am Soc Nephrol 2002; 13: 2570–6.

Zipitis CS, Augustine T, Tavakoli A, et al. Horseshoe kidney transplantation. Surgeon 2003; 3: 160–3.

SELECTION AND PREPARATION OF THE RECIPIENT

Although today very few conditions represent absolute contraindications to renal transplantation (Table 2.1), the potential risks associated with immunosuppressive therapy necessitate careful selection and preparation of the recipient. The screening of candidates for renal transplantation should include a thorough medical history, physical and psychiatric examination, and immunological evaluation. Attention should also be paid to the age of the patient and to the type of disease responsible for end-stage renal failure. Particularly intensive should be the work-up for cardiovascular disease, infection, and malignancy, which represent the most frequent causes of death after transplantation.

History

A complete medical history of the transplant candidate is important (Table 2.2). The history may be useful to ascertain whether the renal disease has a hereditary or familial origin, information that is particularly important in cases of living-related donation. Patients with a high familial incidence of diabetes mellitus, cardiovascular disease, or neoplasia may be at increased risk for developing these complications after transplantation. The history of the transplantation candidate should also include inquiries about any chronic or recurrent infection, malignancy, gastrointestinal complications, or viral hepatitis. Previous myocardial infarction and/or lower-limb arteriopathy does not always represent a formal contraindication to transplantation, but necessitates a particularly careful evaluation.

The renal history should focus on the nature and duration of the *original renal disease*, the correct diagnosis of which is extremely important to estimate the possible risk of recurrence and to plan particular therapeutic strategies. Whenever possible, the transplant specialist should re-examine clinical documents and the results of renal biopsy of the native kidneys. The severity and duration of *hypertension*, a condition that is usually associated with renal disease, must also be carefully described, since patients with a long history of poor blood pressure control are at greater risk of cardiovascular disease. Adverse reactions to vigorous or prolonged prior immunosuppressive therapy for vasculitis, lupus, rapidly progressive nephritis, or a previous transplant may forecast the events after the planned allograft. To avoid the risk of severe toxicity due to the residual effects of prior immunosuppressants and to permit recovery from a catabolic

Table 2.1   Absolute contraindications to renal transplantation

Short life expectancy (less than 3–5 years)

Recent malignancy
Active infection
Severe pulmonary disease (unless lung and kidney transplantation is indicated)
Severe cardiac failure (unless heart and kidney transplantation is indicated)
Severe liver failure (unless liver and kidney transplantation is indicated)
Uncontrolled psychiatric disorders
Absolute non-compliance in dialysis (?)

Table 2.2   Main data included in transplant candidate history
Hereditary or familial origin of the disease
Previous infections, malignancy, cardiovascular disease, hepatitis
Previous operations
Nature and duration of the original disease
Type and duration of dialysis
Presence of comorbid diseases
Main infections; recent urinary infection
Psychiatric events
Previous transplants; causes of failure, duration of transplant

state induced by steroids, it may be necessary in some cases to postpone a planned transplantation for some months, with the initiation of interim maintenance dialysis.

The *duration of dialysis* is an independent variable associated with outcome. The best results have been reported with pre-emptive transplantation, before dialysis (Meier-Kriesche and Kaplan, 2002a). While dialysis up to 6 months does not have detrimental effect on patient and graft survival (Goldfarb-Rumyantzev et al., 2005a), after this period the longer is the dialysis the poorer is the long-term graft survival (Meier-Kriesche and Kaplan, 2002a). Whether the *type of dialysis* may influence the results of transplantation is still uncertain. Some investigators have reported that delayed graft function is less frequent with peritoneal dialysis while the risk of graft thrombosis is more frequent with hemodialysis (Snyder et al., 2002). However, in other series, patients who had been treated with peritoneal dialysis had a higher risk of graft thrombosis than did patients who had received hemodialysis (Murphy et al., 1994). The worst results were seen in patients who had had to change their regular replacement modalities (Golfarb-Rumyantzev et al., 2005b).

In the past, patients who had failed a previous transplantation have been considered to be at higher risk with *retransplantation,* particularly if they developed high levels of anti-HLA antibodies or had short survival of the previous graft. However, the use of more sensitive crossmatching, better class II HLA matching, and more potent immunosuppressive therapy allowed an improvement of results of the second transplant (Cecka, 2001; Coupel et al., 2003; Meier-Kriesche et al., 2004). In assessing the risk of retransplantation it is important to take into account the period of transplantation, the cause(s) of graft failure, and the longevity of the transplant.

Physical examination

Following the interview, in which a full medical history is obtained, a general screening examination should be conducted. This screening should pay special attention to the exit wound of the peritoneal dialysis catheter or the site of the arteriovenous fistula/graft, either of which represents a potential site of infection. In patients with adult polycystic kidney disease, the size of the kidneys should be evaluated to determine whether nephrectomy is required to afford adequate space for the placement of a renal allograft. In addition to cardiac auscultation, the physician should search for bruits in the carotid arteries, the aorta, and the lower-limb vessels as evidence of arteriosclerotic disease. Evaluation of the dorsalis pedis and posterior tibial pulses may help to discern the better side to place the allograft, with less risk of vascular steal from the distal arterial circulation. To complete the physical examination, men should undergo a rectal examination to detect polypoid neoplasms, as well as a prostate palpation, and women, a gynecological examination. Elderly patients, children, and obese candidates need particular evaluation.

Elderly recipients

As the mean age of the dialysis population is progressively increasing and the results of transplantation are improving, many centers now accept transplantation candidates aged 70 years or more. However, this policy must be tempered with an aggressive diagnostic approach to discover underlying *heart disease* among elderly candidates, since patients ≥ 65 years have a high risk of early-post-transplantation acute myocardial infarction (Kasiske *et al.*, 2006), and since about half of elderly patients who die of a cardiovascular event following transplantation were asymptomatic at the time of their inclusion on the waiting list. Moreover, the screening of elderly patients must include an exhaustive search for and correction of silent *cancer* and *infective* foci. While the risks of cardiovascular, malignant, and infectious complications are higher among elderly patients, the incidence and severity of acute rejection episodes among this group are lower than in younger patients (Meier-Kriesche and Kaplan, 2001). Therefore, immunosuppressive therapy may be tailored to a less vigorous approach, for example by avoidance or prompt withdrawal of steroids and/or minimization of calcineurin inhibitors (Ponticelli, 2005; Segoloni *et al.*, 2005).

Large surveys have shown that graft survival is lower among elderly than among younger transplant recipients (Morris *et al.*, 1999). The difference is mainly accounted for by the higher mortality among older recipients. In fact, death-censored graft survival times among well-selected elderly recipients are comparable to those of young adults (Fabrizii and Horl, 2001; Saudan *et al.*, 2001). Furthermore, if available within a timely period, transplantation may offer substantial clinical benefits in comparison with dialysis to older patients (Cameron, 2000; Jassal *et al.*, 2003).

Many transplant units prefer to use cadaveric donor kidneys from elderly donors for transplants to older recipients. Although the long-term graft survival rates are inferior to those obtained with kidneys from younger donors (Kasiske and Snyder, 2002; Meier-Kriesche *et al.*, 2002b), this strategy can allow the offer of higher probabilities of transplant to older patients and good results (Segoloni *et al.*, 2005). The European Best Practice Guidelines for Renal Transplantation (2002) recommended not to exclude elderly patients from transplantation, because renal transplantation can extend the duration and quality of life also in elderly patients. However, accurate diagnosis and aggressive treatment of cardiovascular disease are recommended because of the high number of deaths with functioning grafts in elderly recipients; immunosuppression must be adapted to avoid both rejections and adverse effects; the high risk of concomitant diseases, such as diabetes mellitus, bone disease, and malignancies, needs special consideration.

Pediatric recipients

Infants (0–1 year) have a high incidence of perioperative problems that result in increased graft loss and mortality (Smith *et al.*, 2002). Therefore, although good results have been reported by single centers in children less than 1 year old (Humar *et al.*, 2001), many pediatricians prefer to maintain infants on a regular dialysis program and to postpone the transplant by 1–2 years until the size of the recipient offers a better chance of success. The results among recipients under 5 years of age are inferior to those observed in pediatric patients above 5 years in the short term, but after the first year the outcome is good (Johnson *et al.*, 2002a). Good results have also been reported in handicapped children (Ohta *et al.*, 2006). Of concern, an American survey showed that adolescents had significantly lower living and cadaveric graft survivals compared with younger recipients (Smith *et al.*, 2002). A likely cause is the lack of compliance (Neu, 2006), which is often associated at least in part with the loss of self-esteem due to the metabolic side-effects of corticosteroids and to the cosmetic toxicities of cyclosporine.

Growth represents a particular problem in children. Several factors can interfere with growth after transplantation. Age is of paramount importance, younger patients exhibiting the greatest immediate catch-up growth (Fine, 2002). The better the graft function, the better the possibility of growing. There is a direct correlation between glomerular filtration rate and level of insulin-like growth factor (Kapila *et al.*, 2001). Despite good renal function, some children do not experience growth catch-up; they remain at the 10th centile of height compared with their peers. To a large extent the problem is due to the administration of steroids, which inhibit growth hormone receptors. Indeed, a reduction in the dose of or complete withdrawal from steroids may facilitate normal growth among children whose epiphyses have not yet closed. Withdrawal of steroids has been reported to expose children to an increased risk of rejection (Klaus et al., 2001). However, with modern immunosuppression, it is possible to avoid steroids completely from the beginning, at least in some children (Sarwal et al., 2001). The administration of growth hormones may also be helpful. Growth rates generally increase by 45% during the first year of hormonal therapy, declining subsequently but remaining above baseline. No major side-effects have been reported in transplanted children (Wuhl et al., 2001). However, the efficacy of growth hormone therapy in transplanted children is lower than that observed in non-transplanted children, once again because of the interference of corticosteroids (Clot et al., 2001). As renal transplantation provides a unique opportunity to reach a reasonable height for many uremic children, attempts to avoid steroids completely from the beginning should be encouraged.

Obesity

Some studies reported poorer results of renal transplantation in obese than in non-obese patients (Holley et al., 1990; Pirsch et al., 1995; Pischon and Sharma, 2001), mainly due to cardiovascular complications and to the proclivity of morbidly overweight patients to develop infective complications. More recent reports, however, did not find different patient and graft survival rates between obese and non-obese recipients, although obese recipients developed diabetes and surgical complications more frequently (Howard et al., 2002; Johnson et al., 2002b; Bennett et al., 2004; Massarweh et al., 2005). Moreover, obese patients who received a renal transplant had a significantly lower mortality than those who remained on the waiting list (Glanton et al., 2003). With the exception of patients with cardiovascular disease, obesity per se does not represent a contraindication to renal transplantation. However, special attention should be paid to preoperative weight-loss programs and to close post-transplant monitoring. Whenever possible, steroid-free immunosuppression should be planned.

Psychological evaluation

Although many candidates exhibit active symptoms of or a predisposition to psychiatric disorders, or have a history of substance abuse, a psychiatric evaluation is generally not an integral part of the screening procedure for transplantation. However, the physician should use his own skills of psychological evaluation during the initial examination to assess the patient's motivation for and likelihood of compliance with the post-transplant regimen.

Poor patient compliance to the post-transplant medical regimen represents one of the most frequent, but underrated, causes of graft loss. Although only a small number of patients display complete non-compliance, which almost inevitably results in graft failure, about 20–50% of patients will admit on post-transplant inquiry that they take some but not all of the prescribed drugs (Laederach-Hofman and Bunzel, 2000). These cases of occasional non-compliance may culminate in late rejection episodes, leading to graft loss. In a meta-analysis of 36 studies, Butler et al. (2004a) reported that the median percentage of patients who did not adhere to treatment was 22%, and the risk of graft failure was 3.6–30 times greater in non-compliant than in compliant patients. The elevated number of pills to take every day is a strong contributor to the poor adherence to treatment. However, non-compliance is particularly frequent in particular subjects, such as black patients (Weng et al., 2005), adolescents (Hsu, 2005), those with a poor income (Chisolm et al., 2005), low believers in transplant medications (Butler et al., 2004b), and patients with social isolation or poor familial support (Rosenberger et al., 2005). Efforts should be made to improve the education of the patient by clearly explaining the benefits and risks of the therapy, to favor contact of the patient with the doctor, and to simplify the therapy whenever possible.

Pre-transplant investigations

A series of laboratory investigations should be performed to complete the evaluation process (Table 2.3). Prior to transplantation, some investigations should be repeated, particularly serum potassium, erythrocyte

Table 2.3 Main investigations for the renal transplant candidate

Hematology
Complete blood count with leukocyte differential
Platelet counts
Bleeding time
Prothrombin time
Partial thromboplastin time
Leiden factor V mutation
Antiphospholipid antibodies

Immunological evaluation
Blood group
HLA tissue typing
Preformed HLA antibodies

Gastrointestinal tract
Stool
Gastroscopy
Serum amylase, lipase
Serum transaminases, bilirubin
Serum cholinesterase
Ultrasonography of liver, gallbladder
Colonoscopy (selected cases)

Metabolic evaluation
Blood sugar (basal, postprandial)
Glycosylated hemoglobin (for diabetics)
Serum cholesterol, triglycerides
Homocysteine (?)
Parathormone levels

Infections
Hepatitis markers (A, B, C)
HBV DNA if HBV-positive; HCV RNA if HCV-positive
Toxotest
Anti-HIV antibodies
Epstein–Barr virus titer
CMV IgG–IgM
Herpes virus titer
Purified protein-derived test

Renal and urological investigations
Serum creatinine
Serum electrolytes

(Continued)

Table 2.3   Continued

Urine culture
Prostate-specific antigen
Kidney and bladder ultrasound
Cystography

Cardiovascular evaluation
Electrocardiogram (12-lead)
Echocardiography
Cardiac scintigraphy (selected cases)
Coronarography (selected cases)
Carotid Duplex study
Peripheral arterial Doppler (selected cases)

Pulmonary evaluation
Chest X-ray
Pulmonary functional test (selected cases)

Gynecological investigations
Pelvic echography
Mammography (>40 years)
Pap test

and leukocyte counts, serum calcemia, blood glucose, liver function tests, and, in selected cases, serum cholinesterase (to avoid the risk of curarization in the case of low levels).

As thrombophilia may contribute to significant morbidity after transplantation, a search for thrombophilic factors in candidates for transplantation is advisable, particularly if a patient has a history of venous thrombosis, is diabetic or atherosclerotic, or, in the case of a woman, is taking an oral contraceptive. The investigation should include factor V mutation, lupus anticoagulant, and antiphospholipid antibodies, which increase significantly the risk of vascular thrombosis and are relatively frequent in uremic patients (Vaidya *et al.*, 2000; Wutrich *et al.*, 2001). A search for deficiency of antithrombin III, protein C, and protein S is generally not necessary, as deficiency of these anticoagulant proteins is quite rare in the general population.

Immunological profile

ABO compatibility

The ABO blood group should be determined once the individual is deemed a transplant candidate. The same criteria as used for blood transfusions may be adopted for renal transplants, with group O being the universal donor and group AB the universal recipient.

Without adequate preparation a transplant between incompatible persons leads to a hyperacute irreversible rejection, sustained by preformed circulating antibodies. However, in contrast to the recent past, ABO-incompatible kidney transplants do not represent a formal contraindication. If anti-A/B antibodies are removed from the blood of the recipient using plasmapheresis (Shimmura *et al.*, 2000) or special immunoadsorptive columns (Tyden *et al.*, 2005) before and in the first days after transplantation, and if the transplant recipient is given aggressive immunosuppression with or without splenectomy, it is possible to obtain long-term allograft survival comparable to that observed with ABO-compatible renal transplants (Shimmura et al., 2005).

Minor ABO incompatibilities may cause hemolytic anemia, which is usually self-limiting, but may be severe and even life-threatening in a few cases (Petz, 2005). Blood group antigens might be implied in the mechanisms of cell rejection. All erythrocyte blood groups are not only demonstrated on red cells. Some of them can be observed on several tissues of the body. However, there is little evidence that minor ABO incompatibilities influence the graft outcome (Sienko et al., 2003). Theoretically, also the Rh system could play a role in the process of graft rejection. Bryan et al. (1998) reported that Rh identity allowed a better graft survival at 7 years, but no impact on long-term outcome of the Rh system could be seen in a more recent series (Osman et al., 2004). It is likely that modern immunosuppression may minimize the impact of these minor incompatibilities on allograft outcome.

HLA histocompatasibility

There is ample evidence that the results of renal transplantation are influenced by the number of HLA A, B, DR mismatches. However, with newer immunosuppressive agents, the impact of HLA mismatches on graft outcome is diminished. Still, fully-HLA matched recipients have a much better probability of long-term graft survival than that of mismatched patients both in cadaveric (Takemoto et al., 2000) and in living renal transplants (Cecka, 2002). This evidence has led several national and international organizations to assign cadaveric kidneys to six-antigen-matched patients as an absolute priority. Otherwise, the various combinations of mismatch have a lesser impact on transplant results (Figure 2.1). With the exception of HLA-identical siblings also with living transplants, the impact of HLA compatibility is much lower than in the past. Kidney allografts from unrelated living donors have the same long-term allograft survival as that obtained with kidney transplants from haploidentical siblings or from parents (Gjertson and Cecka, 2000).

Preformed antibodies

In addition to estimating the extent of preformed cytotoxic antibodies at the time of acceptance for transplantation, sera should be collected at least every 2 months thereafter, both to ascertain the state of sensitization and to have materials on hand for crossmatch testing against a potential donor. Patients who have more than 50% antibodies against a panel have significantly poorer graft survival than non- or less-sensitized patients. In cadaveric renal transplant recipients, the graft half-life is 8.2 years for the above patients, it is 10.6 years for patients with antibodies between 1 and 50%, and it is 11.1 years for patients without antibodies (Cecka, 2002).

A major problem for highly sensitized patients is represented by the difficulty of being transplanted, as they may present specific antibodies againts the lymphocytes of recipients that result in a positive crossmatch with exclusion from transplantation. Glotz et al. (2002) treated 15 highly pre-sensitized patients with intravenous immunoglobulins (IVIG), 2 g/kg body weight, for 3 months. Desensitization was obtained in 13 patients, who were transplanted immediately. One patient lost the graft from thrombosis, and another from rejection. Nine patients experienced no rejection, and still had graft functioning after 1 year or more. The benefit of IVIG in highly sensitized patients has been confirmed by further experiences (Jordan et al., 2006). A significant reduction of preformed anti-HLA antibodies can also be obtained with the anti-CD20 monoclonal antibody rituximab (Vieira et al., 2004). A comparison between plasmapheresis plus low-dose IVIG and anti-CD20 antibody versus high-dose IVIG in patients with positive T-cell crossmatch showed that IVIG decreased donor-specific alloantibodies in all treated patients, but only 38% achieved a negative crossmatch. In contrast, a negative crossmatch was achieved in 84% of plasmapheresed patients and in 88% when antithymoglobulins were added before transplantation to plasmapheresis, low-dose IVIG, and anti-CD20 monoclonal antibody. The rejection rate in patients with a negative crossmatch was significantly higher in patients who received high-dose IVIG than in patients treated with plasmapheresis (Stegall et al., 2006).

Crossmatch

Before transplantation, a crossmatch between the serum of the recipient and the lymphocytes of the donor is mandatory. A positive crossmatch indicates the presence of antibodies in the recipient directed specifically against the donor's antigen. This may result in hyperacute irreversible rejection. The fluocytometry technique appears to be more sensisitve than cytotoxic tests. While there is agreement that transplants should not be performed in the case of a positive T crossmatch, there is more controversy about the significance of B crossmatch. UNOS (United Network for Organ Sharing) data reported that a positive B crossmatch reduced the 5-year graft survival by 4–6% (Cho and Cecka, 2002). In a large retrospective review, no significant difference between B-negative and B-positive crossmatch in the 1-, 5-, and 10-year graft survival rates was found. However, graft survival was significantly reduced comparing an IgG anti-B cell with a B-negative group, as well as for IgG compared with IgM. Thus, only a B-positive crossmatch due to IgG decreases graft survival. However, this possibility is uncommon, at around 0.9% (Fagundes et al., 2005).

Immunological reactivity

Although we are still awaiting a reliable test to identify the immunological reactivity of a transplant candidate, there is some evidence that patients with high serum levels of CD30, a Th2 activation marker, have lower graft survival than that in patients with low serum levels (Susal et al., 2002), the difference being particularly striking in patients with poor HLA matching (Susal et al., 2003). Treatment with tacrolimus has been suggested to offer better protection from chronic rejection in patients with elevated levels of CD30 and neopterin (Weimer et al., 2005).

Previous kidney transplant

Patients who are retransplanted have a higher probability of graft failure than recipients of a first transplant. According to the UNOS registry, the 5-year cadaveric graft survival of first, second, and multiple kidney transplants was 66%, 62%, and 56%, respectively (Cecka, 2001). However, the results of retransplantation may depend on the timing and cause of graft failure. Until recently, there was evidence that patients who lost their prior graft because of *early rejection* had a lower probability of maintaining a functional second cadaveric transplant than patients whose first graft functioned long-term (Rigden et al., 1999). However, in the past few years, the risk of acute rejection in retransplanted patients has lowered significantly (Coupel et al., 2003), and the expected graft half-life of second transplants has improved to about 6 years (Meier-Kriesche et al., 2004).

Patients who have experienced graft failure due to recurrent primary *glomerulonephritis atypical hemolytic uremic syndrome* or *metabolic disease* are at high risk of recurrence after a second transplant.

Patients who have lost their graft because of *polyoma BK* virus or interstitial nephritis are at high risk of recurrence, although successful cases of retransplantation have been reported (Poduval et al., 2002; Ginevri et al., 2003; Ramos et al., 2004; Womer et al., 2006). Most patients receive the same immunosuppression as used with the first transplant. Hirsch and Ramos (2006) recommended: (1) to allow enough time to mount an antiviral response before retransplantation, (2) to remove the primary allograft to deplete BK virus-specific immune effectors, and (3) to screen patients after transplantation carefully.

Finally, the *source of the donor* kidney may influence the outcome of the second transplant. In the case of retransplantation, a living donor should be sought whenever possible, since these transplants yield results far superior to those obtained using cadaveric grafts (Rigden et al., 1999).

Evaluation of infections

Candidates for renal transplant must be screened for the presence of infection. Obviously, the discovery of a potentially life-threatening infection represents a formal contraindication to transplantation. One important occult site of infection is the *teeth*: poor dental hygiene may present an immediate and ongoing risk; the repair of dental caries and necessary tooth extractions prior to transplantation are recommended. While Panorex views of the jaws are useful, they seem to be unnecessary when the patient has undergone a thorough examination by a dentist. Active infections at *access sites* for hemodialysis are also considered as possible exclusions from transplantation, pending completion of at least a 2-week course of antibiotics and, in resistant cases, removal of the infected graft. Although it is generally recommended that immuno-suppression be withheld from dialysis patients who have experienced peritonitis within the previous 3–4 weeks (Kasiske, 1998), candidates for well-matched organs have been successfully transplanted despite recent episodes of cured peritonitis.

Until recently, *HIV-positive* patients were disqualified from transplantation. Even today, most centers con-sider HIV status as a contraindication, since immunosuppressive therapy places them at elevated risk of mor-bidity and mortality. On the other hand, the progress in antiretroviral therapy has decreased the incidence of opportunistic infections, and some initial trials have shown that HIV+ patients can tolerate immunosup-pression and have allograft survival comparable to that of HIV– patients. An American survey (Swanson *et al.*, 2002) reported that in 32 HIV-positive patients who received renal transplant from 1987 to 1997, the 3-year graft survival was lower than in other transplant recipients (53% vs. 73%), while patient survival (83% vs. 88%) was almost comparable. These data led some investigators to consider HIV infection not a formal contraindication to transplantation (Roland and Stock, 2003; Wyatt and Murphy, 2005).

Tuberculosis (TB) is not rare after transplantation, and can be life-threatening. Whether transplant candi-dates should receive tuberculin skin testing (TST) to identify carriers of latent TB is still a matter of debate. Although TST is the most reliable test for identifying persons with TB infection, there are two issues regarding TST. First, patients who have received the BCG vaccine may show a positive reaction to TST. Second, dialysis patients are often anergic, and may display a false-negative reaction to TST (European Best Practice Guidelines for Renal Transplantation, 2002). Patients with a previous history of TB and those with a positive TST should be considered for specific chemoprophylaxis with isoniazid. The recommended dose in dialysis patients is 15 mg/kg twice a day (Korzets and Gafter, 1999) for 9 months. In dialysis patients, chemoprophylaxis is usually well tolerated, but mild hepatic dysfunction is common (Vikrant *et al.*, 2005).

Transplant candidates should be screened for *hepatitis B* surface antigen (HBsAg). Vaccination for HBsAG-negative dialysis patients is recommended, since it affords effective protection in most patients (Tong *et al.*, 2005). After transplantation, HBV-positive patients may remain asymptomatic for years, but serial liver biopsies reveal that most individuals show a progression of their histologic lesions (Fornairon *et al.*, 1996), leading in the long term to death from cirrhosis or extrahepatic sepsis (Younossi *et al.*, 1999; Aroldi *et al.*, 2005). A few patients may even develop fibrosing cholestatic hepatitis and terminal liver failure within a few months after transplantation (Tóth *et al.*, 1998). It is generally agreed that HBsAg-positive patients with biochemically active hepatitis and serologic evidence of active viral replication (pos-itive HBV DNA and e antigen) are at high risk for the development of cirrhosis, and should be rejected as candidates for transplantation (Figure 2.2). Patients free of evidence of viral replication (HBV DNA-negative), but displaying increased levels of liver transaminases, require a liver biopsy to determine their status. While some centers do not recommend a liver biopsy for patients with normal transaminase val-ues, a negative HBsAg, and a negative HBV DNA despite a long history of HBV infection (Morales, 1998; European Best Practice Guidelines for Renal Transplantation, 2002), other investigators (Vosnides, 1997) believe that a biopsy must be performed regardless of blood chemistries, since liver enzymes are poor markers of disease activity in uremic patients. Only if the liver biopsy discloses a picture of low-activity hepatitis (Figure 2.3) should the patient be accepted for renal transplantation (Kasiske, 1998); otherwise, the patient should be considered a poor candidate and renal transplantation discouraged. It has been recommended that HBV-infected dialysis patients receive lamivudine for at least 18–24 months after trans-plantation (Roth, 1999) or until suppression of HBV DNA (Chan *et al.*, 2002). Responders may be recon-sidered for transplantation provided that a new biopsy shows an improvement of the histologic picture. If resistance to lamivudine develops, rescue treatment with adefovir may be tried (Gane and Pilmore, 2002; Fontaine *et al.*, 2005). It should be noted, however, that natural immunity to HBV may not protect against reactivation in patients undergoing immunosuppressive therapy (Berger *et al.*, 2005).

Hepatitis C virus (HCV) infection is becoming increasingly common among dialysis patients. Although patients on dialysis have less severe hepatitis C than matched controls without renal disease (Cotler *et al.*,

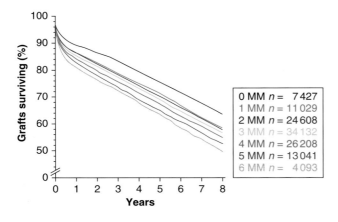

Figure 2.1 Renal allograft survival rates according to HLA A, B, DR mismatches (MM). Data from the Collaborative Transplant Study: first cadaver kidney transplants 1985–2004

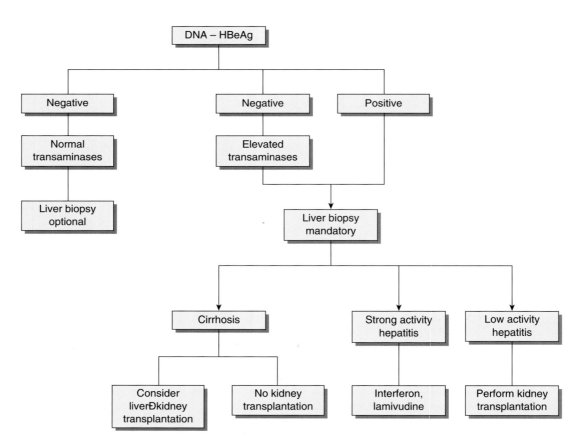

Figure 2.2 Algorithm for evaluating the suitability of a HBsAg+ transplant candidate

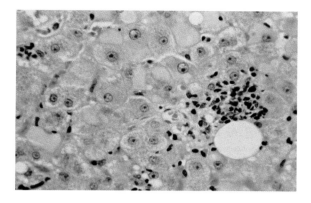

Figure 2.3 A 30-year-old male carrier of HBV. Liver biopsy shows a mild lobular hepatitis, with foci of spotty necrosis and several ground-glass hepatocytes. H&E × 75. (Courtesy of Dr MF Donato, Ospedale Maggiore, Milan, Italy.)

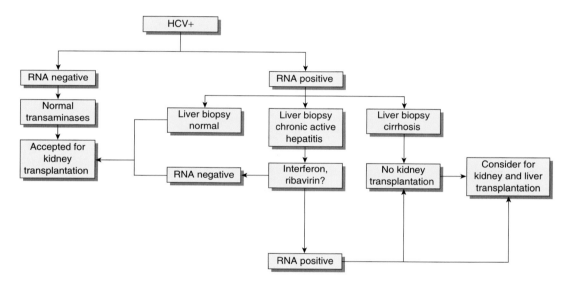

Figure 2.4 Algorithm for evaluating the suitability of a HCV+ transplant candidate

2002), a prospective study reported a better long-term survival rate for transplant patients than for those who remained on dialysis (Pereira and Levey, 1997). After renal transplantation, many HCV-positive patients remain asymptomatic for 5 years or more (Roth, 1995), but repeated biopsies reveal that more than 50% of these transplant recipients display chronic liver disease within 10 years (Vosnides, 1997). HCV-positive status of the recipient increases the risk of graft failure (Fabrizi et al., 2005) and mortality (Batty et al., 2001; Morales et al., 2004; Fabrizi et al., 2005). Cirrhosis, extrahepatic sepsis, and cardiovascular disease are the most frequent causes of death. There is agreement that HCV-positive patients who do not have evidence of severe liver disease are considered good candidates for transplantation. Because the histologic severity of liver disease is the best predictor of hepatic failure and death after renal transplantation, all HCV-positive patients, including those with normal liver enzymes, should undergo a RNA viral charge and ideally a hepatic biopsy to assess disease severity before acceptance as a renal transplant candidate (Figure 2.4). Patients with mild activity may be considered good candidates (Figure 2.5), while the presence of chronic active hepatitis or cirrhosis should be considered a formal contraindication to isolated kidney transplantation. To reduce the risk of liver failure after transplantation, it has been

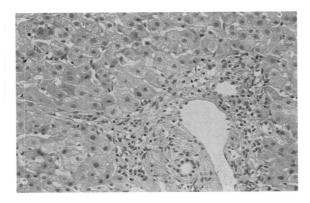

Figure 2.5 A 51-year-old man with HCV-positive hepatitis, showing no signs of activity; mild enlarged portal tract with fibrosis and scanty inflammatory cells; no evidence of periportal necrosis; and pleiomorphic hepatocytes. H&E × 75. (Courtesy of Dr MF Donato, Ospedale Maggiore, Milan, Italy.)

suggested that dialysis patients with evidence of disease undergo therapy with interferon-α. This treatment is usually poorly tolerated by dialysis patients, but can give excellent results in selected cases (Bunnapradist et al., 2002). Unfortunately, most individuals tend to relapse after the cessation of therapy. The addition of ribavirin is very effective in non-renal patients, but it causes a dose-dependent hemolytic anemia which generally precludes its use in dialysis patients (Pol et al., 2002).

Hepatitis G virus (HGV) is caused by GBV-C virus, which is closely related to HCV. HGV is highly prevalent among dialysis patients. A study in renal transplant recipients, however, showed that HGV infection carries a low risk of chronic liver disease even in the long term. Low levels of HCV RNA found in HGV carriers suggest an interaction between these two viruses in transplanted patients (De Filippi et al., 2001). Renal transplantation should not be discouraged solely on the basis of a positive test for GBV-C virus.

Evaluation of cancer

The initial evaluation of the transplant candidate should include an exhaustive history or present stigmata of cancer. In addition to the aforementioned radiological and echographic investigations, the pre-transplant screening should include guaiac (Hemoccult®) testing of the stool and neoplasia markers, particularly prostate-specific antigen in elderly men. Women over 40 years of age or with a family history of breast carcinoma should undergo mammography. Female candidates of all ages must undergo a pelvic examination and a Pap test (cervical smear); men over the age of 50 years should be screened for prostate carcinoma.

The decision whether to consider transplantation for a candidate with a previous history of malignancy but without current evidence of active disease is difficult. Patients may be readily accepted if their neoplasm was a non-invasive basal-cell carcinoma, fully excised squamous-cell carcinoma, or *in situ* bladder neoplasia. In other instances, it is difficult to determine the risk with certainty, since immunosuppressive therapy produces a variable degree of reduction of immunosurveillance, possibly favoring the development and certainly favoring the progression of occult cancer. Penn (1997) estimated the risk of recurrence of neoplastic disease to be 54% of patients if the transplant is performed within 2 years, 33% if performed at 25–60 months, and 13% if performed more than 5 years after apparent recovery from neoplasia.

The length of waiting time may depend on the type of cancer (Table 2.4). It is difficult to decide whether and when to accept women who have had breast cancer; in most cases the cancer recurs after more than 3 years. A waiting time of at least 5 years is desirable for most cases of carcinoma of the breast. For patients with *in situ* bladder cancer, a 1-year wait prior to transplantation may be sufficient, but at least 5 years should pass before considering apparently disease-free patients with a history of diffuse or invasive bladder cancers. In cases of an isolated malignant nodule of the prostate, a wait of 1–2 years may be sufficient, while transplantation should be avoided in cases of diffuse prostatic cancer. A waiting time of at least

Table 2.4   Suggested waiting time before transplantation after apparent cure of the tumor, based on studies of Dr Israel Penn (1997)

No waiting time (low risk of recurrence)
Non-invasive skin basal-cell carcinoma
Fully excised squamous-cell carcinoma
In situ bladder carcinoma
Incidentally discovered small renal carcinoma
Thyroid carcinoma

At least 2 years (intermediate risk of recurrence)
Renal carcinoma
Wilm's tumor
Urothelioma
In situ uterus carcinoma

At least 5 years (high risk of recurrence)
Invasive uterus carcinoma
Melanoma
Breast carcinoma
Diffuse bladder carcinoma
Colorectal carcinoma
Sarcoma
Myeloma

5 years is recommended in cases of lymphoma and carcinomas of the colon or rectum, while a 2–year wait is usually sufficient for patients with other cancers. No waiting period is necessary for incidentally discovered carcinomas, *in situ* carcinomas, and possibly tiny focal neoplasma (Penn, 1997).

Renal-cell carcinoma

The relative risk for cancer of the kidney is increased 3.6-fold in dialysis patients (Stewart *et al.*, 2003). About one-quarter of renal-cell carcinomas are discovered incidentally during medical evaluation for other disorders, during nephrectomy, or during surgery for other reasons (Penn, 1998). Small, non-metastasized, incidentally discovered carcinomas usually do not recur (Penn, 1997). The search for renal carcinomas should be particularly intensive for patients with *analgesic nephropathy* and/or *Balkan nephropathy*, which are frequently associated with urothelial malignancies (Stewart *et al.*, 2003). Another frequent cause of cancer in native kidneys is *acquired cystic disease*, a condition that may occur in about one-third of dialysis patients, being particularly frequent in long-term dialysis patients (Denton *et al.*, 2002). Carcinomas caused by acquired cystic disease are frequently of the papillary type and multifocal (Peces *et al.*, 2004). It is recommended that long-term dialysis recipients be screened by kidney ultrasonography and/or CT prior to their acceptance as candidates for transplantation. The risk of recurrence of renal cancer after transplantation is around 19%, similar to the range expected for general population. Waiting time of less than 2 years, 2–5 years, and more than 5 years did not correlate with recurrence rates (Hanaway *et al.*, 2005). The risk is mainly related to the size of the tumor and its external spread. Although no clear size cut-off exists, a 2-year wait has been suggested (Penn, 1997). As Rapamune® can prolong the survival of mice inoculated with renal cancer (Luan *et al.*, 2002), immunosuppression based on mTOR (mammalian target of rapamycin) antagonists may be suggested for patients at risk of post-transplant renal-cell carcinoma.

Carcinomas of the uterus

The risk for recurrence of uterine cervical and body cancers is related to the spread of tumor outside the uterus and into regional lymph nodes. *In situ* carcinomas display a low risk of recurrence after excision either by core biopsy or by hysterectomy. However, a waiting time of 2 years from cancer treatment to transplant is recommended to minimize the risk of disseminated disease. In contrast, women with invasive carcinomas should wait at least 4–5 years before becoming a transplant candidate (Penn, 1997).

Evaluation of specific systems

Gastrointestinal evaluation

An *abdominal ultrasound* scan is recommended for patients who are symptomatic, diabetic, or aged more than 45 years in order to exclude abnormal masses or signs of metastasis.

In view of the risk of post-transplant peptic ulcer disease, *gastroscopy* is routinely conducted by many, but not all, centers. Patients with *colonic disease,* those aged above 60 years, or carriers of polycystic kidney disease, which is often associated with colonic complications (Dominguez Fernandez *et al.*, 1998), should be evaluated by barium enema and, if indicated, by colonoscopy. In the case of repeated or severe bouts of *diverticulitis,* which once again is more frequent and dangerous in patients with polycystic kidney disease (Lederman *et al.*, 2000), pre-emptive surgical resection may be indicated. Although little information is available about strategies for candidates who have previously experienced *pancreatitis,* problems due to lipid disorders or to alcohol abuse should be corrected prior to transplantation. It should be remembered that, in the absence of a history of acute or chronic pancreatitis or polycystic pancreatic disease, many uremic patients display elevated serum amylase levels or lipase values, without evidence of lesions either by computerized tomography scan or by endoscopic retrograde pancreatography (Tsianos *et al.*, 1994). Exclusion, by endoscopic retrograde cholangiopancreatography, of a precipitating disease within the biliary tree or of abnormalities of the pancreatic ductal tree may be necessary prior to acceptance for transplantation. In view of the possible association between severe hyperparathyroidism and pancreatitis, careful screening should be done in patients with a long history of uremia or with clinical and biochemical signs of hyperparathyroidism. Efforts should be made to avoid hypercalcemia, which seems to be an important factor predisposing to pancreatitis (Carnaille *et al.*, 1998).

Similar to the indications for cholecystectomy in surgical practice on non-end-stage renal-disease patients, the presence of *gallstones per se* is usually not a sufficient cause for operative intervention (Kao *et al.*, 2005). However, in transplant candidates or post-transplant patients, the occurrence of just one bout of acute cholecystitis represents a sufficient indication for operative intervention, particularly if accompanied by cholangitis, biliary colic, and/or gallstone pancreatitis. In contradistinction to most other medical conditions in dialysis patients, gallstone disease is likely to be exacerbated post-transplantation, since both calcineurin inhibitor and mTOR inhibitor agents, as well as their metabolites, are excreted in and increase the lithogenicity of bile. Whereas in the pre-transplant period the gallstones tend to be large and solitary, or, at most, modest in number and readily visualized by abdominal ultrasonography, in the post-transplant period new stones tend to be formed as small fragments of mixed composition.

Urological investigations

A thorough evaluation of the urinary tract prior to renal transplantation is mandatory to avoid unforeseen problems occurring post-transplantation. While the patient history generally guides investigations of the urinary apparatus, several diagnostic tools can be exploited to assess the urological risks in transplant candidates (Table 2.5). An abdominal computerized tomography or an ultrasonographic investigation

Table 2.5 Urological work-up in a candidate for transplantation

All patients
History
Abdominal ultrasound
Urine and urine culture (if possible)

Lower urinary tract abnormalities
Voiding cystourethrography
Urodynamic studies
Cystoscopy

Candidates over 50 years and/or with long-term dialysis
Computerized tomography or magnetic resonance
If man: rectal digital examination and prostate echography
If woman: gynecological examination

Analgesic abuse or Balkan nephropathy
Search for malignant tumor cells in the urine
Cystoscopy
Computerized tomography or magnetic resonance

may reveal nephrolithiasis versus abnormal renal masses or acquired cystic disease. Although the utility of routine voiding cystourethrograms has been challenged due to the cost and potential morbidity associated with the procedure, it affords useful information about the presence and extent of vesicoureteral reflux, the size of the bladder (and anomalies such as trabeculations or diverticula of its surface), and post-void residua. In some cases, this study may provide the information that guides a pre-transplant bilateral nephroureterectomy, bladder augmentation, bladder-neck revision, prostrate resection, or intermittent self-catheterization program, respectively. Cystography has been recommended by some workers only for patients with pyuria, massive crystalluria, a positive urine culture, or previously diagnosed urological abnormalities. Males over 45 years should receive a digital rectal examination and prostate echography to exclude benign hyperplasia or cancer of the prostate. A close urological work-up is recommended in children who suffer from frequent lower urinary tract abnormalities (Van der Weide et al., 2006). Surgical reparative techniques ensuring voiding and adequate control of urinary infections are mandatory in children with severe bladder dysfunction. Augmentation cystoplasty and intermittent catheterization are appropriate techniques currently used for achieving this outcome (Mendizabal et al., 2005).

Cardiovascular evaluation

Cardiovascular disease represents the leading cause of mortality after renal transplantation, accounting for more than 50% of deaths (Briggs, 2001; Cecka, 2003). Thus, a careful work-up of the cardiovascular system and appropriate treatment of abnormalities before admitting a candidate to an active waiting-list are of paramount importance to prevent post-transplant morbidity and mortality.

Cardiac evaluation requires careful preoperative screening. The depth of the investigation depends on the estimated cardiac risk of the candidate (Table 2.6). *Low-risk patients* may be screened simply with an

Table 2.6   Risk factors for post-transplant cardiac events

Low risk	Intermediate risk	High risk
Age <50 years	Age 51–69 years	Age ≥70 years
No smoking	Light smoker	Heavy smoker
Normal ECG	Moderate LVH	Severe LVH
Controlled or no hypertension	Moderate hypertension	Severe hypertension
No diabetes	No diabetes	Diabetes mellitus
Dialysis <3 years	Dialysis 3–6 years	Dialysis >5 years
No previous cardiac events	No previous cardiac events	Previous cardiac infarct
		Unstable angina
		Congestive heart failure

ECG, electrocardiogram; LVH, left ventricular hypertrophy

electrocardiogram (ECG) and echocardiography, which may discover valvular disease, cardiomyopathy, pericardial disease and/or cardiac wall movement. In *intermediate-risk patients,* resting ECG may be predictive of coronary events, while the exercise ECG has a sensitivity of only 35% (Sharma *et al.*, 2005). These patients may require myocardial perfusion studies. There is no consensus as to the preferred study in this setting. Thallium scintigraphy, dipyridamole thallium (or sestamibi) testing, dobutamine echocardiography, and/or dipyridamole echocardiography have a sensitivity between 70 and 80% and a specificity between 85 and 95% (Kasiske *et al.*, 2000). A meta-analysis reported that dialysis patients with a positive test for impaired myocardial perfusion had a significantly greater risk for cardiac infarct and cardiac death compared with patients with a negative test (Rabbat *et al.*, 2003). High-risk patients, even when asymptomatic, should undergo coronary angiography. Treatment should be based on the extent of the underlying coronary artery disease. Multislice computerized tomography, particularly with 16-slice technology, allows good coronary stenosis identification. It is now possible to detect coronary heart disease with this technology, which can replace or help a coronary angiogram in some but not all indications (Vembar *et al.*, 2006). Patients with stenoses greater than 70% are at high risk of a cardiac event. However, there are no data to suggest that coronary revascularization in the absence of symptoms of ischemia is better than medical treatment with beta-blockers, ACE inhibitors, low-dose aspirin, and statins. Rather, coronary revascularization is needed in symptomatic patients (Pilmore, 2006). High-risk symptomatic patients who are not candidates for revascularization should not be accepted on the waiting list (Figure 2.6). Because even a patient who undergoes surgical intervention may not improve sufficiently to be a suitable candidate, we recommend repeat echocardiography 6 months after the procedure in order to assess its benefits.

A *peripheral vascular* examination helps to determine the site for and the technical feasibility of transplantation. The presence of pelvic vessel disease is an important risk factor for surgery. Placement of the allograft constitutes an appreciable vascular 'steal' from the extremity, particularly in the presence of an ipsilateral arteriovenous graft (Zeier and Ritz, 2002). The abdominal X-ray may show calcifications in the iliac vessel, a condition that may pose challenges for the vascular anastomoses. Echography may be useful to exclude aortic aneurysms as well as abdominal masses or abnormal liver parenchyma. Echo color Doppler study of the lower limbs should be performed not only in patients with initial claudicatio intermittens but also in diabetics, heavy smokers, and older patients.

Cerebrovascular complications are more frequent in patients with severe hypertension, diabetes mellitus, long-term dialysis, and advanced age and in heavy smokers. In these cases, carotid artery ultrasonography is advisable. Color Doppler study of the carotid is mandatory for patients who have experienced a previous stroke or transient ischemic attacks, as well as in patients with carotid bruit. Indications to

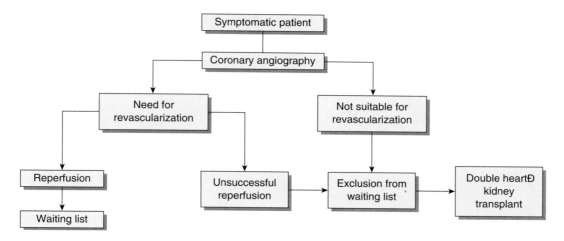

Figure 2.6 Algorithm for inclusion on the waiting list of a symptomatic transplant candidate at high cardiovascular risk

perform angio-magnetic resonance in patients with autosomal dominant polycystic kidney diseases are usually limited to those patients with a family history of intracranial aneurysm or in the case of new-onset severe headache.

Pulmonary evaluation

The risk of postoperative respiratory complications has markedly decreased since doses of steroids have been considerably reduced. However, pneumonia is a not-uncommon complication in the postoperative period, and may become life-threatening. To reduce the incidence and severity of pneumonitis, patients who smoke should be advised to stop prior to transplantation. Patients with bronchiectasis or repeated pulmonary infections are at high risk of severe pneumonia, and should be excluded from transplantation unless a complete and prolonged sterilization can be obtained with antibiotic prophylaxis, frequently combined with either segmentectomy or lobectomy of a particularly virulent nidus of lung parenchyma.

Original renal or systemic disease

Primary glomerulonephritis

All forms of glomerulonephritis may recur after transplantation and may lead to graft failure, but the risks of disease recurrence and its consequences differ among the various subtypes of glomerulonephritis (Table 2.7). Although patients with recurrence have a poorer long-term graft survival than that of standard transplant recipients (Hariharan et al., 1999), this effect may be diluted by many other factors influencing the success of renal transplantation. In our experience (Ponticelli et al., 2002a), patients who have received a kidney transplant because of primary glomerulonephritis have the same probability of long-term graft survival as transplant recipients with other causes of end-stage renal disease (Figure 2.7).

Focal and segmental glomerulosclerosis

Of all the forms of glomerulonephritis, focal and segmental glomerulosclerosis (FSGS) is associated with the highest rate of graft failure, particularly in children. The rate of recurrence varies from 20 to 40% and is higher among children (Tejani and Stablein, 1992). The risk of FSGS recurrence is particularly increased among recipients of second renal transplants (Baum et al., 2001). Many patients with recurrent disease display massive proteinuria within a few days after transplantation. Graft failure with early recurrence

Table 2.7 Risk of recurrence and relative risk of graft failure in patients with recurrent primary renal disease

Primary renal disease	Risk of recurrence (%)	Relative risk of graft loss in patients with recurrence
Focal glomerulosclerosis	20–40	2.25
Membranous GN	6–30	?
Membranoproliferative GN	~10 (3–48)	2.4–2.6
IgA mesangial GN	~35 (9–60)	1.0 up to 10 years
Anti-GBM GN	10–30	1.0 if no circulating anti-GBM antibodies
SLE nephritis	<5–30	~1.0
Henoch–Schönlein	20	?
Hemolytic uremic syndrome	8–56	5.4

GN, glomerulonephritis; GBM, glomerular basement membrane; SLE, systemic lupus erythematosus

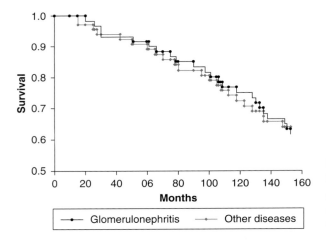

Figure 2.7 Probability of graft survival in 374 renal transplant recipients with glomerulonephritis and in 490 patients with other causes of end-stage renal failure. Modified from Ponticelli *et al.*, 2002

approaches 30% at 3 years (Koushik and Matas, 2005). Late recurrence is more rare, and has an insidious presentation and a less aggressive course.

Unfortunately, it is difficult to predict which patients will show recurrent FSGS (Table 2.8). *Onset in childhood* (Tejani and Stablein, 1992), *rapid progression* to uremia, and the presence of *diffuse mesangial* expansion in native kidneys (Cameron, 1991) have been considered potential risk factors for recurrence. In a pediatric study, the presence of a permeability factor in plasma was predictive of recurrence after transplantation (Dall'Amico *et al.*, 1999). Theoretically, patients with familial FSGS associated with *mutations in podocin* should not have recurrence after transplantation. In fact, proteinuria in these cases will be caused by an altered glomerular permselectivity due to the mutation of podocin, a protein of the podocyte involved in the anchorage of nephrin. However, recent data showed a high rate of recurrence in patients with FSGS associated with mutations of podocin, suggesting a multifactorial etiopathogenesis in this disease (Bertelli *et al.*, 2003).

Table 2.8 Risk factors for FSGS recurrence

Previous graft loss due to recurrence
Pediatric age
Rapidly progressive course
Diffuse mesangial expansion in the native kidney
Living donation?
Permeability factor?

Despite the risk of recurrence and the bad prognosis for recurrent cases, FSGS is not considered a contraindication to cadaveric renal transplantation. Use of a living donor may be associated with some reservations (Baum et al., 2001), although a survey of American data reported an excellent graft outcome for zero HLA-mismatch living-transplant recipients (Cibrik et al., 2003). Nevertheless, the possibility of FSGS recurrence, which could destroy the allograft, must be discussed extensively with both the donor and the recipient.

Pre-emptive *plasmapheresis* before transplantation has been shown to reduce the risk of recurrence in some patients (Ohta et al., 2001). In the case of recurrence, early implementation of aggressive plasmapheresis or immunoadsorption with protein A columns could reduce the degree of proteinuria in more than half of patients (Bosch and Wendler, 2001; Valdivia et al., 2005). In a number of responders, however, further relapses of nephrotic proteinuria can occur, and prolonged use of plasmapheresis may be necessary (Ponticelli et al., 2002b). Good results have been reported in children with intravenous cyclosporine (Salomon et al., 2003).

Membranous nephropathy

Membranous nephropathy (MN) recurs after renal transplantation in 20–30% of cases (Montagnino et al., 1989; Odorico et al., 1996; Briganti et al., 2002). No clinical or histologic findings are available to allow prediction of which patients will show recurrence. The prognosis of recurrent MN is difficult to assess. In a large series of 30 cases of MN recurrence, 38% lost their grafts at 5 years and 52% at 10 years (Cosyns et al., 1998). Cases of spontaneous remission of proteinuria have occurred (Marcen et al., 1996). The issue is obfuscated by the observation that some transplant patients develop *de novo* MN (Hariharan et al., 1999), a condition which is almost indistinguishable from recurrent MN. At present, the renal failure etiology of MN is not considered a contraindication to renal transplantation.

Membranoproliferative glomerulonephritis

An analysis of the ERA–EDTA (European Renal Association–European Dialysis and Transplant Association) Registry database reported a 6% rate of recurrence for *type I membranoproliferative glomerulonephritis* (MPGN) (Briggs and Jones, 1999), similar to the 11% reported by the Australia and New Zealand Dialysis and Transplant Registry (Briganti et al., 2002). Some single-center series have reported higher rates of recurrence, up to 48% in adults (Andresdottir et al., 1997). As for other glomerulonephritis, the risk of recurrence of MPGN increases with the time of observation after transplantation. No clinical features seem to predict the recurrence of type I MPGN, except for ethnicity: the recurrence of MPGN is exceptional in Japanese patients (Shimizu et al., 1998). The recurrence of type I MPGN increases the risk of graft failure by 2.4–2.6-fold (Hariharan et al., 1999; Briganti et al., 2002).

Although in most cases histopathologic evaluations of transplanted kidneys displaying recurrence of *type II MPGN* show intramembranous dense deposits (Cameron, 1991; Andresdottir et al., 1999), clinical evidence of recurrent disease is less frequent. Up to one-quarter of adults with type II MPGN lost their grafts in a single-center experience (Andresdottir et al., 1999). In children, the risk of post-transplant recurrence ranges between 48% (Little et al., 2006) and 68% (Braun et al., 2005). Graft survival is poorer in

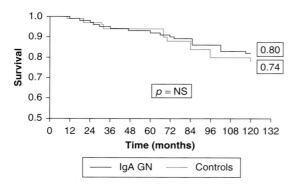

Patients at risk: 12m 24m 36m 48m 60m 72m 84m 96m 108m 120m
IgA   76   70   68   51   42   32   24   20   17   14
Controls   164 140 127 105   90   71   58   44   41   36

Figure 2.8 Probability of long-term graft survival in 76 transplant patients with IgA glomerulonephritis (GN) and in 164 transplant controls transplanted immediately before and immediately after patients with IgA glomerulonephritis. Modified from Ponticelli *et al.*, 2001

patients with recurrence. Younger age at initial diagnosis and the presence of crescents on the original biopsy are independently associated with recurrence on multivariate analysis, suggesting that the severity of the original disease increases the risk of post-transplant recurrence (Little *et al.*, 2006).

In summary, the risk of recurrence of MPGN type I and II is still poorly defined. In spite of an increased risk of graft failure for patients with recurrence, neither type I nor type II MPGN is considered a contraindication to renal transplantation.

IgA nephritis

The recurrence of mesangial deposits of IgA in the renal allograft of patients with IgA nephropathy (IgAGN) ranges around 35% (Ponticelli *et al.*, 2001), but depends largely on the time of transplant biopsy, being more frequent in patients with long-term graft function. As is the case for other primary glomerulonephritis, no clinical or histologic factors have been identified that predict the risk of post-transplant recurrence of IgAGN, although women (Soler *et al.*, 2005) and younger patients (Ponticelli *et al.*, 2001) seem to be more susceptible to recurrence. Whether recurrence is more frequent in living-related transplant recipients is still controversial (Kim *et al.*, 2001; Wang *et al.*, 2001).

Nevertheless, patients with IgAGN are generally considered good candidates for renal transplantation. In a large series (Ponticelli *et al.*, 2001), we could not find any difference in the 10-year graft survival rates between patients with and without IgAGN or between patients with or without recurrence (Figure 2.8).

Anti-GBM glomerulonephritis

Linear glomerular deposits of IgG may occur in 10–30% of transplant patients with anti-GBM (antiglomerular basement membrane) glomerulonephritis (anti-GBM GN; Glassock, 1997). Clinical disease is rare and usually mild, but graft failure occurs in at least a small fraction of patients (Borza *et al.*, 2005). Among patients who do not display circulating anti-GBM antibodies at the time of transplantation, the recurrence of anti-GBM GN is exceptional. Thus, it is recommended that the blood of potential recipients be tested for anti-GBM antibodies, and that renal transplantation be delayed until they have completely disappeared – a process that usually takes 6–12 months.

Systemic diseases

Systemic lupus erythematosus (SLE)

The graft survival rates of patients with lupus nephritis are similar to those of patients with other primary renal diseases, both in adults (Clark and Jevnikar, 1999; Moroni *et al.*, 2005) and in children (Gipson *et al.*, 2003). However, different centers report wide variations in the outcome of allografts, probably due to differing criteria for the selection of transplant recipients. The risk of recurrent lupus nephritis has been reported to range around 30% in a single-center analysis (Goral et al., 2003), but was extremely low, around 2–3%, in large surveys (Stone et al., 1997; Grimbert et al., 1998), and the histologic lesions in transplant patients with recurrent disease tend to be mild (Nyberg et al., 1992; Goral et al., 2003).

The major post-transplant problems in lupus patients are not caused by a recurrence of SLE in the graft, but by extrarenal complications related either to the disease itself or to previous steroid and/or other immunosuppressive drug treatments. Cardiovascular disease frequently occurs, and represents a leading cause of morbidity and mortality. In addition to the traditional risk factors, SLE patients frequently suffer from cardiac valvular disease, and may be carriers of antiphospholipid antibodies, which increase the risk of thrombotic events (Moroni et al., 2004) as well as of cardiac and cerebral complications (Brey et al., 2002). It is also likely that inflammation processes strongly contribute to the increased risk of accelerated atherogenesis in SLE patients (Sander and Giles, 2002). Pre-transplant and post-transplant corticosteroid therapy may further exacerbate cardiovascular complications, as well as produce severe osteoporosis, diabetes mellitus, myopathy, and cataracts, which impair the quality of life of these patients. Also, infections are more frequent and severe in patients who have received a long and vigorous immunosuppression before transplantation, and represent the major cause of death in children (Bartosh et al., 2001). Finally, patients with SLE seem to be exposed to an increased risk of malignancy, particularly non-Hodgkin's lymphoma, although the available results are difficult to interpret definitively (Bernatsky et al., 2002).

For these reasons, the evaluation of transplant candidates must accurately describe the disease and complications, particularly the cardiovascular conditions, possible existence of an underlying infection or cancer, and bone mineral density, of patients with a long history of SLE. While the activity of lupus is alleviated under dialysis therapy, frequently allowing complete cessation of steroid treatment, other patients stabilize only when treated with daily doses of 5–10 mg prednisone. For more frail patients, we recommend a 1–2-year waiting period before transplantation for stabilization and recovery from the metabolic and toxic effects of steroids and other immunosuppressive agents (Ponticelli and Moroni, 2005).

Henoch–Schönlein purpura

The short-term results in patients transplanted after a primary renal disease of Henoch–Schönlein purpura are similar to those obtained with other diseases (Briggs and Jones, 1999). While histologic evidence of the recurrence of mesangial deposits containing IgA may occur in about half of these patients, clinical recurrence has been reported in fewer than 20% of cases (Meulders et al., 1994). However, the risk of recurrence is probably higher in the long term. In fact, cases of recurrence have been reported after 20 years of renal replacement therapy (Piccoli et al., 2001). Clinically, recurrence may present with hematuria, proteinuria, and hypertension. Histologic recurrence is characterized by focal and segmental necrotizing glomerulonephritis and mesangial IgA deposits. Graft survival of patients with recurrence is 57% at 2 years (Briggs and Jones, 1999).

Amyloidosis

Amyloidosis is a systemic disease that may involve several organs (Figure 2.9), and may lead to death due to infections, cardiovascular disease, or progressive cachexia. Moreover, the risk of recurrence of disease in the kidney transplant is approximately 25% (Harrison et al., 1993). Thus, transplantation should be discouraged for patients with severe sequelae of amyloidosis (Kasiske et al., 1995). However, individuals affected by familial Mediterranean fever may be exempt from this exclusion, since early and regular administration of colchicine can prevent intrarenal deposits of amyloid substances (Sever et al., 2001), allowing a long-term outcome similar to that of the general transplant population (Sherif et al., 2003). In addition, acceptable results of renal transplantation have also been obtained in young patients with concomitant rheumatoid arthritis (Emiroglu et al., 2005).

Hemolytic uremic syndrome/thrombotic thrombocytopenic purpura

The risk of recurrence of hemolytic uremic syndrome (HUS) ranges between 8% (Quan et al., 2001) and 56% (Lahlou et al., 2000). A review of USRDS (United States Renal Data System) data (Reynolds et al., 2003)

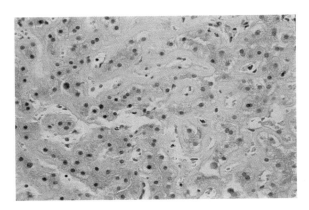

Figure 2.9 Hepatic amyloidosis. Perisinusoidal deposition of amyloid in the space of Disse. Hematoxylin and eosin stain (H&E) × 75. (Courtesy of Dr MF Donato, Ospedale Maggiore, Milan, Italy.)

reported a recurrence of thrombotic microangiopathy in 29% of patients transplanted because of HUS or thrombotic thrombocytopenic purpura (TTP). While patients who have the typical HUS associated with diarrhea do not show a recurrence after transplantation (Ferraris *et al.*, 2002), the risk of recurrence is elevated for patients with non-diarrheal and familial forms of HUS (Ruggenenti, 2002). Approximately 50% of these patients have mutations in one of the complement control proteins: factor H, factor I, or membrane cofactor protein (MCP). In the presence of mutations of these factors, the alternative pathway of complement cannot be underregulated and can contribute to the development of HUS/TTP. Patients with factor H or factor I mutation have a risk of recurrence approaching 80–100%, while MCP deficiency can be corrected in part by renal transplantation. In transplant candidates who have developed renal failure because of HUS or TTP, it has been suggested to perform antigenic screening for factor H and factor I deficiency and to look for low levels of MCP (CD46) expression using flow cytometry (Atkinson *et al.*, 2005). Hypertension must be treated vigorously. Bilateral nephrectomy should be considered in cases of hypertension refractory to treatment. In a series, anephric patients were less prone to HUS recurrence than were patients with native kidneys (Lahlou *et al.*, 2000). The use of calcineurin inhibitors, mTOR antagonists, or antilymphocyte antibodies should be avoided in transplanted patients with sporadic or familial HUS, since these agents may favor the recurrence of HUS. The recurrence of HUS has a relative risk of graft failure of 5.4 in comparison with other renal diseases (Hariharan *et al.*, 1999). The risk of graft loss due to recurrence is particularly elevated in children with familial HUS (Kaplan and Leonard, 2000) and in adults (Artz *et al.*, 2003).

Vasculitis

Polyarteritis

After transplantation, patients with polyarteritis displayed lower 3-year patient survival (77% vs. 91%) and graft survival rates (60% vs. 69%) compared with patients with other primary renal diseases (Briggs and Jones, 1999). Cardiovascular complications accounted for 54% of the deaths. Since only three of 112 patients lost their allograft due to recurrent disease, the inferior outcomes have been attributed to the older mean age, longer period of pre-transplant immunosuppressive therapy, and widespread small-vessel involvement among patients with polyarteritis. Thus, renal transplantation may be successful for well-selected recipients affected with polyarteritis. However, patients who have received vigorous immunosuppression prior to the onset of end-stage renal disease should wait several months before being transplanted, and must be carefully evaluated for concomitant cardiovascular disorders.

Wegener's granulomatosis

Neither patient nor graft survival rates at 3 years differed significantly between 115 transplant patients with Wegener's granulomatosis compared with transplant patients with other primary renal diseases

(Briggs and Jones, 1999). No case of recurrence was seen in some series (Rostaing et al., 1997), while others found a recurrence in 17% of patients (Nachman et al., 1999). Good results were even obtained (Deegens et al., 2003) among antineutrophil cytoplasmic antibody (ANCA)-positive patients with symptoms of acute disease. Despite these good results, however, caution is required, since Wegener's is a multisystem disease that can cause severe involvement of various organs, particularly the lungs. Moreover, most of these patients have received intensive steroid and immunosuppressive therapy before dialysis, rendering them more susceptible to infections, cardiovascular disease, and neoplasia after transplantation. Therefore, a thorough evaluation must be performed before accepting a patient with Wegener's vasculitis as a transplant candidate.

Cryoglobulinemia nephritis

Little information is available about the outcome of cryoglobulinemia nephritis after transplantation. Although there was a high rate of recurrence among a few patients transplanted because of this disease, a recurrence did not seem to jeopardize the outcome of the allograft (Tarantino et al., 1994). Since most patients who develop the disease due to hepatitis C virus-(HCV) related cryoglobulinemia die from vascular complications, liver failure, or infections, a careful evaluation of these systems must be performed and hypertension strictly controlled prior to transplantation. Treatment with interferon is recommended before transplantation in order to eradicate the HCV or at least reduce the viral load (Pol et al., 2002).

Miscellaneous

Analgesic nephropathy

A European review reported the results of renal transplantation among 798 patients with analgesic nephropathy (Briggs and Jones, 1999). Although the mean age of patients affected by this disease was slightly older for patients with other primary renal diseases, the 8-year graft survival rates (51% vs. 47%) and the patient survival rates (81% vs. 77%, respectively) were similar. On the other hand, a survey of UNOS data reported that the mortality rate was more than twice for transplant patients with analgesic nephropathy (Bleyer et al., 2001).

This disorder does not represent a contraindication to transplantation, provided that the patient stops taking analgesic drugs. However, it should be remembered that dialysis patients with analgesic nephropathy have a high risk of kidney and/or bladder cancer (Stewart et al., 2003), and death from neoplasia, particularly urothelial tumors which account for most of the cancers, is three times more frequent among patients with analgesic nephropathy (Kliem et al., 1996). During the evaluation, the patient should undergo cystoscopy and retrograde ureteropyeloscopy with washing and brushing. A bilateral nephroureterectomy should be considered prior to transplantation to prevent the development of urothelioma in the native upper tracts, and the transplant procedure should be performed using antireflux techniques to reduce the risk of colonization of malignant cells in the allograft. After transplantation, the urine should be regularly examined for the presence of malignant cells. Cystoscopy and radiological imaging to diagnose upper-tract transitional-cell carcinoma should be checked annually (Swindle et al., 1998).

Waldenström's macroglobulinemia

Very few patients with Waldenström's macroglobulinemia have undergone renal transplantation (Bradley et al., 1988), due to a major risk of death from sepsis. Recurrences have been reported, and about half of the grafts are lost. Thus, patients with Waldenström's macroglobulinemia are poor candidates for renal transplantation.

Light-chain deposition disease/myeloma

Only a few patients afflicted with light-chain deposition disease/myeloma have been transplanted, because it is generally recognized that the risk of death caused by the original disease or its treatment is high. The risk of recurrence is also elevated (Short et al., 2001). In the experience of the Mayo Clinic, seven patients with light-chain deposition disease (LCDD) have received a kidney transplantation. One died a few months later because of progressive myeloma, and five other patients had a recurrence of LCDD on average 33 months after transplantation. Four of them died, and the fifth patient remained on dialysis. Only one patient was still alive with allograft functioning 13 years after transplantation (Leung et al., 2004). Theoretically, the best indication for kidney transplantation in patients with LCDD/myeloma is represented by those patients receiving a bone marrow transplantation after ablative chemotherapy.

Sickle-cell disease

Although infrequent, chronic renal failure may be one of the complications of this disease. Patients with sickle-cell nephropathy have a worse survival than diabetics on dialysis, and have little chance of receiving a renal transplant (Abbott et al., 2002). The incidences of delayed graft function and acute rejection are similar to those observed for other renal diseases, but the patient and graft survival rates are poorer than in patients with other renal diseases (Ojo et al., 1999). Even among the few successful cases, patients experience more complications and persistence of painful crises that may produce erythrocyte sickling in the allograft (Ataga and Orringer, 2001). Thus, renal transplantation must be undertaken with great caution and only in the absence of recent sickling crises (Ribot, 1999). Special preparation prior to the transplant procedure must include the transfusion of 4–6 units of hemoglobin AA blood (with recipient phlebotomy as necessary) and the liberal use of sodium bicarbonate to maintain the blood at an alkaline pH, thus reducing proclivity to sickling. Consideration should be given to bone marrow or stem cell transplantation in selected patients (Iannone et al., 2002). On the other hand, a hemoglobin sickle cell disease patient who experienced severe vaso-occlusive crises did not show any further crisis for 16 years after a successful renal transplantation, suggesting a protective role of immunosuppression (Chies et al., 2005).

Paroxysmal hemoglobinuria

Paroxysmal hemoglobinuria is a clonal hematopoietic disorder, characterized by nocturnal hemoglobinuria, hemolytic anemia, and thrombosis. Renal failure may develop due to vascular thrombosis or iron overload. Sporadic cases of renal transplantation have been reported (Vanwalleghem et al., 1998; Verswijvel et al., 1999). The long-term risks of malignancy or of allograft deterioration remain unknown.

Medullary cystic disease/nephronophthisis

Medullary cystic disease or nephronophthisis does not pose any particular problem for transplant candidacy.

Scleroderma

The overall results of renal transplantation for patients with scleroderma are considerably worse than those observed in other renal diseases (Bleyer et al., 2001). On the other hand, transplantation confers a better survival than dialysis (Gibney et al., 2004). In the UNOS registry, the 5-year graft survival was 47% for cyclosporine-treated transplant patients with systemic sclerosis (Chang and Spiera, 1999). Skin thickening, anemia, and cardiac complications may predict recurrence of the disease after transplantation (Pham et al., 2005).

Angiotensin-converting enzyme inhibitors seem to be superior to angiotensin receptor blockers for treating recurrent scleroderma crises (Cheung et al., 2005). Patients afflicted with cardiac, pulmonary, or gastrointestinal involvement should not be considered for transplantation. Since many affected patients have severe hypertension, pre-transplant bilateral nephrectomy is recommended for suitable candidates.

Schistosomiasis

The overall results of renal transplantation in patients with healed schistosomiasis are similar to those obtained with other renal diseases (Mahmoud et al., 2001). However, schistosomal patients suffer from a higher incidence of urinary tract infections, and may need the correction of bladder disturbances or even bilateral nephrectomy to eradicate infection before transplantation (Barsoum, 2003). Reinfection with Schistosoma haematobium may occur in endemic areas. Thus, prophylaxis with praziquantel may be suggested.

Fibrillary glomerulopathy

Fibrillary glomerulonephritis is an idiopathic condition characterized by polyclonal immune deposits with restricted gamma isotypes. Most patients present with significant renal insufficiency and have a poor outcome despite immunosuppressive therapy (Brady et al., 1998). Recurrence of the disease after transplantation may occur in almost half of cases. However, only rarely does recurrence lead to rapid graft loss (Palanichamy et al., 1998). In other recurrent cases, graft failure occurred after 4 years or more (Pronovost et al., 1996; Samaniego et al., 2001).

COACH syndrome

The COACH syndrome is a very rare disorder with cerebellar vermis hypoplasia, oligophrenia, ataxia, coloboma, and hepatic fibrosis, and in some cases renal failure. Neurologic abnormalities are the first symptoms in most cases. Portal hypertension, esophageal varices, and gastrointestinal bleeding are the major causes of morbidity and mortality. Liver and kidney transplantation can achieve long-term success if the neurologic conditions remain stable and patients have an excellent support system (Uemura et al., 2005).

Metabolic diseases (Table 2.9)

Diabetes mellitus

Diabetes mellitus is among the most frequent causes of end-stage renal disease (ESRD) in Western countries.

Surprisingly, among patients on the waiting list for renal transplantation, the prevalence of diabetes and the number of patients with diabetic nephropathy are notably underdiagnosed (Hergesell and Zeier, 2003). Transplantation poses several additional problems in these patients: (1) an increased risk of *infection*, above that already engendered by immunosuppressive therapy; (2) exacerbation of the metabolic disorder as well as its common complications of hypertension and hyperlipidemia, which augment the risk of *cardiovascular disease*, by calcineurin inhibitor and steroid immunosuppressive drugs; (3) *recurrence of nephropathy* in the transplanted allograft, a risk that increases progressively over time; (4) hazards of reduced *quality of life* due to extrarenal complications, such as retinopathy, peripheral vascular disease, and neuropathy, even in the presence of a well-functioning kidney allograft; (5) a *risk of death* more than twice in comparison with patients transplanted because of other renal diseases (Bleyer et al., 2001).

Despite these potential problems, renal transplantation is considered the treatment of choice for many diabetics with end-stage renal failure, the overall graft survival being similar for patients with type I or type II diabetes (Kronson et al., 2000). The results are particularly good with pre-emptive transplantation (Becker et al., 2006). However, the pre-transplant investigations, particularly cardiovascular examinations of these patients, must be thorough, since atherosclerotic complications are more common and severe among diabetics. Patients with an ejection fraction below 30% or severe peripheral arteriopathy should be excluded from consideration for transplantation, since the risk of mortality is exceedingly high. Of interest, however, the risk of acute coronary syndrome in diabetics is lower after transplantation than when on dialysis (Hypolite et al., 2002).

Excellent results with a good quality of life and high degree of rehabilitation have been reported in large series with simultaneous pancreas and kidney transplantation. Although this double transplant may expose patients to an increased risk of infection and acute rejection it may obtain normalization of blood glucose metabolism and an improvement in blood pressure control. This may result in better long-term graft survival (Bunnapradist et al., 2003; Reddy et al., 2003) and lower cardiovascular complications (La Rocca et al., 2001) when compared with kidney transplantation alone. A decision analysis indicated that living kidney transplantation is associated with the greatest life expectancy and quality-adjusted life expectancy for type I diabetic patients with renal failure. For patients without living donors, simultaneous kidney–pancreas transplantation is associated with greater life expectancy compared with kidney transplantation alone, and should be considered particularly for patients with frequent metabolic complications of diabetes (Knoll and Nichol, 2003).

Table 2.9   Indications for renal transplantation in metabolic and inherited diseases

Diabetes types I and II	Yes, but risk of recurrence and cardiovascular disease
	Simultaneous kidney and pancreas transplant may
	reduce the risk of cardiovascular disease and/or recurrence
Type 1 hyperoxaluria	Yes, but only in the few patients with pyridoxine sensitivity
	Simultaneous liver and kidney transplant in all other cases
Cystinosis	Yes, but cystine accumulation continues
Fabry's disease	Yes – enzyme replacement is needed
Lipoprotein glomerulopathy	Doubtful. Most patients show recurrence and poor outcome
Alagille's syndrome	Yes if liver and pulmonary functions are normal
	Otherwise a double transplant should be considered
Alport's syndrome	Yes
	Low risk of anti-GBM glomerulonephritis
Polycystic kidneys	Yes
	Possible indication for double kidney and liver transplantation
	in a few patients

Type 1 primary hyperoxaluria

Type 1 primary hyperoxaluria is a rare autosomal recessive error of oxalate metabolism, caused by the partial or complete deficiency of alanine glyoxalate aminotransferase (AGT) in liver cells. A lack of AGT leads to the accumulation of glyoxalate, which is then oxidized to oxalate or reduced to glycolate, resulting in hyperglycolic hyperoxaluria. In infancy, the increased oxalate load leads to nephrocalcinosis and ultimately to renal failure. The disease is usually characterized by progressive nephrolithiasis resulting in renal failure within the first two decades or, in milder cases, even later in life (Marangella, 1999).

The initial experience with kidney transplantation for patients afflicted with this disorder was extremely disappointing, due to the almost invariable recurrence of the disease leading to early graft loss (Figure 2.10). Therefore, oxalosis was considered an absolute contraindication to renal transplantation alone, the only possibility being a simultaneous kidney and liver transplant to correct the deficiency of AGT. Today, the attitude has partially changed, because it has been recognized that more than 20% of cases show pyridoxine sensitivity. In these patients, pyridoxine supplementation coupled with forced diuresis during the early post-transplantation period may prevent or delay progression to renal failure. Thus, before deciding whether a patient should be considered for liver plus kidney transplantation or for kidney transplantation alone, the candidate should undergo a challenge with pyridoxine supplementation (5–10 mg/kg per day). If this treatment restores oxalate and glycolate levels to normal within a few weeks, the patient is deemed pyridoxine-sensitive. The measurement of plasma oxalate concentrations *per se* may also indicate whether liver plus kidney transplantation is necessary. Plasma oxalate levels exceeding 50 μmol/l are usually associated with an elevated risk of calcium oxalate accumulation (Marangella, 1999).

Thus, renal transplantation alone may be indicated for the few patients with pyridoxine sensitivity and relatively low plasma levels of oxalate. The best results tend to be obtained when transplantation is performed with *forced diuresis* and with early administration of *pyridoxine* to convert glyoxalate to glycine, to reduce the degree of oxalate deposition in the allograft. For patients with more severe disease, preemptive *liver–kidney transplantation* is the treatment of choice. In fact, in contrast to dialysis treatments, which do not prevent the accumulation of oxalate crystals in heart or bone, liver transplantation corrects

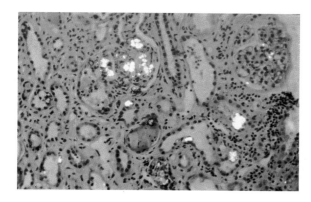

Figure 2.10 Renal biopsy taken 10 days after transplantation, showing recurrence of oxalosis in an 11-year-old child with primary oxalosis

the enzyme defect (Detry *et al.*, 2002) and facilitates excellent graft survival (Cibrik *et al.*, 2002; Jamieson *et al.*, 2005) (Figure 2.11).

Cystinosis

Cystinosis is a rare, autosomal recessive, metabolic defect affecting the specific lysosomal system that transports cystine outside cells. The early administration of cysteamine may delay the onset of end-stage renal failure (Gahl *et al.*, 2002). In contrast to some concerns, children with cystinosis do not appear to be at increased risk for graft failure or graft thrombosis (Langlois *et al.*, 2000), and renal allograft survival in patients with cystinosis is similar to that observed in patients with other primary renal diseases, at least in the short term (Raine *et al.*, 1992). However, after successful transplantation, cystine continues to accumulate in other organs, including the eye and brain, as well as in muscle tissue. To prevent or limit the deleterious consequences of cystine accumulation, early and continuous administration of cysteamine is recommended.

Fabry's disease

Fabry's disease is an X-linked recessive glycosphingolipidosis characterized by the accumulation of glycosphingolipids in most tissues. Affected males may show cloudiness of the cornea, reddish-purple angiokeratomas on their skin, pain in the hands and feet, and gastrointestinal hyperactivity. Patients may suffer from heart attacks or stroke. Hypertension and renal failure are late complications, generally occurring during the fourth or fifth decade. In the past few years, an enzyme replacement therapy has been made commercially available, thus enabling improved care of these patients. Although histologic recurrence after transplantation may occur rarely (Sessa *et al.*, 2004), good graft survival has been reported (Mignani *et al.*, 2001; Inderbitzin *et al.*, 2005). Today, Fabry's disease *per se* is not considered a contraindication to renal transplantation.

Lipoprotein glomerulopathy

Lipoprotein glomerulopathy (LPG) is a glomerular disease characterized by the intracapillary deposition of lipoproteins producing proteinuria, ranging from mild degrees to nephrotic levels, and eventually leading to chronic renal failure, hypercholesterolemia, coronary artery disease, and Alzheimer's disease. Affected patients display a mutant phenotype due to a genetic increase in apolipoprotein E (Saito *et al.*, 1999) with enhanced glomerular binding (Sam *et al.*, 2006). The gene encoding this protein is located on chromosome 19; its polymorphism can result in six possible phenotypes. Most of the described cases have been observed in Japanese patients. Recurrence can occur within a few months after transplantation. In most cases, the recurrence was associated with a poor outcome of the allograft. Treatment with ACE inhibitors and lipid-lowering agents has been advised to slow the progression to renal failure (Mourad *et al.*, 1998).

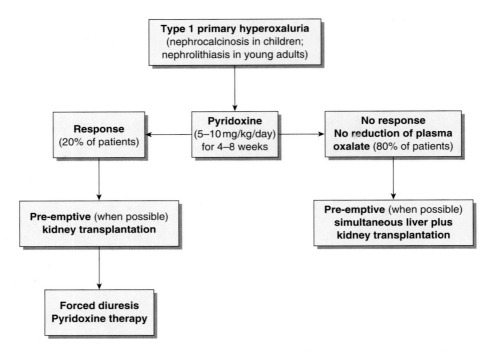

Figure 2.11   Indications to kidney transplantation or simultaneous liver and kidney transplantation in patients with type 1 primary hyperoxaluria

Inherited diseases

Alport's syndrome

Alport's syndrome is an X-linked hereditary disease transmitted in a dominant pattern resulting from the mutation of the COL4A5 gene, which encodes the protein α_5-chain of type IV collagen. This protein is a major, tissue-specific constituent of glomerular basement membrane (GBM). Following transplantation, the new kidney, bearing a normal glomerular basement membrane, may elicit the production of tissue-specific antibodies directed against the normal collagen chain. Although these antibodies occur in about one-third of cases, they generally have no clinical effect on the graft as only rare cases of rapidly progressive glomerulonephritis have been reported (Rutgers *et al.*, 2000). In a large series, the incidence of *anti-GBM disease* in male transplant patients with Alport's syndrome was 3% (Byrne *et al.*, 2002). The overall outcome of renal transplants in patients afflicted with Alport's does not differ from that of recipients not affected by the disease. Thus, patients with Alport's syndrome are generally considered good candidates for renal transplantation.

Bartter's syndrome

Bartter's syndrome is a tubular disorder which is inherited as an autosomal trait. Clinically the disease is characterized by hypokalemia, metabolic alkalosis, polyuria, and resistance to the pressor effect of angiotensin II. The main defect consists of an impaired reabsorption of NaCl at the level of the ascending limb of the Henle's loop. The clinical features are extremely variable, and are related in part to the gene defect involved (Peters *et al.*, 2002). A few patients may enter end-stage renal disease due to superimposed interstitial nephritis. Successful transplantation may fully correct the abnormalities (Takahashi *et al.*, 1996; Calo *et al.*, 2003).

Thin basement membrane nephropathy (TBMN)

There is little information on the post-transplant outcome of the few patients with TBMN who enter end-stage renal failure. A practical problem is the differential diagnosis between TBMN and Alport's syndrome with thinned membranes, as the latter disease might render the recipient more susceptible to develop anti-GBM antibodies after transplantation (Ierino and Kanellis, 2005).

Autosomal polycystic kidney disease

The outcomes of renal transplants in adult recipients afflicted with autosomal dominant polycystic kidney disease are good. Because most patients are older than 50 years, they must be carefully screened for cardiac and neoplastic diseases. Due to the possibilities of intracystic hemorrhage, infections, stone formation, and severe hypertension, bilateral native nephrectomy is often indicated, preferably before rather than after transplantation. In a few patients with giant enlargement of the liver due to cysts, a combined liver and kidney transplantation is indicated (Arnold and Harrison, 2005). Cranial aneurysms are more frequent in patients with polycystic kidney disease than in the general population. In the absence of a family history of aneurysm and with no symptoms or signs of intracranial disease, no diagnostic radiographic tests are usually recommended. However, a family history of cerebral aneurysm or new-onset headache, or signs of intracranial disease, require a rapid evaluation with angio-magnetic resonance imaging. Among patients with polycystic kidney disease, intestinal diverticulosis is frequent and may expose them to an increased risk of colonic perforation after transplantation (Dominguez Fernandez et al., 1998; Lederman et al., 2000).

In children with autosomal recessive polycystic kidney disease the results of renal transplantation are good, but most patients suffer from complications of congenital liver fibrosis, cholangitis, and portal hypertension. About 30% of these patients die (Khan et al., 2002). A careful work-up is necessary in patients with this disease.

Alagille's syndrome

Alagille's syndrome, also known as arteriohepatic dysplasia (Alagille et al., 1987), is the leading cause of cholestatic icterus neonatorum. It is an autosomal dominant disease with a variable expression and random inheritance of a deletion on the short arm of chromosome 20. A characteristic triangular face with a prominent forehead, straight nose, and pointed chin is the most common feature. The clinical findings include butterfly vertebrae, posterior embryotoxon, pulmonary artery stenosis, and a paucity of intrahepatic ducts. Liver transplantation for hepatic failure is often required (MacBride Emerick, 2002). Isolated instances of renal and urinary tract involvement have been reported, such as agenesis of the kidney, vesicoureteral reflux, tubulointerstitial nephritis, or IgA nephritis, although none of these disorders is diagnostic for the disease. Progression to renal failure is common in children with full expression of the gene. In contrast, underdiagnosis is possible in adult patients. Patients with Alagille's syndrome who are referred for renal transplantation require a careful evaluation of liver function and of the vascular system, with particular attention to the pulmonic valve and the iliac arteries.

Conclusions

Only a few conditions represent absolute contraindications to renal transplantation; however, careful selection and preparation of the recipient is necessitated by the growing shortage of donor organs and the risks associated with immunosuppressive therapy. Although the evaluation of candidates for kidney transplantation is a difficult and sometimes subjective process, a thorough investigation of the medical history of the candidate, as well as complete clinical assessment, can alert the transplant team to potential complications, and increased risks of poor clinical outcome. The presence of immunological, infectious, gastrointestinal, pulmonary, and urological conditions must be identified before a patient is considered for transplant. Other factors to be evaluated prior to transplant include elderly or pediatric age, obesity, the presence or a history of cancer; liver, metabolic, inherited, or systemic diseases; and a variety of other disorders. These indications may either suggest poor candidacy for transplantation, or necessitate that special measures be taken to prepare the recipient prior to transplantation and provide appropriate follow-up treatment.

The range of complicating conditions seen in patients desiring renal transplantation necessitates a broad evaluation of urologic, gastrointestinal, and vascular conditions to assess the risk of concomitant conditions and formulate therapeutic strategies to prepare the patient optimally not only for the operation, but also for the consequences of immunosuppressive therapy. An aggressive surgical approach to serious problems enhances the chance of an excellent outcome of transplantation; a delay in surgical intervention until the postoperative period may increase the risks of morbidity and/or graft loss. Among the surgical interventions frequently required are nephrectomy (and ureterectomy) in cases of infection, malignant hypertension, and neoplastic disease; parathyroidectomy in patients with hypercalcemia and serious bone disease; biliary procedures in patients with cholangitis; splenectomy to raise cell counts and thereby increase tolerability to immunosuppressive drugs; aortocoronary bypasses for serious coronary artery disease; and/or aortoiliac vascular grafts for arterial insufficiency. Owing to the advent of hemodialysis without anticoagulation, complex surgical procedures can now be performed with an added degree of safety in ESRD patients.

References

Abbott KC, Hypolite IO, Agodoa LY. Sickle cell nephropathy at end-stage renal failure disease in the United States: patient characteristics and survival. Clin Nephrol 2002; 58: 9–15.

Alagille D, Estrada A, Hadchouel M, et al. Syndromic paucity of intralobular bile ducts (Alagille syndrome or arteriohepatic dysplasia): review of 80 cases. J Pediatr 1987; 110: 195–200.

Andresdottir MB, Assman KJ, Hoitsma AJ, et al. Recurrence of type I membranoproliferative glomerulonephritis after renal transplantation: analysis of the incidence, risk factors and impact on graft survival. Transplantation 1997; 63: 1628–33.

Andresdottir MB, Assman KJ, Hoitsma AJ, et al. Renal transplantation in patients with dense deposit disease: morphologic characteristics of recurrent disease and clinical outcome. Nephrol Dial Transplant 1999; 14: 1723–31.

Arnold HL, Harrison SA. New advances in evaluation and management of patients with polycystic liver disease. Am J Gastroenterol 2005; 100: 2569–82.

Aroldi A, Lampertico P, Montagnino G, et al. Natural history of hepatitis B and C in renal allograft recipients. Transplantation 2005; 79: 1132–6.

Artz MA, Steenbergen EJ, Hoitsma AJ, et al. Renal transplantation in patients with hemolytic uremic syndrome: high rate of recurrence and increased incidence of acute rejection. Transplantation 2003; 76: 821–6.

Ataga KI, Orringer EP. Renal abnormalities in sickle cell disease. Am J Hematol 2000; 63: 205–11.

Atkinson JP, Liszewski MK, Richards A, et al. Hemolytic uremic syndrome: an example of insufficient complement regulation on self-tissue. Ann NY Acad Sci 2005; 1056: 144–52.

Barsoum RS. Schistosomiasis and the kidney. Semin Nephrol 2003; 23: 34–41.

Bartosh SM, Fine RN, Sullivan EK. Outcome after transplantation of young patients with systemic lupus erythematosus: a report of the North American pediatric renal transplant cooperative study. Transplantation 2001; 1: 973–8.

Batty DS Jr, Swanson SI, Kirk AD, et al. Hepatitis C virus seropositivity at the time of renal transplantation in the United States: associated factors and patient survival. Am J Transplant 2001; 1: 179–84.

Baum MA, Stablein DM, Panzarino VM, et al. Loss of living donor renal allograft advantage in children with focal segmental glomerulosclerosis. Kidney Int 2001; 59: 328–33.

Becker BN, Rush SH, Dykstra DM, et al. Preemptive transplantation for patients with diabetes-related kidney disease. Arch Intern Med 2006; 166: 44–8.

Bennett WM, McEvoy KM, Henell KR, et al. Morbid obesity does not preclude successful renal transplantation. Clin Transplant 2004; 18: 89–93.

Berger A, Preiser W, Kachel HG, et al. HBV reactivation after kidney transplantation. J Clin Virol 2005; 32: 162–5.

Bernatsky S, Clarke A, Ramsey-Goldman R. Malignancy and systemic lupus erythematosus. Curr Rheumatol Rep 2002; 4: 351–8.

Bertelli R, Ginevri F, Caridi G, et al. Recurrence of focal glomerulosclerosis after renal transplantation in patients with mutations of podocyn. Am J Kidney Dis 2003; 41: 1314–21.

Bleyer AJ, Donaldson LA, McIntosh M, Adams PL. Relationship between underlying renal disease and renal transplant outcome. Am J Kidney Dis 2001; 37: 1152–61.

Borza DB, Chedid MF, Colon S, et al. Recurrent Goodpasture's disease secondary to a monoclonal IgA1-kappa antibody autoreactive with the alpha1/alpha2 chains of type IV collagen. Am J Kidney Dis 2005; 45: 397–406.

Bosch T, Wendler T. Extracorporeal plasma treatment in primary and recurrent focal segmental glomerular sclerosis: a review. Ther Apher 2001; 5: 155–60.

Bradley JR, Thiru S, Balallan N, Evans DB. Renal transplantation in Waldenström's macroglobulinemia. Nephrol Dial Transplant 1988; 3: 214–16.

Brady HR. Fibrillary glomerulopathy. Kidney Int 1998; 53: 1421–9.

Braun MC, Stablein DM, Hamiwka LA, et al. Recurrence of membranoproliferative glomerulonephritis type II in renal allografts: the North American Pediatric Renal Transplant Cooperative Study experience. J Am Soc Nephrol 2005; 16: 2225–33.

Brey RL, Stallworth CL, McGlasson DL, et al. Antiphospholipid and stroke in young women. Stroke 2002; 33: 2396–401.

Briganti EM, Russ GR, McNeil JJ, et al. Risk of renal allograft loss from recurrent glomerulonephritis. N Engl J Med 2002; 347: 102–9.

Briggs JD. Cardiocvascular complications in renal transplantation. Nephrol Dial Transplant 2001; 16(Suppl 6): 156–8.

Briggs JD, Jones E. Renal transplantation for uncommon diseases. Nephrol Dial Transplant 1999; 14: 570–5.

Bryan CF, Mitchell SI, Lin HM, et al. Influence of the Rh (D) blood group system on graft survival in renal transplantation. Transplantation 1998; 165: 588–92.

Bunnapradist S, Fabrizi F, Vierling J, et al. Hepatitis C therapy with long term remission after renal transplantation. Int J Artif Organs 2002; 25: 1189–93.

Bunnapradist S, Cho YW, Cecka JM, et al. Kidney allograft and patient survival in type I diabetic recipients of cadaveric kidney alone versus simultaneous pancreas/kidney transplants: a multivariate analysis of the UNOS dotabase. J Am Soc Nephrol 2003; 14: 208–13.

Butler JA, Roderick P, Mullee M, et al. Frequency and impact of nonadherence to immunosuppressants after renal transplantation: a systematic review. Transplantation 2004a; 277: 769–76.

Butler JA, Peveler RC, Roderick P, et al. Modifiable risk factors for non-adherence to immunosuppressants in renal transplant recipients: a cross-sectional study. Nephrol Dial Transplant 2004b; 19: 3144–9.

Byrne M, Budisauljevic MN, Fan Z, et al. Renal transplant in patients with Alport's syndrome. Am J Kidney Dis 2002; 39: 769–79.

Calo LA, Marchini F, Davis PA, et al. Kidney transplant in Gitelman's syndrome. Report of the first case. J Nephrol 2003; 1: 144–7.

Cameron JS. Recurrence of primary disease and de novo nephritis following renal transplantation. Pediatr Nephrol 1991; 5: 412–21.

Cameron JS. Renal transplantation in the elderly. Int Urol Nephrol 2000; 32: 193–201.

Carnaille B, Oudar C, Pattou F. Pancreatitis and primary hyperparathyroidism: forty cases. Aust NZ J Surg 1998; 68: 117–19.

Cecka JM. The UNOS transplant registry. In Cecka JM, Terasaki PI, eds. Clinical Transplants 2001. Los Angeles: UCLA, 2002: 1–18.

Cecka JM. The OPT/UNOS Renal Transplant Registry 2003. Clin Transplant 2003: 1–12.

Chan TM, Fang GX, Tang CS, et al. Preemptive lamivudine therapy based on HBV DNA level in HBsAg-positive kidney allograft recipients. Hepatology 2002; 36: 1041–5.

Chang YJ, Spiera H. Renal transplantation in scleroderma. Medicine (Baltimore) 1999; 78: 382–5.

Cheung WY, Gibson IW, Rush D, et al. Late recurrence of scleroderma renal crisis in a renal transplant recipient despite angiotensin II blockade. Am J Kidney Dis 2005; 45: 930–4.

Chies JA, Dresch C, Cruz MS, et al. Immunosuppressive therapy for kidney transplant prevents vaso-occlusive crisis in a haemoglobin SC disease patient. Med Hypotheses 2005; 64: 174–6.

Chisolm MA, Lance CE, Mulloy LL. Patient factors associated with adherence to immunosuppressant therapy in renal transplant recipients. Am J Health Syst Pharm 2005; 62: 1775–81.

Cho YW, Cecka JM. Cross-match tests – an analysis of UNOS data from 1991–2000. In Cecka JM, Terasaki PI, eds. Clinical Transplants 2001. Los Angeles: UCLA, 2002: 237–46.

Cibrik DM, Kaplan B, Arndorfer JA, Meier-Kriesche HU. Renal allograft survival in patients with oxalosis. Transplantation 2002; 15: 707–10.

Cibrik DM, Kaplan B, Campbell DA, Meier-Kriesche HU. Renal allograft survival in transplant recipients with focal segmental glomerulosclerosis. Am J Transplant 2003; 3: 64–7.

Clark WF, Jevnikar AM. Renal transplantation for end-stage renal disease caused by systemic lupus erythematosus nephritis. Semin Nephrol 1999; 19: 77–85.

Clot JP, Crosnier H, Guest G, et al. Effects of growth hormone or growth factors after renal transplantation. Pediatr Nephrol 2001; 16: 397–403.

Cosyns JP, Couchoud C, Pouteil-Noble C, et al. Recurrence of membranous nephropathy after renal transplantation: probability, outcome and risk factors. Clin Nephrol 1998; 50: 144–53.

Cotler SJ, Diaz G, Gundlapalli S, et al. Characteristics of hepatitis C in renal transplant candidates. J Clin Gastroenterol 2002; 35: 191–5.

Coupel S, Giral-Classe M, Karam G, et al. Ten-year survival of second kidney transplants: impact of immunologic factors and renal function at 12 months. Kidney Int 2003; 64: 674–80.

Dall'Amico R, Ghiggeri G, Carraro M, et al. Prediction and treatment of recurrent focal segmental glomerulosclerosis after renal transplantation in children. Am J Kidney Dis 1999; 6: 1048–55.

Deegens JK, Artz MA, Hoitsma AJ, Wetzels JF. Outcome of renal transplantation in patients with pouci-immune small vessel vasculitis or anti-GBM disease. Clin Nephrol 2003; 59: 1–9.

De Filippi F, Lampertico S, Soffredini R, et al. High prevalence, low pathogenicity of hepatitis G virus in kidney transplant recipients. Dig Liver Dis 2001; 33: 477–9.

Denton MD, Magee CC, Ovuworie C, et al. Prevalence of renal cell carcinoma in patients with ESRD pre-transplantation: a pathologic analysis. Kidney Int 2002; 61: 2201–9.

Detry O, Honore P, De Roover A, et al. Reversal of oxalosis cardiomyopathy after combined liver and kidney transplantation. Transpl Int 2002; 15: 50–2.

Dominguez Fernandez E, Albrecht KH, Heemann U, et al. Prevalence of diverticulosis and incidence of bowel perforation after kidney transplantation in patients with polycystic kidney disease. Transpl Int 1998; 11: 28–31.

EBPG Expert Group on Renal Transplantation. European best practice guidelines for renal transplantation. Nephrol Dial Transplant 2002; 17 (Suppl 4): 1–67.

Emiroglu R, Basaran O, Pehlivan S, et al. Effect of amyloidosis on long-term survival in kidney transplantation. Transplant Proc 2005; 37: 2967–8.

Fabrizi F, Martin P, Dixit V, et al. Hepatitis C virus antibody status and survival after renal transplantation: meta-analysis of observational studies. Am J Transplant 2005; 5: 1452–61.

Fabrizii V, Horl WH. Renal transplantation in the elderly. Curr Urol 2001; 11: 159–63.

Fagundes I, Michelon T, Schoroeder RJ, et al. Immunoglobulin G-positive in B-cell cross-match decreases kidney allograft survival. Transplant Proc 2005; 37: 2753–4.

Ferraris JR, Ramirez JA, Ruiz S, et al. Shiga toxin-associated hemolytic uremic syndrome: absence of recurrence after renal transplantation. Pediatr Nephrol 2002; 17: 809–14.

Fine RN. Growth following solid-organ transplantation. Pediatr Transplant 2002; 6: 47–52.

Fontaine H, Vallet-Pichard A, Chaix ML, et al. Efficacy and safety of adefovir dipivoxil in kidney recipients, hemodialysis patients, and patients with renal insufficiency. Transplantation 2005; 80: 1086–92.

Fornairon S, Pol S, Legendre C, et al. The long-term virologic and pathologic impact of renal transplantation on chronic hepatitis B infection. Transplantation 1996; 62: 297–9.

Gahl WA, Thoene JG, Schneider JA. Cystinosis. N Engl J Med 2002; 347: 111–21.

Gane E, Pilmore H. Management of chronic viral hepatitis before and after transplantation. Transplantation 2002; 74: 427–37.

Gibney EM, Parikh CR, Jani A, et al. Kidney transplantation for systemic sclerosis improves survival and may modulate disease activity. Am J Transplant 2004; 12: 2027–31.

Ginevri F, Pastorino N, De Santis R, et al. Retransplantation after kidney allograft loss due to polyoma BK virus nephropathy: successful outcome without original allograft nephrectomy. Am J Kidney Dis 2003; 42: 821–5.

Gipson DS, Ferris ME, Dooley MA, et al. Renal transplantation in children with lupus nephritis. Am J Kidney Dis 2003; 41: 455–63.

Gjertson DW, Cecka JM. Living unrelated donor kidney transplantation. Kidney Int 2000; 58: 491–9.

Glanton CW, Kao TC, Cruess D, et al. Impact of renal transplantation on survival in end-stage renal disease patients with elevated body mass index. Kidney Int 2003; 63: 647–53.

Glassock RJ. Optimizing disease management in the next 25 years. Semin Nephrol 1997; 17: 387–90.

Glotz D, Antoine C, Julia P, et al. Desensitization and subsequent kidney transplantation of patients using intravenous immunoglobulins (IVIg). Am J Transplant 2002; 2: 758–60.

Goldfarb-Rumyantzev A, Hurdle JF, Scandling J, et al. Duration of end stage renal disease and kidney transplant outcome. Nephrol Dial Transplant 2005a; 20: 167–75.

Goldfarb-Rumyantzev A, Hurdle JF, Scandling J, et al. The role of pretransplantation renal replacement therapy modality in kidney allograft and recipient survival. Am J Kidney Dis 2005b; 46: 537–49.

Goral S, Ynares C, Shappell SB, et al. Recurrent lupus nephritis revisited: it is not rare. Transplantation 2003; 75: 651–6.

Grimbert P, Frappier J, Bedrossian J, et al. Long-term outcome of kidney transplantation in patients with systemic lupus erythematosus: a multicenter study. Groupe Cooperative de Transplantation d'Ile de France. Transplantation 1998; 66: 1000–3.

Hanaway MJ, Weber S, Buell JF, et al. Risk for recurrence and death from preexisting cancers after transplantation. Transplant Rev 2005; 19: 151–63.

Hariharan S, Adams MB, Brennan DC, et al. Recurrent and de novo glomerular disease after renal transplantation: a report from Renal Allograft Disease Registry (RADR). Transplantation 1999; 68: 635–41.

Harrison KL, Alpers LE, Davis CL. De novo amyloidosis in a renal allograft: a case report and review of the literature. Am J Kidney Dis 1993; 22: 468–76.

Hergesell O, Zeier M. Underdiagnosis of diabetes mellitus in chronic dialysis patients on the renal transplant waiting list. Transplant Proc 2003; 35: 1287–9.

Hirsch HH, Ramos E. Retransplantation after polyomavirus-associated nephropathy: just do it? Am J Transplant 2006; 6: 7–9.

Holley JL, Shapiro R, Lopatin WB, et al. Obesity as a risk factor following cadaveric renal transplantation. Transplantation 1990; 49: 387–9.

Howard RJ, Thai VB, Patton PR, et al. Obesity does not portend a bad outcome for kidney transplant recipients. Transplantation 2002; 73: 53–5.

Hsu DT. Biological and psychological differences in the child and adolescent transplant recipient. Pediatr Transplant 2005; 9: 416–21.

Humar A, Arrazola L, Mauer M, et al. Kidney transplantation in young children: should there be a minimum age? Pediatr Nephrol 2001; 16: 941–5.

Hypolite IO, Bucci J, Hshieh P, et al. Acute coronary syndromes after renal transplantation in patients with end-stage renal disease resulting from diabetes. Am J Transplant 2002; 2: 274–81.

Iannone R, Chen AR, Casella JF. Commentary on 'Summary of Symposium: The Future of Stem Cell Transplantation for Sickle Cell Disease'. J Pediatr Hematol Oncol 2002; 24: 515–17.

Ierino FL, Kanellis J. Thin basement membrane nephropathy and renal transplantation. Semin Nephrol 2005; 25: 184–7.

Inderbitzin D, Avital I, Largiader F, et al. Kidney transplantation improves survival and is indicated in Fabry's disease. Transplant Proc 2005; 37: 4211–14.

Jamieson NV; European PHI Transplantation Study Group. A 20-year experience of combined liver/kidney transplantation for primary hyperoxaluria (PH1): the European PH1 transplant registry experience 1984–2004. Am J Nephrol 2005; 25: 282–9.

Jassal SV, Krahn MD, Naglie G, et al. Kidney transplantation in the elderly: a decision analysis. J Am Soc Nephrol 2003; 14: 187–96.

Johnson RJ, Armstrong S, Belger MA, et al. The outcome of pediatric renal transplantation in the UK and Eire. Pediatr Transplant 2002a; 6: 367–77.

Johnson DW, Isbel NM, Brown AM, et al. The effect of obesity on renal transplant outcomes. Transplantation 2002b; 74: 675–81.

Jordan SC, Vo AA, Peng A, et al. Intravenous gammaglobulin (IVIG): a novel approach to improve transplant rates and outcomes in highly HLA-sensitized patients. Am J Transplant 2006; 6: 459–66.

Kao LS, Flowers C, Flum DR. Prophylactic cholecystectomy in transplant patients: a decision analysis. J Gastrointest Surg 2005; 9: 965–72.

Kapila P, Jones J, Rees L. Effect of chronic renal failure and prednisolone on the growth hormone-insulin-like growth factor axis. Pediatr Nephrol 2001; 16: 1099–104.

Kaplan BS, Leonard MB. Autosomal dominant hemolytic uremic syndrome : variable phenotypes and transplant results. Pediatr Nephrol 2000; 14: 464–8.

Kasiske BL. The evaluation of prospective renal transplant recipients and living donors. Surg Clin North Am 1998; 78: 27–39.

Kasiske BL, Ramos EL, Gaston RS, et al. The evaluation of renal transplant candidates: clinical practice guidelines, Patient Care and Education Committee of the American Society of Transplant Physicians. J Am Soc Nephrol 1995; 6: 1–34.

Kasiske BL, Vazquez MA, Harmon WE, et al. Recommendation for the outpatient surveillance of renal transplant recipients. American Society of Transplantation. J Am Soc Nephrol 2000; 11 (Suppl 15): S1–86.

Kasiske BL, Snyder J. Matching older kidneys with older patients does not improve graft survival. J Am Soc Nephrol 2002; 13: 1067–72.

Kasiske BL, Maclean JR, Snyder JJ. Acute myocardial infarction and kidney transplantation J Am Soc Nephrol 2006; 17: 900–7.

Khan K, Schwarzenberg SJ, Sharp HL, et al. Morbidity from congenital hepatic fibrosis after renal transplantation for autosomal recessive polycystic kidney disease. Am J Transplant 2002; 2: 360–5.

Kim YS, Moon JI, Jeong HJ, et al. Live donor renal allograft in end-stage renal failure patients from immunoglobulin A nephropathy. Transplantation 2001; 71: 233–8.

Klaus G, Jeck N, Konrad M, et al. Risk of steroid withdrawal in pediatric renal transplant patients with suspected steroid toxicity. Clin Nephrol 2001; 56: S37–42.

Kliem V, Thon W, Krautzig S, et al. High mortality from urothelial carcinoma despite regular tumor screening in patients with analgesic nephropathy after renal transplantation Transpl Int 1996; 9: 231–5.

Knoll GA, Nichol G. Dialysis, kidney transplantation, or pancreas transplantation for patients with diabetes mellitus and renal failure: a decision analysis of treatment options. J Am Soc Nephrol 2003; 14: 500–15.

Korzets A, Gafter U. Tuberculosis prophylaxis for the chronically dialysed patients – yes or no? Nephrol Dial Transplant 1999; 14: 2857–9.

Koushik R, Matas AJ. Focal segmental glomerular sclerosis in kidney allograft recipients: an evidence-based approach. Transplant Rev 2005; 19: 78–87.

Kronson JW, Gillingham KJ, Sutherland DE, Matas AJ. Renal transplantation for type II diabetic patients and patients over 50 years old: a single center experience. Clin Transplant 2000; 14: 226–34.

Laederach-Hofmann K, Bunzel B. Noncompliance in organ transplant recipients: a literature review. Gen Hosp Psychiatry 2000; 22: 412–24.

Lahlou A, Lang P, Charpentier B, et al. Hemolytic uremic syndrome: recurrence after renal transplantation. Groupe Cooperatif de l'Ile de France (GLIF) Medicine (Baltimore) 2000; 79: 90–102.

Land W, Messmer K. The impact of ischemia/reperfusion injury on specific and non-specific early and late chronic events after organ transplantation. Transplant Rev 1996; 10: 108–27.

Langlois V, Geary D, Murray L, et al. Polyuria and proteinuria in cystinosis have no impact on renal transplantation. A report of the North American Pediatric Renal Transplant Cooperative Study. Pediatr Nephrol 2000; 15: 7–10.

La Rocca E, Fiorina P, di Carlo V, et al. Cardiovascular outcomes after kidney–pancreas and kidney alone transplantation. Kidney Int 2001; 60: 1964–71.

Lederman ED, McCoy G, Conti DJ, Lee EC. Diverticulitis and polycystic kidney disease. Am Surg 2000; 66: 200–3.

Leung N, Lager DJ, Gertz MA, et al. Long-term outcome of renal transplantation in light-chain deposition disease. Am J Kidney Dis 2004; 43: 147–53.

Little MA, Dupont P, Campbell E, et al. Severity of primary MPGN, rather than MPGN type, determines renal survival and post-transplantation recurrence risk. Kidney Int 2006; 69: 504–11.

Luan FL, Hojo M, Yamaji K, Suthantiran M. Rapamycin blocks tumor progression: unlinking immunosuppression from antitumor efficacy. Transplantation 2002; 73: 1565–72.

MacBride Emerick K. Outcome of liver disease in children with Alagille syndrome: a study of 163 patients. J Pediatr Gastroenterol Nutr 2002; 35: 103–4.

Mahmoud KM, Sobh MA, El-Agroudy AE, et al. Impact of schistosomiasis on patient and graft outcome after renal transplantation: 10 years' follow-up. Nephrol Dial Transplant 2001; 16: 2214–21.

Marangella M. Transplantation strategies in type 1 primary hyperoxaluria: the issue of pyridoxine responsiveness. Nephrol Dial Transplant 1999; 14: 301–3.

Marcen R, Mampso F, Tervel JL, et al. Membranous nephropathy: recurrence after kidney transplantation. Nephrol Dial Transplant 1996; 11: 1129–33.

Massarweh NN, Clayton JL, Mangum CA, et al. High body mass index and short- and long-term renal allograft survival in adults. Transplantation 2005; 80: 1430–4.

Meier-Kriesche HU, Kaplan B. Immunosuppression in elderly renal transplant recipients: are current regimens too aggressive? Drugs Aging 2001; 18: 751–9.

Meier-Kriesche HU, Kaplan B. Waiting time on dialysis as the strongest modifiable risk factor for renal transplant outcomes. Transplantation 2002a; 74: 1377–81.

Meier-Kriesche HU, Cibrik DM, Ojo AO, et al. Interaction between donor and recipient age in determining the risk of chronic renal allograft failure. J Am Geriatr Soc 2002b; 50: 14–17.

Meier-Kriesche HU, Schold JD, Kaplan B. Long-term renal allograft survival: have we made significant progress or is it time to rethink our analytic and therapeutic strategies? Am J Transplant 2004; 8: 1289–95.

Mendizabal S, Estornell F, Zamora I, et al. Renal transplantation in children with severe bladder dysfunction. J Urol 2005; 173: 226–9.

Meulders Q, Pirson Y, Cosyns JP, et al. Course of Henoch–Schönlein nephritis after renal transplantation. Transplantation 1994; 58: 1172–86.

Mignani R, Gerra D, Maldini L, et al. Long-term survival of patients with renal transplantation in Fabry's disease. Contrib Nephrol 2001; 136: 229–36.

Montagnino G, Colturi C, Banfi G, et al. Membranous nephropathy in cyclosporine-treated renal transplant recipients. Transplantation 1989; 47: 725–7.

Montgomery R, Zibari G, Hill GS, Ratner RE. Renal transplantation in patients with sickle cell nephropathy. Transplantation 1994; 58: 618–20.

Morales JM. Renal transplantation in patients positive for hepatitis B or C (pro). Transplant Proc 1998; 5: 2064–9.

Morales JM, Campistol GM, Dominguez-Gil B. Hepatitis C virus infection and kidney transplantation. Semin Nephrol 2002; 22: 365–74.

Morales JM, Dominguez-Gil B, Sanz-Guajardo D, et al. The influence of hepatitis B and hepatitis C virus infection in the recipient on late renal allograft failure. Nephrol Dial Transplant 2004; 19 (Suppl 3): iii72–6.

Moroni G, Ventura D, Riva P, et al. Antiphospholipid antibodies are associated with an increased risk for chronic renal insufficiency in patients with lupus nephritis. Am J Kidney Dis 2004; 43: 28–36.

Moroni G, Tantardini F, Gallleli B, et al. The long-term prognosis of renal transplantation in patients with lupus nephritis. Am J Kidney Dis 2005; 45: 903–11.

Morris PJ, Johnson RJ, Fuggle SV, et al. Analysis of factors that affect outcome of primary cadaveric renal transplantation in the UK. Lancet 1999; 354: 1147–52.

Mourad G, Djamali A, Turc-Baron C, Cristol JP. Lipoprotein glomerulopathy: a new case of nephrotic syndrome after transplantation. Nephrol Dial Transplant 1998; 13: 1292–4.

Murphy BG, Hill CM, Middleton D, et al. Increased renal allograft thrombosis in CAPD patients. Nephrol Dial Transplant 1994; 9: 1165–9.

Nachman PH, Segelmark M, Westman K, et al. Recurrent ANCA-associated small vessel vasculitis after transplantation: a pooled analysis. Kidney Int 1999; 56: 1544–50.

Neu AM. Special issues in pediatric kidney transplantation. Adv Chronic Kidney Dis 2006; 13: 62–9.

Nyberg G, Blohmé I, Persson H, et al. Recurrence of SLE in transplanted kidneys: a follow-up transplant biopsy study. Nephrol Dial Transplant 1992; 7: 1116–23.

Odorico JS, Knechtle SJ, Rayhill SC, et al. The influence of native nephrectomy on the incidence of recurrent disease following renal transplantation for primary glomerulonephritis. Transplantation 1996; 6: 228–34.

Ohta T, Kawaguchi H, Hattori M, et al. Effect of pre- and postoperative plasmapheresis on posttransplant recurrence of focal segmental glomerulosclerosis in children. Transplantation 2001; 71: 628–33.

Ohta T, Motoyama O, Takahashi K, et al. Kidney transplantation in pediatric recipients with mental retardation: clinical results of a multicenter experience in Japan. Am J Kidney Dis 2006; 47: 518–27.

Ojo AO, Govaerts TC, Schmouder RL, et al. Renal transplantation in end-stage sickle cell nephropathy. Transplantation 1999; 67: 291–5.

Osman Y, El-Husseini A, Sheashaa H, et al. Impact of Rh(D) blood group system on graft function and survival in live-donor kidney transplantation: a single-institution experience. Transplantation 2004; 78: 1693–6.

Palanichamy V, Saffarian N, Jones B, et al. Fibrillary glomerulonephritis in a renal allograft. Am J Kidney Dis 1998; 32: E4.

Peces R, Martinez-Ara J, Miguel J, et al. Renal cell carcinoma co-existent with other renal disease: clinico-pathological features in pre-dialysis patients and those receiving dialysis or renal transplantation. Nephrol Dial Transplant 2004; 19: 2789–96.

Penn I. Evaluation of transplant candidates with pre-existing malignancies. Ann Transplant 1997; 2: 14–17.

Penn I. De novo malignances in pediatric organ transplant recipients. Pediatr Transplant 1998; 2: 56–63.

Pereira BJG, Levey AS. Hepatitis C virus infection in dialysis and renal transplantation. Kidney Int 1997; 51: 981–99.

Peters M, Jeck N, Reinalter S, et al. Clinical presentation of genetically defined patients with hypokalemic salt-losing tubulopathies. Am J Med 2002; 112: 183–90.

Petz LD. Immune hemolysis associated with transplantation. Semin Hematol 2005; 42: 145–55.

Pham PT, Pham PC, Danovitch GM, et al. Predictors and risk factors for recurrent scleroderma renal crisis in the kidney allograft: case report and review of the literature. Am J Transplant 2005; 5: 2565–9.

Piccoli G, Iacuzzo G, Vischi M, et al. Henoch–Schonlein purpura after 20 years of renal replacement therapy. J Nephrol 2001; 14: 307–11.

Pilmore H. Cardiac assessment for renal transplantation. Am J Transplant 2006; 6: 659–65.

Pirsch JD, Armbrust MJ, Knechtle ST, et al. Obesity as a risk factor following renal transplantation. Transplantation 1995; 59: 631–3.

Pischon T, Sharma AM. Obesity as a risk factor in renal transplant patients. Nephrol Dial Transplant 2001; 16: 14–17.

Poduval RD, Meehan SM, Woodle ES, et al. Successful retransplantation after renal allograft loss to polyoma virus interstitial nephritis. Transplantation 2002; 73: 1166–9.

Pol S, Vallet-Pichard A, Fontaine H, Lebray P. HCV infection and hemodialysis. Semin Nephrol 2002; 22: 331–9.

Ponticelli C. Steroid-sparing strategies. Transplant Proc 2005; 37: 3597–9.

Ponticelli C, Moroni G. Renal transplantation in lupus nephritis. Lupus 2005; 14: 95–8.

Ponticelli C, Traversi L, Feliciani A, et al. Kidney transplantation in patients with IgA mesangial glomerulonephritis. Kidney Int 2001; 60: 1948–54.

Ponticelli C, Villa M, Cesana B, et al. Risk factors for late alograft failure. Kidney Int 2002a; 62: 1848–54.

Ponticelli C, Campise M, Tarantino A. The different patterns of response to plasmapheresis of recurrent focal and segmental glomerulosclerosis. Transplant Proc 2002b; 34: 3069–71.

Pronovost PH, Brady HR, Gunning ME, et al. Clinical features, predictors of disease progression and results of renal transplantation in fibrillary/immunotactoid glomerulopathy. Nephrol Dial Transplant 1996; 11: 837–42.

Quan A, Sullivan EK, Alexander SR. Recurrence of hemolytic uremic syndrome after renal transplantation in children: a report of the North American Pediatric Renal Transplant Cooperative Study. Transplantation 2001; 72: 742–5.

Rabbat CG, Treleavan DJ, Russell JD, et al. Prognostic value of myocardial perfusion studies in patients with end-stage renal disease assessed for kidney or kidney–pancreas transplantation. A meta-analysis. J Am Soc Nephrol 2003; 14: 431–9.

Raine AE, Margreiter R, Brunner PF, et al. Report on management of renal failure in Europe, XXII, 1991. Nephrol Dial Transplant 1992; 7 (Suppl 2): 7–35.

Ramos E, Vincenti F, Lu WX, et al. Retransplantation in patients with graft loss caused by polyoma virus nephropathy. Transplantation 2004; 77: 131–3.

Reddy KS, Stablein D, Taranto S, et al. Long-term following simultaneous kidney–pancreas transplantation versus kidney transplantation alone in patients with type 1 diabetes mellitus and renal failure. Am J Kidney Dis 2003; 41: 464–70.

Reynolds JC, Agodoa LY, Yuan CM, Abbott KC. Thrombotic microangiopathy after renal transplantation in the United States. Am J Kidney Dis 2003; 42: 1058–68.

Ribot S. Kidney transplant in sickle cell nephropathy. Int J Artif Organs 1999; 22: 61–3.

Rigden S, Mehls O, Gellert R, on behalf of the Scientific Advisory Board of the ERA-EDTA. Registry Factors influencing second renal allograft survival. Nephrol Dial Transplant 1999; 14: 566–9.

Roland ME, Stock PG. Review of solid-organ transplantation in HIV-infected patients. Transplantation 2003; 75: 425–9.

Rosenberger J, Geckova AM, van Dijk JP, et al. Prevalence and characteristics of noncompliant behaviour and its risk factors in kidney transplant recipients. Transpl Int 2005; 18: 1072–8.

Rostaing L, Modesto A, Oksman F, et al. Outcome of patients with antineutrophil cytoplasmic autoantibody-associated vasculitis following cadaveric kidney transplantation. Am J Kidney Dis 1997; 29: 96–102.

Roth D. Hepatitis C virus: the nephrologist's view. Am J Kidney Dis 1995; 25: 3–16.

Roth D. Hepatitis in non-hepatic transplantation. Graft 1999; 2 (Suppl III): S104–7.

Ruggenenti P. Post-transplant hemolytic–uremic syndrome kidney. Kidney Int 2002; 62: 1093–104.

Rutgers A, Meyers KE, Canziani G, et al. High affinity of anti-GBM antibodies for Goodpasture and transplanted alport patients to alpha 3 (IV) NC1 collagen. Kidney Int 2000; 58: 115–22.

Saito T, Oikawa S, Sato H, et al. Lipoprotein glomerulopathy: significance of lipoprotein and ultrastructural features. Kidney Int 1999; 71: S37–41.

Salomon R, Gagnadoux MF, Niaudet P. Intravenous cyclosporine therapy in recurrent nephritic syndrome after renal transplantation in children. Transplantation 2003; 75: 810–14.

Sam R, Wu H, Yue L, et al. Lipoprotein glomerulopathy: a new apolipoprotein E mutation with enhanced glomerular binding. Am J Kidney Dis 2006; 47: 539–48.

Samaniego M, Nadasdy GM, Laszik Z, Nadasdy T. Outcome of renal transplantation in fibrillary glomerulonephritis. Clin Nephrol 2001; 55: 159–66.

Sander GE, Giles TD. Cardiovascular complications of collagen vascular disease. Curr Treat Options Cardiovasc Med 2002; 4: 151–9.

Sarwal MM, Yorgin PD, Alexander S, et al. Promising early outcomes with a novel, complete steroid advoidance immunosuppression protocol in pediatric transplantation. Transplantation 2001; 72: 13–21.

Saudan P, Berney T, Leski M, et al. Renal transplantation in the elderly: a long-term single center experience. Nephrol Dial Transplant 2001; 16: 824–8.

Segoloni G, Messina M, Squiccimarro G, et al. Preferential allocation of marginal kidney allografts to elderly recipients combined with modified immunosuppression gives good results. Transplantation 2005; 80: 953–8.

Sessa A, Meroni M, Battini G, et al. Chronic renal failure, dialysis, and renal transplantation in Anderson–Fabry disease. Semin Nephrol 2004; 24: 532–6.

Sever MS, Turkmen A, Battini G. Renal transplantation in systemic amyloidosis secondary to familial Mediterranean fever. Transplant Proc 2001; 33: 3392–3.

Sharma R, Pellerin D, Gaze DC, et al. Dobutamine stress echocardiography and the resting but not exercise electrocardiograph predict severe coronary artery disease in renal transplant candidates. Nephrol Dial Transplant 2005; 20: 2207–14.

Sherif AM, Refail AF, Sobh MA, et al. Long-term outcome of live donor kidney transplantation for renal amyloidosis. Am J Kidney Dis 2003; 42: 370–5.

Shimizu T, Tanabe K, Oshima T, et al. Recurrence of membranoproliferative glomerulonephritis in renal allografts. Transplant Proc 1998; 30: 3910–13.

Shimmura H, Tanabe K, Ishikawa N, et al. Role of anti-A/B antibody titers in results of ABO-incompatible kidney transplantation. Transplantation 2000; 70: 1331–5.

Shimmura H, Tanabe K, Ishida H, et al. Lack of correlation between results of ABO-incompatible living kidney transplantation and anti-ABO blood type antibody titers under our current immunosuppression. Transplantation 2005; 80: 985–8.

Short AK, O'Donoghue DJ, Riad HN, et al. Recurrence of light chain nephropathy in a renal allograft. A case report and review of the literature. Am J Nephrol 2001; 21: 237–40.

Sienko J, Wisniewska M, Ostrowski M, et al. Factors that impact on immediate graft function in patients after renal transplantation. Transplant Proc 2003; 35: 2153–4.

Smith JM, Ho PL, Mc Donald RA. Renal transplant outcomes in adolescents: a report of the North American Pediatric Renal Transplant Cooperative Study. Pediatr Transplant 2002; 6: 493–9.

Snyder JJ, Kasiske BL, Gilbertson T, Collins AJ. A comparison of transplant outcomes in peritoneal and hemodialysis patients. Kidney Int 2002; 62: 1423–30.

Soler MJ, Mir M, Rodriguez E, et al. Recurrence of IgA nephropathy and Henoch–Schonlein purpura after kidney transplantation: risk factors and graft survival. Transplant Proc 2005; 37: 3705–9.

Stegall MD, Gllor J, Winters JL, et al. A comparison of plasmapheresis versus high-dose IVIG desensitization in renal allograft recipients with high levels of donor specific antibodies. Am J Transplant 2006; 6: 346–51.

Stewart JH, Buccianti G, Agodoa L, et al. Cancers of the kidney and urinary tract in patients on dialysis for end-stage renal disease: analysis of data from the United States, Europe, and Australia and New Zealand. J Am Soc Nephrol 2003; 14: 197–207.

Stone JH, Amend WJ, Criswell LA. Outcome of renal transplantation in systemic lupus erythematosus. Semin Arthritis Rheum 1997; 1: 17–26.

Susal C, Pelzl S, Dohler B, Opelz G. Identification of highly responsive kidney transplant recipients using soluble CD30. J Am Soc Nephrol 2002; 13: 1650–6.

Susal C, Pelzl S, Opelz G. Strong human leukocyte antigen matching effect in nonsensitized kidney transplant recipients with high pretransplant soluble CD30. Transplantation 2003; 16: 1231–2.

Swanson SJ, Kirk AD, Ko CW, et al. Impact of HIV seropositivity on graft and patient survival after cadaveric renal transplantation in the United States in the pre highly active antiretroviral therapy (HAART) era: an historical cohort analysis of the United States Renal Data System. Transpl Infect Dis 2002; 4: 144–7.

Swindle P, Falk M, Rigby R, et al. Transitional cell carcinoma in renal transplant recipients: the influence of compound analgesics. Br J Urol 1998; 81: 229–33.

Takahashi M, Yanagida N, Okano M. A first report: living related kidney transplantation on a patient with Bartter's syndrome. Transplant Proc 1996; 3: 1588.

Takemoto SK, Terasaki PI, Gjertson DW, Cecka JM. Twelve years' experience with national sharing of HLA-matched cadaveric kidneys for transplantation. N Engl J Med 2000; 343: 1078–84.

Tarantino A, Moroni G, Banfi G, et al. Renal replacement therapy in cryoglobulinemic nephritis. Nephrol Dial Transpl 1994; 9: 1426–30.

Tejani A, Stablein DH. Recurrence of focal segmental glomerulosclerosis post-transplantation: a special report of the North America Pediatric Renal Transplant Cooperative Study. J Am Soc Nephrol 1992; 2 (Suppl): S258–61.

Tong NK, Beran J, Kee SA, et al. Immunogenicity and safety of an adjuvanted hepatitis B vaccine in pre-hemodialysis and hemodialysis patients. Kidney Int 2005; 68: 2298–303.

Tóth M, Réti V, Gondos T. Effects of recipients' peri-operative parameters on the outcome of kidney transplantation. Clin Transplant 1998; 12: 511–17.

Tsianos EV, Dardamanis MA, Elisaf M, et al. The value of alpha-amylase and isoamylase determination in chronic renal failure patients. Int J Pancreatol 1994; 15: 105–11.

Tyden G, Kumlien G, Genberg H, et al. ABO-incompatible kidney transplantation and rituximab. Transplant Proc 2005; 37: 3286–7.

Uemura T, Sanchez EQ, Ikegami T, et al. Successful combined liver and kidney transplant for COACH syndrome and 5-yr follow-up. Clin Transplant 2005; 19: 717–20.

Vaidya S, Sellers R, Kimball P, et al. Frequency, potential risk and therapeutic intervention in ESRD patients with antiphospholipid antibody syndrome. A multicenter study. Transplantation 2000; 69: 1348–52.

Van der Weide MJ, Cornelissen EA, Van Achterberg T, et al. Lower urinary tract symptoms after renal transplantation in children. J Urol 2006; 175: 297–302.

Valdivia P, Gonzalez Roncero F, Gentil MA, et al. Plasmapheresis for the prophylaxis and treatment of recurrent focal segmental glomerulosclerosis following renal transplant. Transplant Proc 2005; 37: 1473–4.

Vanwalleghem J, Zachée P, Kuypers D, et al. Renal transplantation for end-stage renal disease due to paroxysmal nocturnal hemoglobinuria. Nephrol Dial Transplant 1998; 13: 3250–2.

Vembar M, Walker MJ, Johnson PC. Cardiac imaging using multislice computed tomography scanners: technical considerations. Coron Artery Dis 2006; 17: 115–23.

Verswijvel G, Vanbeckevoort D, Maes B, Oyen R. Paroxysmal nocturnal hemoglobinuria. MRI of renal cortical hemosiderosis in two patients including one renal transplant. Nephrol Dial Transplant 1999; 14: 1586–9.

Vieira EA, Agarwal A, Book BK, et al. Rituximab for reduction of anti-HLA antibodies in patients awaiting renal transplantation: safety, pharmacodynamics, and pharmacokinetics. Transplantation 2004; 77: 542–8.

Vikrant S, Agarwal SK, Gupta S, et al. Prospective randomized control trial of isoniazid chemoprophylaxis during renal replacement therapy. Transpl Infect Dis 2005; 7: 99–108.

Vosnides GG. Hepatitis C in renal transplantation. Kidney Int 1997; 3: 843–61.

Wang AY, Lai FM, Yu AW, et al. Recurrent IgA nephropathy in renal transplant allografts. Am J Kidney Dis 2001; 38: 588–96.

Weimer R, Susal C, Yildiz S, et al. sCD30 and neopterin as risk factors of chronic renal transplant rejection: impact of cyclosporine A, tacrolimus, and mycophenolate mofetil. Transplant Proc 2005; 37: 1776–8.

Weng FL, Joffe MM, Feldman HI, Mange KC. Rates of completion of the medical evaluation for renal transplantation. Am J Kidney Dis 2005; 46: 734–45.

Womer KL, Meier-Kriesche HU, Patton PR, et al. Preemptive retransplantation for BK virus nephropathy: successful outcome despite active viremia. Am J Transplant 2006; 6: 209–13.

Wuhl E, Haffner D, Offner G, et al. Long-term treatment with growth hormone in short children with nephropathic cystinosis. J Pediatr 2001; 138: 880–7.

Wutrich RP, Cicvara-Muzar S, Body C, et al. Heterozygosity for the factor V Leiden (G1691A) mutation predisposes renal transplant recipients to thrombotic complications and graft loss. Transplantation 2001; 72: 549–50.

Wyatt CM, Murphy B. Kidney transplantation in HIV-infected patients. Semin Dial 2005; 18: 495–8.

Younossi ZM, Braun WE, Protiva DE, et al. Chronic viral hepatitis in renal transplant recipients with allograft functioning for more than 20 years. Transplantation 1999; 67: 272–5.

Zeier M, Ritz E. Preparation of the dialysis patient for transplantation. Nephrol Dial Transplant 2002; 17: 552–6.

3 DELAYED GRAFT FUNCTION

Definition

The *definition* of delayed graft function (DGF) varies among transplant centers, although most of them classify under the term DGF those cases who require dialysis in the first week after transplantation. This definition has at least two main drawbacks: (1) there are different criteria for dialysis prescription among nephrologists, and (2) it includes both reversible and irreversible cases of acute graft failure, such as acute tubular necrosis, acute rejection, cortical necrosis, primary non-function, and hyperacute rejection. Some investigators proposed defining DGF on the basis of prognostic predictors. Park *et al.* (2002) found that graft survival is consistently lower in patients with a slow reduction of creatinine levels during the first 2 weeks after transplant than in patients with an immediate resumption of graft function Govani *et al.* (2002) proposed defining immediate graft function and DGF on the basis of the creatinine reduction ratio and 24-hour creatinine excretion from post-transplant day 1 to day 2. These criteria were validated by Rodrigo *et al.* (2004), who found a good correlation between the creatinine reduction ratio at post-transplant day 2 and renal function throughout the first year.

Nevertheless, even if inappropriate, the most used definition adopted by the transplant community remains that based on the need for dialysis, so that the term DGF encompasses most cases of early post-transplant renal failure. Accordingly, DGF may occur in 8–50% of cadaveric renal transplant recipients (Ojo *et al.*, 1997; Halloran and Hunsicker, 2001; Brier *et al.*, 2003). Improvements in medical and surgical strategies reduced the incidence of this complication (Shoskes *et al.*, 2001). On the other hand, the shortage of donors has led to a widening of the criteria for donor acceptance in recent years, with the potential risk of increasing the incidence of DGF (Irish *et al.*, 2003; Woo *et al.*, 2005).

Causes of acute graft failure

Several different causes may account for acute kidney allograft failure (Table 3.1).

Pre-renal failure

Renal hypoperfusion

Reduced renal perfusion of the transplanted kidney can be responsible for oliguria and renal failure which may be promptly reversed by the appropriate administration of salt and water and/or by renal vasodilators. Cases of functional renal failure due to *hypovolemia* have been found to be more frequent in patients treated with hemodialysis than in those treated with peritoneal dialysis (Bleyer *et al.*, 1999), probably because of the stronger dehydration induced by hemodialysis preceding transplantation. Sometimes, hypovolemia may be caused by massive polyuria in the first post-transplant hours, not compensated by adequate infusion of salt and water. Pre-renal failure may also be caused by the profound *vasoconstriction* of pre-glomerular arterioles induced by cyclosporine or tacrolimus, often used at high doses in the first post-transplant period. An exception is represented by oligoanuria in cases of *acute heart failure*, often caused by salt and water retention.

Renal vascular thrombosis (see also Chapter 18)

Vascular thrombosis of the renal artery or vein after a kidney transplant is an infrequent but devastating complication. Apart from cases of technical error or surgical complications, often no cause is identified. In

Table 3.1   Main causes of delayed graft function

Pre-renal	Parenchymal	Post-renal

Functional
  hypotension hypovolemia
	Acute tubular necrosis
	  ischemia–reperfusion,
	  drug nephrotoxicity
		Intrinsic ureteral obstruction
		  ureteral stenosis, blood clots

Vascular obstruction
  arterial thrombosis,
  venous thrombosis
	Rejection
	  hyperacute, acute
		Extrinsic ureteral obstruction
		  lymphocele, hematoma,
		  ureteral kinking

	Thrombotic microangiopathy
	  calcineurin inhibitors, mTOR
	  inhibitors
		Urine leakage
		urinary fistula

	Recurrence of original
	  disease
	  focal segmental
	  glomerulosclerosis, hemolytic
	  uremic syndrome, primary
	  hyperoxaluria	

a number of incidences, vascular thrombosis may be triggered by a *hypercoagulable state* associated with early recurrence of nephrotic syndrome, or by coagulation abnormalities, such as the presence of antiphospholipid antibodies (Forman *et al.*, 2004) or a deficit in antithrombin III (Hara and Naito, 2005) or a pro-thrombin mutation (Irish, 2004). Other predisposing factors include *vessel size discrepancy* in small children, *en bloc* use of pediatric kidneys, atherosclerosis of the donor and/or recipient vessels, a kidney with multiple arteries, and vessel lesions during kidney removal. Rarely, renal artery thrombosis may develop after the administration of *OKT3* which, together with cyclosporine or high-dose intravenous methylprednisolone, may produce a procoagulant effect (Abramowicz *et al.*, 1996; Shankar *et al.*, 2001).

Parenchymal acute renal failure

Non-viable kidney   The use of *marginal donors* and of *non-heart-beating donors* may be associated with a higher risk of irreversible post-transplant non-function caused by non-viable kidneys (Irish *et al.*, 2003). It is difficult to estimate the incidence of post-transplant non-function as these cases are often not reported in publications of large clinical trials.

De novo thrombotic microangiopathy   This may occur early after transplantation, being favored by the use of *calcineurin inhibitors* (Lin *et al.*, 2003) or *mTOR* (mammalian target of rapamycin) *inhibitors* (Reynolds *et al.*, 2003), or by a *virus infection* (Waiser *et al.*, 1999). It does not usually lead to a dramatic onset of acute renal failure, but is rather characterized by a subacute or slow progression. However, in patients with marginal kidneys, pre-existing endothelial lesions may rapidly progress to thombotic microangiopathy under treatment with sirolimus, which may impair repair of the endothelium by inhibiting endothelial growth factor (Pelle *et al.*, 2005).

Hyperacute rejection   This leads to fulminant graft failure.

Acute and accelerated rejection   This may also cause acute renal failure that may be reversible but which raises a number of problems, diagnosis and treatment being difficult in oliguric patients.

Recurrent diseases   These do not usually cause early graft failure, with some possible exceptions. *Primary hyperoxaluria type* I generally develops in children. After renal transplantation there is a high risk

Table 3.2 Factors predisposing to post-transplant acute tubular necrosis

Hypovolemia
Calcineurin inhibitors
mTOR inhibitors
Nephrotoxic agents
Brain death
Prolonged warm and/or cold ischemia time
Older age of the donor

of rapid graft destruction due to massive oxalate precipitation in the kidney, especially in patients with post-transplant oligoanuria. *Hemolytic uremic syndrome* may recur immediately after renal transplantation with rapid graft failure, particularly in patients with a deficiency of complement factor H or in familial forms (Ruggenenti, 2002). A few cases of anuria requiring dialysis have been described in children with recurrent *focal glomerular sclerosis* (Saleem et al., 2000).

Acute tubular necrosis (ATN)   This is by far the most frequent cause of DGF. Several factors may contribute to the development of ATN (Table 3.2). Preparation of the recipient may be important, as *hypovolemic recipients* are more exposed to ATN. The use of high-dose *cyclosporine* or *tacrolimus* may render the kidney more susceptible to ATN, particularly when these agents are combined with other *nephrotoxic drugs* such as aminoglycosides, non-steroidal anti-inflammatory drugs, cidofovir, foscarnet, amphotericin B, or sulfonamides. However, experimental studies showed that pharmacological preconditioning with low-dose cyclosporine or tacrolimus may reduce the subsequent ischemia–reperfusion injury in the kidney (Yang et al., 2001). The mTOR inhibitors *sirolimus* and *everolimus* can also exert a dose-dependent tubular toxicity, either by inhibiting the proliferation of tubular epithelial cells (Pallet et al., 2005) or by inducing proinflammatory or antiapoptotic pathways (Loverre et al., 2004). In combination with calcineurin inhibitors, sirolimus may lead to a form of cast nephropathy indistinguishable from myeloma cast nephropathy (Smith et al., 2003). The *source of donors* is particularly important. It is a common experience that ATN is more rare in living than in cadaveric kidney transplant recipients. The difference is mainly accounted for by cytokine release, and by hemodynamic instability associated with *brain death*. A massive release of cytokines and growth factors can cause injury, ischemia, and inflammation (Takada et al., 1997), which can concur with the consequences of hemodynamic instability in producing ATN. After brain death, persistent hypotension, coagulopathy, pulmonary changes, hypothermia, and electrolyte disturbances can occur. Intense sympathetic stimulation, either from direct neural activity or from endogenous catecholamines, and activation of the renin system (Blumenfeld et al., 2001), can markedly decrease organ perfusion. Simultaneously, there is a sudden increase in cytosol calcium, which in turn activates enzymes detrimental to the cell, thereby contributing to organ failure (Novitzky, 1997; Van der Hoevon et al., 1998). *Older age* may also play an important role. The requirement for dialysis within the first week was 17% when the donor was aged 15–20 years, but it was more than 40% when the donor was aged 65 or older (Cecka, 2000).

Poor perfusion of the donor kidney before removal, coupled with warm ischemia during the disconnection of kidney vessels from the donor's circulation and cold ischemia after refrigeration and perfusion, may cause an *ischemia–reperfusion syndrome*. Cell hypoxia leads to activation of the endothelium, increased permeability, and the expression of adhesion molecules. Transcription factors are activated, leading to enhanced expression of inflammatory genes. The endothelial cells lose their antiadhesive capacity and develop a thrombogenic surface. The reinstitution of blood flow increases endothelial cell permeability, while adherent leukocytes enter the subendothelial space by releasing cytokines and reactive oxygen species. Therefore, the syndrome is characterized by the inability of physiologic enzymes to hold within tight

Table 3.3 Alterations caused by ischemia–reperfusion

Activation of endothelium and transcription factors (such as NFκB). Endothelial cells lose their antiadhesive properties
After reperfusion, PMN cells and platelets adhere and cause increased permeability and cell activation with enhanced expression of inflammatory genes
ATP is broken down to hypoxanthine. Increased activation of lytic enzymes. Loss of cell energy
Increased production of intracellular free iron. Increased reactions generating oxygen radicals
Overproduction of reactive oxygen species and cytokines
Derangement of ionic homeostasis. Cell death

limits the intracellular concentration of reactive oxygen species (Table 3.3). The oxygen deprivation is followed by cell tubular dysfunction, of variable severity, until ATN (Edelstein *et al.*, 1997, Bellos *et al.*, 2005).

Post-renal failure

This is mainly a result of urinary obstruction or extravasation.

Intrinsic ureteral obstruction may be caused by clots or edema at the ureterovesical anastomosis, or by a technical error causing ureteral stenosis.

Extrinsic ureteral obstruction may occur with lymphocele, hematoma, urinoma, or abscess lesions.

Extravasation may occur in the case of inadequate blood supply to the ureter. Too short a ureter may create tension at the anastomosis and favor the production of a ureteral fistula; too long a ureter may lead to an insufficient blood supply, with consequent necrosis and extravasation. Thus, in removing the donor kidney, great attention should be paid to preserving the branches in the renal hilum to maintain ureteral viability. The ureter should be short, but tension at the anastomosis should be avoided.

Etiological diagnosis

As the possibility of reversing a renal artery or vein *thrombosis* depends strongly on a prompt diagnosis, the most urgent maneuvers in a case of sudden anuria should be addressed to evaluate the patency of renal vessels. Echo color Doppler can show a poor or absent renal vascularization. The diagnosis may be confirmed by scintigraphy, arteriography, or angio-magnetic resonance.

The possibility of a *bladder obstruction* should be ascertained either by urethral catheterization or by ultrasonography. Echography is also important to identify *uretero-pyelectasia* and/or the presence of an obstructive mass or fluid collection (Figure 3.1). It should be noted, however, that a spontaneously reversible low-grade dilatation of the collecting system is not unusual in the early postoperative period. On the other hand, in cases of concomitant urinary obstruction and acute tubular necrosis, dilatation may be lacking, making the diagnosis particularly difficult. In doubtful cases, the percutaneous insertion of a cannula into the renal pelvis with the perfusion of a few milliliters of contrast can help to define the presence and location of a urological obstruction.

After excluding a macrovascular or urological cause, it is important to know the type and reversibility of the parenchymal damage. In fact, early diagnosis of the irreversible nature of DGF – cortical necrosis, hyperacute rejection, or non-viable kidney – can avoid useless immunosuppression, which may be dangerous in an anuric patient. Irreversible cases can be easily recognized by an isotopic scan and/or echo color Doppler. Renal biopsy may confirm the existence of irreversible lesions (Figure 3.2), or may show the presence of rejection, interstitial nephritis, acute nephrotoxicity, or acute tubular necrosis (Figure 3.3), although the typical histological findings may be absent in some cases of ATN.

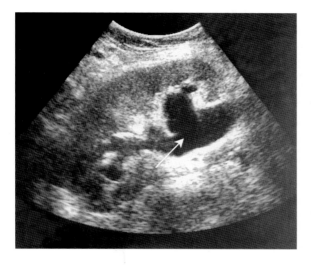

Figure 3.1 Ultrasound of transplant kidney with hydronephrosis arising from ureteral obstruction. The arrow shows the dilated transplant renal pelvis.

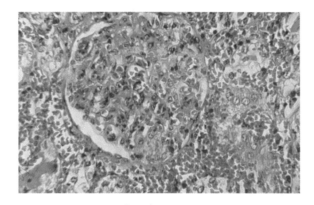

Figure 3.2 Histologic appearance of a renal allograft showing interstital hemorrhage due to accelerated rejection (hematoxylin and eosin (H&E × 25) (Courtesy of Dr G. Banfi, Ospedale Maggiore Milano)

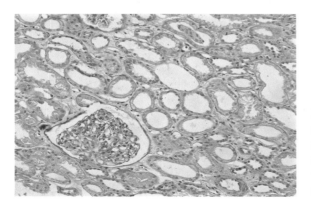

Figure 3.3 'Acute tubular necrosis'. Tubuli show diffuse flattening of the epithelial cells. Some lumina are filled with clumps of necrotic epithelial cells. Scanty inflammatory infiltrates are present in the interstitium. (PAS × 160) (Courtesy of Dr G. Banfi, Ospedale Maggiore Milano)

Table 3.4   The role of ischemia–reperfusion injury in inducing non-antigen-dependent rejection

Overproduction of reactive oxygen species (ROS)
ROS activate innate immunity (complement, polymorphonuclear cells, natural killer cells, toll-like receptors (TLR)
TLR of host origin (heat shock proteins) interact with and activate TLR4-bearing dendritic cells that mature
Matured dendritic cells activate T helper 1 cells and induce *adaptive alloimmune response*
Adaptive alloimmune response may trigger *acute rejection*

Early consequences of delayed graft function

Reactive oxygen species, endothelial activation, and the release of chemoattractants, chemokines, and cytokines mediate the recruitment and activation of circulating factors responsible for acute tubular necrosis often associated with oligoanuria. In turn, the ischemic–reperfusion injury initiates a series of events that may trigger counter-adaptive immunity. Cell damage and the production of reactive oxygen species stimulate the innate immunity of the donor and the recipient (Kim *et al.*, 2005), with the activation of polymorphonuclear cells, complement, natural killer cells, and toll-like receptors (TLR), which cause a proinflammatory state favoring the maturation of dendritic cells (Mazouz *et al.*, 2005). While immature dendritic cells are tolerogenic and may prolong allograft survival (Steinman *et al.*, 2003), mature dendritic cells, after forming a ligand with TLR, may activate antigen-specific Th1 effector cells (Pasare and Medzhitov, 2004), thus inducing adaptive alloimmunity (Land, 2005; Boros and Bromberg 2006). Ischemia–reperfusion not only may give way to a T-cell-dominant milieu (Hoffmann *et al.*, 2002; Land 2005), but also may upregulate incompatible MHC class II antigens leading to increased immunogenicity of grafts (Lu *et al.*, 1999), eventually resulting in an increased rate of *early rejection* (Table 3.4).

The occurrence of DGF may require dialysis, may prolong hospitalization, increases the complexity of the therapeutic approach, facilitates infections, and impairs patient rehabilitation. More important, in patients with DGF, acute rejection or other insults to the graft may remain undiagnosed.

Late consequences of delayed graft function

In non-transplanted patients, ATN is not usually associated with long-term consequences for renal function. Moreover, in syngeneic grafts, ischemic injury does not produce chronic lesions (Paul, 1999). However, the impact of ischemia–reperfusion injury and ATN on allograft kidneys is different. In a review of UNOS (United Network for Organ Sharing) data, Cecka (2000) found that DGF reduced the 5-year graft survival rate by 10–15% and shortened the half-life by about 2 years. However, it is possible that some cases with post-transplant DGF had irreversible renal failure, caused by cortical necrosis, graft thrombosis, or acute rejection superimposed on ATN. In single-center studies, some investigators reported no impact of DGF on long-term graft survival in the absence of acute rejection (Troppmann *et al.*, 1996; Lehtonen *et al.*, 1997; Marcen *et al.*, 1998; Boom *et al.*, 2000), but others found a deleterious effect of DGF, independent of rejection (Giral-Classe *et al.*, 1998; Pfaff *et al.*, 1998; Shoskes and Cecka, 1998; El-Maghraby *et al.*, 2002). If so, the harmful effects of DGF in the long term might be mediated by cell damage caused by ischemia–reperfusion injury that may lead to inflammation, and eventually interstitial fibrosis and tubular atrophy (Figure 3.4). Moreover, as pointed out above, the cell damage caused by ischemia–reperfusion injury can activate the innate immune response and create a reactive oxygen-mediated proinflammatory state, which may be directly responsible for endothelial lesions and, through the maturation of dendritic cells, may trigger a T-cell-mediated immune response leading to rejection (Land, 2005; Boros and Bromberg 2006). Both mechanisms

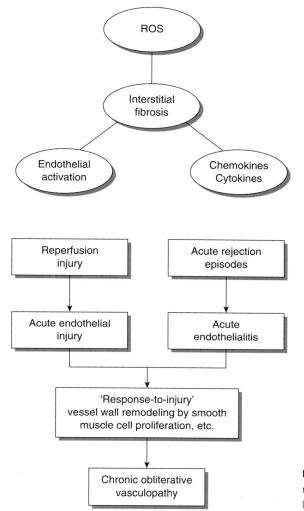

Figure 3.4 Main mechanisms by which ischemia–reperfusion injury may lead to interstitial fibrosis

Figure 3.5 Both reperfusion injury and acute rejection may cause severe vascular lesions eventually leading to chronic obliterative vasculopathy

may concur in the development of obliterative vascular occlusion in the long term (Figure 3.5). Actually, there is general agreement that the combination of DGF with acute rejection is associated with poorer long-term graft survival (Cosio *et al.*, 1997; Geddes *et al.*, 2002; Qureshi *et al.*, 2002).

From a practical point of view, the level of serum creatinine after recovery from DGF is probably the best marker for long-term prognosis. Transplant patients showing only a partial recovery of graft function after DGF are at risk of deleterious long-term consequences. As a matter of fact, retrospective analyses have shown that not only elevated serum creatinine at 1 year after transplantation (Hariharan *et al.*, 2002; Salvadori *et al.*, 2006) but also poor graft function at discharge (Ortiz *et al.*, 2005) are independent variables associated with a poor long-term outcome of the transplanted kidney.

Prevention of delayed graft function

If the response to injury is an important component of DGF and rejection, efforts should be made to decrease injury during the transplant process. This includes optimal management of cadaveric donors,

Table 3.5 Main measures to prevent the onset of delayed graft function

Donor
Normovolemia
Maintain blood pressure
Optimize cardiac output
Adequate kidney perfusion

Kidney perfusion
Intracellular solution
Phosphate-buffered sucrose, hyperosmolar citrate?
CO-releasing molecules?

Cold ischemia time
Maintain < 12–24 h when possible, especially in the case of elderly donors

Ischemia–reperfusion injury
Super-oxide dismutase?
L-arginine?

Recipient
Check volemia
Calcium channel blockers (monitor calcineurin inhibitor blood levels!)
Low-dose dopamine
Loop diuretics

minimizing cold ischemia time, accurate surgical technique, optimizing allograft perfusion during intra- and postoperative periods, and adequate preparation of the recipient (Table 3.5).

Management of organ donors

The goals of management of the donor are to achieve normovolemia, maintain blood pressure, and optimize cardiac output so as to achieve adequate perfusion pressure and blood flow with use of the least amount of vasoactive drug support (Wood *et al.*, 2004). Brain death is generally associated with generalized ischemia due to hyperactivity of the sympathetic system aimed to maintain cerebral perfusion pressure. In spite of this, most donors have profound hypotension. As hypovolemia is a frequent cause of donor hypotension, efforts should be made to restore normal volemia. Hypotonic saline solutions should be preferred, since most donors show hypernatremia. Sodium bicarbonate should be added to correct the concomitant acidosis, and packed red blood cells should be transfused to keep hemoglobin levels >10 g/dl. Antidiuretic hormone should be considered in donors with diabetes insipidus, and insulin in the case of hyperglycemia caused by too-generous administration of glucose solutions. In spite of these measures, most donors remain hypotensive and require vasoactive drugs. The general recommendation is to avoid large use of vasopressor agents. However, some investigators have reported that the use of catecholamines has a not unfavorable impact on graft outcome (Schnuelle *et al.*, 2001). Dopamine is the most frequently used vasopressor, but in a number of cases it must be associated with other vasopressor agents, such as arginine vasopressin or epinephrine, which may help in maintaining renal perfusion (Ueno *et al.*, 2000).

Kidney perfusion solutions

Most preservation solutions have an ionic composition similar to that of intracellular fluid, with a large amount of potassium and phosphate relative to sodium and chloride. Glucose and mannitol are added to provide energy for anaerobic processes and to reduce the osmotic differential between the aqueous medium and the tissue. These solutions represent progress in comparison with the old extracellular formulations, but are not completely effective in preventing molecular alterations. Promising results have been obtained with phosphate-buffered sucrose, hyperosmolar citrate solution, which, in an experimental model, proved to be more effective than an intracellular solution in preventing damage due to prolonged warm ischemia (Ahmad et al., 2006). Low concentrations of carbon monoxide (CO) can protect tissues against ischemia–reperfusion injury. Sandouka et al. (2006) identified a novel class of compounds, CO-releasing molecules (CO-RMs), which exert important pharmacological activities by carrying and delivering CO to biological systems. Kidneys flushed with Celsior solution supplemented with CO-RMs (50 μmol/l) and stored at 4°C for 24 h displayed, at reperfusion, a significantly higher perfusion flow rate, glomerular filtration rate, and sodium and glucose reabsorption rates, compared with control kidneys flushed with Celsior solution alone.

Cold ischemia time

There is agreement that prolonged *cold ischemia* time may represent a major risk factor for DGF, but it is still unclear how short the ischemia time should be to prevent DGF. By reviewing CTS (Collaborative Transplant Study) data, Opelz (1998) found that, up to 36 h, the impact of cold ischemia time does not affect the graft outcome. However, in a retrospective analysis of 816 paired kidneys transplanted from 408 cadaveric donors, the frequency of DGF was 22% in patients with a mean ischemia time of 22 h versus 35% in a group with a mean ischemia time of 28 h (Kyllonen and Salmela, 2000). An analysis of UNOS data showed that the 4-year graft survival rate was decreased by 5% when the cold ischemia time exceeded 42 h (Cecka, 2003). It has been pointed out that the impact of cold ischemia time increases with advancing age (Hetzel et al., 2002). However, efforts to reduce cold ischemia times for cadaveric kidneys have been modestly successful in the USA. The percentage of kidneys transplanted within 12 h increased from 18% in 2001 to 25% in 2003, and the percentage with more than 24 h of cold ischemia fell from 28% in 2001 to 20% in 2003 (Cecka, 2003).

Ischemia–reperfusion injury

In experimental transplantation, several substances have been successfully used in the prevention of ischemia–reperfusion injury. These include: monoclonal antibodies against adhesion molecules (Kelley et al., 1995); antisense oligodesoxynucleotides (Dragun et al., 1998); an endothelin receptor antagonist (Buyukgebiz et al., 1996); allopurinol (Hernandez et al., 1999); trifluoperazine, an inhibitor of the calmodulin–Ca^{2+} complex (Edagawa et al., 1999); induction of the stress protein heme oxygenase-1 by cobalt protoporphyrin (Tullius et al., 2002); polyethylene glycol (Faure et al., 2002); propionyl-L-carnitine (Mister et al., 2002); caspase inhibitors (Jani et al., 2004); glibenclamide (Pompermayer et al., 2005); N-acetylcysteine (de Araujo et al., 2005) ; TNFα inhibitors (Pascher and Klupp, 2005); erdosteine (Erdogan et al., 2006); and trimetazidine (Domanski et al., 2006).

In spite of the experimental evidence that ischemic preconditioning is a powerful method to prevent ischemia–reperfusion damage, there are only a few randomized studies in clinical renal transplantation. Super oxide dismutase (SOD) can strongly decrease the toxic oxygen metabolites released during ischemia–reperfusion injury. In a prospective randomized double-blind placebo-controlled trial, the effect of SOD, at a dose of 200 mg given intravenously during surgery to cadaveric renal transplant recipients, was to reduce significantly acute rejection episodes from 33.3% in controls to 18.5%, as well as early irreversible acute rejection from 12.5% in controls to 3.7%. In the long term there was a significant improvement of the actual 4-year graft survival rate in rhSOD-treated patients to 74% compared with 52% in controls (Land et al., 1994). L-Arginine may stimulate nitric oxide despite saturating the intracellular concentration (arginine 'paradox'). Clinical studies showed that the administration of L-arginine could improve renal graft function, although the effect was mainly observed with kidneys coming from young donors with short cold ischemia times (Schramm et al., 2002).

In summary, inhibition of the production of oxygen radicals and inflammatory cytokines remains the primary goal in preventing ischemia–reperfusion injury. Whether immunosuppressive drugs may be helpful by inhibiting the activation of adaptive immunity, or may be harmful by inhibiting stem cell proliferation and migration, is still a matter of investigation.

Treatment of the recipient

If the recipient needs to be dialyzed before transplantation, it is recommended that dehydration be avoided, unless strictly necessary. Many centers recommend that the central venous pressure of the recipient is maintained in a supranormal range in order to allow satisfactory perfusion of the transplanted kidney. Plasma expanders or hypertonic mannitol may be administered immediately before the vascular connection. The infusion of loop diuretics may be useful, to give an immediate good urine output. The impact of ischemia–reperfusion on the transplanted kidney may be enhanced by the vasoconstrictive effects of calcineurin inhibitors. In patients at higher risk of DGF, such as elderly recipients of older kidneys, the administration of calcineurin inhibitors may be delayed until the serum creatinine falls below 2.0–2.5 mg/dl (Segoloni *et al.*, 2006). Other strategies to attenuate vasospasm and to improve kidney perfusion include the direct injection of a *calcium channel blocker* into the renal artery (Dawidson *et al.*, 1994), or the early administration of oral non-dihydropyridine calcium channel blockers. It should be remembered, however, that the latter agents may increase the blood levels of calcineurin inhibitors. When given at 'renal doses', i.e. 1–3 µg/kg/min, also *dopamine* may produce renal vasodilatation (Dalton *et al.*, 2005). Moreover, dopamine can stimulate the induction of protective enzymes such as heme oxygenase-1 (HO-1), rendering the kidney more resistant to the insult of ischemia–reperfusion and inflammation (Van der Woude *et al.*, 2004). On the other hand, a review of clinical trials in non-transplanted patients showed the lack of efficacy of low-dose dopamine in preventing acute renal failure (Schenarts *et al.*, 2006).

In cases of *heart failure*, the treatment depends on the cause. Loop diuretics or dialysis are needed if cardiac decompensation is caused by salt and water retention. In cases of poor myocardial contractility, diuretic therapy should be associated with digitalis, ACE inhibitors, angiotensin receptor blockers, and/or beta-blockers, such as carvedilol.

References

Abramowicz D, De Pauw L, Le Moine, et al. Prevention of OKT3 nephrotoxicity after kidney transplantation. Kidney Int 1996; 49: S39–43.

Ahmad N, Pratt JR, Potts DJ, Lodge JP. Comparative efficacy of renal preservation solutions to limit functional impairment after warm ischemic injury. Kidney Int 2006; 69: 884–93.

Bellos JK, Perrea DN, Vlachalos D, Kostakis AI Chronic allograft nephropathy: the major problem in long-term survival: review of etiology and interpretation. Transplant Rev 2005: 138–44.

Bleyer AJ, Burkart JM, Russel GB, Adams PL Dialysis modality and delayed graft function after cadaveric renal transplantation. J Am Soc Nephrol 1999; 10: 154–9.

Blumenfeld JD, Catanzaro DF, Kinkhabwala M, Renin system activation and delayed graft function of the renal transplant. Am J Hypertens 2001; 14: 1270–4.

Boom H, Mallat MJK, DeFijter JW, et al. Delayed graft function influences renal function but not survival. Kidney Int 2000; 58: 859–66.

Boros P, Bromberg JS. New cellular and molecular immune pathways in ischemia/reperfusion injury. Am J Transplant 2006; 6: 652–8.

Brier ME, Ray PC, Klein JB. Prediction of delayed renal allograft function using an artificial neural network. Nephrol Dial Transplant 2003; 18: 2655–9.

Buyukgebiz O, Aktan AO, Haklar G, et al. BQ-123, a specific endothelin (ETA) receptor antagonist, prevents ischemia–reperfusion injury in kidney transplantation. Transpl Int 1996; 9: 201–7.

Cecka M. The UNOS Scientific Renal Transplant Registry. In Cecka JM, Terasaki PI, eds. Clinical Transplants 1999. Los Angeles, CA: UCLA Tissue Typing Laboratory, 2000: 1–18.

Cecka M. The OPTN/UNOS Renal Transplant Registry 2003. Clin Transpl 2003: 1–12.

Cosio FG, Pelletier PR, Falkenhain ME, et al. Impact of acute rejection and early allograft function on renal allograft survival. Transplantation 1997; 63: 1611–15.

Dalton RS, Webber JN, Cameron C, et al. Physiologic impact of low-dose dopamine on renal function in the early post renal transplant period. Transplantation 2005; 79: 1561–7.

Dawidson I, Ar'Rajab A, Dickerman R, et al. Perioperative albumin and verapamil improve early outcome after cadaver renal transplantation.Transplant Proc 1994; 26: 3100–1.

De Araujo M, Andrade L, Coimbra TM, et al. Magnesium supplementation combined with N-acetylcysteine protects against postischemic acute renal failure. J Am Soc Nephrol 2005; 16: 3339–49.

Domanski L, Sulikowski T, Safranow K, et al. Effect of trimetazidine on the nucleotide profile in rat kidney with ischemia–reperfusion injury. Eur J Pharm Sci 2006; 27: 320–7.

Dragun D, Tullius GS, Park KJ, et al. ICAM-1 antisense oligodesoxynucleotides prevent perfusion injury and enhance immediate graft function in renal transplantation. Kidney Int 1998; 54: 590–602.

Edagawa M, Yoshida E, Matsuzaki Y, et al. Reduction of post-ischemic lung reperfusion injury by fibrinolytic activity suppression. Transplantation 1999; 67: 944–9.

Edelstein CL, Ling H, Schrier RW. The nature of cell injury. Kidney Int 1997; 51: 1341–51.

El-Maghraby TA, Boom K, Campos JA Delayed graft function is characterized by reduced functional mass measured by (99m) T-technetium-mercaptoacetyltriglycine renography. Transplantation 2002; 74: 203–8.

Erdogan H, Fadillioglu E, Yagmurca M, et al. Protein oxidation and lipid peroxidation after renal ischemia–reperfusion injury: protective effects of erdosteine and N-acetylcysteine. Urol Res 2006; 34: 41–6.

Faure JP, Hauet T, Han Z, et al. Polyethylene glycol reduces early and long-term cold ischemia–reperfusion and renal medulla injury. J Pharmacol Exp Ther 2002; 302: 861–70.

Forman JP, Lin J, Pascual M, et al. Significance of anticardiolipin antibodies on short and long term allograft survival and function following kidney transplantation. Am J Transplant 2004; 4: 1786–91.

Geddes CC, Woo YM, Jardine AC The impact of delayed graft function on the long-term outcome of renal transplantation. J Nephrol 2002; 15: 17–21.

Giral-Classe M, Hourmant M, Cantavorich D, et al. Delayed graft function of more than six days strongly decreases long-term survival of transplanted kidneys. Kidney Int 1998; 54: 972–8.

Govani MV, Kwon O, Batiuk TD, et al. Creatinine reduction ratio and 24-hour creatinine excretion on posttransplant day two: simple and objective tools to define graft function. J Am Soc Nephrol 2002; 13: 1645–9.

Halloran PF, Hunsicker LG. Delayed graft function: state of the art, November 10–11, 2000. Summit meeting, Scottsdale, Arizona, USA. Am J Transplant 2001; 1: 115–20.

Hara T, Naito K. Inherited antithrombin deficiency and end stage renal disease. Med Sci Monit 2005; 11: 346–54.

Hariharan S, Johnson CP, Bresnahan BA, et al. Improved graft survival after renal transplantation in the United States, 1988 to 1996. N Engl J Med 2000; 342: 605–12.

Hariharan S, McBride MA, Cherich WS, et al. Post-transplant renal function in the first year predicts long-term kidney transplant survival. Kidney Int 2002; 62: 311–18.

Hernandez A, Light AJ, Barhyte YD, et al. Ablating the ischemia–reperfusion injury in non-heart-beating donor kidneys. Transplantation 1999; 67: 200–6.

Hetzel GR, Klein B, Brause M, et al. Risk factors for delayed graft function after renal transplantation and their significance for long-term clinical outcome. Transpl Int 2002; 15: 10–16.

Hoffmann SC, Kamper RL, Amur S, et al. Molecular and immunohistochemical characterization of the onset and resolution of human renal allograft ischemia–reperfusion injury. Transplantation 2002; 74: 916–23.

Irish A. Hypercoagulability in renal transplant recipients. Identifying patients at risk of renal allograft thrombosis and evaluating strategies for prevention. Am J Cardiovasc Drugs 2004; 4: 139–49.

Irish WD, McCollum DA, Tesi RJ, et al. Nomogram for predicting the likelihood of delayed graft function in adult cadaveric renal transplant recipients. J Am Soc Nephrol 2003; 14: 2967–74.

Jani A, Ljubanovic D, Faubel S, et al. Caspase inhibition prevents the increase in caspase-3, -2, -8 and -9 activity and apoptosis in the cold ischemic mouse kidney. Am J Transplant 2004; 4: 1246–54.

Kelley KJ, Williams WW Jr, Colvin RB, Bonventre JV Antibodies to intercellular adhesion molecule 1 protect the kidney against ischemic injury. Proc Natl Acad Sci USA 1995; 91: 812–16.

Kim BS, Lim SW, Li C, et al. Ischemia–reperfusion injury activates innate immunity in rat kidneys. Transplantation 2005; 79: 1370–7.

Kyllonen L, Salmela K. Transplantation of both kidneys from 408 donors; comparison of results. Transpl Int 2000; 13 (Suppl 1): S95–8.

Land W, Schneeberger H, Schleibner S, et al. The beneficial effect of human recombinant superoxide dismutase on acute and chronic rejection events in recipients of cadaveric renal transplants. Transplantation 1994; 57: 211–17.

Land W. The role of postischemic reperfusion injury and other nonantigen-dependent inflammatory pathways in transplantation. Transplantation 2005; 79: 505–14.

Lehtonen SRK, Isoniemi HM, Salmela KT, et al. Long-term graft outcome is not necessarily affected by delayed onset of graft function and early rejection. Transplantation 1997; 64: 103–7.

Lin CC, King KL, Chao YW, et al. Tacrolimus-associated hemolytic uremic syndrome: a case analysis. J Nephrol 2003; 16: 580–5.

Loverre A, Ditonno P, Crovace A. Ischemia–reperfusion induces glomerular and tubular activation of proinflammatory and antiapoptotic pathways: differential modulation by rapamycin. J Am Soc Nephrol 2004; 15: 2675–86.

Lu C, Penfield JG, Kielar M, et al. Does the injury of transplantation initiate acute rejection? Graft 1999; 2 (Suppl II): S36–41.

Marcen R, Orofino L, Pascual J, et al. Delayed graft function does not reduce the survival of renal transplant allografts. Transplantation 1998; 66: 461–6.

Mazouz N, Detournay O, Buelens C, et al. Immunostimulatory properties of human dendritic cells generated using IFN-beta associated either with IL-3 or GM-CSF. Cancer Immunol Immunother 2005; 54: 1010–17.

Mister M, Noris M, Szymczuk J, et al. Propionyl-L-carnitine prevents renal function deterioration due to ischemia/reperfusion. Kidney Int 2002; 6: 1064–78.

Novitzky D. Detrimental effects of brain death on the potential organ donor. Transplant Proc 1997; 29: 3770.

Ojo AO, Wolfe RA, Held PJ, et al. Delayed graft function: risk factors and implications for renal allograft survival. Transplantation 1997; 63: 968–74.

Opelz G. Cadaver kidney graft outcome in relation to ischemia time and HLA match. Collaborative Transplant Study. Transplant Proc 1998; 30: 4294–6.

Ortiz F, Paavonen T, Tornrorth T, et al. Predictors of renal allograft histologic damage progression. J Am Soc Nephrol 2005; 16: 817–24.

Pallet N, Thervet E, Le Corre D, et al. Rapamycin inhibits human renal epithelial cell proliferation: effect on cyclin D3 mRNA expression and stability. Kidney Int 2005; 67: 2422–33.

Park JH, Yang CW, Kim YS, et al. Comparison of clinicopathological correlations between immediate and slow graft function in renal transplant recipients. Clin Transplant 2002; 16: 18–23.

Pasare C, Medzhitov R. Toll-like receptors: linking innate and adaptive immunity. Microbes Infect 2004; 6: 1382–7.

Pascher A, Klupp J. Biologics in the treatment of transplant rejection and ischemia/reperfusion injury: new applications for TNFα inhibitors? BioDrugs 2005; 19: 211–31.

Paul LC. Chronic allograft nephropathy. Kidney Int 1999; 56: 783–93.

Pelle G, Xu Y, Khoury N, et al. Thrombotic microangiopathy in marginal kidney after sirolimus use. Am J Kidney Dis 2005; 46: 1124–8.

Pfaff WW, Howard RJ, Pattorn PR, et al. Delayed graft function after transplantation. Transplantation 1998; 65: 219–23.

Pompermayer K, Souza DG, Lara GG, et al. The ATP-sensitive potassium channel blocker glibenclamide prevents renal ischemia/reperfusion injury in rats. Kidney Int 2005; 67: 1785–96.

Qureshi F, Rabb H, Kasiske BL. Silent acute rejection during prolonged delayed graft function reduces kidney allograft survival. Transplantation 2002; 74: 1400–4.

Reynolds JC, Agodoa LY, Yuan CM, Abbott KC. Thrombotic microangiopathy after renal transplantation in the United States. Am J Kidney Dis 2003; 42: 1058–68.

Rodrigo E, Ruiz JC, Pinera C, et al. Creatinine reduction ratio on post-transplant day two as criterion in defining delayed graft function. Am J Transplant 2004; 4: 1163–9.

Ruggenenti P. Post-transplant haemolytic–uremic syndrome. Kidney Int 2002; 62: 1093–104.

Saleem MA, Ramanan AV, Rees L. Recurrent focal segmental glomerulosclerosis in grafts treated with plasma exchange and increased immunosuppression. Pediatr Nephrol 2000; 14: 361–4.

Salvadori M, Rosati A, Bock A, et al. Estimated one-year glomerular filtration rate is the best predictor of long-term graft function following renal transplant. Transplantation 2006; 81: 202–6.

Sandouka A, Fuller BJ, Mann BE, et al. Treatment with CO-RMs during cold storage improves renal function at reperfusion. Kidney Int 2006; 69: 239–47.

Schenarts PJ, Sagraves SG, Bard MR, et al. Low-dose dopamine: a physiologically based review. Curr Surg 2006; 63: 219–25.

Schnuelle P, Berger S, De Boer J, et al. Effects of catecholamine application to brain-dead donors on graft survival in solid organ transplantation. Transplantation 2001; 72: 455–63.

Schramm L, La M, Heidelbreder E, et al. L-arginine deficiency and supplementation in experimental acute renal failure and in human kidney transplantation. Kidney Int 2002; 61: 1423–32.

Segoloni G, Messina M, Squiccimarro G, et al. Preferential allocation of marginal kidney allografts to elderly recipients combined with modified immunosuppression gives good results. Transplantation 2006; 80: 953–8.

Shankar R, Bastani B, Salinas-Madrigal L, Sudarshan B. Acute thrombosis of the renal transplant artery after a single dose of OKT3. Am J Nephrol 2001; 21: 141–4.

Shoskes DA, Cecka JM. Deleterious effects of delayed graft function in cadaveric renal transplant recipients independent of acute rejection. Transplantation 1998; 66: 1697–701.

Shoskes DA, Shahed AR, Kim S. Delayed graft function. Influence on outcome and strategies for prevention. Urol Clin North Am 2001; 28: 721–32.

Smith KD, Wrenshall LE, Nicosia RF, et al. Delayed graft function and cast nephropathy associated with tacrolimus plus rapamycin use. J Am Soc Nephrol 2003; 14: 1037–45.

Steinman RM, Hawiger D, Nussenzweig MC. Tolerogenic dendritic cells. Annu Rev Immunol 2003; 21: 685–711.

Takada M, Nadeau KC, Shaw DG, Tilney LN. Prevention of late renal changes after initial ischemia/reperfusion injury by blocking early selectin binding. Transplantation 1997; 64: 1520–5.

Troppmann C, Gillingham KJ, Guessner RW, et al. Delayed graft function in the absence of rejection has no long-term impact. A study of cadaver kidney recipients with good graft function at 1 year after transplantation. Transplantation 1996; 61: 1331–7.

Tullius SG, Nieminen-Kelha M, Buelow R, et al. Inhibition of ischemia/reperfusion injury and chronic graft deterioration by a single-donor treatment with cobalt-protoporphyrin for the induction of heme-oxygenase-1. Transplantation 2002; 74: 591–8.

Ueno T, Zhi-Li C, Itoh T. Unique circulatory responses to exogenous catecholamines after brain death. Transplantation 2000; 70: 430–6.

Van der Hoevon JAB, Postema F, Van Suylichem PTR, et al. Effects of brain death on donor organ quality: endothelial cell activation and predisposition for ischemia/reperfusion damage in transplantation. Transplantation 1998; 65: 95–9.

Van der Woude FJ, Schnuelle P, Yard BA. Preconditioning strategies to limit graft immunogenicity and cold ischemic organ injury. J Invest Med 2004; 52: 323–9.

Waiser J, Budde K, Rudolph B, et al. De novo haemolytic uremic syndrome postrenal transplant after cytomegalovirus infection. Am J Kidney Dis 1999; 34: 556–9.

Woo YM, Gill JS, Johnson N, et al. The advanced age deceased kidney donor: current outcomes and future opportunities. Kidney Int 2005; 67: 2407–14.

Wood KE, Becker BN, McCartney JG, et al. Care of the potential organ donor. N Engl J Med 2004; 351: 2730–9.

Yang CW, Ahn HJ, Han HJ, et al. Pharmacological preconditioning with low-dose cyclosporine or FK506 reduces subsequent ischemia/reperfusion injury in rat kidney. Transplantation 2001; 72: 1726–7.

4

ACUTE REJECTION

The nature of alloantigen disparity between recipient and donor is considered a barrier to engraftment. The recipient responds to this challenge by mounting an immune response involving both the cellular (T cell) and humoral (B cell) arms of the immune response. There are three main patterns diagnosed on the basis of time of onset, pathogenetic mechanisms (humoral or cellular immunity), and clinical and histologic features: *hyperacute*, *acute*, and *chronic* or *late* rejection. The last form is discussed in Chapter 5 ('Chronic allograft nephropathy'), often being indistinguishable from other causes of late graft dysfunction.

Hyperacute rejection

Hyperacute rejection is the term used to describe an irreversible antibody-mediated rejection that generally occurs within minutes or hours after transplantation. It is initiated by preformed donor-specific antibodies present in the serum of the recipient at the time of transplantation and produced by previous pregnancies, blood transfusions, or renal allografts. Hyperacute rejection may also occur in non-preconditioned ABO-incompatible kidney transplants. The graft is damaged by the binding of preformed antibodies to donor endothelium and by complement activation.

Hyperacute rejection is very rare nowadays, because a *crossmatch* between the serum of the recipient and the lymphocytes of the donor is regularly performed before transplantation. The modern crossmatching techniques, such as flow cytometry crossmatch, are capable of revealing donor-relevant antibody specificities in the recipient which may not be detected by the standard complement-dependent cytotoxic technique (Cole *et al.*, 2002).

In its typical form, hyperacute rejection may be recognized by the surgeon in the operating theater. Immediately following the completion of vascular anastomoses, or a few minutes later, the graft appears flaccid and blue, instead of having the normal firm, pink appearance. There is no urine formation. At histology, the most striking features are seen in the small vessels (Figure 4.1). At an early stage there is intense engorgement affecting both glomerular and peritubular capillaries, with the clumping of red blood cells. These changes rapidly involve the small arteries, in particular the afferent glomerular arterioles. Somewhat later, interstitial hemorrhages are seen most markedly at the corticomedullary junction, while there is an infiltration of neutrophils. After 24 hours or more, tubular necrosis, thrombosis, and fibrinoid necrosis of small vessels with complete cortical necrosis can be seen.

Differential diagnosis

Hyperacute rejection must be distinguished from acute tubular necrosis (ATN), thrombosis of the renal artery or vein, or ureteric obstruction or disruption. Investigations should include a perfusion scan, echo color Doppler, and an angiogram if necessary. Graft biopsy can confirm the diagnosis of hyperacute rejection. A repeat crossmatch may be performed after graft nephrectomy to confirm the diagnosis.

Prevention

Some trials have been conducted in order to prevent hyperacute rejection in *highly sensitized patients*. Plasma exchange or immunoadsorption can reduce the concentration of panel-reactive antibodies and allow long-term graft survival in hyperimmunized renal transplant recipients (Higgins *et al.*, 1996; Hickstein *et al.*, 2002). A different approach may consist of the infusion of high-dose intravenous immunoglobulins (Glotz *et al.*, 2002; Jordan *et al.*, 2006). Once desensitization is obtained, patients should be immediately transplanted in order to avoid a possible rebound of antibodies.

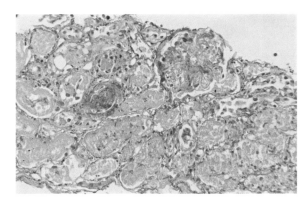

Figure 4.1 Complete necrosis and thrombosis of a small preglomerular arteriole and glomerular thrombosis characterize severe vascular ('accelerated') rejection. (AFOG ×160)

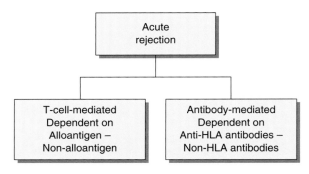

Figure 4.2 Different types of acute rejection

A number of similar techniques have been proposed to prevent hyperacute rejection in *ABO-incompatible* kidney transplants. The removal of preformed antibodies by plasmapheresis (Shimmura *et al.*, 2000) or immunoadsorption (Tyden *et al.*, 2005) with (Shimmura *et al.*, 2005) or without splenectomy, the administration of intravenous immunoglobulins (Segev *et al.*, 2005) or rituximab (Tyden *et al.*, 2005), and strong immunosuppression initiated a few days before transplantation (Mannami and Mitsuhata, 2005) have proved capable of preventing hyperacute rejection in ABO-incompatible transplants and allowing good kidney allograft function also in the long term (Shimmura *et al.*, 2005).

There is no effective therapy for hyperacute rejection. Graft nephrectomy may be mandatory when severe systemic toxicity from necrotic renal tissue and consumption coagulopathy develop.

Acute rejection

Most cases of acute rejection are sustained by a T-cell immune response, triggered by direct recognition of donor antigens of the major histocompatibility complex (MHC). However, acute rejection may also be triggered by non-alloantigen-driven pathways. Kidney transplant recipients who develop donor-specific antibodies or non-HLA antibodies may develop an antibody-mediated form of rejection, also called humoral rejection (Figure 4.2).

T-cell-mediated rejection

The alloantigen-dependent pathway

Mounting rejection needs the co-operation of a number of cells and cellular factors. The activation, progression, proliferation, and differentiation of T cells require three signals (Kahan and Stepkowski, 2000; Halloran, 2004).

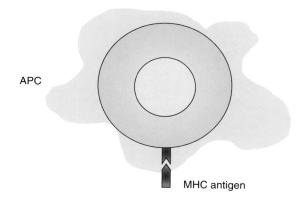

Figure 4.3 Antigen-presenting cell (APC) is a dendritic cell of the donor which has the function of recognizing antigens of the major histocompatibility complex (MHC) and presenting them to T cells in the form of peptides

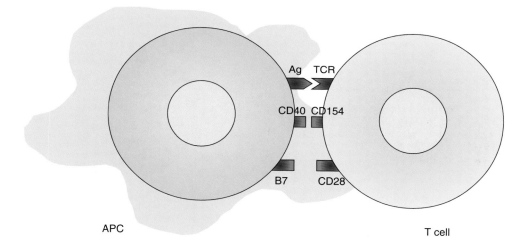

Figure 4.4 The activation of T cells from APC requires two signals. Signal 1 is given by contact of the peptides of the MHC with a specific T cell receptor. Signal 2 (co-stimulatory signal) is given by contact of adhesion molecules located on the surface of APC (B7, CD40) and on the surface of T cells (CD154, CD28)

Signal 1 The first cells to be involved are the so-called antigen-presenting cells (APC), which are mostly represented by dendritic cells of the donor. The APC recognize and engage the MHC antigens, and present them in the form of peptides to central memory T lymphocytes, which recirculate between lymphoid compartments without having access to peripheral tissues (Von Andrian and MacKay, 2000), and to alloantigen-reactive T cells (Figure 4.3).

Signal 2 The activation of T cells requires two steps. The first step is the direct contact of the APC with the T cell receptor. When a lymphocyte is stimulated by an antigen, via APC, the T cell obtains an initial activation signal as well as an anergic/apoptotic signal. A second step, called co-stimulation, is needed to rescue the T cell from apoptosis and to activate it (Figure 4.4). *Co-stimulation* requires contact between adhesion molecules located on the surface of the APC (CD40, B7-1, B7-2) and on the surface of the T lymphocyte (CD28, CD154, CTLA-4). Therefore, the blockage of co-stimulation will drive all graft-activated cells toward anergy and/or apoptosis, which leads to selective unresponsiveness to the graft. Once the T lymphocyte is activated, there is a large influx of Ca^{2+} ions into the cytoplasm leading to the activation of a system of phosphatases called *calcineurin*. Calcineurin dephosphorylates a family of proteins called

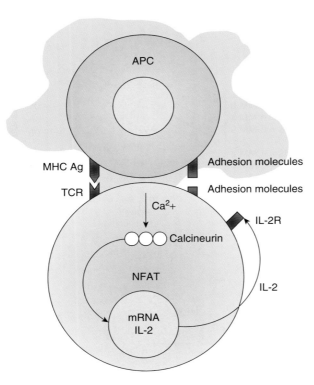

Figure 4.5 After contact of the T cell receptor with antigen presented by APC and co-stimulation by adhesion molecules, there is a large influx of calcium ions into the T lymphocyte which activates a system of phosphatases called calcineurin. Calcineurin dephosphorylates a family of proteins called nuclear factor-activating T cells (NFAT), thus allowing its entrance into the nucleus where it encodes interleukin 2 (IL-2) and other cytokines

nuclear factor-activating T cells (NFAT), thus allowing its entrance into the nucleus where it participates in the encoding and synthesis of interleukin-2 (IL-2) and other cytokines (Figure 4.5). Contact with APC also activates the mitogen-activated protein kinase pathway, and the protein kinase C-nuclear factor-κB (NFκB) pathway. The result is *activation of IL-2*, IL-2 receptor, and NFκB, and further activation of APC.

Signal 3   IL-2 binds to to its receptor (CD25), and together with IL-15 and probably other cytokines activates a kinase known as Janus kinase (Jak 3), and delivers growth signals through a family of kinases governed by phosphatidylinositol 3 kinase (PI3k) and its companion Akt (Figure 4.6). The downstream effector of PI3k/Akt is a serine-threonine kinase, called *FRAP* or *mTOR*, which plays a key regulatory role in protein translation by modulating through phosphorylation other kinases necessary for lymphocyte proliferation (Ponticelli, 2004). Nucleotide synthesis is also required for the proliferation of T lymphocytes. Proliferation and differentiation generate a large number of *effector T cells* (Figure 4.7) directed against MHC antigens, located mainly on tubular (tubulitis) and endothelial cells (endothelial arteritis). Although T cells play a major role in cell-mediated rejection, B cells, which are activated when APC engage the antigens, may contribute to tissue damage by producing alloantibodies against MHC antigens.

Recent evidence has shown that *tubular epithelial cells* may play an active role in acute rejection. These cells may produce chemokines that favor the migration of CD8+ lymphocytes; moreover, they may create a microenvironment of cytokines and growth factors that stimulate αβ integrins, necessary to stabilize interactions between T cells and E-cadherin, leading in turn to interstitial changes up to fibrosis. Finally, IL-15 produced by tubular epithelial cells can support the long-term survival of antigen-specific memory-like CD8+ cells, promoting tubulointerstitial changes and interstitial fibrosis (Robertson and Kirby, 2001). Specific effector T cells directly kill targets via tumor necrosis factor, perforin, and granzyme. Moreover, cytokines recruit polymorphonuclear granulocytes, macrophages, and incompetent T cells to attack the graft. B cells may directly attack graft cells by activating complement, or may activate macrophages.

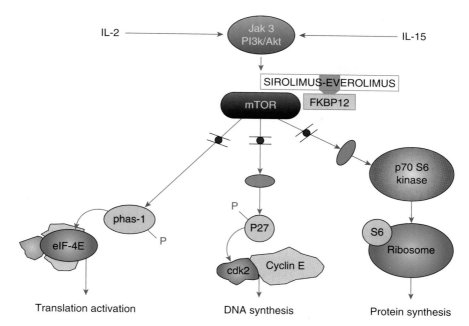

Figure 4.6   Interleukin 2 and interleukin 15 may activate Janus kinase 3 (Jak 3) and phosphatidylinositol 3 kinase (PI3k) that through its downstream effector mammalian target of rapamycin (mTOR) activates a cascade of kinases through different steps of phosphorylation. These kinases provide the signals for proliferation to activated T lymphocytes. This pathway may be inhibited by the mTOR antagonists sirolimus and everolimus

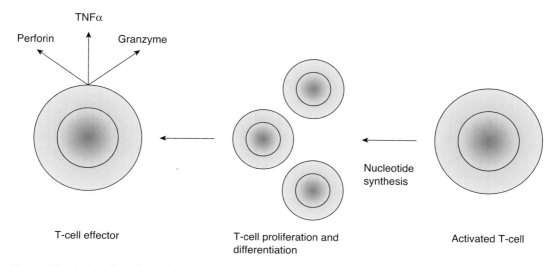

Figure 4.7   Activated T cells need nucleotide synthesis to proliferate and differentiate into T-cell effectors that attack the target cells

Non-alloantigen-dependent pathways

All vertebrates have inborn defense mechanisms that constitute *innate immunity*. Polymorphonuclear cells, complement, natural killer cells, macrophages, and dendritic cells are important components of innate immunity, which is mainly directed towards defense against bacterial attack. Polymorphonuclear cells may produce chemokines (Molesworth-Kenyon *et al.*, 2005) that can activate effector function and T cell proliferation (Segerer and Nelson, 2005). Macrophages and dendritic cells incorporate a set of transmembrane receptors called toll-like receptors (TLR) that identify different types of molecular patterns. Mammals have 12 different TLR, each of which specializes – often with the aid of accessory molecules – in a subset of pathogen-associated molecular pattern. Which TLR it binds to will determine what the response will be. In this way, the TLR identify the nature of the pathogen and turn on an effector response appropriate for dealing with it. These signaling cascades lead to the expression of various cytokine genes. In transplant recipients, the innate immunity may be activated by *viral* or *bacterial infection* as well as by *cell damage*, with the overproduction of reactive oxygen species. TLR bind to TLR4-binding dendritic cells that, in the proinflammatory environment created by activated innate immunity, may mature (Land, 2005). Chemokines and cell adhesion facilitate dendritic and T-cell trafficking between lymph nodes and the transplant. This results in a specific and acquired alloimmune response mediated by T cells. Subsequently, T cells and cells from the innate immune system function synergistically to reject the allograft through non-exclusive pathways, including contact-dependent T cell cytotoxicity, granulocyte activation by either Th1- or Th2-derived cytokines, NK cell activation, alloantibody production, and complement activation (Le Moine *et al.*, 2002). The blockade of individual pathways generally does not prevent allograft rejection, and long-term allograft survival is achieved only after the simultaneous blockade of several of them.

Antibody-mediated humoral rejection

Significant advances in the diagnosis of antibody-mediated graft rejection have led to the re-evaluation of humoral alloreactivity in organ transplantation. Rejection that is caused by antibody is mediated by different mechanisms compared with rejection that is caused by T cells.

Anti-HLA alloantibody

Antibodies against donor alloantigens target the capillary endothelium, but not the arterial endothelium, with *fixation of complement*, resulting in tissue injury and coagulation. Complement activation also recruits macrophages and neutrophils, causing additional endothelial injury, and induces gene expression by endothelial cells, which remodels arteries and basement membranes, leading to fixed and irreversible anatomic lesions that permanently compromise graft function (Colvin and Smith, 2005). The role of complement activation can be demonstrated by the abundant presence in peritubular capillaries of C4d – a terminal component of the complement cascade which persists in graft tissue (Feucht *et al.*, 1991). This finding is today considered a reliable marker of humoral rejection (Mauiyyedi *et al.*, 2001; Regele *et al.*, 2002; Feucht 2003), and has been incorporated in the Banff classification (Racusen *et al.*, 2003). This form of acute humoral rejection most frequently occurs in sensitized patients or in those with a history of previous failed allograft (Moll and Pascual, 2005).

Non-anti-HLA antibodies

The allograft endothelium may also be the target of non-HLA antibodies (Le Bas Bernadet *et al.*, 2003). Dragun *et al.* (2005) reported the absence of anti-HLA antibodies in 16 of 33 transplant patients with vascular rejection and malignant hypertension. Activating IgG antibodies targeting the angiotensin II type 1 receptor (AT1) were detected in sera of these patients. The authors suggested that these antibodies may attack the endothelial cells which have one AT1 receptor and activate a downstream signaling cascade, mimicking the action of angiotensin II and inducing damage to the allograft.

Clinical diagnosis

With improved immunosuppression, acute rejection has become less frequent and severe than in the past. Acute rejection is more frequent in the early post-transplant period but it can occur at any time, particularly when immunosuppressive therapy is changed, or in the case of infection.

The typical presentation of acute rejection is characterized by fever, graft tenderness, oliguria, and proteinuria. However, these findings are not at all specific and are becoming more and more rare after the advent of cyclosporine (CsA) and other powerful immunosuppressants. In clinical practice, acute rejection is suspected whenever there is acute graft dysfunction, which is usually detected by a rapid *increase in plasma creatinine*. How much plasma creatinine should increase for a diagnosis of rejection is still controversial, however. Some clinicians consider diagnostic an absolute increase in plasma creatinine of 0.3 mg/dl or more. Such an approach exposes the patient to the risk of overdiagnosis in the case of elevated basal levels of plasma creatinine. Monitoring the percentage increase in plasma creatinine is probably more accurate. However, a mild increase can give good sensitivity but poor specificity, while a large increase may offer good specificity but poor sensitivity. Considering the elevated coefficient of variability of plasma creatinine, which may also expose the patient to the risk of an incorrect diagnosis, a percentage increase of 30% over baseline may be considered a reasonable compromise (Ponticelli and Campise, 1997). It has to be pointed out, however, that some rejections may show no relevant clinical test or biochemical abnormalities and may be difficult to recognize by renal biopsy (Rush *et al.*, 1999).

Another major problem is that a number of causes other than rejection can produce an increase in plasma creatinine (Table 4.1). *Non-invasive imaging* is helpful in this setting. Radionuclide imaging, ultrasonography, and/or echo color Doppler can detect the presence of lymphocele or urological complications and can give information on the vascularization and viability of the allograft. However, in spite of initial enthusiasm, the value of Doppler imaging for a confirmatory diagnosis of acute rejection is questionable. Neither grading of the vascularity resistance index measurement nor the combination of these methods is an accurate means of detecting rejection (Chow *et al.*, 2001). Power Doppler sonography is superior to duplex Doppler sonography in screening patients with acute parenchymal renal dysfunction post-transplant. However, a normal examination does not exclude the presence of acute rejection (Datta *et al.*, 2005). A number of clinicians feel that while imaging techniques are very important for assessing whether the allograft is viable and for diagnosing urological and/or vascular complications, they provide information little better than that obtained by careful clinical observation for the diagnosis of acute rejection.

Particularly difficult is the diagnosis of acute rejection in patients with *delayed graft function*, as in most cases rejection may be completely silent. As in oligoanuric transplant recipients, silent acute rejection has been found to occur in more than 50% of protocol biopsies; repeat biopsies and early treatment of acute rejection are recommended in the case of prolonged oligoanuria (Qureshi *et al.*, 2002). The differential diagnosis between *acute rejection* and *toxicity* caused by calcineurin inhibitors may be difficult. Some clinical data may orientate the diagnosis (Table 4.2), but in more difficult cases a renal biopsy may be needed. Even difficult can be clinical diagnosis when an increase in plasma creatinine occurs months or years after transplantation. In *late acute rejection* the increase in plasma creatinine is usually slow, and is not associated with other clinical findings, with the possible exception of proteinuria and hypertension. Late acute rejection should be suspected if a patient is poorly compliant or if immunosuppression was reduced days or weeks before the increase in plasma creatinine.

A number of *immunological tests* have been proposed for the early confirmation of acute rejection. However, these tests are either expensive or time-consuming, or have low sensitivity or specificity. It has been reported that urinary levels of perforin mRNA and granzyme B mRNA may predict rejection with a sensitivity of 83% and a specificity of 83% (Li *et al.*, 2001). However, in other studies the expression of these cytotoxic effector molecules in graft biopsies showed considerable variability (Muthukumar *et al.*, 2005; Graziotto *et al.*, 2006). Waiting for simple, cheap, and reproducible tests, most clinicians still base the clinical diagnosis of rejection on the exclusion of other causes of graft dysfunction. An important exception is represented by the search for *circulating antibodies* directed against donor HLA or other endothelial antigens. There is

Table 4.1   Main causes of an acute increase in plasma creatinine after renal transplantation

False results
Laboratory error (double check!)
Drugs (trimethoprim, flucytosine, vitamin C)

Extra-renal causes
Hypovolemia
Lymphocele
Urinary tract obstruction
Urine extravasation
Vascular occlusion
Infection (any site)

Renal damage
Acute rejection
Acute tubular necrosis
Cyclosporine, tacrolimus
Other nephrotoxicity drugs (aminoglycosides, amphotericin B, ciprofloxacin, etc.)
Thrombotic microangiopathy
Recurrence of primary renal disease
Cholesterol embolization
Acute interstitial nephritis
Acute pyelonephritis

Table 4.2   Clinical clues for the differential diagnosis between acute rejection and toxicity of calcineurin inhibitors

	Rejection	Toxicity
Calcineurin inhibitor blood levels	Normal/low	High
C-reactive protein levels	Elevated	Normal
Fever	May be present	Absent
Oliguria	May be present	Absent
Increase in plasma creatinine	Rapid	Slow
Graft palpation	May be enlarged and painful	Normal

evidence that circulating donor-specific antibodies are frequently associated with humoral rejection and can help in distinguishing graft dysfunction due to immunological and non-immunological causes (McKenna *et al.*, 2000). Preformed antibodies against carbohydrates have been described in humoral rejection occurring in ABO-incompatible renal transplants (Holgersson *et al.*, 2005). As pointed out above, *de novo* antibodies directed against AT1 receptors can also be responsible for humoral rejection (Dragun *et al.*, 2005).

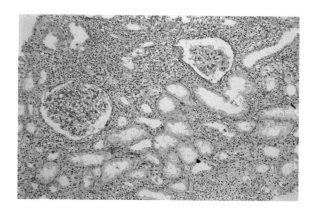

Figure 4.8 Acute cellular rejection. A dense and diffuse infiltrate of mononuclear cells occupies the interstitial space and focally invades tubular structures. (PAS × 160) (Courtesy of Dr G Banfi, Ospedale Maggiore, Milan, Italy)

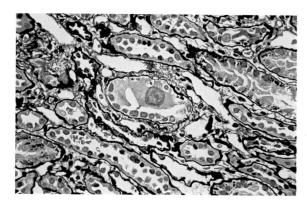

Figure 4.9 Peritubular capillary congestion and focal erythrocyte extravasation into the interstitium may accompany severe cellular rejection. (AFOG × 250) (Courtesy of Dr G Banfi, Ospedale Maggiore, Milan, Italy)

Pathology

Renal biopsy is helpful not only for correct diagnosis but also for assessing the prognosis and establishing the treatment of acute rejection. Obviously, the sample of kidney tissue should be adequate. One artery with endothelialitis is sufficient for the diagnosis of acute rejection, but a portion of cortex with minimal infiltrate does not exclude acute rejection even if many glomeruli are present. Medulla alone is insufficient for a correct diagnosis. Finally, subcapsular specimens, which usually show inflammation and fibrosis, are not useful (Colvin, 1996).

The typical histologic features in acute rejection are a pleiomorphic *interstitial infiltrate* of mononuclear cells (Figure 4.8) associated with interstitial edema, and a variable amount of hemorrhage in the most severe cases (Figure 4.9). The infiltrating cells are mainly represented by T cells. Macrophages are often present, sometimes being predominant. Mononuclear cells invade tubules and insinuate between tubular epithelial cells. This '*tubulitis*' (Figure 4.10) has been regarded a reliable marker of acute rejection (Racusen *et al.*, 1999), although it can be seen even in other forms of acute interstitial nephritis (Colvin, 1996). While the intensity of the interstitial infiltrate has no correlation with the outcome of acute rejection, the presence and the intensity of interstitial hemorrhage and interstitial fibrosis correlate with a poor long-term graft outcome (Banfi *et al.*, 1981; Matas *et al.*, 1983; Visscher *et al.*, 1991). A high density of eosinophils in the infiltrate is rare, but may predict a poor graft outcome (Hongwei *et al.*, 1994).

Endarteritis is another characteristic feature of acute rejection. The infiltration of mononuclear cells under the arteriolar endothelium (*endothelialitis*) is considered to be pathognomonic (Figure 4.11). More

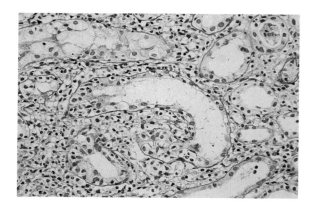

Figure 4.10 Cellular rejection. Some tubular segments show 'tubulitis': several inflammatory mononuclear cells have crossed the tubular basement membrane and lie beneath epithelial cells (arrows). (PAS × 400) (Courtesy of Dr G Banfi, Ospedale Maggiore, Milan, Italy)

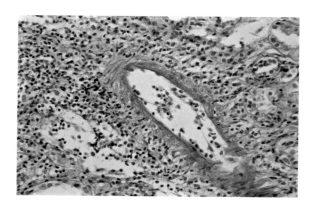

Figure 4.11 Mild endoarteritis ('endothelialitis'). Inflammatory mononuclear cells not only stick to the endothelium but also have penetrated underneath, lifting it up. (PAS × 250) (Courtesy of Dr G Banfi, Ospedale Maggiore, Milan, Italy)

uncertain is the significance of lymphocytes on the surface of the endothelium (Colvin, 1996). However, endothelialitis is seen in only about half the cases of acute rejection. The media of the artery usually shows few changes (Figure 4.12), but in severe cases the cellular infiltration may cause medial necrosis and thrombosis. The response to anti-rejection therapy is related to the severity of intimal arteritis, being relatively good in patients with mild–moderate lesions while being poor in cases with severe arteritis, particularly when associated with severe arteritis (Haas et al., 2002). A more severe vascular lesion is *necrotizing arteritis* (Figure 4.13), which, unlike cellular arteritis, does not show a mononuclear infiltrate within and around the artery. *Thrombotic vasculopathy* may also occur. The prognosis of necrotizing arteritis and of arterial thrombi is severe, although some cases may be reversible.

Glomeruli are usually spared, or show only mild changes in acute rejection. Rarely, an *acute glomerulopathy* may develop, characterized by hypercellularity, injury and enlargement of endothelial cells, and glomerular infiltration of mononuclear cells (Figure 4.14). The prognosis of this form of acute rejection, which in the past was thought to be associated with cytomegalovirus infection, is severe (Richardson et al., 1981).

Several types of classification and categorization of acute rejection have been proposed. The 1997 revised *Banff classification* (Racusen et al., 1999) has generally been used for scoring and classifying rejection in kidney transplant biopsies (Table 4.3). However, this classification does not consider antibody-mediated rejection as a possible component of acute rejection. The recent identification of *peritubular capillary staining with C4d* has led to a modification of the previous schema (Racusen et al., 2004) by renaming the prior categories of rejection using the terms acute/active cellular rejection and antibody-mediated rejection (Table 4.4). In kidney allografts with *humoral rejection*, deposits of C4d are detected

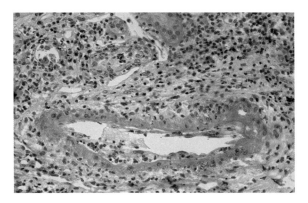

Figure 4.12 Moderate endoarteritis of an interlobular artery. Inflammatory cells infiltrate the subendothelial space and the intima which irregularly proliferates with partial luminal narrowing. Some inflammatory cells are also present in the deeper muscular layer and in the adventitia. (PAS × 250) (Courtesy of Dr G Banfi, Ospedale Maggiore, Milan, Italy)

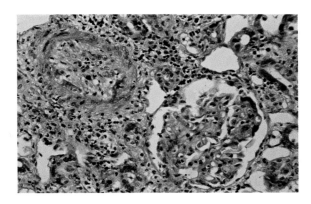

Figure 4.13 Severe endoarteritis. The lumen of an interlobular artery is completely obliterated by a messy myointimal proliferation and by infiltrating inflammatory cells. Lumpy fibrinoid insudates lean upon the lamina elastica which appears focally disrupted (arrow). (PAS × 250) (Courtesy of Dr G Banfi, Ospedale Maggiore, Milan, Italy)

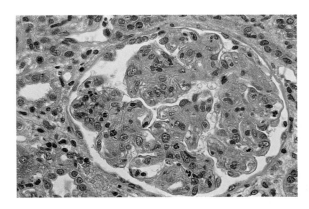

Figure 4.14 Acute transplant glomerulitis. Capillary lumina are severely narrowed by endothelial swelling and infiltrating inflammatory mononuclear cells. Capillary walls appear markedly thickened showing 'double contour' appearance. (Masson trichrome × 400)

in the peritubular capillaries (Figure 4.15). The C4d molecules are located at the luminal surface of peritubular endothelial cells, or between endothelial cells and the luminal surface of peritubular endothelial cells (Regele *et al.*, 2002). Although some authors consider only diffuse capillary C4d staining as a significant clue, focal capillary staining might also be of clinical relevance (Magil and Tinckam, 2006). Certain histologic features may help in diagnosing humoral rejection. All cases of humoral rejection

Table 4.3   Banff 1997 diagnostic categories for renal allograft biopsies: update

1. Normal, see Definitions

2. Antibody-mediated rejection
    Rejection due, at least in part, to documented anti-donor antibody ('suspicious for' if antibody not demonstrated)
    Type (grade)
    I   ATN-like C4d+, minimal inflammation
    II   Capillary margination and/or thromboses, Ig, and/or C4d+
    III   Transmural arteritis and/or arterial fibrinoid change and medial smooth muscle necrosis, Ig, and/or C4d+

3. Bordeline changes: 'Suspicious' for acute cellular rejection
    This category is used when no intimal arteritis is present, but there are foci of mild tubulitis (1–4 mononuclear cells/tubular cross-section) and at least 10–25% of parenchyma inflamed

4. Acute/active cellular rejection

Type (grade)	Histopathological findings
IA	Cases with significant interstitial infiltration (>25% of parenchyma affected) and foci of moderate tubulitis (>4 mononuclear cells/tubular cross-section or group of 10 tubular cells)
IB	Cases with significant interstitial infiltration (>25% of parenchyma affected) and foci of severe tubulitis (>10 mononuclear cells/tubular cross-section or group of 10 tubular cells)
IIA	Cases with mild to moderate intimal arteritis
IIB	Cases with severe intimal arteritis comprising >25% of the luminal area
III	Cases with 'transmural arteritis and/or arterial fibrinoid change and necrosis of medical smooth muscle cells with accompanying inflammation'

5. Chronic/sclerosing allograft nephropathy

Grade	Histopathological findings
Grade I (mild)	Mild interstitial fibrosis and tubular atrophy without (a) or with (b) specific changes suggesting chronic rejection
Grade II (moderate)	Moderate interstitial fibrosis and tubular atrophy (a) or (b)
Grade III (severe)	Severe interstitial fibrosis and tubular atrophy and tubular loss (a) or (b)

6. Other   Changes not considered to be due to rejection

present vascular lesions, type II or more frequently type III according to the Banff classification. Glomerulitis with neutrophils or monocyte infiltration is also suggestive of humoral rejection (Moll and Pascual, 2005). On electron microscopy an intracapillary exudate composed mainly of monocytes can be seen (Liptak *et al.*, 2005).

If renal biopsy remains the more valid tool for correct diagnosis and for therapeutic decision it must be pointed out that there are also limits with this technique (Table 4.5). The *time* of the biopsy (too early a renal biopsy may fail to assess the severity of rejection), the *poor specificity* of some lesions, and the *difficulty of classifying* some acute rejections (a biopsy section may contain hundreds of tubular cross-sections with different severities of infiltration) are the main limits. Moreover, the *grading* of acute rejection relies

Table 4.4   Diagnostic criteria for humoral rejection according to Banff 2003 criteria. From Racusen et al., 2004

C4d deposits in peritubular capillaries
One of the following
    neutrophils in the peritubular capillaries and glomeruli
    arterial fibrinoid necrosis
    acute tubular injury
Circulating donor-specific antibodies

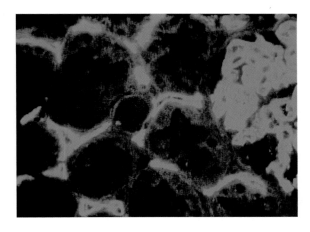

Figure 4.15 Deposits of C4d in peritubular capillaries in a case of humoral rejection

heavily on the presence of arterial vessels. This implies that graft biopsies without representative arteries should be considered inadequate. Finally, there is large *interobserver variation* in interpreting the results of a graft biopsy. Furness and Taub (2001) circulated 55 graft biopsies around pathologists of 22 major European transplant units. For every feature studied, some pathologists consistently under-graded or over-graded. No single feature permitted a reliable diagnosis of acute rejection.

DNA microarray is a microhybridization-based assay that is used to study the expression of thousands of genes. Acute rejections that are indistinguishable on conventional histologic analysis may show extensive differences in gene expression, which are associated with different immunological pattern and clinical course. The presence of dense clusters of B cells in a biopsy sample is strongly associated with severe graft rejection, suggesting a pivotal role of infiltrating B cells in acute rejection (Sarwal *et al.*, 2003). The analysis of gene expression patterns can have a profound impact on the diagnosis, prognosis, and treatment of renal allograft rejection (Zhang and Reed, 2006). However, the technique is expensive, and has not been adopted in routine clinical practice.

In summary, the clinical diagnosis of acute rejection is mainly a diagnosis of exclusion. Renal biopsy is very useful, as it can confirm the diagnosis or discover rejection in asymptomatic patients (Rush *et al.*, 1999). Moreover, the identification of antibody-mediated rejection and the severity of arteritis may help in choosing the type of anti-rejection therapy. Nevertheless, even histology may be misleading in a few cases.

Consequences of acute rejection

The occurrence of acute rejection may have several consequences both in the short and in the long term. At onset, the *severity* of acute rejection may be difficult to assess on clinical grounds. It may be regarded as

Table 4.5   Limits of kidney allograft biopsy in acute rejection

Time
Too early a biopsy may fail to assess the severity
Too late a biopsy does not allow prompt therapeutic intervention

Specificity
Interstitial infiltrate and tubulitis are not specific

Grading
It is difficult to assess the severity of tubulitis as the tubular infiltrate of lymphocytes may vary in different tubular sections
Not all samples contain arterial vessels

Interpretation
Large variations in interpreting the diagnostic and prognostic features among experts

Table 4.6   Prognostic factors for long-term consequences of acute rejection

Reversibility
Complete reversibility of rejection usually has little impact on long-term graft survival

Number
The higher the number of rejections the worse the long-term graft survival

Time
Poor prognosis for late rejections

Histology
Rough correlation between Banff grade of rejection and long-term prognosis
Intimal arteritis often associated with poor prognosis

severe if the peak plasma creatinine level reaches 5 mg/dl or more. It may also be considered severe if it does not reverse after five consecutive intravenous steroid pulses. Renal biopsy may help in assessing the severity. The presence of severe intimal arteritis or transmural arteritis, fibrinoid necrosis, and/or interstitial hemorrhage indicates a more severe prognosis. Severe cases require more aggressive and prolonged treatment. Although a few rejections are irreversible, today most rejections respond to adequate treatment, and the risk of graft failure due to acute rejection has become low (Briganti *et al.*, 2002; Ponticelli *et al.*, 2002). In some cases, however, particularly in anuric patients (Qureshi *et al.*, 2002), diagnosis may be delayed, leading to an incomplete recovery of graft function. In other patients, the heavy immunosuppression used for handling acute rejection may result in infection or other life-threatening complications. To overcome these complications, immunosuppression often has to be reduced or stopped, with consequent damage of the allograft.

Acute rejection can also influence the *long-term outcome* (Table 4.6). Acute rejection has been found to correlate with the risk of chronic rejection (Flechner *et al.*, 1996); the graft half-life has been found to be longer in patients who have never experienced acute rejection (Hariharan *et al.*, 2000). It seems, however, that fully reversible acute rejection does not have a deleterious impact on long-term graft function. An analysis of the Collaborative Transplant Study showed that the 6-year graft survival was significantly lower in patients who needed anti-rejection treatment (60% vs. 75%), but patients with acute rejection whose graft function returned to normal after treatment (serum creatinine lower than 1.5 mg/dl) had a 6-year graft survival only 2% lower than patients without acute rejection (Opelz, 1997). The *number* of rejections can influence the graft outcome. The long-term graft survival is better in patients who have had a single episode of acute rejection than in patients with two or more episodes (Dickenmann *et al.*, 2002; Pascual *et al.*, 2002). The *time* of rejection is also important. Sijpkens *et al.* (2003) reported that the 10-year graft survival censored by death was 86% for patients who rejected within the third post-transplant month and 45% for patients who had an acute rejection after the third month. A significant association between the revised Banff 1997 classification and graft outcome was observed in a number of studies (Mueller *et al.*, 2000; Tanaka *et al.*, 2004; Kaminska *et al.*, 2006). *Intimal arteritis* was the main significant predictor of poor survival probability. *Glomerular monocyte* infiltration has also been found to be an independent variable associated with a poor outcome (Tinckam *et al.*, 2005). Muthukumar *et al.* (2005) found that the urinary mRNA levels for *FOXP3*, a functional marker of T regulatory cells, were inversely correlated with the risk of graft loss at 6 months. These data provide a further marker to predict the prognosis of acute rejection and suggest that the outcome depends on the balance between the activation of T effector cells, which have the function of destroying the graft, and the activation of T regulatory cells, which have a graft-protective function.

Treatment of acute rejection

The three most-used approaches for treating acute rejection are high-dose steroids, antithymocyte globulins (ATG), and OKT3. Each of these treatments may lead to severe complications, and some precautions should be taken to reduce the incidence and severity of side-effects (Table 4.7).

High-dose steroids prevent the release of IL-1 by macrophages, block IL-2-mediated synthesis by T helper cells, and inhibit tumor necrosis factor-α (TNFα) and eicosanoids. These agents may be given orally (100–200 mg/24 h prednisone gradually tapered over 1–3 weeks) or intravenously (0.25–2 g/24 h methylprednisolone (MP) for 3–5 days). Exceptionally, the administration of high-dose MP may cause seizures, anaphylaxis, and even sudden death. These complications are more likely to occur when MP is injected rapidly or through a central venous line. Some patients may suffer from ventricular arrhythmias, others complain of flushing, tremor, or nausea. Hyperglycemia is frequent after MP infusion, and some patients may develop diabetes. Most centers use intravenous MP pulses at a dose of 0.5 g every 24 h for 3–5 days. About 75% of primary acute rejection episodes are reversible after treatment with MP. It should be borne in mind, however, that acute rejection may be associated with tubular lesions that may require as long as 10 days to disappear (Mazzucchi *et al.*, 1999). As a consequence, even serum creatinine returns to previous values slowly. Persisting with the administration of MP pulses in these cases is useless, and may lead to infections or the development of diabetes.

Intravenous ATG lyse circulating T cells and perhaps favor the production of T suppressor cells. The available ATG are purified, pasteurized immunoglobulins obtained by the immunization of rabbits with human thymocytes. ATG have been claimed to be more effective than MP in reversing rejection and in preventing a second episode of acute rejection. The efficacy of ATG depends on the animal source. Rabbit ATG proved to be superior to horse ATG in reversing acute rejection and in preventing recurrent rejection (Gaber *et al.*, 1998). Among the available ATG, thymoglobulins have been shown to protect against recurrent rejection and return to dialysis better than Atgam® (Schnitzler *et al.*, 2000). Treatment with ATG is expensive, may require hospitalization (ATG should be administered in a central vein, needs premedication with MP, and should be infused in at least 4–6 h), and may render the patient more susceptible to viral infection The use of ATG is generally limited to acute rejection episodes that do not respond to steroids, or to episodes with vascular involvement.

The *monoclonal antibody OKT3* blocks the antigen receptor complex CD3 and prevents antigen recognition. It is administered intravenously, usually at a dose of 5 mg/day for 7–14 days. OKT3 is significantly more effective than steroids in reversing the first acute rejection episode, and can also reverse a number

Table 4.7 Some suggestions to reduce the side-effects of anti-rejection treatment

Intravenous methylprednisolone (MP)	ATG	OKT3
Abnormal plasma K$^+$ levels should be corrected before infusion	Premedication with intravenous MP (0.5 g), acetaminophen (650 mg orally) and/or an antihistaminic drug	Hydrosaline excess should be corrected by dialysis or diuretics
MP should be infused in a peripheral vein over 30 min (60 min in an elderly patient)	Infusion using a high-flow vein	Intravenous MP (0.25 g) 6 h and 1 h before OKT3
Patients with pre-existing cardiac lesions should have electrocardiographic monitoring during infusion	Duration of infusion at least 6 h for the first administration 4 h on subsequent days	Infuse the first dose over 2 h
Outpatients should stay in hospital for at least 2 h after MP infusion	Anti-CMV prophylaxis	Infuse half-dose (2.5 mg) for the first injection
Glycemia should be checked in the following days	Treatment should not exceed 7–14 days	Reduce or stop CsA, tacrolimus or MMF during treatment
No more than five consecutive MP pulses should be administered		Anti-CMV prophylaxis
		Limit treatment to 7–14 days

of steroid-resistant acute rejection episodes. The efficacy of OKT3 in reversing rejection seems to be similar to that of rabbit ATG (Mariat et al., 1998). In a study, no significant difference was seen between the two agents in graft survival and in major side-effects even at 10 years (Stippel et al., 2002). The first injection of OKT3 exposes the patient to the so-called cytokine release syndrome (chills, hyperpyrexia, tremor, sudden rise in plasma creatinine), to pulmonary edema in overhydrated patients, and rarely to aseptic meningitis (Hopkins and Jolles, 2005) or vascular thrombosis (Abramowicz et al., 1996). Severe hepatitis has also been reported (Go and Bumgardner, 2002). Before administration of OKT3 several precautions should be taken. Patients with overhydration should be treated with high-dose furosemide or with dialysis in order to avoid the bronchospasm and pulmonary edema that can follow the first injection. Premedication with intravenous MP may be useful in order to reduce the effects of the massive release of cytokines. The dose of MP should not exceed 8 mg/kg, as higher doses could concur with OKT3 in producing a procoagulant effect, with the risk of arterial thrombosis (Abramowicz et al., 1996). A slow infusion of OKT3, over 2 h, has been found to reduce the intensity of cytokine release syndrome (Ten Berge et al., 1996). Nevertheless, a controlled trial did not confirm the beneficial effect of pentoxifyllin (Vincenti et al., 1996) in preventing the side-effects of OKT3. It has also been demonstrated that the use of a half-dose of OKT3 is as effective as the full dose, and may also reduce side-effects (Midtvedt et al., 1996; Machado et al., 2002).

Both ATG and OKT3 can expose the patient to viral infection and to an increased risk of lymphoproliferative disorders (Opelz and Dohler, 2004). Moreover, in patients treated with antilymphocyte antibodies, there is increased mortality in the short and the long term, because of infection and malignancy, respectively (Meier-Kriesche et al., 2002). Thus, whenever antilymphocyte antibodies are used, the duration of treatment should be limited to 7–10 days, maximum 14 days, basic immunosuppression should be reduced, and antiviral agents such as ganciclovir or acyclovir should be administered.

Campath®-1H or alemtuzumab is a humanized monoclonal antibody directed against CD52. It has been used successfully as rescue therapy in a few patients with steroid-resistant rejection, with mild and self-limited side-effects (Csapo et al., 2005). On the other hand, Basu et al. (2005) treated with alemtuzumab 29 steroid-resistant rejections and 11 rejections more severe than the IB Banff classification. Rejection reversed in 25 cases, but a high rate of serious infections (35%) was noted and two patients died.

Intravenous immunoglobulins (0.5 g/kg per day for 7 days) have been shown to be as effetive as OKT3 (5 mg/kg per day for 14 days) in steroid-resistant rejection (Casadei et al., 2001). Also, in patients with ATG-resistant rejection, a course of intravenous immunoglobulins (total 2 g/kg over 2–10 days) could obtain reversal of rejection in most cases (Luke et al., 2001). Their administration also proved to be beneficial in some cases of antibody-mediated rejection (Jordan et al., 2006).

Plasmapheresis or immunoadsorption may remove antibodies produced by B cells. These techniques proved capable of reversing some cases of severe acute humoral rejection (Sayegh and Colvin, 2003). A combination of plasmapheresis and intravenous immunoglobulins proved to be particularly effective in this setting, allowing the rescue of 70–78% of allografts (Ibernon et al., 2005; Lehrich et al., 2005).

References

Abramowicz D, De Pauw L, Le Moine A, et al. Prevention of OKT3 nephrotoxicity after kidney transplantation. Kidney Int 1996; 49 (Suppl 53): S39–43.

Banfi G, Imbasciati E, Tarantino A, Ponticelli C. Prognostic value of renal biopsy in acute rejection of kidney transplantation. Nephron 1981; 28: 222–6.

Basu A, Ramkumar M, Tan HP, et al. Reversal of acute cellular rejection after renal transplantation with Campath-1H. Transplant Proc 2005; 37: 923–6.

Briganti EM, Russ GR, McNeil JJ, et al. Risk of renal allograft loss from recurrent glomerulonephritis. N Engl J Med 2002; 347: 103–9.

Casadei DH, del C Rial M, Opelz G, et al. A randomized and prospective study comparing treatment with high-dose intravenous immunoglobulin with monoclonal antibodies for rescue of kidney grafts with steroid-resistant rejection. Transplantation 2001; 71: 53–9.

Chow L, Sommer FG, Huang J, Li KC. Power Doppler imaging and resistance index measurement in the evaluation of acute renal transplant rejection. J Clin Ultrasound 2001; 29: 483–90.

Cole J, Wortley A, Stoves J, Clark B. Laboratory investigations following an unexpectedly positive crossmatch result in a patient awaiting renal transplantation. J Clin Pathol 2002; 55: 627–8.

Colvin RB. The renal allograft biopsy. Kidney Int 1996; 50: 1069–82.

Colvin RB, Smith RN. Antibody-mediated organ-allograft rejection. Nat Rev Immunol 2005; 5: 807–17.

Csapo Z, Benavides-Viveros C, Podder H, et al. Campath-1H as rescue therapy for the treatment of acute rejection in kidney transplant patients. Transplant Proc 2005; 37: 2032–6.

Datta R, Sandhu M, Saxena AK, et al. Role of duplex Doppler and power Doppler sonography in transplanted kidneys with acute renal parenchymal dysfunction. Australas Radiol 2005; 49: 15–20.

Dickenmann MJ, Nikeleit V, Tsinalis D, et al. Why do kidney grafts fail? A long-term single center eperience. Transpl Int 2002; 15: 508–14.

Dragun D, Muller DN, Brasen JH, et al. Angiotensin II type 1 receptor activating antibodies in renal allograft rejection. N Engl J Med 2005; 352: 558–69.

Feucht HE, Felber E, Gokel MJ, et al. Vascular deposition of complement-split products in kidney allografts with cell-mediated rejection. Clin Exp Immunol 1991; 86: 464–70.

Feucht HE. Complement C4d in graft capillaries – the missing link in the recognition of humoral alloreactivity. Am J Transplant 2003; 3: 646–52.

Flechner SM, Modlin CS, Serrano DP, et al. Determinants of chronic renal allograft rejection in cyclosporine-treated recipients. Transplantation 1996; 62: 1235–41.

Furness P, Taub N. International transplant biopsies: report of CERTPAP project. Kidney Int 2001; 60: 1998–2012.

Gaber AO, First MR, Tesi R, et al. Results of the double-blind, randomized, multicenter, phase III clinical trial of thymoglobulin versus ATGAM in the treatment of acute graft rejection episodes after renal transplantation. Transplantation 1998; 66: 29–37.

Glotz D, Antoine C, Julia P, et al. Desensitization and subsequent kidney transplantation of patients using intravenous immunoglobulins. Am J Transplant 2002; 2: 758–60.

Go MR, Bumgardner GL. OKT3 (muromonab CD3) associated hepatitis in a kidney transplant recipient. Transplantation 2002; 73: 1957–9.

Graziotto R, Del Prete D, Rigotti P, et al. Perforin, granzyme B, and fas ligand for molecular diagnosis of acute renal-allograft rejection: analyses on serial biopsies suggest methodological issues. Transplantation 2006; 81: 1125–32.

Haas M, Kraus ES, Samaniego-Picota M, et al. Acute renal failure allograft rejection with intimal arteritis: histologic predictors of response to therapy and graft survival. Kidney Int 2002; 61: 1516–26.

Halloran PF. Immunosuppressive drugs for kidney transplantation. N Engl J Med 2004; 351: 2715–29.

Hariharan S, Johnson CP, Bresnahan BA, et al. Improved graft survival after renal transplantation in the United States. N Engl J Med 2000; 342: 605–12.

Hickstein H, Korten G, Bast R, et al. Immunoadsorption of sensitized kidney transplant candidates immediately prior to surgery. Clin Transplant 2002; 16: 97–101.

Higgins RM, Bevan DJ, Carey BS, et al. Prevention of hyperacute rejection by removal of antibodies to HLA immediately before renal transplantation. Lancet 1996; 2: 1208–11.

Holgersson J, Gustafsson A, Breimer ME. Characteristics of protein–carbohydrate interactions as a basis for developing novel carbohydrate-based antirejection therapies. Immunol Cell Biol 2005; 83: 694–708.

Hongwei W, Nanra RS, Stein A, et al. Eosinophils in acute renal allograft rejection.Transpl Immunol 1994; 12: 41–6.

Hopkins S, Jolles S. Drug-induced aseptic meningitis. Expert Opin Drug Saf 2005; 4: 285–97.

Ibernon M, Gil-Vernet S, Carrera M, et al. Therapy with plasmapheresis and intravenous immunoglobulin for acute humoral rejection in kidney transplantation. Transplant Proc 2005; 37: 3743–5.

Kahan BD, Stepkowski SM. Immunobiology of allograft rejection. In Kahan BD, Ponticelli C, eds. Principle and Practice of Renal Transplantation. London: Martin Dunitz, 2000: 41–87.

Kaminska D, Bernat B, Mazanowska O, et al. Predictive value of Banff score of early kidney allograft biopsies for 1-year graft survival. Transplant Proc 2006; 38: 59–61.

Jordan SC, Vo AA, Peng A, et al. Intravenous gammaglobulin (IVIG): a novel approach to improve transplant rates and outcomes in highly HLA-sensitized patients. Am J Transplant 2006; 6: 459–66.

Land W. The role of postischemic reperfusion injury and other nonantigen-dependent inflammatory pathways in transplantation. Transplantation 2005; 79: 505–14.

Le Bas Bernadet S, Hourmant M, Coupel S, et al. Non HLA-type endothelial cell reactive alloantibodies in pre-transplant sera of kidney recipients trigger apoptosis. Am J Transplant 2003; 3: 167–77.

Le Moine A, Goldman M, Abramowicz D. Multiple pathways to allograft rejection. Transplantation 2002; 73: 1373–81.

Lehrich RW, Rocha PN, Reinsmoen N, et al. Intravenous immunoglobulin and plasmapheresis in acute humoral rejection: experience in renal allograft transplantation. Hum Immunol 2005; 66: 350–8.

Li B, Hartono C, Ding R, et al. Renal allograft surveillance by mRNA profiling of urinary cells. Transplant Proc 2001; 33: 3280–2.

Liptak P, Kemeny E, Morvay Z, et al. Peritubular capillary damage in acute humoral rejection: an ultrastructural study on human renal allografts. Am J Transplant 2005; 5: 2870–6.

Luke PPW, Scantlebury VP, Jordan ML, et al. Reversal of steroid- and antilymphocyte antibody-resistant rejection using intravenous immunoglobulin (IVIG) in renal transplant recipients. Transplantation 2001; 72: 419–22.

Machado PG, Tedesco HS, Silva RG, et al. Use of reduced dose of OKT3 (2.5 mg) after renal transplantation. Transplant Proc 2002; 34: 104.

Magil AB, Tinckam KJ. Focal peritubular capillary C4d deposition in acute rejection. Nephrol Dial Transplant 2006; 21: 1382–8.

Mannami M, Mitsuhata N. Improved outcomes after ABO-incompatible living-donor kidney transplantation after 4 weeks of treatment with mycophenolate mofetil. Transplantation 2005; 79: 1756–8.

Mariat C, Alamartine E, Dial N, et al. A randomised prospective study comparing low-dose OKT3 to low-dose ATG for the treatment of acute steroid-resistant episodes in kidney transplant recipients. Transpl Int 1988; 11: 231–6.

Matas AJ, Sibley R, Mauer M, et al. The value of needle renal allograft biopsy. I. A retrospective study of biopsies performed during rejection episodes. Ann Surg 1983; 197: 226–37.

Mauiyyedi S, Pelle PD, Saidman S, et al. Chronic humoral rejection. Identification of antibody-mediated chronic allograft rejection by C4d deposits in peritubular capillaries. J Am Soc Nephrol 2001; 12: 574–82.

Mazzucchi E, Lucon AM, Nahas WC, et al. Histological outcome of acute cellular rejection in kidney transplantation after treatment with methylprednisolone. Transplantation 1999; 67: 430–4.

McKenna RM, Takemoto SK, Terasaki PI. Anti-HLA antibodies after solid organ transplantation. Transplantation 2000; 69: 319–26.

Meier-Kriesche HU, Arndorfer JA, Kaplan B. Association of antibody induction with short- and long-term cause-specific mortality in renal transplant recipients. J Am Soc Nephrol 2002; 13: 769–72.

Midtvedt K, Tafjord AB, Hartmann A, et al. Half dose of OKT3 is efficient in treatment of steroid-resistant renal allograft rejection. Transplantation 1996; 62: 38–42.

Molesworth-Kenyon SJ, Oakes JE, Lausch RN. A novel role for neutrophils as a source of T cell-recruiting chemokines IP-10 and Mig during the DTH response to HSV-1 antigen. J Leukoc Biol 2005; 77: 552–9.

Moll S, Pascual M. Humoral rejection of organ allografts. Am J Transplant 2005; 5: 2611–15.

Mueller A, Schnuelle P, Walherr R, van der Woude FJ. Impact of the Banff '97 classification for histological diagnosis of rejection on clinical outcome and renal function parameters after kidney transplantation. Transplantation 2000; 69: 1123–7.

Muthukumar T, Dadhania D, Ding R, et al. Messenger RNA for FOXP3 in the urine of renal-allograft recipients. N Engl J Med 2005; 353: 2342–51.

Opelz G, for the Collaborative Transplant Study. Critical evaluation of the association of acute with chronic graft rejection in kidney and heart transplant recipients. Transplant Proc 1997; 29: 73–6.

Opelz G, Dohler B. Lymphomas after solid organ transplantation: a collaborative transplant study report. Am J Transplant 2004; 4: 222–30.

Pascual M, Theruvath T, Kawai T, et al. Strategies to improve long-term outcomes after renal transplantation. N Engl J Med 2002; 346: 580–90.

Ponticelli C. The pleiotropic effects of mTor inhibitors. J Nephrol 2004; 17: 762–6.

Ponticelli C, Campise M. Appropriate endpoints for renal transplantation. Drug Inform J 1997; 31: 207–12.

Ponticelli C, Villa M, Cesana B, et al. Risk factors for late kidney allograft failure. Kidney Int 2002; 62: 1848–54.

Qureshi F, Rabb H, Kasiske BL. Silent acute rejection during prolonged delayed graft function reduces kidney allograft survival. Transplantation 2002; 74: 1400–4.

Racusen LC, Solez K, Colvin RB. The Banff 97 working classification of renal allograft pathology. Kidney Int 1999; 55: 713–23.

Racusen LC, Colvin RB, Solez K, et al. Antibody-mediated rejection criteria. An addition to the Banff '97 classification of renal allograft rejection. Am J Transplant 2003; 3: 708–14.

Racusen LC, Halloran PF, Solez K. Banff 2003 meeting report: new diagnostic insights and standards. Am J Transplant 2004; 4: 1562–6.

Regele H, Bohmig GA, Habicht A, et al. Capillary deposition of complement split product C4d in renal allograft is associated with basement membrane injury in peritubular and glomerular capillaries: a contribution of humoral immunity to chronic allograft rejection. J Am Soc Nephrol 2002; 13: 2371–80.

Richardson WP, Colvin RB, Cheeseman SH, et al. Glomerulopathy associated with cytomegalovirus viremia in renal allografts. N Engl J Med 1981; 305: 57–62.

Robertson H, Kirby JA. Renal allograft rejection: the development and function of tubulitis. Transplant Rev 2001; 15: 109–28.

Rush D, Grimm P, Jeffrey J, et al. Predicting rejection. Graft 1999; 2 (Suppl 2): S31–5.

Sarwal M, Chua MS, Kambham N, et al. Molecular heterogeneity in acute renal allograft rejection identified by DNA microarray profiling. N Engl J Med 2003; 349: 125–38.

Sayegh MH, Colvin RB. Case records of the Massachusetts General Hospital. N Engl J Med 2003; 348: 1033–44.

Schnitzler MA, Woodward RS, Lowell JA, et al. Economics of the antithymocyte globulins thymoglobulin and Atgam in the treatment of acute renal transplant rejection. Pharmacoeconomics 2000; 17: 287–93.

Segerer S, Nelson PJ. Chemokines in renal diseases. Sci World J 2005; 5: 835–44.

Segev DL, Simpkins CE, Warren DS, et al. ABO incompatible high-titer renal transplantation without splenectomy or anti-CD20 treatment. Am J Transplant 2005; 5: 2570–5.

Shimmura H, Tanabe K, Ishikawa N, et al. Role of anti-A/B antibody titers in results of ABO-incompatible kidney transplantation. Transplantation 2000; 70: 1331–5.

Shimmura H, Tanabe K, Ishida H, et al. Lack of correlation between results of ABO-incompatible living kidney transplantation and anti-ABO blood type antibody titers under our current immunosuppression. Transplantation 2005; 80: 985–8.

Sijpkens YW, Doxiadis JJ, Mallat MJ, et al. Early versus late acute rejection episodes in renal transplantation. Transplantation 2003; 75: 204–8.

Stippel DL, Arns W, Pollak M, et al. ALG versus OKT3 for treatment of steroid-resistant rejection in renal transplantation. Ten year follow-up results of a randomized trial. Transplant Proc 2002; 34: 2201–2.

Tanaka T, Kyo M, Kokado Y, et al. Correlation between the Banff '97 classification of renal allograft biopsies and clinical outcome. Transpl Int 2004; 17: 59–64.

Ten Berge RJM, Buysmann S, van Diepen FNJ, et al. Consequence of OKT3 administration via continuous infusion as compared to bolus infusion. Transplant Proc 1996; 28: 3217–20.

Tinckam KJ, Djurdjev O, Magil AB. Glomerular monocytes predict worse outcomes after acute renal allograft rejection independent of C4d status. Kidney Int 2005; 68: 1866–74.

Tyden G, Kumlien G, Genberg H, et al. ABO-incompatible kidney transplantation and rituximab. Transplant Proc 2005; 37: 3286–7.

Vincenti F, Danovich GM, Neylan JF, et al. Pentoxifylline does not prevent cytokine induced first dose reaction following OKT3: a randomized double-blind placebo-controlled study. Transplantation 1996; 61: 573–7.

Visscher D, Carey I, Oh H, et al. Histologic and immunophenotypic evaluation of pre-treatment renal biopsies in OKT3-treated allograft rejections. Transplantation 1991; 51: 1023–8.

Von Andrian UH, MacKay CR. T-cell function and migration: two sides of the same coin. N Engl J Med 2000; 343: 1020–34.

Zhang O, Reed EF. Array-based methods for diagnosis and prevention of transplant rejection. Expert Rev Mol Diagn 2006; 6: 165–78.

5 CHRONIC ALLOGRAFT NEPHROPATHY

In the past few years there has been a tremendous improvement in short-term renal allograft survival, but no corresponding improvement in the long-term results (Meier-Kriesche *et al.*, 2004). The main cause of late graft failure is represented by the development of progressive graft dysfunction, eventually leading to graft loss. Renal biopsy usually shows fibrosing changes which may be caused by chronic rejection as well as by a number of non-immunological factors. Since these conditions are difficult to differentiate morphologically, the term *chronic allograft nephropathy* (CAN) has been adopted to indicate progressive graft dysfunction associated with fibrosing changes (Racusen *et al.*, 1999).

Clinical diagnosis

Clinically, CAN is characterized by a slowly progressive increase in serum creatinine, often associated with proteinuria and hypertension. Proteinuria commonly ranges from 0.4 to 2 g/day, but nephrotic proteinuria can be observed in the presence of transplant glomerulopathy (Banfi *et al.*, 2005).

CAN may be diagnosed only in the absence of other identifiable complications responsible for late and progressive allograft dysfunction (Table 5.1). To rule out urological or vascular disorders, ultrasonography and echo color Doppler are useful. With the novel parameter tissue perfusion index, differences between compromised and well-functioning transplants and significant changes of transplant perfusion at various points of the post-transplantation time-scale may be seen (Scholbach *et al.*, 2006). This may allow prompt detection of a defect in renal perfusion, but a graft biopsy is often required to rule out causes of late renal dysfunction other than CAN. Even with biopsy, however, the differential diagnosis between immunological and non-immunological causes of CAN, in particular between rejection and nephrotoxicity caused by calcineurin inhibitors (CNI), is difficult.

Predictors of outcome

Attempts have been made to predict as early as possible whether a patient will progress to end-stage renal failure, and the rate of progression. Kasiske *et al.* (2002a) found that a decrease in the level of inverse serum creatinine less than 30% is an excellent predictor of graft failure. Salvadori *et al.* (2006) found that glomerular filtration rate (GFR) at 1 year is the most relevant predictor of graft function at 5 years. Hariharan *et al.* (2003) proposed combining graft function at 1 year with the chronicity Banff score as a composite end-point for renal transplant outcome. A renal resistance index of 80 or higher measured by echo Doppler at least 3 months after transplantation has also been found to be associated with a poor graft outcome (Radermacher *et al.*, 2003), but others found that the resistance index was less predictive than serum creatinine (de Vries *et al.*, 2006). The concomitant development or worsening of proteinuria (Arias *et al.*, 2005) and hypertension (Opelz and Dohler, 2005) is also a prognostic indicator for graft failure.

Pathology

Histologically, CAN is characterized by interstitial fibrosis, tubular atrophy, glomerular sclerosis, and vascular obliteration. Both alloantigen-dependent and alloantigen-independent stimuli may cause mononuclear inflammation. The inflammation primarily involves the interstitium, with consequent peritubular capillary ischemia, *tubular atrophy*, and *fibrosis* (Racusen *et al.*, 2002). It is likely that the process of fibrosis follows different steps, including cell activation, a fibrogenic signaling phase, a fibrogenic phase, and eventually

Table 5.1   Possible causes of late kidney allograft dysfunction other than chronic allograft nephropathy

Renal artery stenosis
Ureteral obstruction
BK virus nephropathy
Late acute rejection
De novo glomerular disease
Recurrent glomerulonephritis
Recurrent vasculitis
Recurrent diabetic nephropathy
Interstitial nephritis
Cholesterol embolization
Thrombotic microangiopathy

Table 5.2   Banff classification of the severity of chronic allograft nephropathy. The severity of glomerular, mesangial matrix, and vascular changes is not integrated in the grading system. From Racusen et al., 1999

Grade I	Mild fibrosis of the interstitium (6–25% of the cortical area)
	Mild atrophy of the tubules (≤25% of tubules in the cortical area)
Grade II	Moderate interstitial fibrosis (26–50% of the cortical area)
	Moderate tubular atrophy (26–50% of tubules in the cortical area)
Grade III	Severe interstitial fibrosis (>50% of the cortical area)
	Severe tubular atrophy (>50% of tubules in the cortical area)

the obliteration of tubules and capillaries (Eddy, 2001). The Banff conference (Racusen *et al.*, 1999) proposed grading the severity of chronic allograft nephropathy on the basis of the extent of interstitial fibrosis and tubular atrophy, without integrating in the grading system the severity of glomerular and vascular changes (Table 5.2). Many efforts have been made to determine whether chronic rejection causes specific lesions. Attention has mainly focused on vascular, glomerular, and, more recently, peritubular capillary changes.

Arterial changes associated with chronic rejection are characterized by intimal proliferation and thickening, with intimal lymphocytes, and splintering and disruption of the elastica, with formation of neomedia and neointima (Mihatsch *et al.*, 1999). The lesions of chronic vascular rejection evolve at varying rates. The earlier lesion, called *endothelialitis,* may consist of subendothelial inflammation, with little intimal thickening (Figure 5.1). This lesion may lead at a later stage to pronounced intimal thickening, calcification, and cholesterol clefts, with or without subendothelial inflammation (Figure 5.2), until complete occlusive vasculopathy (Figure 5.3). However, while most patients with chronic rejection show arteriopathy with fibrointimal hyperplasia, in about a quarter of cases it is impossible to classify the nature of CAN because of the absence of adequate vessels in the biopsy sample (Cosio *et al.*, 1999).

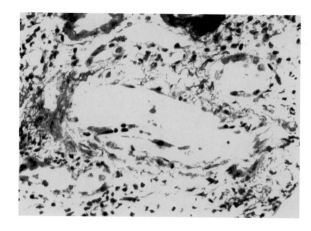

Figure 5.1 Endothelialitis: infiltration of mononuclear cells under the endothelium (Courtesy of Dr G Banfi, Ospedale Maggiore, Milan, Italy)

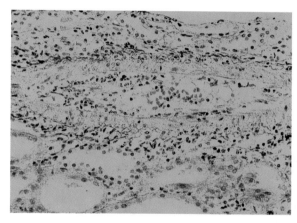

Figure 5.2 Intimal proliferation with subocclusion of vascular lumen (Courtesy of Dr G Banfi, Ospedale Maggiore, Milan, Italy)

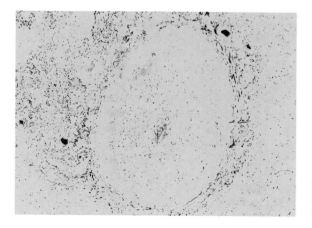

Figure 5.3 Severe occlusive vasculopathy (Courtesy of Dr G Banfi, Ospedale Maggiore, Milan, Italy)

About 5–6% of renal transplant recipients (Banfi *et al.*, 2005) may show a peculiar pattern of glomerular changes called *allograft glomerulopathy* (AGP), which is considered an expression of chronic rejection. The histologic picture of AGP is different from that of recurrent or *de novo* glomerulonephritis. Three stages of AGP lesions have been recognized (Richardson *et al.*, 1981; Maryniak *et al.*, 1985;

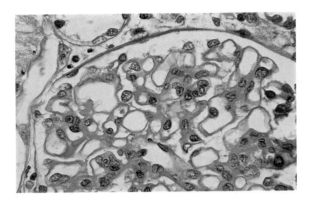

Figure 5.4 Chronic allograft glomerulopathy (initial phase). A slight but diffuse thickening of the capilliary walls gives to the glomerulus a 'membranous nephropathy-like' appearance. (PAS × 400) (Courtesy of Dr G Banfi, Ospedale Maggiore, Milan, Italy)

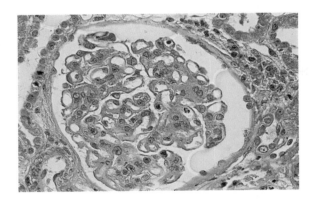

Figure 5.5 Chronic allograft glomerulopathy (advanced phase). Capillary walls show severe thickening and 'double contour' appearance. Cellular component is preserved while mesangial matrix is irregularly and moderately expanded. (Masson trichrome × 400) (Courtesy of Dr G Banfi, Ospedale Maggiore, Milan, Italy)

Habib and Broyer, 1993). The *early stage* has been described in biopsy specimens obtained 8–83 days after transplantation. It is characterized by the swelling of endothelial and mesangial cells which, together with the presence of monocyte–macrophages in the mesangial areas, results in a diminished patency of the capillary lumina. On electron microscopy endothelial cells show abundant cytoplasm, and capillary lumina are occluded or significantly reduced. The glomerular basement membrane (GBM) is not affected, or may show a slight and diffuse thickening, giving a 'membranous nephropathy-like' aspect (Figure 5.4). The *intermediate stage* is characterized by enlarged glomeruli, mesangiolysis, and glomerular capillary enlargement with microaneurysm formation. GBM may occasionally show partial reduplication (Figure 5.5). A spongy appearance of the expanded mesangial zone can be seen. In the *advanced stage* there is a prominent reduplication of GBM with vacuolization and reticulation. Electron microscopy shows a widening of the subendothelial zone associated with electron-lucent thickening of the lamina rara interna (Figure 5.6), which may contain inclusions of cytoplasmic organelles, remnants of erythrocytes, and mesangial interposition. In advanced stages a thin membrane similar to lamina densa appears in the subendothelial space. Immunofluorescence is usually negative or may show non-specific IgM deposits.

Peritubular capillaries may show, on electron microscopy, features consistent with the splitting and multilayered duplication of the basement membranes (Figure 5.7). These changes, analogous to those seen in the glomerular capillaries of transplant glomerulopathy, have been considered typical of chronic rejection by some investigators (Monga et al., 1992; Drachenberg et al., 1997). An important clue for the diagnosis of chronic rejection is the peritubular staining for C4d in frozen tissue, a finding which is now considered sensitive and specific for antibody-mediated rejection (Mauiyyedi et al., 2001; Regele et al., 2002).

The main limitation of graft biopsy in patients with CAN is represented by the lack of specificity of the histologic features. In most cases of CAN there are fibrotic changes that may be caused either by nephrotoxic

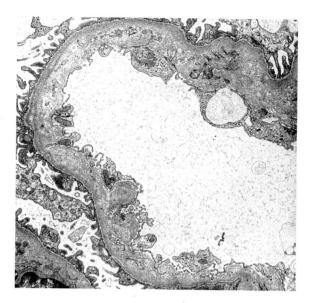

Figure 5.6 At electron microscopy chronic allograft glomerulopathy is characterized by a progressive widening of the lamina rara interna without cellular interposition and/or protein deposits. ($\times$ 6800)

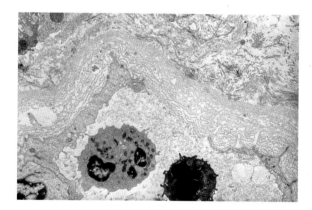

Figure 5.7 A peritubular capillary wall shows splitting of the basement membrane in multiple layers. ($\times$ 14000. By courtesy of Professor G Mazzucco, University of Turin, Italy)

drugs, such as calcineurin inhibitors, or by ongoing chronic rejection. However, the use of immunohistology and electron microscopy may shed some light. It is reasonable to think that the presence of C4d deposits in the peritubular capillaries indicates an antibody-mediated immunological activity; AGP also indicates an immunological origin; while the absence of C4d staining and/or AGP may indicate the prevalence of non-immunological mechanisms in the etiopathogenesis of CAN. A possible biomarker for CNI nephrotoxicity is the tissue factor, the promoter of coagulation. Its staining in the tubular brush border was found to be significantly higher in transplanted kidneys with acute cyclosporine nephrotoxicity than in normal kidneys or in those with acute rejection (Osterholm *et al.*, 2005).

Risk factors

Even if alloantigen-dependent mechanisms probably play a major role in initiating chronic rejection and late graft failure, there is evidence that both immune-mediated and non-immune mechanisms may contribute to the development and progression of chronic allograft nephropathy (Table 5.3). For the sake of clarity we consider immune and non-immune factors separately, although there is often an interaction between them.

Table 5.3 Factors involved in the etiopathogenesis of chronic allograft nephropathy

Alloantigen-dependent	Alloantigen-independent
HLA match	Donor age
Anti-HLA antibodies	Donor comorbidity
Subclinical rejection	Donor source
Acute rejection	Recipient age
Under-immunosuppression	Ischemia–reperfusion
Poor compliance	Body mass index
Variable bioavailability	Viral infections
CXCL10 serum levels	Hyperlipidemia
High serum CD30 levels	Hypertension

Table 5.4 Impact of type of acute rejection on long-term allograft outcome

	Prognosis	
	Good	Poor
Reversibility	Complete	Partial
Number	One	Two or more
Histology	Banff I, IIa	Banff IIb–III
C4d deposits	Negative	Positive
Time of onset	<3 months post-transplant	>3 months post-transplant

Immune-mediated factors

Immune-mediated factors might favor a continuous low-level host immune response to alloantigens expressed by the allograft. The importance of alloantigen-dependent factors is supported by several pieces of evidence.

HLA compatibility

Although the impact of HLA compatibility is decreasing under the influence of modern immunosuppression, nevertheless the analysis of large registries based on tens of thousands of transplants has shown a stepwise decrease in graft survival rate and in graft half-life as the number of HLA mismatches increases (Feucht and Opelz, 1996; Cecka, 2000), probably because HLA incompatibility triggers a continuous, subclinical, immunological aggression against the allograft.

Previous rejection

Acute rejection has been recognized as one of the most important risk factors for chronic rejection (Hariharan *et al.*, 2000). The long-term impact of chronic rejection may depend on a number of factors

(Table 5.4; see also Chapter 4). By reviewing data of the Collaborative Transplant Study, Opelz (1997) showed that patients with rejection had a worse outcome than those who did not have rejection. However, 'rejecting' patients who showed complete reversal of renal function after rejection had a similar 5-year graft survival to that of non-rejecting patients. Mueller et al. (2000) found that the more severe was the histologic picture of rejection, the poorer was the long-term graft survival. Recent reports have pointed out that severe tubulitis may have an unfavorable outcome, approaching that seen in cases of mild intimal arteritis (Minervini et al., 2000; Robertson and Kirby, 2001). Humoral antibody-mediated rejection has the poorest prognosis not only in the short term but also in the long term (Moll and Pascual, 2005). Also, the time of acute rejection has a prognostic importance. Sijpkens et al. (2003) found that the 10-year death-censored graft survival was 84% for patients who had rejection within the third month versus 45% for those who rejected later. The mechanisms by which acute rejection causes progressive damage may be different. An irreversible loss of nephrons may be followed by glomerular hyperfiltration and hypertension that trigger a vicious circle eventually leading to graft failure. On the other hand, tubular epithelial cells damaged by T cell infiltration may produce IL-15, which can support the long-term survival of a donor-specific memory-like population of CD8+, thus promoting tubulointerstitial changes including fibrosis and, in the long term, chronic graft dysfunction (Robertson and Kirby, 2001). The endothelial damage, coupled with factors of progression such as hypertension, diabetes, CMV infection, etc., may eventually lead to occlusive vasculopathy.

Subclinical rejection has been postulated to be responsible for CAN (Rush et al., 2004), and is an independent predictor of poor graft survival when associated with CAN (Moreso et al., 2006).

Circulating antibodies

The deleterious long-term impact of cytotoxic anti-HLA antibodies developed after transplantation is another factor supporting immunological involvement in chronic rejection (Abe et al., 1997; Lee et al., 2002; Terasaki and Ozawa 2005). The presence of C4d in peritubular capillaries of biopsies from patients with CAN, which is now considered an expression of a previous attack from antibodies leading to complement activation, supports the role of humoral immunity at least in some patients (Mauiyyedi et al., 2001).

Immunosuppression

The role of immunosuppressive therapy has also been investigated. Two randomized trials showed a significantly higher 10-year graft survival in patients assigned to receive cyclosporine (CsA) than in those assigned to receive azathioprine (Beveridge and Calne, 1995; Ponticelli et al., 1996). Neoral® and tacrolimus allowed better long-term graft survival than did the old formulation of CsA (Meier-Kriesche and Kaplan, 2002), while the addition of mycophenolate mofetil (MMF) reduced the incidence of early (Halloran et al., 1997) and late rejection (Meier-Kriesche et al., 2003). On the other hand, the withdrawal of MMF may be followed by the development of late C4d-positive humoral rejection (Sun et al., 2005). The variable bioavailability of oral CsA also correlates with chronic rejection (Kahan et al., 1996; Stoves and Newstead, 2002).

Compliance

Poor compliance is an underrated cause of graft failure. It is not easy to determine the true rate of poor compliance by interviewing the patient. In a meta-analysis of the available studies, Butler et al. (2004) found that a median of 22% of transplant recipients were non-adherent to medical prescriptions, and a median of 35% of graft failures occurred in patients with poor compliance. The odds of graft failure increased seven-fold in non-adherent subjects compared with adherent subjects. Some patients are at particular risk of non-compliance (Table 5.5).

Immune reactivity

We still do not have good markers of immune reactivity. However, preliminary data indicate that some markers might be useful in predicting the risk of rejection after transplantation. Pre-transplant patients with a high serum content of CD30, a marker for the activation state of the Th2-type cytokine-producing

Table 5.5 Patients at risk of poor compliance
The more complex the treatment the lower the compliance
Adolescents
Patients with poor compliance to dialysis
Patients with esthetic disfiguration
Patients with social isolation

T cell, showed more rejections and more long-term graft failures than patients with low serum CD30 levels (Susal et al., 2002). However, a good HLA match may neutralize the deleterious effect of high pre-transplant serum CD30 levels (Matinlauri et al., 2005). Also, pre-transplant serum levels of the chemokine *CXCL10* greater than 150 pg/ml confer an increased risk of early, severe acute rejection and subsequent CAN, finally resulting in renal allograft failure (Lazzeri et al., 2005). These data support a major role for immune-mediated mechanisms in the development of chronic rejection.

Non-immune mechanisms

Alloantigen-independent mechanisms may cause a number of injuries that could increase the risk of late renal allograft failure. The most important factors are probably older age of the donor, delayed graft function after transplantation, the source of the donor, and recipient-related factors.

Donor age

Older age is considered to be one of the strongest predictors of poor long-term survival. By reviewing the UNOS data, Cecka (2000) reported that donor age over 55 years reduced the 3-year cadaveric renal graft survival from 78 to 65%. The deleterious effect of age may be attributed to a number of factors. It is well known that glomerular filtration rate and renal function reserve tend to decrease with age, although at least one-third of older subjects maintain normal renal function over time (Macias-Nunez and Cameron, 2005). The phenomenon of *replicative senescence* increases with age. Normal somatic cells have a finite replicative capacity. With each cell division the telomere (end of the linear chromosome) shortens, until a critical length is reached at which it enters clonal exhaustion, or replicative senescence. It has been hypothesized that the development of CAN may be related to replicative senescence (Halloran et al., 1999). Supporting this hypothesis, a strong association between replicative senescence markers and CAN has been found in some studies (Ferlicot et al., 2003; Joosten et al., 2004). Moreover, the older kidney is more *vulnerable* to injury. Thus, it is particularly susceptible to damage caused by delayed graft function and by calcineurin inhibitors (Feutren and Mihatsch, 1992).

Comorbidity

Comorbidity in the donor can also influence the outcome of the allograft. Most donors die from cerebrovascular events, which are frequently caused by underlying hypertension, diabetes, and/or atherosclerosis that may also involve the kidney (Gourishankar et al., 2002). The effect of donor hypertension or diabetes is not evident in the short term, but the 3-year graft survival is diminished in renal transplants from donors with these diseases (Ojo et al., 2000). The importance of comorbidity of the donor is also stressed by the data of the Collaborative Transplant Study (2005) for living donors. Patients who received a kidney from a living donor aged 65 years or more had the same 5-year graft survival of 78% as patients who received a kidney from donors aged between 16 and 40 years. These data suggest that the absence of comorbidity in elderly living donors may overcome the drawbacks associated with elderly cadaver donors.

Ischemia–reperfusion

Ischemia–reperfusion injury may be responsible for delayed graft function, and can also be associated with late graft dysfunction particularly when it is combined with acute rejection (Geddes et al., 2002; Hetzel et al., 2002b). In this context, it is noteworthy to recall that ischemia–reperfusion injury may activate toll-like receptors (Andrade et al., 2005) and innate immunity (Kim et al., 2005), thus creating an inflammatory state that may directly damage the kidney, or favor the maturation of dendritic cells that induce the adaptive alloimmune response leading to rejection (Land, 2005). Moreover, ischemic lesions in cadaver kidneys may upregulate the expression of HLA-DR antigens and cell adhesion molecules on tubular cells (Koo et al., 1999), hence favoring the development of rejection.

Source of the kidney

The source of the kidney is another major factor. The better results observed with living-unrelated donors than with cadaveric HLA-matched donors (Gjertson and Cecka, 2000) have been explained by the fact that living donor kidneys are healthy, without a reduced nephron mass and/or pre-existing diseases. Moreover, brain death causes severe hypotension, coagulopathy, hypothermia, and electrolyte disorders which, coupled with increased sympathetic activity, lead to generalized and renal ischemia. Finally, the kidney of a living donor does not suffer the heavy consequences of ischemia–reperfusion mentioned above. Brain death is often associated with severe hypotension, an increase in catecholamines, electrolyte abnormalities, and intracranial hypertension that can favor the overproduction of cytokines and growth factors leading to overexpression of alloantigens on tubular and endothelial cells (Pratschke et al., 2001).

Nephron underdosing

An elevated body mass index is significantly associated with worse graft survival independent of patient survival (Meier-Kriesche et al., 2002a). In particular, large patients who receive a kidney from small donors have a 43% increased risk of late graft failure compared with medium-size patients receiving a kidney from medium-size donors (Kasiske et al., 2002b). It is still unclear, however, whether the worse graft survival in obese patients is actually caused by nephron underdosing or by comorbidity, such as diabetes and hypertension, which can have a deleterious effect on graft function.

Clinical status of the recipient

The *age* of the recipient is another factor that can deleteriously influence the results. As expected, the older is the recipient, the higher is the risk of death after transplantation (Cecka, 2000). Moreover, older patients are often given the kidney of an older donor. This may increase the risk of late graft failure (Meier-Kriesche et al., 2002b), although good results have been obtained with the 'old-to-old' allocation, by avoiding the use of calcineurin inhibitors in the first post-transplant period and minimizing the use of steroids in maintenance (Segoloni et al., 2005).

After transplantation, *proteinuria* (Braun et al., 2001; Roodnat et al., 2001), *hyperlipidemia* (Roodnat et al., 2000; Ponticelli et al., 2002), *oxidative stress* (Cristol et al., 1998), and *hypertension* (Opelz et al., 1998) have been found to be independent variables associated with the risk of late graft failure. However, it is still unclear whether these abnormalities represent a cause or an effect of late graft failure. *Nephrocalcinosis* in patients with severe hyperparathyroidism is also predictive of CAN (Schwarz et al., 2005).

Cytomegalovirus infection

Cytomegalovirus infections also have a deleterious influence on late graft function (Tong et al., 2000), both because viruses may increase neointima formation (Kloppenburg et al., 2005), particularly when HLA incompatibility between recipient and donor is present (Li et al., 1998), and because they may trigger rejection (Geddes et al., 2003) and enhance the detrimental effects of rejection (Kosisken et al., 1999).

Calcineurin inhibitors

Calcineurin inhibitors are considered the main factor responsible for progressive graft dysfunction by many investigators. There is no doubt that these agents are nephrotoxic (see Chapter 6) and can lead to the development of chronic nephropathy. Some investigators found that chronic interstitial fibrosis was more frequent in patients treated with cyclosporine (CsA) than in those treated with tacrolimus (Nankivell et al., 2004). However, a review of USRDS (United States Renal Data System) data reported a similar outcome for renal transplant recipients given a microemulsion of CsA and those given tacrolimus (Meier-Kriesche and Kaplan, 2002), and a randomized study with protocol biopsies could not find any difference in the fibrogenic response between the two drugs (Roos-van Groningen et al., 2006). In one study, kidney and pancreas transplant recipients treated with CNI were followed for 10 years and received a protocol renal biopsy every year. At 10 years, nephrotoxicity was almost universal; severe chronic allograft nephropathy was present in 58.4% of patients, with sclerosis in 37.3% of glomeruli. Tubulointerstitial and glomerular damage, once established, was irreversible, resulting in declining renal function and graft failure (Nankivell et al., 2003). However, in the same study, the authors reported an astonishing 95% renal graft survival at 10 years, by far the best data ever obtained. Protocol biopsies have shown that there is an increase of glomerular volume after transplantation and that a larger glomerular volume at 4 months is associated with a better glomerular filtration rate. This adaptation mechanism may be impaired with high CsA levels (Seron et al., 2005). On the other hand, Lipkowitz et al. (1999) followed 91 renal transplant recipients for up to 7–9 years, and performed kidney graft biopsy on all grafts that had failed as well as in the majority of patients with deteriorating renal function. As measured by iothalamate clearances, 65% of the patients exhibited absolutely stable renal function despite the maintenance of cyclosporine levels of more than 200 ng/ml for 7–9 years. Furthermore, none of the patients with declining renal function or with a failed graft showed any evidence of nephrotoxicity on biopsy. The authors concluded that chronic cyclosporine nephrotoxicity may be a cause of declining function or graft loss with renal transplant recipients, but if so, it is exceedingly rare. Other investigators also reported that in CsA-treated transplant recipients, plasma creatinine levels remained stable for up to 12–14 years (Matas et al., 1995; Ponticelli et al., 1999). Since many CsA-treated patients did not reveal any decline in renal function, it therefore follows that they did not experience severe chronic cyclosporine nephrotoxicity. In some cases, plasma creatinine may improve years after transplantation if CsA is stopped or reduced (Mourad et al., 1998), showing that even in the long term CsA-induced nephropathy may be functional, dose-related, and potentially reversible. Finally, repeat renal biopsies demonstrated the histologic reversibility of arteriolopathy after the reduction or discontinuation of CsA (Mihatsch et al., 1995). In summary, there is no doubt that CNI are actually nephrotoxic and can lead to progressive kidney graft dysfunction; on the other hand, CNI may be given for many years without necessarily leading to graft failure, if their doses are adjusted on the basis of blood levels, renal function, and clinical features. Caution should be exercised before relinquishing these agents from the therapeutic armamentarium of renal transplantation.

Preventive measures

On the basis of the available knowledge, some strategies to prevent long-term graft dysfunction may be adopted.

Living donation offers better results than cadaveric transplantation, not only in patients with good HLA compatibility but also in HLA-incompatible patients. The preferential use of living donors (related or unrelated) seems therefore to be justified. Whenever possible the kidney of a cadaver donor should be assigned to the recipient with the best *HLA compatibility*, unless this is associated with an exceedingly long cold ischemia time.

Every effort should be made to prevent *ischemia–reperfusion injury* (Table 5.6). Appropriate care of the donor, trying to avoid profound hypotension while sparing vasoconstrictor agents, is of paramount importance. Warm and cold ischemia times should be kept as short as possible. The use of intracellular solutions for perfusion has improved results. Newer, promising solutions are under investigation. Good

Table 5.6   Main measures to prevent ischemia–reperfusion injury

Optimize care of the donor
Minimize warm ischemia
Keep cold ischemia time as short as possible
Optimize renal perfusion
Use intracellular preservation solution (Phosphate sucrose? CO releaser?)
Antioxidant agents (Super Oxide Dismutase?) Allopurinol? CO+biliverdin? Acetylcysteine?)
Antiapoptotic agents (Trimetazidine? Dopamine? Caspase inhibitors?)

results have also been obtained in experimental studies with antioxidant and/or antiapoptotic agents (see Chapter 3). In CMV-negative patients who receive a kidney from a *CMV-positive* patient, close monitoring of pp65 antigen or CMV DNA is strongly recommended, and pre-emptive treatment with intravenous ganciclovir or with oral valganciclovir should be scheduled whenever there is a suspicion of CMV infection. Any viral or bacterial infection should be diagnosed and treated promptly.

The treatment of *hyperlipidemia* and *hypertension* is also warranted to prevent both progressive graft dysfunction and cardiovascular disease (El-Amm *et al.*, 2006). *Angiotensin-converting enzyme* (ACE) *inhibitors* and *angiotensin receptor blockers* (ARB) can oppose the production of cytokines and growth factors in experimental models of chronic rejection (Szabo *et al.*, 2000; Ziai *et al.*, 2000). When given together with MMF, ARB protected fully against chronic rejection in a rat model (Noris *et al.*, 2001). In renal transplant recipients these agents can reduce blood pressure and proteinuria (Ersoy *et al.*, 2002; Zeier *et al.*, 2001). In a retrospective study, it was observed that renal transplant recipients treated with ACE inhibitors or ARB had a significantly better 10-year graft survival than did patients without these agents (Heinze *et al.*, 2006). On the other hand, in stable renal transplant patients, a controlled trial failed to show any difference in graft function at 5 years between patients assigned to an ACE inhibitor or to a beta-blocker. There was stable proteinuria in the first group and a significant but mild increase in the second group (Suwelack *et al.*, 2003).

To improve *compliance,* the physician should maximize the education of the patient, by clearly explaining the reasons for prescribing that particular type of drug(s) and the possible consequences of poor adherence to the prescription. It is also important that a good relationship between the doctor and the patient is established. The doctor should be available to answer the many questions or deal with problems that the patient may have. The compliance of the patient should be checked at any follow-up visit. Finally, treatment should be as simple as possible, trying to reduce the number of pills and minimize doses of steroids and other agents that may cause esthetic side-effects (Table 5.7).

Adequate immunosuppression plays the most important role. In the past few years the incidence and severity of acute rejection have been considerably reduced by the use of modern immunosuppressive agents, including monoclonal antibodies against the IL-2 receptor. Moreover, the use of powerful polyclonal or monoclonal antilymphocyte antibodies, and/or intravenous immunoglobulins, may obtain the reversal of severe acute rejection. This should result in a longer graft half-life. Whether calcineurin inhibitors should be avoided or used at low doses in order to reduce the risk of long-term nephrotoxicity is still a matter of controversy. Good results have been reported with the discontinuation of cyclosporine and its replacement by azathioprine (Hollander *et al.*, 1995). In a multicenter randomized trial, renal transplant recipients treated with CsA, sirolimus, and steroids for 3 months were randomized to continue triple therapy or to withdraw CsA while increasing the dose of sirolimus. After 4 years, the glomerular filtration rate was significantly better in patients treated with sirolimus and steroids, independent of baseline graft function (Russ *et al.*, 2005).

Table 5.7 Some recommendations for improving adherence to prescriptions

Maximize patient education
Establish partnership with the patient
Check compliance regularly at each folow-up visit
Try to simplify the treatment

However, the control arm continued to receive standard doses of CsA, while it is known today that the dose of CsA should be considerably reduced when given in combination with anti-mTOR (mammalian target of rapamycin) agents, in order to prevent nephrotoxicity (Nashan *et al.*, 2004; Lorber *et al.*, 2005). On the other hand, similar acute rejection rates, graft survival, and renal function at 1–2 years after transplantation were seen in a randomized trial comparing a regimen comprising sirolimus, MMF, and prednisone with a regimen based on tacrolimus, MMF, and prednisone (Larson *et al.*, 2006). A CNI-free immunosuppression based on sirolimus, mycophenolate mofetil, and steroids appeared to be effective, but the available studies have only a short follow-up (Kreis *et al.*, 2000; Flechner *et al.*, 2002). Thus, whether is it worthwhile and safe to avoid the use of calcineurin inhibitors is still doubtful (Meier-Kriesche and Hricik, 2006). Even reduction of the dosage of calcineurin inhibitors should be done with caution. A European survey showed that doses of cyclosporine lower than 3 mg/kg per day in the first year gave poorer graft survival than that obtained with doses ranging between 3 and 6 mg/kg per day (Opelz and Dohler, 2001). However, a randomized study showed that a 50% reduction of CsA at 1 year in renal transplant patients with stable graft function was safe, and improved renal function (Pascual *et al.*, 2003).

Therapeutic approaches

There is no effective treatment for established CAN.

Little information is available on the role of *ACE inhibitors* and *ARB* in altering the progressive course of CAN. Some studies reported the capacity of these agents in reducing the production of TGFβ1 in renal transplant recipients (Campistol *et al.*, 1999; Hetzel *et al.*, 2002a). In a retrospective study in 63 patients with biopsy-proven CAN, 32 patients treated for at least 6 months with ACE inhibitors or ARB showed a trend of slowing renal insufficiency when compared with 31 patients given other antihypertensive agents (Lin *et al.*, 2002). On the other hand, in another study, nifedipine was found to be more effective than the ACE inhibitor lisinopril in obtaining a sustained improvement of graft function (Midtvedt *et al.*, 2001). The problem is rendered even more complex by experimental studies in Fischer rats with kidney transplants, showing that prolonged treatment with ACE inhibitors may cause severe intimal hyperplasia of renal arteries. This paradoxical effect of ACE inhibitors may be explained by the fact that Fischer rats have a higher ACE activity than do other strains. This is comparable to the human DD/II genotype. Thus, it may be speculated that renal transplant recipients with the DD genotype may be more vulnerable to vascular changes when treated with ACE inhibitor blockers (Smit-van Oosten *et al.*, 2003).

The early introduction of *statins* was associated with an improved 1-year graft outcome in renal transplant recipients treated with cyclosporine, MMF, and steroids (Masterson *et al.*, 2005). It is unclear whether this beneficial effect was due to a reduction of cholesterol, to the immunomodulating activity, or to endothelial protection by statins.

While adequate *immunosuppression* is important to prevent either immunological activation or nephrotoxicity caused by excessive doses of calcineurin inhibitors, it is still unclear whether changes in immunosuppression in patients with CAN are of any benefit. *Mycophenolate mofetil* (MMF), which inhibits lymphocyte

Table 5.8   Some clues for identifying the main cause of chronic allograft nephropathy

Late (chronic) rejection	Nephrotoxicity–non-immunological factors
Peritubular C4d deposits	Absence of C4d deposits
Arteritis	CNI arteriolopathy
Transplant glomerulopathy	Positive tissue factor on tubular brush border
HLA–non-HLA circulating antibodies	Absence of circulating antibodies
Poor compliance	Good compliance

proliferation, adhesion molecule glycosylation, and smooth muscle proliferation, proved to be effective in preventing chronic vascular rejection in experimental models (Raisanen-Sokolowski et al., 1995). These results encouraged the use of MMF in patients with established chronic rejection in kidney transplantation. In one study (Glicklich et al., 1998), the replacement of azathioprine with MMF showed no advantage. In contrast, another study (Weir et al., 2001) reported a beneficial effect of MMF in 118 transplant recipients with progressive deterioration of renal function. In all patients, CsA was reduced or withdrawn. Renal function improved in most patients, particularly in the 18 who stopped CsA. It is not clear, however, whether the benefit of this change in immunosuppression was related to the reduced dose of CsA or to a specific effect of MMF. Other studies reported an improvement in graft function after replacing cyclosporine with MMF, but this therapeutic maneuver implied a risk of biopsy-proven acute or chronic rejection (Smak Gregoor et al., 2000). In another study, patients were followed for 5 years after the withdrawal of CsA from an MMF-containing immunosuppressive regimen. An increased risk for acute rejection and graft loss was found, while creatinine clearance improvement was maintained at 5 years (Abramowicz et al., 2005).

In a pilot study in 22 patients with progressive graft dysfunction, azathioprine or MMF was replaced by leflunomide, while leaving unchanged the dosage of CsA. After 6 months serum creatinine was reduced from 3.0 to 2.8 mg/dl (Hardinger et al., 2002). No information on the long-term outcome is available.

Conversion from CsA to sirolimus may benefit some patients with CAN, but may aggravate proteinuria and renal function in other patients. In a study, 19 patients with CAN were rapidly converted from CsA to sirolimus. Six months after conversion, amelioration of renal function was found in 36%, stabilization in 21%, and continuous deterioration in 43% (Citterio et al., 2003). In another study (Diekmann et al., 2004), 59 patients with CAN were gradually converted from CNI to sirolimus. A significant improvement of serum creatinine was seen in 54% of patients and a significant deterioration in the other 46%. Baseline proteinuria, histologic grade of CAN, grade of vascular fibrous intimal thickening, and number of acute rejections before conversion differed significantly between responders and non-responders; at multivariate analysis, proteinuria below 800 mg/day was the only independent predictor for a positive outcome in the conversion from CNI to sirolimus. In a randomized, prospective, open-label, single-center study, 84 consecutive transplant patients with biopsy-proven CAN were randomized to receive either a 40% CNI reduction plus MMF or immediate withdrawal of CNI and sirolimus introduction (Stallone et al., 2005). After 24 months, in patients without CNI, graft survival was significantly better; in the few patients who received a second biopsy the alpha-smooth muscle actin protein expression was dramatically reduced; however, mean serum creatinine variations at the end of follow-up did not differ between the two groups. On the other hand, Boratynska et al. (2006) reported progressive graft dysfunction and the onset of nephrotic proteinuria in patients with CAN who were switched from CsA to sirolimus.

A main issue in planning treatment is to know whether CAN has been mainly caused by non-immunological factors or by ongoing immunological activity (Table 5.8). It is likely that in patients with

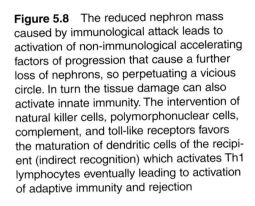

Ongoing immunological attack

Figure 5.8 The reduced nephron mass caused by immunological attack leads to activation of non-immunological accelerating factors of progression that cause a further loss of nephrons, so perpetuating a vicious circle. In turn the tissue damage can also activate innate immunity. The intervention of natural killer cells, polymorphonuclear cells, complement, and toll-like receptors favors the maturation of dendritic cells of the recipient (indirect recognition) which activates Th1 lymphocytes eventually leading to activation of adaptive immunity and rejection

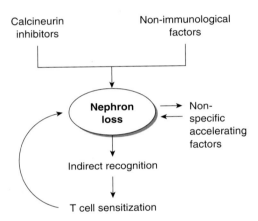

Figure 5.9 The nephron loss caused by non-immunological factors perpetuates a further reduction of nephrons through non-specific factors of progression. Moreover, the tissue damage triggers innate immunity, a proinflammatory environment, and maturation of dendritic cells of the recipient, with T cell activation leading to rejection and further tissue damage

circulating anti-HLA antibodies and/or C4d staining and/or arteritis in graft biopsy there is antibody-mediated immunological activity. The reinforcement of immunosuppression with tacrolimus and MMF (Theruvath et al., 2001; Mauiyyedi et al., 2001) and/or therapeutic attempts with *plasmapheresis*, *immunoadsorption*, *intravenous immunoglobulins*, or *rituximab* may be tried in these cases. However, there is no evidence that these attempts can actually lead to an improvement of graft function in patients with CAN. Transplant glomerulopathy is also an expression of chronic rejection. Even in this case we do not have any effective treatment (Suri et al., 2000). The major problem with the treatment of CAN caused initially by immunological factors is that the loss of nephrons activates a vicious circle of glomerular hyperfiltration and hypertension which, in association with proteinuria, hyperlipidemia, and atherosclerosis, leads to further nephron loss. Moreover, cell damage may also activate innate immunity and create a proinflammatory environment, so favoring the maturation of dendritic cells, and the activation of Th1 lymphocytes with consequent activation of adaptive immunity, through indirect recognition (Figure 5.8).

If biopsy does not show C4d deposits, arteritis, or transplant glomerulopathy, it is possible to speculate that non-immunological factors are prevailing in the etiopathogenesis of CAN. In these cases a careful reduction of calcineurin inhibitors and the aggressive treatment of non-alloantigen-dependent factors of progression may be tried. Even in these cases, however, a vicious circle can occur, leading to progressive graft dysfunction through the continuous damage produced by accelerating non-immune factors coupled with the activation of innate immunity and indirect recognition (Figure 5.9).

At any rate, it must be outlined that renal allografts as well as native kidneys have a 'point of no return'. Interstitial fibrosis and glomerular sclerosis are irreversible lesions which may favor irreversible progression even when the initial events are eliminated. Thus, the failure of therapeutic interventions may be caused not only by the fact that they are tried 'blind', without knowing the cause of CAN, but also because they are started too late.

References

Abe M, Kawai T, Fatatsuyama K, et al. Postoperative production of anti-donor antibody and chronic rejection in renal transplantation. Transplantation 1997; 63: 1616–19.

Abramowicz D, Del Carmen Rial M, Vitko S, et al. Cyclosporine withdrawal from a mycophenolate mofetil-containing immunosuppressive regimen: results of a five-year, prospective, randomized study. J Am Soc Nephrol 2005; 16: 2234–40.

Andrade CF, Waddell TK, Keshavjee S, Liu M. Innate immunity and organ transplantation: the potential role of toll-like receptors. Am J Transplant 2005; 5: 969–75.

Arias M, Fernandez-Fresnedo G, Rodrigo E, et al. Non-immunologic intervention in chronic allograft nephropathy. Kidney Int 2005; 99 (Suppl): S118–23.

Banfi G, Villa M, Cresseri D, Ponticelli C. The clinical impact of transplant glomerulopathy in the cyclosporine era. Transplantation 2005; 80: 1392–7.

Beveridge T, Calne RY, for the European Multicentre Trial Group. Cyclosporine (Sandimmun) in cadaveric renal transplantation: ten-year follow-up of a multicentre trial. Transplantation 1995; 59: 1568–9.

Boratynska M, Banasik M, Watorek E, et al. Conversion to sirolimus from cyclosporine may induce nephrotic proteinuria and progressive deterioration of renal function in chronic allograft nephropathy patients. Transplant Proc 2006; 38: 101–4.

Braun N, Bachmann F, Horch B, et al. Newly developing proteinuria but not blood pressure is an independent risk factor for chronic graft dysfunction following renal transplantation in patients with well-controlled blood pressure. Transplant Proc 2001; 33: 3361–2.

Butler JA, Roderick P, Mullee M, et al. Frequency and impact of nonadherence to immunosuppressants after renal transplantation: a systematic review. Transplantation 2004; 77: 769–76.

Campistol JM, Iñigo P, Jimenez W, et al. Losartan decreases plasma levels of TGF-β1 in transplant patients with chronic allograft nephropathy. Kidney Int 1999; 56: 714–19.

Cecka M. The UNOS Scientific Renal Transplant Registry. In Cecka JM, Terasaki PI, eds. Clinical Transplants 1999. Los Angeles, CA: UCLA Tissue Typing Laboratory, 2000: 1–18.

Citterio F, Scata MC, Violi P, et al. Rapid conversion to sirolimus for chronic progressive deterioration of the renal function in kidney allograft recipients. Transplant Proc 2003; 35: 1292–4.

Cosio FG, Pelletier PR, Sedmak DD, et al. Pathologic classification of chronic allograft nephropathy: pathogenic and prognostic implications. Transplantation 1999; 67: 690–7.

Cristol J, Vela C, Maggi M, et al. Oxidative stress and lipid abnormalities in renal transplant recipients with or without chronic rejection. Transplantation 1998; 65: 1322–8.

CTS Collaborative Transplant Study. CTS Newslett 2005; 1.

de Vries AP, van Son WJ, van der Heide JJ, et al. The predictive value of renal vascular resistance for late renal allograft loss. Am J Transplant 2006; 6: 364–70.

Diekmann F, Budde K, Oppenheimer F, et al. Predictors of success in conversion from calcineurin inhibitor to sirolimus in chronic allograft dysfunction. Am J Transplant 2004; 4: 1869–75.

Drachenberg CB, Steinberger E, Hoehn-Saric E, et al. Specificity of intertubular capillary changes: comparative ultrastructural studies in renal allografts and native kidneys. Ultrastruct Pathol 1997; 21: 227–33.

Eddy A. Molecular basis of fibrosis. Pediatr Nephrol 2001; 15: 290–301.

El-Amm JM, Haririan A, Crook ED. The effects of blood pressure and lipid control on kidney allograft outcome. Am J Cardiovasc Drugs 2006; 6: 1–7.

Ersoy A, Dilek K, Usta M, et al. Angiotensin II receptor antagonist losartan reduces microalbuminuria in renal transplant recipients. Clin Transplant 2002; 16: 202–5.

Ferlicot S, Durrbach A, Ba N, et al. The role of replicative senescence in chronic allograft nephropathy. Hum Pathol 2003; 34: 924–8.

Feucht HE, Opelz G. The humoral immune response towards HLA class II determinants in renal transplantation. Kidney Int 1996; 50: 1464–75.

Feutren G, Mihatsch MJ. Risk factors for cyclosporine-induced nephropathy in patients with autoimmune diseases. International Kidney Biopsy Registry of Cyclosporine in Autoimmune Diseases. N Engl J Med 1992; 326: 1654–60.

Flechner SM, Goldfarb D, Modlin C, et al. Kidney transplantation without calcineurin inhibitor drugs: a prospective, randomized trial of sirolimus versus cyclosporine. Transplantation 2002; 74: 1070–6.

Geddes CC, Woo YM, Jardine AC. The impact of delayed graft function on the long-term outcome of renal transplantation. J Nephrol 2002; 15: 17–21.

Geddes CC, Church CC, Collidge T, et al. Management of cytomegalovirus infection by weekly surveillance after renal transplant: analysis of cost, rejection and renal function. Nephrol Dial Transplant 2003; 18: 1891–8.

Gjertson DW, Cecka JM. Living unrelated kidney transplantation. Kidney Int 2000; 58: 491–9.

Glicklich D, Gupta B, Schurter-Frey G, et al. Chronic renal allograft rejection. No response to mycophenolate mofetil. Transplantation 1998; 66: 398–9.

Gourishankar S, Melk A, Halloran P. Nonimmune mechanisms of injury in renal transplantation. Transplant Rev 2002; 16: 73–86.

Habib R, Broyer M. Clinical significance of allograft glomerulopathy. Kidney Int 1993; 44 (Suppl 43): 595–8.

Halloran PF, Mathew T, Tomlanovich S, et al. Mycophenolate mofetil in renal allograft recipients: a pooled efficacy analysis of three randomized, double-blind, clinical studies in prevention of rejection. The International Mycophenolate Mofetil Renal Transplant Study Group. Transplantation 1997; 63: 39–47.

Halloran PF, Melk A, Barth C. Rethinking chronic allograft nephropathy: the concept of accelerated senescence. J Am Soc Nephrol 1999; 10: 167–81.

Hardinger KL, Wang CD, Schnitzler MA, et al. Prospective, pilot, open-label, short-term study of conversion to leflunomide reverses chronic renal allograft rejection. Am J Transplant 2002; 2: 867–71.

Hariharan S, Johnson CP, Bresnahan BA, et al. Improved graft survival after renal transplantation in the United States. N Engl J Med 2000; 342: 605–12.

Hariharan S, McBride MA, Cohen EP. Evolution of end-points for renal transplant outcome. Am J Transplant 2003; 8: 933–41.

Heinze G, Mitterbauer C, Regele H, et al. Angiotensin-converting enzyme inhibitor or angiotensin II type 1 receptor antagonist therapy is associated with prolonged patient and graft survival after renal transplantation. J Am Soc Nephrol 2006; 17: 889–99.

Hetzel GR, Hemsen D, Hohfeld T, et al. Effects of candesartan and perindopril on renal function, TGF beta 1 plasma levels and excretion of prostaglandins in stable renal allograft recipients. Clin Nephrol 2002a; 57: 296–302.

Hetzel GR, Klein B, Brause M, et al. Risk factors for delayed graft function after renal transplantation and their significance for long-term clinical outcome. Transpl Int 2002b; 15: 10–16.

Hollander AA, Van Saase JL, Kootte AM, et al. Beneficial effects of conversion from cyclosporin to azathioprine after kidney transplantation. Lancet 1995; 345: 610–14.

Joosten SA, van Kooten C, Sijpkens YW, et al. The pathobiology of chronic allograft nephropathy: immune-mediated damage and accelerated aging. Kidney Int 2004; 65: 1556–9.

Kahan BD, Welsh M, Shoenberg L, et al. Variable oral absorption of cyclosporine: a biopharmaceutical risk factor for chronic renal allograft rejection. Transplantation 1996; 62: 599–606.

Kasiske BL, Andany MA, Danielson B. A thirty percent chronic decline in inverse serum creatinine is an excellent predictor of late graft failure. Am J Kidney Dis 2002a; 39: 762–8.

Kasiske BL, Snyder JJ, Gilbertson D. Inadequate donor size in cadaveric kidney transplantation. J Am Soc Nephrol 2002b; 13: 2152–9.

Kim BS, Lim SW, Li C, et al. Ischemia–reperfusion injury activates innate immunity in rat kidneys. Transplantation 2005; 79: 1370–7.

Kloppenburg G, de Graaf R, Herngreen S, et al. Cytomegalovirus aggravates intimal hyperplasia in rats by stimulating smooth muscle cell proliferation. Microbes Infect 2005; 7: 164–70.

Koo DDH, Welsh KI, McLaren J, et al. Cadaver versus living donor kidneys: impact of donor factors on antigen induction before transplantation. Kidney Int 1999; 56: 1551–9.

Kosisken PK, Kallio EA, Tikkanen JM, et al. Cytomegalovirus infection and cardiac allograft vasculopathy. Transpl Infect Dis 1999; 1: 115–26.

Kreis H, Cisterne JM, Land W. Sirolimus in association with mychophenolate mofetil induction for the prevention of acute rejection in renal allograft recipients. Transplantation 2000; 69: 1252–60.

Land W. The role of postischemic reperfusion injury and other nonantigen-dependent inflammatory pathways in transplantation. Transplantation 2005; 79: 505–14.

Larson TS, Dean PG, Stegall MD, et al. Complete avoidance of calcineurin inhibitors in renal transplantation: a randomized trial comparing sirolimus and tacrolimus. Am J Transplant 2006; 6: 514–22.

Lazzeri E, Rotondi M, Mazzinghi B, et al. High CXCL10 expression in rejected kidneys and predictive role of pretransplant serum CXCL10 for acute rejection and chronic allograft nephropathy. Transplantation 2005; 79: 1215–20.

Lee PC, Terasaki PI, Takemoto SK, et al. All chronic rejection failures of kidney transplants were preceded by the development of HLA antibodies. Transplantation 2002; 74: 1192–4.

Li F, Yin M, Van Dam JG, et al. Cytomegalovirus enhances the neointima formation in rat aortic allografts. Transplantation 1998; 65: 1298–304.

Lin J, Valeri AM, Markowitz GS. Angiotensin converting enzyme inhibition in chronic allograft nephropathy. Transplantation 2002; 73: 783–8.

Lipkowitz GS, Madden RL, Mulhern J, et al. Long-term maintenance of therapeutic cyclosporine levels leads to optimal graft survival without evidence of chronic nephrotoxicity. Transpl Int 1999; 12: 202–7.

Lorber MI, Ponticelli C, Whelchel J, et al. Therapeutic drug monitoring for everolimus in kidney transplantation using 12-month exposure, efficacy, and safety data. Clin Transplant 2005; 19: 145–52.

Macias-Nunez J, Cameron JS. The ageing kidney. In Davison A, Cameron JS, Grunfeld JP, et al., eds. Oxford Textbook of Clinical Nephrology. Oxford: Oxford University Press, 2005; I: 73–87.

Maryniak RK, First MR, Weiss MA. Transplant glomerulopathy: evolution of morphologically distinct changes. Kidney Int 1985; 27: 799–806.

Masterson R, Hewitson T, Leikis M, et al. Impact of statin treatment on 1-year functional and histologic renal allograft outcome. Transplantation 2005; 80: 332–8.

Matas AJ, Almond PS, Moss A, et al. Effect of cyclosporine on renal function in kidney transplant recipients: a 12-year follow-up. Clin Transplant 1995; 9: 450–3.

Matinlauri IH, Kyllonen LE, Salmela KT, et al. Serum sCD30 in monitoring of alloresponse in well HLA-matched cadaveric kidney transplantations. Transplantation 2005; 80: 1809–12.

Mauiyyedi S, Pelle PD, Saidman S, et al. Chronic humoral rejection. Identification of antibody-mediated chronic allograft rejection by C4d deposits in peritubular capillaries. J Am Soc Nephrol 2001; 12: 574–82.

Meier-Kriesche HU, Kaplan B. Cyclosporine microemulsion and tacrolimus are associated with decreased chronic allograft failure and improved long-term graft survival as compared with sandimmune. Am J Transplant 2002; 2: 100–4.

Meier-Kriesche HU, Arndorfer JA, Kaplan B. The impact of body mass index on renal transplant outcomes: a significant independent risk factor for graft failure and patient death. Transplantation 2002a; 73: 70–4.

Meier-Kriesche HU, Cibrik DM, Ojo AO, et al. Interaction between donor and recipient age in determining the risk of chronic allograft failure. J Am Geriatr Soc 2002b; 50: 14–17.

Meier-Kriesche HU, Steffen BJ, Hochberg AM, et al. Long-term use of mycophenolate mofetil is associated with a reduction in the incidence and risk of late rejection. Am J Transplant 2003; 3: 68–73.

Meier-Kriesche HU, Schold JD, Kaplan B. Long-term renal allograft survival: have we made significant progress or is it time to rethink our analytic and therapeutic strategies? Am J Transplant 2004; 4: 1289–95.

Meier-Kriesche HU, Hricik DE. Are we ready to give up on calcineurin inhibitors? Am J Transplant 2006; 6: 445–6.

Midtvedt K, Tafjord AB, Hartmann A, et al. Half dose of OKT3 is efficient in treatment of steroid-resistant renal allograft rejection. Transplantation 1996; 62: 38–42.

Mihatsch MJ, Morozumi K, Strom EH, et al. Renal transplant morphology after long-term therapy with cyclosporine. Transplant Proc 1995; 27: 39–42.

Mihatsch MJ, Nickeleit V, Gudat F. Morphologic criteria of chronic renal allograft rejection. Transplant Proc 1999; 31: 1295–7.

Minervini MI, Torbenson M, Scantlebury V, et al. Acute renal allograft rejection with severe tubulitis (Banff 1997 class IB). Am Surg Pathol 2000; 24: 533–8.

Moll S, Pascual M. Humoral rejection of organ allografts. Am J Transplant 2005; 5: 2611–18.

Monga G, Mazzucco G. Messina M, et al. Intertubular capillary changes in kidney allografts: a morphologic investigation on 61 renal specimens. Mod Pathol 1992; 5: 125–30.

Moreso F, Ibernon M, Goma M, et al. Subclinical rejection associated with chronic allograft nephropathy in protocol biopsies as a risk factor for late graft loss. Am J Transplant 2006; 6: 747–52.

Mourad G, Vela C, Ribstein J, Mimran A. Long-term improvement after cyclosporine reduction in renal transplant recipients with histologically proven chronic cyclosporine nephropathy. Transplantation 1998; 65: 661–7.

Mueller A, Schnuelle P, Waldherr R, van der Woude FJ. Impact of the Banff '97 classification for histological diagnosis of rejection on clinical outcome and renal function parameters after kidney transplantation. Transplantation 2000; 69: 1123–7.

Nankivell BJ, Borrows RJ, Fung CL, et al. The natural history of chronic allograft nephropathy. N Engl J Med 2003; 349: 2326–33.

Nankivell BJ, Borrows RJ, Fung CL, et al. Delta analysis of posttransplantation tubulointerstitial damage. Transplantation 2004; 78: 434–41.

Nashan B, Curtis J, Ponticelli C, et al. Everolimus and reduced-exposure cyclosporine in de novo renal-transplant recipients: a three-year phase II, randomized, multicenter, open-label study. Transplantation 2004; 78: 1332–40.

Noris M, Azzolini N, Pezzotta A, et al. Combined treatment with mycophenolate mofetil and angiotensin II receptor antagonist fully protects fom chronic rejection in a rat model of renal allograft. J Am Soc Nephrol 2001; 12: 1937–46.

Ojo AO, Leichtman AB, Punch JD, et al. Impact of preexisting donor hypertension and diabetes mellitus on cadaveric renal transplant outcomes. Am J Kidney Dis 2000; 36: 153–9.

Opelz G. Critical evaluation of the association of acute with chronic graft rejection in kidney and heart transplant recipients. The Collaborative Transplant Study. Transplant Proc 1997; 29: 73–6.

Opelz G, Wujciak T, Ritz E. Association of chronic kidney graft failure with recipient blood pressure. Kidney Int 1998; 53: 217–22.

Opelz G, Dolher B. Cyclosporine and long-term kidney graft survival. Transplantation 2001; 72: 1267–73.

Opelz G, Dohler B. Collaborative Transplant Study. Improved long-term outcomes after renal transplantation associated with blood pressure control. Am J Transplant 2005; 5: 2725–31.

Osterholm C, Veress B, Simanaitis M, et al. Differential expression of tissue factor (TF) in calcineurin inhibitor-induced nephrotoxicity and rejection – implications for development of a possible diagnostic marker. Transpl Immunol 2005; 15: 165–72.

Pascual M, Curtis J, Delmonico FL, et al. A prospective, randomized clinical trial of cyclosporine reduction in stable patients greater than 12 months after renal transplantation. Transplantation 2003; 75: 1501–5.

Ponticelli C, Civati G, Tarantino A, et al. Randomized study with cyclosporine in kidney transplantation: 10-year follow-up. J Am Soc Nephrol 1996; 7: 792–7.

Ponticelli C, Aroldi A, Elli A, et al. The clinical status of cadaveric renal transplant patients treated for 10 years with cyclosporine therapy. Clin Transplant 1999; 13: 324–9.

Ponticelli C, Villa M, Cesana B, et al. Risk factors for late kidney allograft failure. Kidney Int 2002; 62: 1848–54.

Pratschke J, Wilhelm MJ, Laskowski I, et al. Influence of donor brain on chronic rejection of renal transplants in rats. J Am Soc Nephrol 2001; 12: 2474–81.

Racusen LC, Solez K, Colvin RB. The Banff 97 working classification of renal allograft pathology. Kidney Int 1999; 55: 713–23.

Racusen LC, Solez K, Colvin RB. Fibrosis and atrophy in the renal allograft: interim report and new directions. Am J Transplant 2002; 2: 203–6.

Radermacher J, Mengel M, Ellis S, et al. The renal arterial resistance index and renal allograft survival. N Engl J Med 2003; 349: 115–24.

Raisanen-Sokolowski A, Vuoristo P, Myllarnierni M, et al. Mycophenolate mofetil inhibits inflammation and smooth muscle cell proliferation in rat aortic allografts. Transpl Immunol 1995; 3: 342.

Regele H, Bohmig GA, Habicht A, et al. Capillary deposition of complement split product C4d in renal allografts is associated with basement membrane injury in peritubular and glomerular capillaries: a contribution of humoral immunity to chronic allograft rejection. J Am Soc Nephrol 2002; 13: 2371–80.

Richardson WP, Colvin RB, Cheeseman SH, et al. Glomerulopathy associated with cytomegalovirus viremia in renal allografts. N Engl J Med 1981; 305: 57–62.

Robertson H, Kirby JA. Renal allograft rejection: the development and function of tubulitis. Transplant Rev 2001; 15: 109–28.

Roodnat JI, Mulder PG, Zietse R, et al. Cholesterol as an independent factor of outcome after renal transplantation. Transplantation 2000; 69: 1704–10.

Roodnat JI, Mulder PG, Rischen-Vos J, et al. Proteinuria after renal transplantation affects not only graft survival but also patient survival. Transplantation 2001; 72: 438–44.

Roos-van Groningen M, Scholten EM, Lelieveld PM, et al. Molecular comparison of calcineurin inhibitor-induced fibrogenic responses in protocol renal transplant biopsies. J Am Soc Nephrol 2006; 17: 881–8.

Rush D; Winnipeg Transplant Group. Insights into subclinical rejection. Transplant Proc 2004; 36 (Suppl): 71S–3S.

Russ G, Segoloni G, Oberbauer R, et al. Superior outcomes in renal transplantation after early cyclosporine withdrawal and sirolimus maintenance therapy, regardless of baseline renal function. Transplantation 2005; 80: 1204–11.

Salvadori M, Rosati A, Bock A, et al. Estimated one-year glomerular filtration rate is the best predictor of long-term graft function following renal transplant. Transplantation 2006; 81: 202–6.

Scholbach T, Girelli E, Scholbach J. Tissue pulsatility index: a new parameter to evaluate renal transplant perfusion. Transplantation 2006; 81: 751–5.

Schwarz A, Mengel M, Gwinner W, et al. Risk factors for chronic allograft nephropathy after renal transplantation: a protocol biopsy study. Kidney Int 2005; 67: 341–8.

Segoloni G, Messina M, Squiccimarro G, et al. Preferential allocation of marginal kidney allografts to elderly recipients combined with modified immunosuppression gives good results. Transplantation 2005; 80: 953–8.

Seron D, Fulladosa X, Moreso F. Risk factors associated with the deterioration of renal function after kidney transplantation. Kidney Int 2005; 99 (Suppl): S113–17.

Sijpkens YW, Doxiadis II, Mallat MJ, et al. Early versus late acute rejection episodes in renal transplantation. Transplantation 2003; 75: 204–8.

Smak Gregoor PJ, van Gelder T, van Besouw NM, et al. Randomized study on the conversion of treatment with cyclosporine to azathioprine or mycophenolate mofetil followed by dose reduction. Transplantation 2000; 70: 143–8.

Smit-van Oosten A, Stegeman CA, van Goor. RAS blockade in experimental renal transplantation. Benefits and limitations. Curr Drug Targets Cardiovasc Haematol Disord 2003; 3: 73–9.

Stallone G, Infante B, Schena A, et al. Rapamycin for treatment of chronic allograft nephropathy in renal transplant patients. J Am Soc Nephrol 2005; 16: 3755–62.

Stoves J, Newstead CG. Variability of cyclosporine exposure and its relevance to chronic allograft nephropathy: a case-control study. Transplantation 2002; 74: 1794–7.

Sun Q, Tang Z, Chen J, et al. Late developing C4d-positive humoral renal allograft rejection associated with withdrawal of mycophenolate mofetil. Transplant Proc 2005; 37: 4244–5.

Suri D, Tomlanovich SJ, Olson JL, Meyer TW. Transplant glomerulopathy as a cause of late graft loss. Am J Kidney Dis 2000; 35: 674–80.

Susal C, Pelzl S, Dohler B, Opelz G. Identification of highly responsive kidney transplant recipients using CD30. J Am Soc Nephrol 2002; 13: 1650–6.

Suwelack B, Kobelt V, Erfmann M, et al. Long-term follow-up of ACE-inhibitor versus β-blocker treatment and their effects on blood pressure and kidney function in renal transplant recipients. Transpl Int 2003; 16: 313–20.

Szabo A, Lutz J, Schleimer K, et al. Effect of angiotensin-converting enzyme inhibition on growth factor mRNA in chronic allograft rejection in the rat. Kidney Int 2000; 57: 982–91.

Terasaki PI, Ozawa M. Predictive value of HLA antibodies and serum creatinine in chronic rejection: results of a 2-year prospective trial. Transplantation 2005; 80: 1194–7.

Theruvath TP, Saidman SL, Mauiyyedi S, et al. Control of antidonor antibody production with tracrolimus and mychophenolate mofetil in renal allograft recipients with chronic rejection. Transplantation 2001; 72: 77–83.

Tong CY, Bakran A, Peiris JS, et al. The association of viral infection and chronic allograft nephropathy with graft dysfunction after renal transplantation. Transplantation 2002; 74: 576–8.

Weir MR, Ward MT, Blahut SA, et al. Long-term impact of discontinued or reduced calcineurin inhibitor in patients with chronic allograft nephropathy. Kidney Int 2001; 59: 1567–73.

Zeier M, Dikow R, Ritz E. Blood pressure after renal transplantation. Ann Transplant 2001; 6: 21–4.

Ziai F, Nagano H, Kusaka M, et al. Renal allograft protection with Losartan in Fischer Lewis rats: hemodynamics, macrophages and cytokines. Kidney Int 2000; 57: 2618–25.

6 IMMUNOSUPPRESSIVE DRUG-RELATED COMPLICATIONS

The main goal of immunosuppressive therapy is the prevention of rejection while favoring the development of an immunological adaptation. More potent and specific immunosuppressive agents have allowed a significant reduction in the incidence and severity of rejection. However, all the available drugs are associated with a number of side-effects. Their interference with the inflammatory and immune response render the transplant patient more susceptible to *infection* and *neoplasia*, which are described in Chapters 9 and 11, respectively. In this chapter, some other specific drug-related complications are described.

Calcineurin inhibitors

The first calcineurin inhibitor used in renal transplantation was *cyclosporine* (CsA). CsA is a peptide derived from the soil fungus *Tolypocladium inflatum Gams*. Following reports of its immunosuppressive properties, first described in the early 1970s, cyclosporine was approved as an anti-rejection agent in the early 1980s. A few years later, *tacrolimus* (TAC) was approved, a macrolactone derived from the fungus *Streptomyces tsukubaensis* discovered on Mount Fuji.

Mechanisms of action

Both CsA and TAC are lipophylic prodrugs that need to bind to cytoplasmic receptors, known as immunophilins, to gain pharmacological activity. The receptor for CsA is called cyclophilin, and that for TAC is called FK-binding protein 12 (FKBP-12). After binding to the respective cyclophilin, calcineurin inhibitors (CNIs) inhibit the activity of a complex of phosphatases called calcineurin. The activity of calcineurin is important because it phosphorylates a family of proteins termed nuclear factor-activating T cells (NFAT), thus allowing its entrance into the nucleus, where NFAT encodes interleukin-2 (IL-2) and other cytokines (Figure 6.1). Therefore, CNI suppress the immune response by downregulating the transcription of various cytokine genes, of which the most significant is IL-2, which serves as the major activation factor for T cells in numerous immunological processes. Although the major effect of CNI is the inhibition of cytokine production from T helper cells (Th1 and Th2), these agents also have an inhibitory effect on antigen-presenting cells, which are the first agents involved in T cell stimulation. A further effect of IL-2 inhibition is a reduction in B cell activation and subsequent antibody production (Kahan and Ponticelli, 2000). Owing to the similar mechanisms of action, it is not surprising that CsA and tacrolimus can exert similar side-effects, including reversible acute renal function deterioration, hemolytic–uremic syndrome, and chronic renal insufficiency (Table 6.1).

Acute renal toxicity

Acute nephrotoxicity of calcineurin inhibitors may manifest with variable severity, which is usually, but not always, dose-dependent.

Tubular toxicity

In the milder forms of toxicity, there is a slight reduction of glomerular filtration rate and renal blood flow associated with sodium retention, hypomagnesemia, hyperuricemia, hyperkalemia, and hyperchloremic acidosis. Interestingly, no signs of proximal tubular dysfunction are seen. These functional changes are caused by *afferent arteriolar vasoconstriction*, which can be sustained by increased sympathetic nervous activity, activation of the renin–angiotensin system, increased production of thromboxane A_2, impaired production

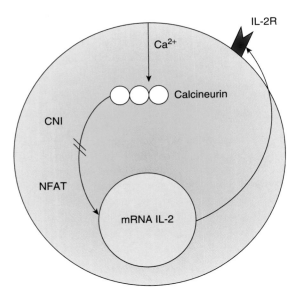

Figure 6.1 After contact with the antigen-presenting cell and co-stimulation, there is a large influx of calcium ions (Ca^{2+}) in the cytoplasm of the T cell. Calcium ions activate a complex of phosphatases called calcineurin. Calcineurin dephosphorylates a family of proteins called nuclear factor-activating T cells (NFAT). NFAT enters the nucleus and encodes the synthesis of interleukin-2 (IL-2) and other cytokines. Calcineurin inhibitors (CNI) bind to their cystoplasmic receptors (FKBP-12 for tacrolimus, cyclophilin for cyclosporine) and inhibit the activity of calcineurin, thus impeding the synthesis of IL-2

Table 6.1	Main side-effects of calcineurin inhibitors	
	TAC	**CsA**
Nephrotoxicity	+++	+++
Neurotoxicity	++	+
Diabetes	++	+
GI toxicity	+	±
Hypertension	++	+++
Hyperlipidemia	±	++
Hypertrichosis	—	++
Gum hyperplasia	—	++

of vasodilating prostaglandins, excessive renal synthesis of endothelin-1, and reduced production of nitric oxide (Olyaei *et al.*, 2001). Studies in experimental animals showed that CNI-related tubular toxicity may be prevented by endothelial growth factor (Alvarez Arroyo *et al.*, 2002). In several cases there are no morphologic abnormalities, but more often *tubular lesions* can be seen, such as isometric vacuolization, giant mitochondria, and microcalcification (Figures 6.2 and 6.3). These lesions are not pathognomonic although they are particularly frequent in patients treated with CsA or tacrolimus. Although these abnormalities are not particularly severe, they may be a sign of general cytotoxicity that can also occur in endothelial cells. Both the functional and morphologic changes may be reversible if the doses of calcineurin inhibitor are reduced (Mihatsch *et al.*, 1995).

Arteriolar toxicity

More severe nephrotoxicity may lead to an important increase in plasma creatinine. This condition is often associated with an *arteriolopathy*, characterized by focal myocyte necrosis in the media of small arteries (Figures 6.4 and 6.5), in the absence of intimal changes (Mihatsch *et al.*, 1995). Differential diagnosis

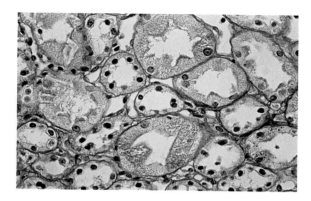

Figure 6.2 Cyclosporine tubular toxicity. Tubular cells show fine isometric vacuolization of the cytoplasm. (AFOG ×400) (Courtesy of Professor MJ Mihatsch, University of Basel)

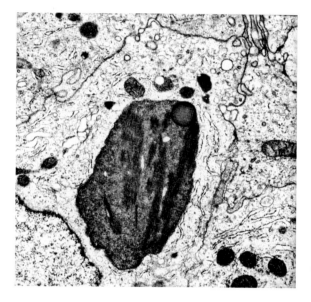

Figure 6.3 Giant mitochondria in a case of cyclosporine toxicity. (EM ×25 000) (Courtesy of Professor MJ Mihatsch, University of Basel)

from acute rejection may be difficult. Usually, acute rejection occurs earlier, the increase in plasma creatinine is higher and more rapid in acute rejection, and fever and proteinuria are absent in the case of nephrotoxicity. Some investigators have suggested that the measurement of C-reactive protein (CRP) may help in the differential diagnosis. CRP does not change in the case of renal toxicity, while it increases during acute rejection (Reek *et al.*, 2001). Renal biopsy shows the typical interstitial infiltrate, tubulitis, and cellular arteritis in the case of acute rejection. These findings are usually absent in the case of CsA or tacrolimus nephrotoxicity (Table 6.2). Decreasing the doses of calcineurin inhibitors can reverse renal dysfunction and morphologic changes.

Thrombotic microangiopathy

The most severe form of acute toxicity is represented by thrombotic microangiopathy, which has been described both in CsA-treated and in TAC-treated renal transplant patients (Burke *et al.*, 1999; Pham *et al.*, 2002). Some 60% of these cases show a typical picture of *hemolytic–uremic syndrome* with acute renal failure, hypertension, microangiopathic hemolytic anemia, and thrombocytopenia. In the remaining patients systemic signs and symptoms may be absent and patients have thrombotic microangiopathy

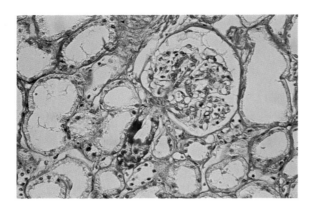

Figure 6.4 Cyclosporine arteriolopathy. A preglomerular arteriole shows severe nodular hyalinosis of the wall. (AFOG ×250) (Courtesy of Dr G Banfi, Ospedale Maggiore, Milan, Italy)

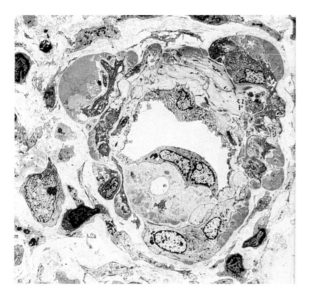

Figure 6.5 Cyclosporine ateriolopathy. At electron microscopy myocytes of a small arteriole show necrosis and cytoplasma filled with lumpy amorphous material. (×4800) (Courtesy of Professor M Mihatsch, University of Basel, Switzerland

localized to the graft (Schwimmer *et al.*, 2003). It should be noted that in the absence of extra-renal signs and symptoms the diagnosis may be missed or delayed (Ruggenenti, 2002). *Histologically*, the character-istic features of thrombotic microangiopathy can be seen. Interlobular arteries, arterioles, and glomeruli show mucinoid intimal thickening, necrosis of the wall, thrombi, and narrowed lumens. The lesions may have a patchy distribution and variable severity (Figure 6.6).

The precise *pathogenesis* of calcineurin inhibitor-associated hemolytic–uremic syndrome is unknown. It is possible that the endothelial damage caused by ischemia–reperfusion injury (Land, 2005), viral infec-tion (Guetta *et al.*, 2001), and/or rejection may be amplified by the endothelial injury caused by CNI. The concomitant increased platelet aggregation, the anti-fibrinolysis induced by the increased expression of plasminogen activator inhibitor (Olyaei *et al.*, 2001), and the pro-necrotic activity of CNI on endothelial cells (Raymond *et al.*, 2003) may eventually lead to the development of thrombotic microangiopathy. The prognosis is better for patients with localized thrombotic microangiopathy (Schwimmer *et al.*, 2003).

Treatment should first consist of prompt withdrawal of the offending drug. Conversion to sirolimus (Yango *et al.*, 2002), or a switch to another calcineurin inhibitor (Franz *et al.*, 1998) could obtain recovery in some patients; however, such a maneuver should be made with great caution, as all these drugs may be responsible for thrombotic microangiopathy. Plasma infusion and/or plasmapheresis may improve

Table 6.2 Differential histologic diagnosis between rejection and calcineurin inhibitor (CNI) toxicity. Adapted from Mihatsch et al., 1995

	Rejection	CNI toxicity	Common features
Arteries (arcuate, interlobular)	Endarteritis Proliferation, necrosis, subendothelial infiltrates		
Arterioles	Associated with artery changes	CNI arteriolopathy	Arteriolar hyalinosis
Tubules	Tubulitis	Isometric vacuolization Giant mitochondria Microcalcifications	Necrosis, vacuoles
Interstitium	Diffuse cellular infiltrate Interstitial fibrosis in advanced phase	Cell infiltrate Striped interstitial fibrosis Diffuse interstitial infiltrate in advanced phase	Cell infiltrate Interstitial fibrosis
Glomeruli	Acute glomerulopathy (rare)	Thrombosis in cases of hemolytic–uremic syndrome	Glomerulosclerosis in advanced phase

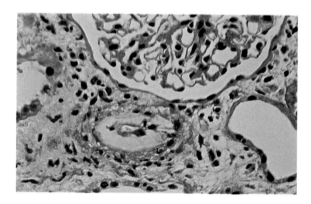

Figure 6.6 Hemolytic-uremic syndrome-like cyclosporine arteriolopathy. A preglomerular arteriole shows mucinoid initimal thickening with severe luminal restriction. (AFOG ×400)

thrombocytopenia, but their role in preventing renal lesions has been challenged (Moake, 2002). However, Karthikeyan *et al.* (2003) reported the recovery of graft function in 23 of 29 cases of post-transplant thrombotic microangiopathy, who stopped calcineurin inhibitors and were treated with plasmapheresis for a mean of 8.5 days. Continuation of the same calcineurin inhibitor may lead to irreversible lesions and eventually to graft failure.

Chronic renal toxicity

The main problem with the use of CNI is the possible development of progressive nephrotoxicity.

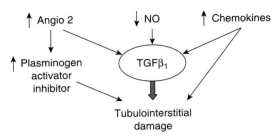

Figure 6.7 Pathogenesis of nephrotoxicity induced by calcineurin inhibitors. Both cyclosporine and tacrolimus cause systemic and renal vasoconstriction, by increasing angiotensin 2 (angio 2) production and endothelin-1 synthesis, and by decreasing nitric oxide (NO) synthesis. Vasoconstriction coupled with endothelial lesions may induce profound ischemia eventually leading to interstitial fibrosis and tubular atrophy. Moreover, angiotensin 2 and the reduced synthesis of NO together with the increased production of chemokines enhance the expression of TGFβ₁ and plasminogen activator inhibitor that may also lead to interstitial fibrosis and tubular atrophy either directly or through the mediation of SMAD

Pathophysiology

The mechanisms responsible for this chronic nephropathy have not been completely elucidated. Both cyclosporine and tacrolimus can cause renal and systemic vasoconstriction, through increased release of endothelin-1, activation of the renin–angiotensin system, increased production of thromboxane A_2, and decreased production of vasodilators such as nitric oxide and prostacyclin (Olyaei *et al.*, 2001). The profound vasoconstriction together with the typical arteriolar lesions may induce ischemia, with consequent tubular atrophy and interstitial fibrosis. However, CNI may also increase the levels of plasminogen activator inhibitor (PAI), an inducer of interstitial fibrosis and tubular atrophy and an inhibitor of matrix degradation (Border and Noble, 1994). PAI may favor the recruitment of interstitial cells (Matsuo *et al.*, 2005), and enhances the expression of mRNA transforming growth factor-β_1 (TGFβ₁), which represents a central mediator of fibrogenic remodeling processes (Figure 6.7). TGFβ is a biologically multipotent regulatory protein implicated in functions that include the regulation of cellular growth, differentiation, extracellular matrix formation, and wound healing. This cytokine may induce transdifferentiation to myofibroblasts and extracellular matrix production either directly (Dai *et al.*, 2003) or through the activation of the signal pathway of several intracellular SMAD proteins that exert different roles in regulating cell growth, differentiation, and apoptosis (Hill, 2006). In response to TGFβ, SMAD 3 increases the expression of connective-tissue factor while SMAD 2 increases the expression of alpha smooth-muscle actin (Phanish *et al.*, 2006). In contrast, SMAD 7 and 8 inhibit the signal pathway (Dai *et al.*, 2003). Therefore, the response to the increased expression of TGF is the result of a complex interplay between different SMAD proteins (Figure 6.8). Important roles are also played by phosphatases, which may inactivate SMAD phosphorylation (Chen *et al.*, 2006), and by the molecular crosstalk between profibrogenic TGFβ and antifibrogenic IFNγ. Overexpression of TGFβ or inadequate contra-regulation enhances the expression of some cytokines such as platelet-derived growth factor (PDGF) and fibroblast growth factor, and of vasoactive proteins such as endothelin, which can lead to cellular proliferation, hypertension, and chronic allograft dysfunction (Sharma *et al.*, 1996; Paul, 1999).

Several *drugs* have been used in experimental models to prevent chronic toxicity. They include a novel antifibrotic compound called pirfenidone (Shihab *et al.*, 2002), melatonin (Longoni *et al.*, 2002), colchicine (Li *et al.*, 2002), carvedilol (Padi and Chopra, 2002), magnesium supplementation (Asai *et al.*, 2002), and high-dose spironolactone (Feria *et al.*, 2003).

Clinical and histologic features

Clinically, the chronic nephropathy caused by calcineurin inhibitors is indistinguishable from chronic rejection, being characterized by a slowly progressive graft dysfunction, hypertension, and mild to moderate proteinuria. At *renal biopsy*, the chronic toxic nephropathy is heralded by *arteriolar lesions* characterized

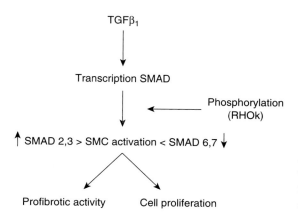

TGFβ$_1$

Transcription SMAD

Phosphorylation (RHOk)

$\uparrow$ SMAD 2,3 > SMC activation < SMAD 6,7 $\downarrow$

Profibrotic activity   Cell proliferation

Figure 6.8 TGFβ$_1$ activates the signal pathway of SMAD proteins by phosphorylation. This pathway may be regulated by phosphatases that inactivate SMAD activity. There is a balance between some SMAD favoring activation of smooth muscle cells and SMAD inhibiting activation. Activated smooth muscle cells induce profibrotic activity and cell proliferation

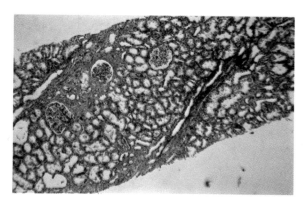

Figure 6.9 'Stripe-fibrosis' of the interstitium suggesting chronic cyclosporine toxicity. (AFOG ×80) (Courtesy of Dr G Banfi, Ospedale Maggiore, Milan Itlay)

by either a mucinoid intimal thickening similar to that seen in hemolytic–uremic syndrome or by nodular hyaline deposits replacing myocytes as seen in malignant hypertension (Mihatsch *et al.*, 1995). At a later stage, scarring of arterioles, glomerular obsolescence, and *striped interstitial fibrosis* (Figure 6.9) may develop, eventually leading to diffuse interstitial fibrosis and glomerular sclerosis. The dimensions of the involved vessels may allow the differentiation of toxic nephropathy from chronic rejection. While only small vessels are affected in the case of renal toxicity, the vascular lesions in chronic rejection can affect not only arterioles but also arcuated and interlobular arteries (Mihatsch *et al.*, 1995). However, in many biopsies, large vessels are not present; in other instances, chronic toxicity and chronic rejection may coexist, so that a firm diagnosis of chronic toxicity caused by CsA or tacrolimus may often be very difficult or even impossible. Although it is possible that chronic rejection and nephrotoxicity may coexist in the same patient, the presence of C4d deposits in peritubular capillaries, which is now considered a marker of antibody-mediated rejection (Racusen *et al.*, 2002), may indicate that immunological factors are prevailing over nephrotoxicity in determining the chronic lesions in that particular case. A small randomized study reported, at 1-year protocol biopsy, a significant increase in interstitial fibrosis in transplant recipients assigned to CsA (Neoral®) compared with those given tacrolimus (Murphy *et al.*, 2003). However, patients with tacrolimus nephrotoxicity exhibited an increased expression of TGFβ and profibrogenic genes, compared with CsA nephrotoxicity (Khanna *et al.*, 2002). Other studies based on sequential graft biopsies showed that TGF expression in the transplanted kidney may progressively increase even in the absence of acute events (Jain *et al.*, 2002).

Impact on long-term graft function

Although nephrotoxicity caused by calcineurin inhibitors remains a major concern for long-term kidney allograft function, its real impact on the long-term graft outcome is still a matter of controversy. Some investigators reported that, in the long term, practically all CsA-treated transplant patients showed histo-logic signs of nephrotoxicity, but in spite of this the 10-year kidney graft survival was 95% (Nankivell et al., 2003). Other groups reported excellent long-term graft survival (Ponticelli et al., 2002; Sijpkens et al., 2003) and stable, although subnormal, graft function, for 12 years or more (Matas et al., 1995; Ponticelli et al., 1999), without histologic signs of nephrotoxicity in patients with deteriorating renal function or graft loss (Lipkowitz et al., 1999). Thus, severe nephrotoxicity is not an inexorable complication of the chronic use of CNI, but largely depends on a number of factors, including the 'quality' of the transplanted kidney, the doses of CNI used, and the concomitant use of other nephrotoxic drugs, or of agents that interfere with the pharmacokinetics of CNI.

Nevertheless, it should be recognized that the use of CNI in a renal transplant recipient is a difficult task. The administration of too-low doses in order to prevent nephrotoxicity exposes the patient to the risk of chronic rejection (Opelz and Dohler, 2001), while the use of high doses to prevent rejection can cause progressive graft dysfunction. As both cyclosporine (Kahan et al., 1996) and tacrolimus (Staatz et al., 2002) have variations in bioavailability and pharmacokinetics, periodic determinations of peak levels or areas-under-the-curve, which are more reliable than trough levels, are necessary to optimize the therapeutic index of these agents. The monitoring of blood levels of CsA 2 h after administration (C2) is now widely adopted as an accurate measurement of drug exposure (Keown, 2002). It should also be pointed out that there is a strong interaction between calcineurin inhibitors and sirolimus (Kelly and Kahan, 2002), which can lead to an enhancement of efficacy but also of renal toxicity.

Prevention and treatment

To *prevent* the potential toxicity of CNI, different approaches have been proposed. A first approach may consist of halving the dose of cyclosporine after 1 year in transplant patients with stable renal function. In a small randomized trial, such a maneuver was not associated with rejection, while renal function significantly improved (Pascual et al., 2003). In patients given CsA–sirolimus and steroids, different strategies have been proposed. In a multicenter randomized trial, renal transplant recipients were randomly allocated to the above regimen or to continue with triple therapy after the third month. Patients were followed for 4 years. The group without cyclosporine showed significantly better creatinine clearance, particularly in patients with creatinine clearance <45 ml/min at randomization. Graft survival was also better in CsA-free patients, but the difference was not significant (Russ et al., 2005).

Another strategy consists of minimizing the dose of CsA in association with everolimus. In a random-ized trial, patients assigned to receive low doses of CsA had significantly less rejection and better creati-nine clearance at 3 years than patients given standard doses of cyclosporine (Nashan et al., 2004).

A third approach is that of completely avoiding the use of calcineurin inhibitors. Grinyo et al. (2005) treated 30 patients with thymoglobulin, mycophenolate mofetil (MMF), and steroids. Seven patients had acute rejection and were given cyclosporine; in nine other patients CsA was added, as MMF had to be reduced to <1 g per day. The patient and graft survival rates at 5 years were, respectively, 79% and 65%. The mean level of serum creatinine at 5 years was 218 µmol/l. Larson et al. (2006) randomized 165 patients to sirolimus–MMF–prednisone or to tacrolimus–MMF–prednisone. At 1 year there was no differ-ence in patient survival, graft survival, iothalamate clearance, clinical acute rejection, and hypertension. Also, the chronicity index at graft biopsy was similar, although there were fewer chronic vascular changes in the sirolimus group. Taken together, these results do not show a particular benefit with calcineurin-free immunosuppression.

If there is a progressive *increase in plasma creatinine*, reduction of the dosage of calcineurin inhibitors may obtain reversal or stabilization of renal dysfunction in some patients (Mourad et al., 1998). A more strik-ing reduction or even discontinuation of cyclosporine after the introduction of MMF have been successfully tried in some patients (Houde et al., 2000; Weir, 2001), but in other patients these maneuvers led to rejection or even to graft loss (Smak Gregoor *et al.*, 2000; Abramowicz *et al.*, 2005). Similar results have been reported after conversion to sirolimus. Better graft function (Dominguez *et al.*, 2000) and graft survival (Stallone *et al.*, 2005) were seen in patients after conversion to sirolimus by some investigators. Others, however, reported that about half of the patients showed an improvement while the remaining patients had a renal function deterioration after switching from calcineurin inhibitors to sirolimus (Citterio *et al.*, 2003; Diekmann *et al.*, 2004), the risk being more elevated in patients with proteinuria. The results were particularly poor in patients with elevated serum creatinine (Boratynska *et al.*, 2006). Therefore, it is recommended that caution should be exercised before completely stopping calcineurin inhibitors. Patients should be closely monitored in order to determine the possible onset of proteinuria or a further increase in serum creatinine.

Neurologic complications (see also Chapter 16)

Calcineurin plays an important role in the diverse functions of the nervous system, as it regulates synaptic transmission, ion channels, and gene transcription (Tan and Robinson, 2006). Tremor, burning paresthesias, headache, and flushing are possible side-effects of CNI. These complications are usually dose-dependent and tend to be more frequent with TAC than with CsA (Margreiter, 2002). A few cases of reversible posterior leukoencephalopathy have been reported, more often in children (Bechstein, 2000). Other severe symptoms include disabling pain syndrome, hallucinations, seizures, cerebellar ataxia, and motor weakness (Ponticelli and Campise, 2005). Sirolimus, but not everolimus, enhances the negative effects of cyclosporine on mitochondrial metabolism in the rat brain (Serkova *et al.*, 2001).

Diabetes

Both CsA and TAC can cause hyperglycemia, by inducing an acquired insulin sensitivity defect (Mora, 2005). Their diabetogenic effect is strongly enhanced by the concomitant administration of corticosteroids. There is agreement that tacrolimus is more diabetogenic than cyclosporine (Gourishankar *et al.*, 2004; Martinez-Castelao *et al.*, 2005; Wong *et al.*, 2005), probably because it also exerts a direct toxicity on islet cells (Tamura *et al.*, 1995). Older patients, obese patients, the carriers of hepatis C virus, and those receiving steroid pulses are at increased risk of developing diabetes (Markell, 2004; Araki *et al.*, 2006).

Gastrointestinal complications

About 10% of patients complain of some gastric symptoms, namely anorexia, nausea, and vomiting. These side-effects are usually mild, but may be aggravated by the concomitant administration of other drugs (Ponticelli and Passerini, 2005).

CNI alter calcium fluxes across hepatocyte cell membranes, elevate bile acids, and decrease bile flow. As a consequence, an elevation in serum bilirubin and/or transaminase levels may occur. Rarely, a cholestatic syndrome may also develop (Ganschow *et al.*, 2006).

Hypertension

Hypertension represents a frequent complication of CNI. It is more frequent and severe with CsA than with TAC (Margreiter, 2002). As pointed out earlier, CNI may cause systemic vasoconstriction, which increases the peripheral vascular resistance. Moreover, the vasoconstrictive effect on afferent preglomerular arterioles enhances the proximal resorption of sodium chloride, with consequent volume expansion. As a result, there is an increased cardiac output and volume-dependent hypertension may develop (Luke, 1991). Although the plasma renin levels are often normal, they may be inappropriately high before volume expansion, and may concur in causing hypertension (Figure 6.10). Calcium channel blockers are probably the most effective drugs for treating CNI-induced hypertension. It should be remembered, however, that non-dihydropyridinic calcium channel blockers may substantially increase the blood levels of CNI.

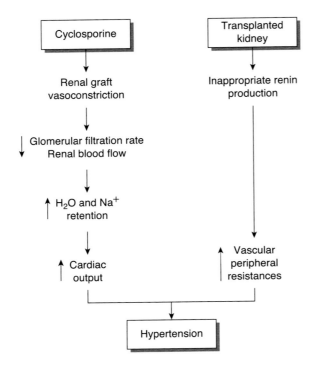

Figure 6.10 Pathogenesis of cyclosporine-induced hypertension

Hyperlipidemia

CNI may increase LDL and VLDL cholesterol levels, VLDL triglyceride levels, and apolipoprotein B and lipoprotein(a). Of note, hypercholesterolemia is significantly less frequent in transplant patients given tacrolimus than in those treated with cyclosporine (Johnson *et al.*, 2000; Artz *et al.*, 2003). CsA may inhibit the enzyme 26-hydroxylase, hence decreasing the synthesis of bile acids from cholesterol and the transport of cholesterol to the intestines. Cyclosporine also binds to the LDL receptor, which results in increased serum levels of LDL cholesterol and impairs the clearance of VLDL and LDL by decreasing lipoprotein lipase activity (Kobashigawa and Kasiske, 1997). Moreover, CsA increases LDL oxidation (Bosmans *et al.*, 2001).

Statins (HMG-CoA reductase inhibitors) are the drugs of choice for treating hypercholesterolemia. Although some investigators reported increased cyclosporine exposure under statin treatment (Lepre *et al.*, 1999), other studies found that the area-under-the-curve of cyclosporine is only slightly influenced by simvastatin, pravastatin, or atorvastatin (Knopp, 1999; Asberg, 2003).

Dermatologic complications (see also Chapter 14)

CsA may cause *hypertrichosis* on the face, arms, shoulders, and back, and is particularly troublesome in young women and children, particularly if dark-haired. This disorder is dose-dependent, and, at least in experimental animals, seems to be related to the inhibition of NFAT in follicular keratinocytes (Gafter-Gvili *et al.*, 2003). CsA may also cause *gingival hyperplasia* by increasing the number of fibroblasts and the production of collagen by them. Scrupulous oral hygiene is necessary to prevent inflammation, which may impair gingival hypertrophy. A 5-day treatment with azithromycin is sufficient to reduce significantly gingival overgrowth (Chand *et al.*, 2004). Both the above disorders may reverse after switching from CsA to TAC (Thorp *et al.*, 2000). *Alopecia* has been reported in women treated with TAC (Tricot *et al.*, 2005).

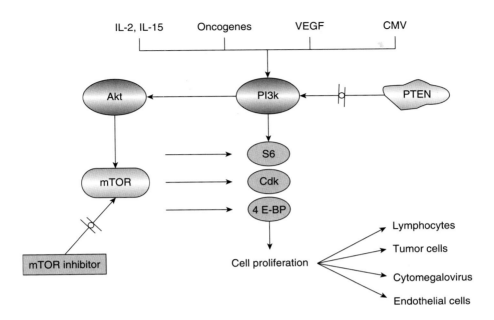

Figure 6.11 A number of factors may stimulate a kinase family governed by phosphatidylinositol 3 kinase (PI3k). In response to IL-2 or IL-5, the Jak 3 kinase is stimulated and PI3k is activated. In turn, PI3k activates a cascade of kinases through different steps of phosphorylation. The final result is a signal of proliferation for lymphocytes. A key role in this cascade of kinases is played by mTOR which is the downstream effector of PI3k. Sirolimus and everolimus enter the cytoplasm and bind to a receptor called FKBP-12. The receptor–drug complex inhibits the activity of mTOR and therefore inhibits the signal for lymphocyte proliferation

mTOR inhibitors

Sirolimus is a macrolide lactone produced naturally by *Streptomyces hygroscopicus*. The drug has a long half-life, about 62 hours, and a high concentration in the brain. Its derivate *everolimus* has a similar chemical structure, but a covalently bound 2-hydroxyethyl group was introduced at position 40 to improve bioavailability and reduce the half-life to about 26 hours (Kovarik et al., 2001; Kovarik, 2004).

Mechanisms of action

After oral administration, mTOR (mammalian target of rapamycin) inhibitors enter the cells and bind to a specific cytoplasmic receptor, FKBP-12, the same receptor as that for tacrolimus. However, different from tacrolimus, the drug–receptor complex does not inhibit the enzymatic activity of calcineurin, but rather blocks the serine-threonine kinase known as mTOR. This kinase is the downstream effector of phosphatidylinositol 3 kinase (PI3k), which, together with a protein kinase B (Akt), governs several signal pathways by activating a cascade of other kinases that provide the signals for cell proliferation. A number of different stimuli – including IL-2, IL-15, oncogenic proteins, vascular endothelial growth factor (VEGF), and CMV – may activate PI3k (Figure 6.11). In response to IL-2 and/or IL-15, PI3k activates a cascade of kinases that provide the signal for T cell proliferation. mTOR antagonists inhibit this pathway, thus interfering with the stimulus leading to T cell proliferation. Besides immunosuppressive activity, these agents show protective effects on the endothelium, and may inhibit CMV proliferation in the host cells (Ponticelli, 2004). Of great importance, mTOR antagonists also exert antitumor activity, either alone or in combination with cytotoxic agents. There are a large number of ongoing clinical trials with these agents

Table 6.3 Types of cancer that may benefit from treatment with mTOR inhibitors

Upstream of mTOR

Loss of PTEN
  glioblastoma
  prostate cancer
  endoimetrial cancer
PI3k/Akt overactivity
  breast cancer
  chronic myeloid leukemia
  ovarian cancer

Downstream of mTOR

Overexpression of mTOR regulators (cyclin D1, Myc)
  mantle cell lymphoma
  breast, kidney cancer
  Burkitt's lymphoma

in lymphoma, prostate cancer, and other types of cancer, caused by an overactivity of PI3k, a deficiency of the physiological inhibitor of PI3k (PTEN), or overexpression of mTOR (Table 6.3).

Both sirolimus and everolimus have important immunosuppressive properties and may synergize with CNI. In fact, while CNI interfere with the synthesis of IL-2 and other cytokines, mTOR antagonists inhibit the response to IL-2 and IL-15. CNI interfere with the cell cycle between G_0 and G_1, while mTOR antagonists inhibit the cell cycle between G_1 and S. There are also pharmacological interactions between CNI and mTOR inhibitors. CsA increases the area-under-the curve of mTOR inhibitors, but not vice versa.

Side-effects

The side-effects of mTOR antagonists are mainly related to their antiproliferative activities (Table 6.4). On the other hand, by inhibiting the signals for cell proliferation, mTOR antagonists can also protect against CMV and other viral infections, can exert antioncogenic activity, and can prevent endothelial cell proliferation and consequent intimal thickening of the vessels (Ponticelli, 2004).

Hyperlipidemia

The most frequent side-effect of mTOR inhibitors is represented by hyperlipidemia. These drugs may increase the serum levels of total cholesterol, LDL cholesterol, triglycerides, and apo C-III. In a study, 80% of renal transplant recipients treated with sirolimus had cholesterolemia higher than 240 mg/dl, and 78% had triglyceridemia higher than 200 mg/dl (Chueh and Kahan, 2003). A similar prevalence has been found for everolimus-treated renal transplant recipients (Kovarik et al., 2002). Of note, the risk of hyperlipidemia is significantly higher in patients with apoliporotein E 3/3 genotype (Maluf et al., 2005), suggesting a contributing role of genetic factors. Lipid abnormalities are probably the result of complex interferences of the class of mTOR inhibitors on lipid metabolism. Experimental and clinical studies showed that everolimus as well as sirolimus may upregulate apolipoprotein C-III (Hoogeveen et al., 2001), reduce the catabolism of VLDL apo B100-containing lipoproteins (Morrissett et al., 2002), alter the insulin signaling pathway with increased hepatic synthesis of triglycerides and increased secretion of VLDL (Deters et al., 2004), and/or

Table 6.4   Potential side-effects of mTOR inhibitors

Metabolic	Hematologic	Renal	Surgical	Miscellaneous
Hypercholesterolemia	Thrombocytopenia	Tubular toxicity	Retarded wound healing	Interstitial pneumonia
Hypertriglyceridemia Diabetes?	Anemia Hemolytic–uremic syndrome	Proteinuria Thrombotic microangiopathy	Lymphocele	Mouth ulcers Joint pain
				Edema

impair bile salt synthesis with consequent hypercholesterolemia (Kirklin *et al.*, 2002; Deters *et al.*, 2004). The co-administration of hyperlipidemic drugs such as cyclosporine and corticosteroids may aggravate lipid abnormalities.

Statins should be part of drug regimen in organ transplant recipients with hypercholesterolemia (Fellstrom *et al.*, 2004). Statins are generally well tolerated, but potential interactions with drugs metabolized by the P450 cytochrome enzymatic system, such as cyclosporine, tacrolimus, and mTOR antagonists, may potentiate the risk of myopathy (Goldberg and Roth, 1996). It is therefore advisable not to exceed daily doses of 40 mg with fluvastatin or 20 mg with simvastatin, pravastatin, or atorvastatin. Studies with sirolimus and with everolimus showed that hyperlipidemia tends to improve over time (Blum, 2002; Nashan *et al.*, 2004; Vitko *et al.*, 2004). Immunosuppressive strategies minimizing doses of cyclosporine and corticosteroids may help in controlling hyperlipidemia. *Fibrates* are effective in reducing hypertriglyceridemia but may expose patients to the risk of myopathy and rhabdomyolysis. These side-effects are dose-dependent, and are more frequent in patients with renal insufficiency, or in those also given HMG-CoA reductase inhibitors. A number of patients may also show an increase in serum creatinine during treatment with fenofibrates, bezafibrates, and ciprofibrates, but not with gemfibrozil (Broeders *et al.*, 2000).

Glucose intolerance

There are conflicting data about the interference of mTOR inhibitors in diabetes. Some studies showed that sustained activation of mTOR signaling is a critical event, rendering the insulin-receptor substrate irresponsive to insulin (Shah *et al.*, 2004). Therefore, mTOR inhibitors should restore the sensitivity of the insulin-receptor substrate to insulin. On the other hand, phosphorylation of proteins plays an important role in regulating insulin secretion. In pancreatic β cells, protein phosphatase 2A changes its activity in the presence of glucose and inhibitors and probably plays a key role in insulin secretion (Parameswara *et al.*, 2005). Thus, the inhibition of the serine–threonine phosphatase mTOR might favor the onset of diabetes. Teutonico *et al.* (2005) reported that conversion from cyclosporine to sirolimus was associated with a 30% increased incidence of impaired glucose tolerance, and with some patients developing new-onset diabetes.

Bone marrow toxicity

Thrombocytopenia and *anemia* may occur in patients treated with mTOR inhibitors, but they are usually mild, unless they occur in the context of a hemolytic–uremic syndrome. However, about 48% of renal transplant recipients were reported to have thrombocytopenia when sirolimus was associated with MMF (Kreis *et al.*, 2000). The late introduction of sirolimus may induce anemia, probably because of a chronic inflammatory state due to defective IL-10-dependent inflammatory autoregulation (Thaunat *et al.*, 2005). When given in combination with MMF, mTOR inhibitors may cause microcytosis, independent from iron depletion (Kim *et al.*, 2006). Rare cases of severe bone marrow hypoplasia have been reported (Joist *et al.*, 2006).

Renal toxicity

Experimental studies showed that sirolimus can cause *tubular toxicity* characterized by tubular collapse, vacuolization, and nephrocalcinosis (Andoh *et al.*, 1996). The drug may also impair the recovery of renal function after ischemia–reperfusion injury, both by increasing the apoptosis of tubular cells and by inhibiting the regenerative response of tubular cells (Lieberthal *et al.*, 2001).

Initial controlled trials showed that, in combination with standard doses of CsA, both sirolimus (Kahan, 2000) and everolimus (Vitko *et al.*, 2004) administration was associated with *increased serum creatinine* when compared with MMF. This effect might be caused by an increased expression of $TGF\beta_1$ when CsA is combined with mTOR agents (Shihab *et al.*, 2004). Clinical studies showed that the risk of nephrotoxicity in patients given a combination of CsA and everolimus was mainly related to blood concentrations of CsA, while the blood levels of everolimus had little impact (Lorber *et al.*, 2005). More recent trials showed that withdrawing CsA after 3 months in patients treated with CsA and sirolimus (Russ *et al.*, 2005), or minimizing the dose of CsA when given in combination with everolimus (Nashan *et al.*, 2004; Vitko *et al.*, 2004), may prevent the increase in serum creatinine without reducing the anti-rejection efficacy.

Up to 30% of renal transplant recipients may develop *proteinuria* within 1 year after conversion from cyclosporine to a mTOR inhibitor (Sennesael *et al.*, 2005). The appearance of proteinuria might be attributable to the fact that a pre-existing proteinuria was masked by cyclosporine, which has a well-known anti-proteinuric effect. However, it is likely that mTOR inhibitors may also cause proteinuria by other mechanisms. Experimental studies showed that mTOR inhibitors may interfere with protein endocytosis in the tubular epithelial cell (Coombes *et al.*, 2005). Accordingly, an impaired tubular resorption of albumin has been demonstrated in a transplant patient treated with sirolimus (Straathof-Galema *et al.*, 2006). On the other hand, Saurina *et al.* (2006) showed that, after conversion from cyclosporine to sirolimus, there is an increase in intraglomerular pressure with a concomitant reduction of renal reserve, suggesting that proteinuria may be caused at least partially by glomerular hyperfiltration.

Whether the administration of mTOR inhibitors may improve or worsen *glomerular lesions* is still unknown. There are different results with different experimental models. Everolimus improved the development of puromycin aminonucleoside nephrosis, while it increased mesangial proliferation in a model of inflammatory glomerular disease (Daniel *et al.*, 2000). Sirolimus caused acute renal failure sustained by intratubular casts in a model of protein overload nephropathy (Coombes *et al.*, 2005), while it protected against tubulointerstitial changes in a model of experimental membranous nephropathy (Bonegio *et al.*, 2005). In a clinical study, four patients developed glomerulonephritis after conversion from CsA to sirolimus. In all cases proteinuria disappeared after sirolimus was stopped and CsA reintroduced. However, it is unclear how sirolimus might have induced different types of glomerulonephritis – IgA nephritis in two patients, membranoproliferative type 1 in another patient, and membranous nephropathy in a fourth patient – and how these chronic diseases improved rapidly after switching to CsA (Dittrich *et al.*, 2004). On the other hand, sirolimus significantly attenuated tubulointerstitial damage in a rat model of renal fibrosis, suggesting that mTOR inhibitors may have the potential to delay the progression of tubulointerstitial renal fibrosis (Wu *et al.*, 2006).

Thrombotic microangiopathy

Cases of *de novo* hemolytic–uremic syndrome caused by thrombotic microangiopathy have been reported in transplant patients given mTOR inhibitors in the context of contemporaneous or contiguous administration of calcineurin inhibitors (Langer *et al.*, 2002; Robson *et al.*, 2003; Saikali *et al.*, 2003; Fortin *et al.*, 2004; Crew *et al.*, 2005). It has been hypothesized that mTOR inhibitors may induce the downregulation of vascular endothelial growth factor, which is required for repairing endothelial damage caused by CNI (Sartelet *et al.*, 2005). However, mTOR inhibitors may also have an antiangiogenic activity that might account for the few cases of thrombotic microangiopathy observed in the marginal kidneys of transplant patients treated with sirolimus alone (Pelle *et al.*, 2005). Usually, withdrawal of the offending drug may obtain resolution of the disease, if the diagnosis is made early.

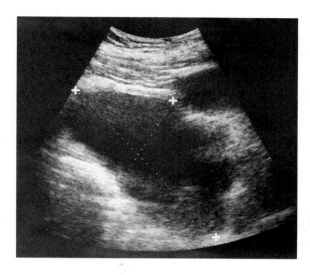

Figure 6.12 Large lymphocele cavity on ultrasonography. The greatest dimension is shown by transecting dotted lines

Wound healing and lymphocele

Retarded wound healing has been noted in patients treated with mTOR inhibitors (Valente *et al.*, 2003), probably as a consequence of their antiproliferative activity. However, a retrospective analysis of 513 renal transplant patients treated with different immunosuppressive therapies did not show any deleterious effects of sirolimus on wound healing. The only factor associated with delayed wound healing was obesity (Flechner *et al.*, 2003). Rather than mTOR inhibitors, the most likely culprits for delayed healing among the immunosuppressive agents used in transplantation are corticosteroids (Wicke *et al.*, 2000). Dietetic counseling of obese patients before transplantation and low-dose corticosteroids after transplantation can minimize the risk of delayed wound healing.

Lymphocele occurred in 6% of renal transplant patients given everolimus at a dose of 1.5 mg per day and in 15% of patients given everolimus at a dose of 3 mg per day (Vitko *et al.*, 2004). In a retrospective analysis, Langer and Kahan (2002) reported that 15.8% of patients treated with sirolimus–cyclosporine–steroids versus 4.4% of patients given cyclosporine and steroids required drainage or surgical procedures for perirenal fluid collections. Lymphocele is caused by the reduced healing of lymphatic vessels that are truncated during surgery. In most cases, lymphocele may resolve spontaneously or after povidone–iodine instillations. Only rarely is surgical intervention necessary (Figure 6.12). The risk of lymphocele is more elevated in patients with a body mass index higher than 30 and/or with acute rejection (Goel *et al.*, 2004). Careful hemostasis and clamping of lymphatics during transplant surgery may minimize the risk of lymphocele.

Interstitial pneumonia

A number of cases of *interstitial pneumonia* caused by sirolimus have been reported. Pham *et al.* (2004) analyzed 43 cases of pulmonary toxicity in patients treated with sirolimus. Although no case treated with everolimus has been reported, it is likely that this antiproliferative agent may also expose the lung to toxicity. Clinically, patients have presented with cough and dyspnea followed by fatigue and fever. Chest X-ray and computed tomography have shown bilateral patchy or diffuse alveolointerstitial infiltrates. Differential diagnosis from lung infection is difficult. Sirolimus discontinuation or reduction led to resolution within 3 weeks in most cases in the above study.

Mouth ulcers

Mouth ulcers have been reported in 24% of patients treated with sirolimus (Montalbano *et al.*, 2004). The development of mouth ulcers seems to be dose-related, as they can improve after dose reduction

(Schaffellner *et al.*, 2005). Painful oral ulcers seem to be particularly frequent and severe in patients given a combination of sirolimus and MMF. This may depend either on over-immunosuppression or on the use of sirolimus in the form of an oral emulsion rather than in the form of tablets (Van Gelder, 2003).

Joint pain

Joint pain has been reported in 23% of patients treated with sirolimus (Montalbano *et al.*, 2004). Pain may be disabling, but usually resolves with dose reduction (Pascual *et al.*, 2005) or drug withdrawal in more severe cases. It is possible that pain is caused by changes of circulation in the bone (Johnson, 2002). The simultaneous administration of cyclosporine may contribute to the development of joint pain, as calcineurin inhibitors may cause intraosseous vasoconstriction (Franco *et al.*, 2004).

Edema

Eyelid and/or leg edema may occur in everolimus-treated patients. These edemas are mild to moderate and usually reverse with low-dose furosemide.

Purine synthesis inhibitors

Activated T lymphocytes require the synthesis of nucleotides to proliferate and differentiate into T cell effectors. There are two main categories of antiproliferative agents that may inhibit the purine synthesis: azathioprine and mycophenolic acid.

Mechanisms of action

Azathioprine

Azathioprine is an *N*-methylnitroimidazole thiopurine which was developed in the early 1950s. It is an orally absorbed prodrug, being a modification of 6-mercaptopurine, which is in turn an analog of the purine basis hypoxanthine. After oral administration, azathioprine is rapidly transformed into 6-mercaptopurine by hepatic and erythrocyte glutathione. Mercaptopurine-containing nucleotides inhibit the synthesis and utilization of precursors of RNA and DNA, thus halting the proliferation of activated lymphocytes. There are two main pathways of degradation: direct oxidation by the enzyme xanthine oxidase, and *S*-methylation.

Mycophenolic acid

Mycophenolic acid is an antipurine that inhibits the enzyme inosine monophosphate dehydrogenase, by which means guanine is synthesized from inosine. As a consequence, the *de novo pathway* of purine synthesis is inhibited (Figure 6.13). Since activated lymphocytes rely more than other cells on *de novo* pathways, T and B cells are preferentially affected by mycophenolic acid, which causes an accumulation of lymphocytes at the G_1–S phase of the cell cycle (Allison *et al.*, 1993). There are two salts of mycophenolic acid, *mycophenolate mofetil* (MMF) and *sodium mycophenolate*.

Side-effects

Because of their immunosuppressive activity, the purine synthesis inhibitors may contribute to rendering the transplant patient more susceptible to infection and neoplasia. Most of the other side-effects are dose-dependent (Table 6.5).

Bone marrow toxicity

In *azathioprine*-treated patients, leukopenia is the most common manifestation of bone marrow toxicity, although thrombocytopenia and anemia with macrocytosis may also occur. These complications are usually dose-dependent, but in some patients with a genetic defect of thiopurine methyltransferase, which mediates *S*-methylation of 6-mercaptopurine, severe myelotoxicity may develop even with standard doses of azathioprine (Chocair *et al.*, 1992). Cases of bone marrow aplasia are rare. However, severe bone marrow suppression, often complicated by sepsis, occurs with the concomitant administration of azathioprine

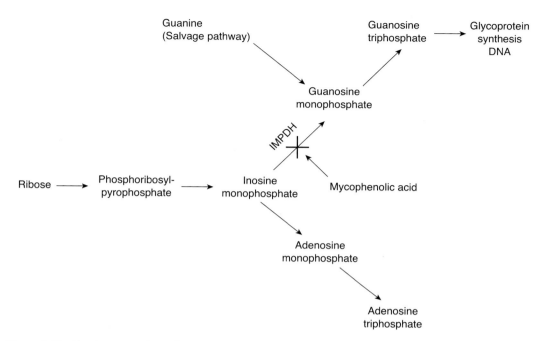

Figure 6.13 The de novo pathway for generation of guanosine monophosphate is dependent upon the conversion of inosine monophosphate by inosine monophosphate dehydrogenase (IMPDH), the site of inhibition by mycophenolic acid

Table 6.5   Potential side-effects of purine synthesis inhibitors

Hematologic	Gastrointestinal (mycophenolic acid)	Liver (azathioprine)	Respiratory (mycophenolic acid)	Inflammation (mycophenolic acid)
Leukopenia	Nausea	Cholestasis	Cough–dyspnea	Fever, arthralgias
Anemia	Vomiting			
Thrombocytopenia	Diarrhea			

and allopurinol, which blocks the xanthine oxidase necessary to oxidize 6-mercaptopurine to inactive metabolites. Whenever allopurinol is introduced, it should be recommended that azathioprine be reduced to one-third of the previous dosage or, even better, that azathioprine be replaced by mycophenolate, which is not degraded by xanthine oxidase.

The risk of leukopenia with *micophenolate salts* is increased in patients with high circulating levels of free mycophenolic acid (Weber *et al.*, 2002). Hypoalbuminemia and renal insufficiency may increase the level of mycophenolic acid, and are associated with hemotoxicity (Borrows *et al.*, 2006). Interaction between mycophenolic acid and valacyclovir may also lead to neutropenia (Royer *et al.*, 2003). Some studies reported that anemia is more frequent with MMF than with azathioprine (Yorgin *et al.*, 2002; Vanrenterghem *et al.*, 2003). Marked erythrocyte microcytosis without persistent anemia has been observed in patients treated with sirolimus and MMF (Kim *et al.*, 2006). Exceptionally, MMF may even cause aplastic anemia (Arbeiter *et al.*, 2000).

Gastrointestinal toxicity

Gastrointestinal discomfort is rare with *azathioprine*. Instead, nausea, vomiting, and diarrhea are relatively frequent in patients treated with *mycophenolic acid* (Behrend, 2001). These complications often require a dose reduction or even discontinuation of the drug. In these cases, an increased incidence of acute rejection has been reported (Knoll *et al.*, 2003; Pelletier *et al.*, 2003). In reviewing the data of the USRDS (United States Renal Data System), Hardinger *et al.* (2004) found that 21% of renal transplant recipients had to withdraw from MMF treatment because of gastrointestinal side-effects. The 4-year graft survival was significantly lower in patients who discontinued MMF than in those who continued the treatment. To mitigate the incidence and the impact of gastrointestinal disturbances, an enteric-coated formulation of mycophenolate sodium, Myfortic®, has been produced. Clinical trials have shown therapeutic equivalence between MMF and Myfortic (Budde *et al.*, 2004; Salvadori *et al.*, 2004).

Hepatic toxicity

Azathioprine may cause cholestasis, which presents with a reversible increase in serum transaminase and bilirubin. A rare but severe complication is represented by veno-occlusive hepatic disease, characterized histologically by the fibrous obliteration of terminal hepatic venules. This condition may cause portal hypertension and death. Early discontinuation of azathioprine may improve the outcome.

Hepatotoxicity with *mycophenolate* is rare. However, cases of increased liver enzymes, which returned to normal levels after reducing the dosage of MMF, have been reported (Balal *et al.*, 2005).

Pulmonary toxicity

In rare cases, MMF may cause dry cough and dyspnea. In most patients, symptoms develop within the third month, and may raise problems of differential diagnosis from pneumonitis. Exceptionally, MMF may lead to pulmonary fibrosis and acute respiratory failure (Gross *et al.*, 1997). The clinical symptoms reverse only after MMF discontinuation (Elli *et al.*, 1998).

Acute inflammatory syndrome

Maes *et al.* (2002) reported a new syndrome characterized by fever, arthralgias, oligoarthritis, and increased levels of C-reactive protein in two patients with Wegener's granulomatosis treated with MMF. After discontinuation of the drug, the symptoms reversed. Recently, a similar acute inflammatory syndrome has been described in a renal transplant recipient. The discontinuation of MMF resulted in complete resolution of the syndrome. The pathogenesis has been attributed to a paradoxical proinflammatory reaction of polymorphonuclear cells (Hochegger *et al.*, 2006).

Corticosteroids

Mechanisms of action

Corticosteroids have ubiquitous actions, affecting virtually every tissue. After dissociation from their plasma carrier protein called transcortin, the fat-soluble glucocorticoids enter the cell and bind to cytosolic receptors that are complexed to heat-shock protein and immunophilin. When the ligand binds, the receptor dissociates from the rest of the complex and translocates to the nucleus, through an allosteric change in conformation. Once having traversed the nuclear membrane, through nucleopores, the activated receptors bind to their acceptor sites and trigger the transcription of DNA to RNA transcripts in order to synthesize new proteins, usually enzymes, which can activate or inhibit the synthesis of some proteins. Thus, the biological mechanisms of corticosteroids largely depend on: (1) the number of available receptors, (2) the affinity for receptors, (3) the process of transcription and translation.

Corticosteroids interfere with each stage of *inflammation* by lowering chemotactic, oxygen burst, and cytotoxic activities, by inhibiting the synthesis of proinflammatory molecules – such as platelet activating factor, prostaglandins, and leukotrienes – and by inhibiting the release of tumor necrosis factor α and stabilizing the membranes of target cells. Corticosteroids also interfere with the *immune response*. These agents may inhibit the co-stimulation pathway by interfering with the expression of CD28 and CD40 ligand, and may also interfere with several other steps of the immune response, cellular immunity being more susceptible than humoral immunity. These effects are mainly mediated by stabilization of the inhibitory factor IκB, which blocks the generation of NFκB, a proinflammatory regulatory factor for cytokine gene transcription. When given at high doses intravenously, corticosteroids may also inhibit the alternative and amplification pathways of complement, may better stabilize the cell membrane, and can alter lymphocyte trafficking, promoting migration of these cells from the circulation (Ponticelli, 1997).

Side-effects

Due to their multiple interferences with the inflammatory and immune responses, it is not surprising that corticosteroids may also be responsible for a large number of side-effects (Table 6.6).

Cardiovascular complications

The sodium and water retention caused by corticosteroids may aggravate *congestive heart failure*.

Experimental (Tauchi *et al.*, 2001) and clinical studies (del Rincon *et al.*, 2004) also suggest the possibility that corticosteroids may be directly responsible for accelerated *atherosclerosis*. Corticosteroids may favor atherosclerosis by causing glucose intolerance, hyperlipidemia, obesity, and hypertension.

Corticosteroids may also produce *hypertension*. Hemodynamic changes, fluid retention, increased arterial contractile sensitivity (Yang and Zhang, 2004), suppression of nitric oxide (Williamson *et al.*, 2005), obesity (Rahmouni *et al.*, 2005), and perhaps a direct hypertensinogen action may concur in the pathogenesis of arterial hypertension.

In order to reduce the cardiovascular morbidity that represents the most frequent cause of death in renal transplant recipients, a number of trials with avoidance of corticosteroids have been performed. Unfortunately, most studies had a short-term follow-up. The only randomized trial with a long-term follow-up showed that renal transplant recipients assigned to receive steroid-free immunosuppression with CsA had significantly less cardiovascular events and a significantly lower mortality than patients assigned to receive steroids together with CsA (Montagnino *et al.*, 2001). Another strategy is based on the withdrawal of corticosteroids after some months. A meta-analysis of trials performed with modern immunosuppression reported that the incidence of acute rejection was significantly higher in patients assigned to steroid-free immunosuppression, but the risk of graft failure was lower. Mean cholesterol levels were significantly lower in patients who stopped corticosteroids (Pascual *et al.*, 2004).

Diabetes

Corticosteroids may cause glucose intolerance by inducing insulin resistance (Weir, 2001) and obesity. The risk of overt diabetes may depend on the dose and duration of steroid treatment, and is increased in patients with familial diabetes, in elderly patients, and in HCV-positive patients (Fabrizi *et al.*, 2005; Martinez-Castelao *et al.*, 2005). Usually, diabetes develops after weeks or months of steroid therapy. Immediately after intravenous high-dose methylprednisolone, severe hyperglycemia can occur. It usually reverses spontaneously, but in a few patients this hyperglycemia heralds the development of severe diabetes.

Obesity

Treatment with corticosteroids stimulates the appetite, and is associated with dose-dependent body-weight gain in many patients. Corticosteroid-induced obesity aggravates other corticosteroid-associated health risks. Insulin therapy in diabetic patients usually increases body weight (Kulkarni and Kaur, 2001).

Hyperlipidemia

Corticosteroids may enhance the activity of acetyl coenzyme A carboxylase and free fatty acid synthetase, may increase hepatic synthesis of VLDL, may downregulate LDL receptor activity of 3-hydroxy-3-methylglutaryl

Table 6.6 Potential side-effects of corticosteroids

Cardiovascular	Hyperlipidemia	Neuropsychiatric	Bone	Skin	Gastric	Muscular	Ocular	Other
Congestive heart failure	Hypercholesterolemia	Pseudotumor cerebri	Osteoporosis	Moon facies	Peptic ulcer	Myopathy	Cataract	Diabetes
Atherosclerosis	Hypertriglyceridemia	Psychiatric reactions	Aseptic necrosis	Buffalo hump		Tendinitis	Glaucoma	Obesity
Hypertension	Reduced HDL	Sleeplessness		Skin thinning				Growth retardation
	Increased VLDL			Bateman's purpura				
				Acne Maculopapulae				

coenzyme A (HMG-CoA) reductase, and may inhibit lipoprotein lipase (Kobashigawa and Kasiske, 1997). The final result is increased levels of VLDL, total cholesterol, and triglycerides and decreased levels of high-density lipoproteins.

Gastrointestinal complications

It is generally thought that corticosteroids increase the risk of peptic ulcer, but this assumption has been challenged by some studies. In a prospective trial it was shown that the increased risk of peptic ulcer in patients taking corticosteroids could be explained by the concomitant use of non-steroidal anti-inflammatory drugs (Piper *et al.*, 1991). Other studies showed that high doses of corticosteroids may contribute, along with stress, toward favoring the development of a peptic ulcer (Messman and Scholmerich, 2000), and a strong association between intravenous high-dose methylprednisolone pulses and development of a peptic ulcer has also been found (Chen *et al.*, 2004).

Neuropsychiatric complications

Pseudotumor cerebri is a well known complication of steroid therapy, which occurs mainly in children but rarely also in adults, after rapid withdrawal of corticosteroids. It is characterized by intracranial hypertension and papilledema, and is probably caused by rapid fluid shifts within the brain, resulting in intracranial hypertension. Pseudotumor cerebri can be managed with lumbar taps or increased doses of steroids.

Psychiatric reactions are not rare, particularly in patients with known psychological difficulties. Lithium carbonate is usually effective, while tricyclic antidepressants may worsen steroid-induced depression.

Sleeplessness is frequent, and may be minimized by using short-acting steroids given in a single-morning administration.

Muscular complications

The typical steroid-induced *myopathy* symmetrically involves proximal muscles of the lower extremities. The first complaint is the inability to climb stairs. Muscle enzymes are normal. Myopathy is not related to age or dosage. Improvement usually occurs when steroids are discontinued.

Tendon rupture is a rare complication, but it may occur more frequently when steroids are given in combination with CNI or fluoroquinolones.

Bone complications

Osteoporosis is a frequent complication of steroid therapy. Corticosteroids may cause osteopenia by decreasing the net intestinal calcium absorption and by increasing urinary calcium excretion. Moreover, steroids inhibit the secretion of growth hormone and decrease the production and/or bioactivity of some skeletal growth factors, such as insulin-like growth factor I and transforming growth factor-β_1. However, the main deleterious effect of corticosteroids is a direct inhibition of bone formation, as they inhibit osteoblast differentiation, induce apoptosis in mature osteoblasts as well as osteocytes (Weinstein *et al.*, 1998; Rojas *et al.*, 2003), and stimulate the proliferation and differentiation of human osteoclast precursors (Hirayama and Athanasou, 2002). While trabecular bone is particularly vulnerable, cortical bone is relatively spared even in long-term therapy.

Aseptic necrosis of hips and more rarely knees or shoulders usually occurs after long-term therapy, but may also develop in the first post-transplant weeks. Unilateral hip pain is the most common initial symptom. Although the cause of aseptic necrosis is still unknown, there are few doubts that corticosteroids are important contributors toward its development (Tang *et al.*, 2000).

Dermatologic effects

The redistribution of subcutaneous fat is responsible for *moon facies*, *buffalo hump*, and irregular adipose tissue accumulation. *Hirsutism, diffuse alopecia, skin thinning, telangiectasia, Bateman's purpura, purplish striae, acne, and maculopapular eruption* are frequent complications. These complications are partly related to effects occurring at the androgen receptor (Wright, 1995).

Ocular complications

Bilateral posterior subcapsular *cataract* is a dose- and time-related complication of steroid therapy.

Glaucoma is a dose-related complication. Patients with diabetes, myopia, or a familial history of glaucoma have an increased risk.

Growth retardation

Corticosteroids impair statural growth in children and adolescents, which is already altered by chronic renal failure. The effect of corticosteroids is probably related to a reduced response of receptors to the stimulation of growth hormone and to a reduced local production of insulin-like growth factor. Successful transplantation with steroid-free immunosuppression may improve catch-up growth and the weight/height index (Ghio *et al.*, 1992).

Recently, recombinant human growth hormone (rhGH) has been made available. A review of North American Pediatric Renal Transplant data showed that recipients who received treatment with rhGH had superior final adult height compared with well-matched untreated controls. No increased incidence of adverse events was noted in the rhGH-treated group. The authors concluded that rhGH is effective and safe for use in growth-retarded pediatric renal allograft recipients (Fine and Stablein, 2005).

Wound-healing retardation

Corticosteroids may be responsible for wound healing retardation, as they decrease $TGF\beta_1$ and IGFI levels and tissue deposition in the wound (Wicke *et al.*, 2000) and interfere with epithelial cell restoration and proliferation (Jung *et al.*, 2001). The use of high doses in the early post-transplant period may enhance these effects.

Withdrawal of corticosteroids

The suppression of ACTH release and cortisol secretion can occur after long-term steroid administration. The dosage should therefore be gradually reduced and discontinued only after reaching minimal doses (i.e. prednisone 2.5 mg per day or, even better, 5 mg every other day). In the case of serious infection, operation, or injury, patients should receive supplementary hormone.

Biological reagents

Antilymphocyte antibodies (ALG)

Xenogenic polyclonal antibodies directed against human lymphocytes were first prepared for clinical use in horses. However, the available products today are antithymocyte globulins (ATG) represented by purified, pasteurized IgG obtained by immunizing rabbits with thymus-derived human lymphocytes. The mechanism of action of ALG/ATG is not completely elucidated. As both of them may result in a profound reduction in the T lymphocyte count, it is possible to speculate that these agents may cause a T cell clearance from the circulation, or modulate T cell activation, or exert a cytotoxic effect. When given at high doses, ATG may also decrease the number of B cells and NK cells (Giebel *et al.*, 2005), and may modify the expression levels of leukocyte adhesion molecules required for cell adhesion (Beiras-Fernandez *et al.*, 2005).

ALG/ATG are strongly irritating for the veins, and should therefore be infused into high-flow veins. Infusion should last at least 6 hours for the first treatment and not less than 4 hours in the following days. The infusion may be complicated by a number of adverse events (Table 6.7). Therefore, some precautions should be taken. They include premedication with methylprednisolone (0.5 g IV), oral acetaminophen, and/or antihistamine drugs, 1 hour before starting the infusion. It is also recommended to start prophylaxis against CMV infection with intravenous ganciclovir or with valganciglovir. In fact, the intense immunosuppression can increase the incidence and severity of *opportunistic infection*, particularly CMV and EBV infections. The most worrying complication is represented by the development of *lymphoproliferative* disorders (Opelz and Dohler, 2004).

Table 6.7   Side-effects of ALG/ATG infusion

Side-effect	%
Fever, chills	63
Leukopenia	57
Pain	46
Headache	40
Diarrhea	37
Hypertension	37
Thrombocytopenia	37
Dyspnea	28
Anaphylactic reaction	1

Anti-CD3 monoclonal antibody (OKT3)

OKT3 is a monoclonal antibody produced by hybridomas generated from the fusion of mouse plasmacy-toma cells and splenic cells that produce an antibody directed against the CD3 receptor. OKT3 has been successfully used either to delay and reduce the incidence of acute rejection or for the treatment of steroid-resistant rejection (Ortho Multicenter Study Group 1985). A recent meta-analysis did not show any benefit of OKT3 over ATG or ALG in reversing rejection (Webster et al., 2006).

A major problem with OKT3 is the *cytokine release syndrome* caused by T cell activation following anti-body binding to the T cell receptor. The first symptoms usually occur within 2 hours after the first intra-venous administration, and may include hyperpyrexia, chills, tremor, dyspnea, chest pain, wheezing, nausea, and vomiting. The more severe complications include pulmonary edema, aseptic meningitis, and blurred vision (Ponticelli and Campise, 2005). Cases of impaired kidney function (Wever et al., 1996) and hemolytic uremic syndrome (Doutrelepont et al., 1992) have also been reported. Several strategies have been sug-gested to prevent this severe syndrome, including premedication with methylprednisolone at doses not higher than 8 mg/kg to prevent hypercoagulation (Abramowicz et al., 1996), low-dose OKT3, i.e. 2 mg instead of 5 mg (Machado et al., 2002), and slow infusion instead of rapid injection. Moreover, it is recom-mended that any possible overhydration be corrected before the first administration either with dialysis or with intravenous furosemide, to prevent the possible development of pulmonary edema (Table 6.8).

Another possible disadvantage of OKT3 is the development of neutralizing antibodies directed against xenogenic immunoglobulins that may render the patient resistant to a second course. In view of the severe side-effects, as well as the increased risk of *viral infection* and *lymphoproliferative* disorders, the use of OKT3 is limited today to a few cases of refractory rejection.

Anti-IL-2 receptor monoclonal antibodies

Upon activation, IL-2 binds to its trimeric $\alpha\beta\gamma$ receptor. The IL-2 receptor is composed of three chains: the α chain (CD25), expressed on activated T cells, the β chain (CD12), which is expressed on resting cells and whose expression increases about three times on activated T cells, and the γ chain (CD 132), expressed on resting T cells and whose expression is only mildly increased (less than three times) on activated T cells.

Two monoclonal antibodies targeting *CD25* are available in renal transplantation: basiliximab and daclizumab. *Basiliximab* is a chimeric monoclonal antibody obtained by grafting the FAB variable regions of a mouse antibody onto the constant regions of human immunoglobulins. *Daclizumab* is a humanized IgG that maintains only the hypervariable antigen-binding sequences of the parent mouse monoclonal antibody.

Table 6.8   Precautions to take with first administration of OKT3

Before administration
Correct overhydration (dialysis or high-dose furosemide)
High-dose IV MP but not more than 8 mg/kg
Diphenhydramine HCL (25–50 mg IV)
Acetominophen (500 mg by mouth)

Administration
Slow infusion over 2 hours
Half-dose of OKT3

Both drugs are administered by direct intravenous injection. Neither drug triggers the cytokine release syndrome that occurs with OKT3 or ATG. Although these monoclonal antibodies cannot prevent immune activation generated by IL-7 and IL-15, a number of randomized controlled trials showed that both basiliximab and daclizumab could significantly reduce the risk of acute rejection either in patients treated with CsA and steroids (Nashan *et al.*, 1999; Kahan *et al.*, 1999) or in patients treated with CsA, azathioprine, and steroids (Vincenti *et al.*, 1998; Ponticelli *et al.*, 2001). Of great importance, no significant difference in the incidence and severity of side-effects could be noted in these randomized trials between patients assigned to receive basiliximab or daclizumab and controls. When compared with antilymphocyte antibodies, the anti-CD25 antibodies show a better profile of tolerance and safety: (1) no cytokine release syndrome, (2) less frequent lukopenia and thrombocytopenia, and (3) reduced risk of CMV infection (Vincenti *et al.*, 2006). Moreover, a meta-analysis of nine randomized trials indicated that the relative risk of malignancy with IL-2 receptor antagonists versus no induction was 0.67 (Webster *et al.*, 2004). The risk of sensitization is low, below 2%.

Anti-CD20 monoclonal antibody

Rituximab is a chimeric human/murine monoclonal antibody with a high affinity for the CD20 antigen, a membrane protein expressed on a subset of B cells. After intravenous injection at a dose of 375 mg/m², rituximab induces the rapid elimination of B cells, by complement-dependent cytotoxicity, by antibody-dependent cellular cytotoxicity, or by stimulation of the apoptotic pathway (Reff *et al.*, 1994).

In renal transplantation, rituximab has been used not only for treating post-transplant lymphoproliferative disorders, which is the main indication for this monoclonal antibody, but also for treating resistant rejection (Becker *et al.*, 2004) and for breaking the immunological barriers posed by preformed anti-HLA or anti-AB antibodies (Magee, 2006).

Side-effects correlate with the number of circulating CD20 cells and are more frequent in patients with tumor. They include fever, chills, rigor, orthostatic hypotension, and bronchospasm. Leukopenia and thrombocytopenia may also develop. In patients with pre-exisiting cardiac morbidity, arrhythmias, angina, and acute respiratory distress syndrome have been reported. However, in renal transplant recipients these side-effects are more rare and less severe, although cough and mild hypotension may occur (Pescovitz, 2006).

Campath®-1H

Campath-1H or alemtuzumab is a humanized monoclonal antibody directed against CD52, which is expressed on both T and B lymphocytes and other lymphoid subsets. It can be administered intravenously or subcutaneously. After intravenous infusion, *cytokine release syndrome* is almost constant. Patients may suffer from chills, fever, rash, rigor, and bronchospasm. These symptoms are less frequent and less severe with subcutaneous injection. After a 30-mg injection there is an almost complete disappearance of circulating lymphocytes. This antibody has been mainly used for treating hematological malignancies. However, there is an increasing use of alemtuzumab in renal transplantation.The profound depletion of lymphocytes may allow immunosuppression to be continued with a single agent, either cyclosporine (Calne, 2004), tacrolimus, or MMF (Malek, 2006), opening up the possibility of prope (near) tolerance. However, the incidence of acute rejection is relatively high, around 30%, and humoral irreversible rejection may occur (Flechner *et al.*, 2005). At present there is no evidence that a degree of tolerance is produced with this agent (Morris and Russel, 2006).

A number of patients may show severe *neutropenia* and *thrombocytopenia*, and some may have prolonged cytopenias including severe *bone marrow hypoplasia*. Trilineage morphological myelodysplasia, with new clonal cytogenetic abnormalities, has also been reported (Gibbs *et al.*, 2005). A case of *acute renal failure* and disseminated intravascular coagulation has been described (Osborne and Lennard, 2005) In neoplastic patients the most significant side-effect of alemtuzumab is predisposition to *infections* related to the associated profound and persisting lymphopenia. In pancreas transplantation, alemtuzumab predis- posed to systemic *fungal infection* (Nath *et al.*, 2005), and there is much concern for fungal infection also in renal transplantation (Singh, 2005). While some investigators reported that the risk of infection appears to be lower than that observed with standard regimens (Malek *et al.*, 2006) or with ATG (Kaufman *et al.*, 2006), others found a high rate of infection, with a fatal outcome in a few patients (Basu *et al.*, 2005).

References

Abramowicz D, De Pauw L, Le Moine A, et al. Prevention of OKT3 nephrotoxicity after kidney transplantation. Kidney Int 1996; 49 (Suppl 53): S39–43.

Abramowicz D, Del Carmen Rial M, Vitko S, et al. Cyclosporine withdrawal from a mycophenolate mofetil-containing immunosuppressive regimen: results of a five-year, prospective, randomized study. J Am Soc Nephrol 2005; 16: 2234–40.

Allison AC, Eugui EM, Sollinger HW. Micophenolate mofetil: mechanism of action and effects in transplantation. Transplant Rev 1993; 7: 129–39.

Alvarez Arroyo MV, Suzuki Y, Yague S, et al. Role of endogenous vascular endothelial growth factor in tubular cell pro- tection against acute cyclosporine toxicity. Transplantation 2002; 74: 1618–24.

Andoh TF, Burdmann EA, Franceschini N, et al. Comparison of acute rapamycin nephrotoxicity with cyclosporine and FK 506. Kidney Int 1996; 54: 1110–17.

Araki M, Flechner SM, Ismail HR, et al. Posttransplant diabetes mellitus in kidney transplant recipients receiving cal- cineurin or mTOR inhibitor drugs. Transplantation 2006; 81: 335–41.

Arbeiter K, Greenbaum L, Balzar E, et al. Reproducible erythroid aplasia caused by mycophenolate mofetil. Pediatr Nephrol 2000; 14: 195–7.

Artz MA, Boots JM, Ligtenberg G, et al. Improved cardiovascular risk profile and renal function in renal transplant patients after randomized conversion from cyclosporine to tacrolimus. J Am Soc Nephrol 2003; 14: 1880–8.

Asai T, Nakatami T, Yamanaka S, et al. Magnesium supplementation prevents chronic cyclosporine nephrotoxicity via renin-angiotensin system independent mechanism. Transplantation 2002; 74: 784–91.

Asberg A. Interactions between cyclosporine and lipid-lowering drugs: implications for organ transplant recipients. Drugs 2003; 663: 367–78.

Balal M, Demir E, Paydas S, et al. Uncommon side effect of MMF in renal transplant recipients. Ren Fail 2005; 27: 591–4.

Basu A, Ramkumar M, Tan HP, et al. Reversal of acute rejection after renal transplantation with Campath-1H. Transplant Proc 2005; 37: 923–6.

Bechstein WO. Neurotoxicity of calcineurin inhibitors: impact and clinical management. Transpl Int 2000; 13: 313–26.

Becker YT, Becker BN, Pirsch JD, Sollinger HW. Rituximab as treatment for refractory kidney transplant rejection. Am J Transplant 2004; 4: 996–1001.

Behrend M. Mycophenolate mofetil: suggested guidelines for use in renal transplantation. Biodrugs 2001; 15: 37–53.

Beiras-Fernandez A, Walther S, Kaczmarek I, et al. In vitro influence of polyclonal anti-thymocyte globulins on leukocyte expression of adhesion molecules. Exp Clin Transplant 2005; 3: 370–4.

Blum CB. Effects of sirolimus in renal allograft recipients: an analysis using the Framingham risk model. Am J Transplant 2002; 6: 551–9.

Bonegio RG, Fuhro R, Wang Z, et al. Rapamycin ameliorates proteinuria-associated tubulointerstitial inflammation and fibrosis in experimental membranous nephropathy. J Am Soc Nephrol 2005; 7: 2063–72.

Boratynska M, Banasik M, Watorek E, et al. Conversion to sirolimus from cyclosporine may induce nephrotic proteinuria and progressive deterioration of renal function in chronic allograft nephropathy patients. Transplant Proc 2006; 38: 101–4.

Border WA, Noble NA. Transforming growth factor-β in tissue fibrosis. N Engl J Med 1994; 331: 1286–92.

Borrows R, Chusney G, Loucaidou M, et al. Mycophenolic acid 12-h trough level monitoring in renal transplantation: association with acute rejection and toxicity. Am J Transplant 2006; 6: 121–8.

Bosmans JL, Holvoet P, Dauwe SE, et al. Oxidative modification of low-density lipoproteins and the outcome of renal allografts at 1½ years. Kidney Int 2001; 59: 2346–56.

Broeders N, Knoop C, Antoine M, et al. Fibrate-induced increase in urea and creatinine: is gemfibrozil the only innocuous agent? Nephrol Dial Transplant 2000; 15: 1993–9.

Budde K, Curtis J, Knoll G, et al. Enteric-coated mycophenolate sodium can be safely administered in maintenance renal transplant patients. Am J Transplant 2004; 4: 237–44.

Burke G, Ciancio G, Cirocco R, et al. Microangiopathy in kidney and simultaneous pancreas/kidney recipients treated with tacrolimus: evidence of endothelin and cytokine involvement. Transplantation 1999; 68: 1336–42.

Calne RY. Prope tolerance – the future of organ transplantation from the laboratory to the clinic. Transpl Immunol 2004; 13: 83–6.

Chand DH, Quattrocchi J, Poe SA, et al. Trial of metronidazole vs. azithromycin for treatment of cyclosporine-induced gingival overgrowth. Pediatr. Transplant 2004; 8: 60–4.

Chen HB, Shen J, Ip YT, Xu L. Identification of phosphatases for Smad in the BMP/DPP pathway. Genes Dev 2006; 20: 648–53.

Chen KJ, Chen CH, Cheng CH, et al. Risk factors for peptic ulcer disease in renal transplant recipients – 11 years of experience from a single center. Clin Nephrol 2004; 62: 14–20.

Chocair PR, Duley JA, Simmonds HA, Cameron JS. The importance of thiopurine methyltransferase activity for the use of azathioprine in transplant recipients. Transplantation 1992; 53: 1051–6.

Chueh SC, Kahan BD. Dyslipidemia in renal transplant recipients treated with a sirolimus and cyclosporine-based immunosuppressive regimen: incidence, risk factors, progression, and prognosis. Transplantation 2003; 76: 375–82.

Citterio F, Scata MC, Violi P, et al. Rapid conversion to sirolimus for chronic progressive deterioration of the renal function in kidney allograft recipients. Transplant Proc 2003; 35: 1292–4.

Coombes JD, Mreich E, Liddle C, Rangan GK. Rapamycin worsens renal function and intratubular cast formation in protein overload nephropathy. Kidney Int 2005; 68: 2599–607.

Crew RJ, Radhakrishnan J, Cohen DJ. De novo thrombotic microangiopathy following treatment with sirolimus: report of two cases. Nephrol Dial Transplant 2005; 20: 203–9.

Dai C, Yang J, Liu Y. Transforming growth factor-beta1 potentiates renal tubular epithelial cell death by a mechanism independent of Smad signaling. J Biol Chem 2003; 278: 12537–45.

Daniel C, Ziswiler R, Frey B, et al. Proinflammatory effects in experimental mesangial proliferative glomerulonephritis of the immunosuppressive agent SDZ RAD, a rapamycin derivative. Exp Nephrol 2000; 1: 52–62.

del Rincon I, O'Leary DH, Haas RW, Escalante A. Effect of glucocorticoids on the arteries in rheumatoid arthritis. Arthritis Rheum 2004; 50: 3813–22.

Deters S, Kirchner G, Koal T, et al. Everolimus/cyclosporine interactions on bile flow and biliary excretion of bile salts and cholesterol in rats. Dig Dis Sci 2004; 49: 30–7.

Diekmann F, Budde K, Oppenheimer F, et al. Predictors of success in conversion from calcineurin inhibitor to sirolimus in chronic allograft dysfunction. Am J Transplant 2004; 4: 1869–75.

Dittrich E, Schmaldienst S, Soleiman A, et al. Rapamycin-associated post-transplantation glomerulonephritis and its remission after reintroduction of calcineurin-inhibitor therapy. Transpl Int 2004; 17: 215–20.

Dominguez I, Mahalati K, Kiberd B, et al. Conversion to rapamycin immunosuppression in renal transplant recipients: report of an initial experience. Transplantation 2000; 70: 1244–7.

Doutrelepont J, Abramowicz D, Flonquin S, et al. Early recurrence of hemolytic uremic syndrome in a renal transplant recipient during prophylactic OKT3 therapy. Transplantation 1992; 53: 1378–83.

Elli A, Aroldi A, Montagnino G, et al. Mycophenolate mofetil and cough [Letter]. Transplantation 1998; 66: 409.

Fabrizi F, Martin P, Dixit V, et al. Post-transplant diabetes mellitus and HCV seropositive status after renal transplantation: meta-analysis of clinical studies. Am J Transplant 2005; 5: 2433–40.

Fellstrom B, Holdaas H, Jardine AG, et al. Effect of fluvastatin on renal end points in the Assessment of Lescol in Renal Transplant (ALERT) trial. Kidney Int 2004; 66: 1549–55.

Feria I, Pichardo I, Juarez P, et al. Therapeutic benefit of spironolactone in experimental chronic cyclosporine A nephrotoxicity. Kidney Int 2003; 63: 43–52.

Fine RN, Stablein D. Long-term use of recombinant human growth hormone in pediatric allograft recipients: a report of the NAPRTCS Transplant Registry. Pediatr Nephrol 2005; 20: 404–8.

Flechner SM, Zhou L, Derweesh I, et al. The impact of sirolimus, mycophenolate mofetil, cyclosporine, azathioprine, and steroids on wound healing in 513 kidney transplant recipients. Transplantation 2003; 76: 1729–34.

Flechner SM, Friend PJ, Brockmann J, et al. Alemtuzumab induction and sirolimus plus mycophenolate mofetil maintenance for CNI and steroid-free kidney transplant immunosuppression. Am J Transplant 2005; 5: 3009–14.

Fortin MC, Raymond MA, Madore F, et al. Increased risk of thrombotic microangiopathy in patients receiving a cyclosporin–sirolimus combination. Am J Transplant 2004; 6: 946–52.

Franco M, Blaimont A, Albano L, et al. Tacrolimus pain syndrome in renal transplant patients: report of two cases. Joint Bone Spine 2004; 71: 157–9.

Franz M, Regele H, Schmaldienst S, et al. Posttransplant hemolytic uremic syndrome in adult retransplanted kidney graft recipients: advantage of FK 506 therapy? Transplantation 1998; 66: 1258–62.

Gafter-Gvili A, Sredni B, Gal R, et al. Cyclosporin A-induced hair growth in mice is associated with inhibition of calcineurin-dependent activation of NFAT in follicular keratinocytes. Am J Physiol Cell Physiol 2003; 284: C1593–603.

Ganschow R, Albani J, Grabhorn E, et al. Tacrolimus-induced cholestatic syndrome following pediatric liver transplantation and steroid-resistant graft rejection. Pediatr Transplant 2006; 10: 220–4.

Ghio L, Tarantino A, Edefonti A, et al. Advantages of cyclosporine as sole immunosuppressive agent in children with transplanted kidneys. Transplantation 1992; 54: 834–8.

Gibbs SD, Westerman DA, McCormack C, et al. Severe and prolonged myeloid haematopoietic toxicity with myelodysplastic features following alemtuzumab therapy in patients with peripheral T-cell lymphoproliferative disorders. Br J Haematol 2005; 130: 87–91.

Giebel S, Dziaczkowska J, Wojnar J, et al. The impact of immunosuppressive therapy on an early quantitative NK cell reconstitution after allogeneic haematopoietic cell transplantation. Ann Transplant 2005; 10: 29–33.

Goel M, Flechner SM, Zhou L, et al. The influence of various maintenance immunosuppressive drugs on lymphocele formation and treatment after kidney transplantation. J Urol 2004; 171: 1788–92.

Goldberg R, Roth D. Evaluation of fluvastatin in the treatment of hypercholesterolemia in renal transplant recipients taking cyclosporine. Transplantation 1996; 62: 1559–64.

Gourishankar S, Jhangri GS, Tonelli M, et al. Development of diabetes mellitus following kidney transplantation: a Canadian experience. Am J Transplant 2004; 4: 1876–82.

Grinyo JM, Gil-Vernet S, Cruzado JM, et al. Calcineurin inhibitors-free immunosuppression based on anti-thymocyte globulin and mycophenolate moferil in cadaveric renal transplantation: results after 5 years. Transplant Int 2005; 16: 820–7.

Gross DC, Sasasky TM, Buick MK, Light JA. Acute respiratory failure and pulmonary. fibrosis secondary to administration of mycophenolate mofetil. Transplantation 1997; 64: 1607–9.

Guetta E, Scarpati EM, Di Corlet PE. Effect of cytomegalovirus immediate early gene. products on endothelial cell gene activity. Cardiovasc Res 2001; 50: 538–46.

Hardinger KL, Brennan DC, Lowell J, Schnitzler MA. Long-term outcome of gastrointestinal complications in renal transplant patients treated with mycophenolate mofetil. Transpl Int 2004; 10: 609–16.

Hill CS. Turning off Smads: identification of a Smad phosphatase. Dev Cell 2006; 10: 412–13.

Hirayama T, Athanasou NA. Effects of corticosteroids on human osteoclast formation and activity. J Endocrinol 2002; 175: 155–63.

Hochegger K, Gruber J, Lhotta K. Acute inflammatory syndrome induced by mycophenolate mofetil in a patient following kidney transplantation. Am J Transplant 2006; 6: 852–4.

Hoogeveen R, Ballantyne CM, Pownall HJ. Effects of sirolimus on the metabolism of apoB100-containing lipoproteins in renal transplant patients. Transplantation 2001; 72: 1244–50.

Houde I, Insering P, Boucher D, et al. Mychophenolate mofetil, an alternative to cyclosporine A for long-term immunosuppression in kidney transplantation. Transplantation 2000; 70: 1251–3.

Jain S, Mohamed MA, Sandford R, et al. Sequential protocol biopsies from renal transplant recipients show an increasing expression of active TGF beta. Transpl Int 2002; 15: 630–4.

Johnson C, Ahsan N, Gonwa T, et al. Randomized trial of tacrolimus (Prograf) in combination with azathioprine or mycophenolate mofetil versus cyclosporine (Neoral) with mycophenolate mofetil after cadaveric kidney transplantation. Transplantation 2000; 69: 834–41.

Johnson RW. Sirolimus (Rapamune) in renal transplantation. Curr Opin Nephrol Hypertens 2002; 11: 603–7.

Joist H, Brennan DC, Coyne D, et al. Anemia in the kidney-transplant patient. Adv Chronic Kidney Dis 2006; 1: 4–10.

Jung S, Fehr S, Harder-d'Heureuse J, et al. Corticosteroids impair intestinal epithelial wound repair mechanisms in vitro. Scand J Gastroenterol 2001; 36: 963–70.

Kahan BD. Efficacy of sirolimus compared with azathioprine for reduction of acute renal allograft rejection: a randomised multicentre study. The Rapamune US Study Group. Lancet 2000; 356: 194–202.

Kahan BD, Welsh M, Shoenberg L, et al. Variable oral absorption of cyclosporine: a biopharmaceutical risk factor for chronic renal allograft rejection. Transplantation 1996; 62: 599–606.

Kahan BD, Rajagopalan PR, Hall M. Reduction of the occurrence of acute cellular rejection among renal allograft recipients treated with basiliximab, a chimeric anti-interleukin-2-receptor monoclonal antibody. United States Simulect Renal Study Group. Transplantation 1999; 67: 276–84.

Kahan BD, Ponticelli C. Immunosuppressive drugs: molecular and cellular mechanisms of action. In Kahan BD, Ponticelli C, eds. Principles and Practice of Renal Transplantation. London: Martin Dunitz, 2000; 314–47.

Karthikeyan V, Parasuraman R, Shah V, et al. Outcome of plasma exchange therapy in thrombotic microangiopathy after renal transplantation. Am J Transplant 2003; 3: 1289–94.

Kaufman DB, Leventhal JR, Gallon LG, Parker MA. Alemtuzumab induction and prednisone-free maintenance immunotherapy in simultaneous pancreas–kidney transplantation comparison with rabbit antithymocyte globulin induction – long-term results. Am J Transplant 2006; 6: 331–9.

Kelly P, Kahan BD. Review: metabolism of immunosuppressant drugs. Curr Drug Metab 2002; 3: 275–87.

Keown PA. New concepts in cyclosporine monitoring. Curr Opin Nephrol Hypertens 2002; 11: 619–26.

Kim MJ, Mayr M, Pechula M, et al. Marked erythrocyte microcytosis under primary immunosuppression with sirolimus. Transpl Int 2006; 1: 12–18.

Kirklin JK, Benza RL, Rayburn BK, McGiffin DC. Strategies for minimizing hyperlipidemia after cardiac transplantation. Am J Cardiovasc Drugs 2002; 2: 377–87.

Knoll GA, MacDonald I, Khan A, Van Walraven C. Mycophenolate mofetil dose reduction and the risk of acute rejection after renal transplantation. J Am Soc Nephrol 2003; 14: 2381–6.

Knopp RM. Treatment of lipid disorders. N Engl J Med 1999; 341: 498–511.

Kobashigawa JA, Kasiske BL. Hyperlipidemia in solid organ transplantation. Transplantation 1997; 63: 331–8.

Kovarik JM. Everolimus. A proliferation signal inhibitor targeting primary causes of allograft dysfunction. Drugs Today 2004; 40: 101–9.

Kovarik JM, Hsu CH, McMahon L, et al. Population pharmacokinetics of everolimus in de novo renal transplant patients: impact of ethnicity and comedications. Clin Pharmacol Ther 2001; 70: 247–54.

Kovarik JM, Kaplan B, Tedesco Silva H, et al. Exposure–response relationships for everolimus in de novo kidney transplantation: defining a therapeutic range. Transplantation 2002; 73: 920–5.

Kreis H, Cisterne JM, Land W. Sirolimus in association with mychophenolate mofetil induction for the prevention of acute rejection in renal allograft recipients. Transplantation 2000; 69: 1252–60.

Kulkarni SK, Kaur G. Pharmacodynamics of drug-induced weight gain. Drugs Today 2001; 37: 559–71.

Land W. The role of postischemic reperfusion injury and other nonantigen-dependent inflammatory pathways in transplantation. Transplantation 2005; 79: 505–14.

Langer RM, Kahan BD. Incidence, therapy, and consequences of lymphocele after sirolimus–cyclosporine–prednisone immunosuppression in renal transplant recipients. Transplantation 2002; 27: 804–8.

Langer RM, Van Buren CT, Katz SM, Kahan BD. De novo hemolytic uremic syndrome after kidney transplantation in patients treated with cyclosporine–sirolimus combination. Transplantation 2002; 73: 756–60.

Larson TS, Dean PG, Stegall MD, et al. Complete avoidance of calcineurin inhibitors in renal transplantation: a randomized trial comparing sirolimus and tacrolimus. Am J Transplant 2006; 6: 514–22.

Lepre F, Rigby R, Hawley C, et al. A double blind controlled trial for the treatment of dyslipidaemia in renal allograft recipients. Clin Transplant 1999; 13: 520–6.

Li C, Yang CW, Ahn HJ, et al. Colchicine decreases apoptotic cell death in chronic cyclosporine nephrotoxicity. J Lab Clin Med 2002; 139: 364–71.

Lieberthal W, Fuhro R, Andry CC, et al. Rapamycin impairs recovery from acute renal failure: role of cell-cycle arrest and apoptosis of tubular cells. Am J Physiol Renal Physiol 2001; 281: F693–706.

Lipkowitz GS, Madden RL, Mulhern J. Long-term maintenance of therapeutic cyclosporine levels leads to optimal graft survival without evidence of chronic nephrotoxicity. Transpl Int 1999; 12: 202–7.

Longoni B, Migliori M, Ferretti A, et al. Melatonin prevents cyclosporine-induced nephrotoxicity in isolated and perfused rat kidney. Free Rad Res 2002; 36: 357–63.

Lorber MI, Ponticelli C, Whelchel J, et al. Therapeutic drug monitoring for everolimus in kidney transplantation using 12-month exposure, efficacy, and safety data. Clin Transplant 2005; 19: 145–52.

Luke RG. Mechanism of cyclosporine-induced hypertension. Am J Hypertens 1991; 4: 468–71.

Machado PG, Tedesco HS, Silva RG, et al. Use of reduced dose of OKT3 (2.5 mg) after renal transplantation. Transplant Proc 2002; 34: 104.

Maes B, Oellerich M, Ceuppens JL, et al. A new acute inflammatory syndrome related to the introduction of mycophenolate mofetil in patients with Wegener granulomatosis. Nephrol Dial Transplant 2002; 17: 923–6.

Magee CC. Transplantation across previously incompatible immunological barriers. Transpl Int 2006; 19: 87–97.

Malek SK, Obmann MA, Gotoff RA, et al. Campath-1H induction and the incidence of infectious complications in adult renal transplantation. Transplantation 2006; 81: 17–20.

Maluf DG, Mas VR, Archer KJ, et al. Apolipoprotein E genotypes as predictors of high-risk groups for developing hyperlipidemia in kidney transplant recipients undergoing sirolimus treatment. Transplantation 2005; 80: 1705–11.

Margreiter R; European Tacrolimus vs Ciclosporin Microemulsion Renal Transplantation Study Group. Efficacy and safety of tacrolimus compared with ciclosporin microemulsion in renal transplantation: a randomised multicentre study. Lancet 2002; 359: 741–6.

Markell M. New-onset diabetes mellitus in transplant patients: pathogenesis, complications, and management. Am J Kidney Dis 2004; 43: 953–65.

Martinez-Castelao A, Hernandez MD, Pascual J, et al. Detection and treatment of post kidney transplant hyperglycemia: a Spanish multicenter cross-sectional study. Transplant Proc 2005; 37: 3813–16.

Matas AJ, Almond PS, Moss A, et al. Effect of cyclosporine on renal transplant recipients: a 12 year follow-up. Clin Transplant 1995; 9: 450–5.

Matsuo S, Lopez-Guisa JM, Cai X, et al. Multifunctionality of PAI-1 in fibrogenesis: evidence from obstructive nephropathy in PAI-1-overexpressing mice. Kidney Int 2005; 67: 2221–38.

Messman H, Scholmerich J. Do adrenal cortical hormones influence the pathogenesis of stress ulcer? Dtsch Med Wochenschr 2000; 125: 99–100.

Mihatsch MJ, Ryffel B, Gudat F. The differential diagnosis between rejection and cyclosporine toxicity. Kidney Int 1995; 48 (Suppl 52): S63–9.

Moake JL. Thrombotic microangiopathies. N Engl J Med 2002; 347: 589–600.

Montagnino G, Tarantino A, Segoloni GP. Long-term results of a randomized study comparing three immunosuppressive schedules with cyclosporine in cadaveric kidney transplantation. J Am Soc Nephrol 2001; 12: 2163–9.

Montalbano M, Neff GW, Yamashiki N et al. A retrospective review of liver transplant patients treated with sirolimus from a single center: an analysis of sirolimus-related complications. Transplantation 2004; 78: 264–8.

Mora PF. Post-transplantation diabetes mellitus. Am J Med Sci 2005; 329: 86–94.

Morris P, Russell NK. Alemtuzumab (Campath-1H): a systematic review in organ transplantation. Transplantation 2006; 1: 1361–7.

Morrissett JD, Abdel-Fattah G, Hoogeveen R, et al. Effects of sirolimus on plasma lipids, lipoprotein levels, and fatty acid metabolism. J Lipid Res 2002; 43: 1170–80.

Mourad G, Vela C, Ribstein J, Mimran A. Long-term improvement in renal function after cyclosporine reduction in renal transplant recipients with histologically proven chronic cyclosporine nephropathy. Transplantation 1998; 65: 661–6.

Murphy GJ, Waller JR, Sandford RS, et al. Randomized clinical trial of the effect of microemulsion cyclosporin and tacrolimus on renal allograft fibrosis. Br J Surg 2003; 90: 680–6.

Nankivell BJ, Borrows RJ, Fung CL. The natural history of chronic allograft nephropathy. N Engl J Med 2003; 349: 2326–33.

Nashan B, Light S, Hardie IR, et al. Reduction of acute renal allograft rejection by daclizumab. Daclizumab Double Therapy Study Group. Transplantation 1999; 67: 110–15.

Nashan B, Curtis J, Ponticelli C, et al. Everolimus and reduced-exposure cyclosporine in de novo renal-transplant recipients: a three-year phase II, randomized, multicenter, open-label study. Transplantation 2004; 78: 1332–40.

Nath DS, Kandaswamy R, Gruessner R, et al. Fungal infections in transplant recipients receiving alemtuzumab. Transplant Proc 2005; 37: 934–46.

Olyaei AJ, De Mattos AM, Bennett WM. Nephrotoxicity of immunosuppressive drugs: new insight and preventive strategies. Curr Opin Crit Care 2001; 7: 384–9.

Opelz G, Dolher B. Cyclosporine and long-term kidney graft survival. Transplantation 2001; 72: 1267–73.

Opelz G, Dohler B. Lymphomas after solid organ transplantation: a collaborative transplant study report. Am J Transplant 2004; 4: 222–30.

Ortho Multicenter Study Group. A randomized clinical trial of OKT3 monoclonal antibody for acute rejection of cadaveric renal transplants. N Engl J Med 1985; 313: 337–42.

Osborne WL, Lennard AL. Acute renal failure and disseminated intravascular coagulation following an idiosyncratic reaction to alemtuzumab (Campath 1H) or fludarabine. Haematologica 2005; 90: ECR05.

Padi SS, Chopra K. Salvage of cyclosporine A-induced oxidative stress and renal dysfunction by carvedilol. Nephron 2002; 92: 685–92.

Parameswara VK, Sule AJ, Esser V. Have we overlooked the importance of serine/threonine protein phosphatases in pancreatic beta-cells? Role played by protein phosphatase 2A in insulin secretion. JOP 2005; 8: 303–15.

Pascual M, Curtis J, Delmonico FL, et al. A prospective, randomized clinical trial of cyclosporine reduction in stable patients greater than 12 months after renal transplantation. Transplantation 2003; 75: 1501–5.

Pascual J, Quereda C, Zamora J, et al. Steroid withdrawal in renal transplant patients on triple therapy with a calcineurin inhibitor and mycophenolate mofetil: a meta-analysis of randomized, controlled trials. Transplantation 2004; 78: 3746–8.

Pascual J, Marcén R, Ortuno J. Clinical experience with everolimus (Certican): optimizing dose and tolerability. Transplantation 2005; 79 (Suppl): S80–4.

Paul LC. Chronic allograft nephropathy. Kidney Int 1999; 56: 783–93.

Pelle G, Xu Y, Khoury N, et al. Thrombotic microangiopathy in marginal kidneys after sirolimus use. Am J Kidney Dis 2005; 46: 1124–8.

Pelletier RP, Kin B, Henry ML, et al. The impact of mycophenolate mofetil dosing patterns on clinical outcome after renal transplantation. Clin Transplant 2003; 17: 200–5.

Pescovitz MD. Rituximab, an anti-CD 20 monoclonal antibody: history and mechanism of action. Am J Transplant 2006; 6: 859–66.

Pham PT, Peng A, Wilkinson A, et al. Cyclosporine- and tacrolimus-associated thrombotic microangiopathy. Am J Kidney Dis 2002; 35: 844–50.

Pham PT, Pham PC, Danovitch G et al. Sirolimus-associated pulmonary toxicity. Transplantation 2004; 77: 1215–80.

Phanish MK, Wahab NA, Colville-Nash P, et al. The differential role of Smad2 and Smad3 in the regulation of pro-fibrotic TGFbeta1 responses in human proximal-tubule epithelial cells. Biochem J 2006; 393: 601–7.

Piper J, Ray WA, Daugherty JR, Griffith MR. Corticosteroid use and peptic ulcer disease: role of nonsteroidal anti-inflammatory drugs. Ann Intern Med 1991; 114: 735–40.

Ponticelli C. Glucocorticoids and immunomodulating agents. In Ponticelli C, Glassock RJ, eds. Treatment of Primary Glomerulonephritis. Oxford: Oxford University Press, 1997: 25–77.

Ponticelli C. The pleiotropic effects of mTor inhibitors. J Nephrol 2004; 17: 762–8.

Ponticelli C, Campise MR. Neurological complications in kidney transplant recipients. J Nephrol 2005; 18: 521–8.

Ponticelli C, Civati G, Tarantino A, et al. Randomized study with cyclosporine in kidney transplantation: 10-year follow-up. J Am Soc Nephrol 1996; 7: 792–7.

Ponticelli C, Aroldi A, Elli A, et al. The clinical status of cadaveric renal transplant patients treated for 10 years with cyclosporine therapy. Clin Transplant 1999; 13: 324–9.

Ponticelli C, Yussim A, Cambi V. A randomized, double-blind trial of basiliximab immunoprophylaxis plus triple therapy in kidney transplant recipients. Transplantation 2001; 72: 1261–7.

Ponticelli C, Villa M, Cesana B, et al. Risk factors for late kidney allograft failure. Kidney Int 2002; 62: 1848–54.

Ponticelli C, Passerini P. Gastrointestinal complications in renal transplant recipients. Transpl Int 2005; 18: 643–50.

Racusen LC, Solez K, Colvin RB. Fibrosis and atrophy in the renal allograft: interim report and new directions. Am J Transplant 2002; 2: 203–6.

Rahmouni K, Correia ML, Haynes WG, Mark AL. Obesity-associated hypertension: new insights into mechanisms. Hypertension 2005; 45: 9–14.

Raymond MA, Mollica L, Vigneault N, et al. Blockade of anti-apoptotic machinery by cyclosporine A redirects cell death toward necrosis in arterial endothelial cells: regulation by reactive oxygen species and cathepsin D. FASEB J 2003; 17: 515–17.

Reek C, Conrad S, Tenscher V, Huland H. Do serum C-reactive protein measurements help to discriminate episodes of renal dysfunction in patients after renal transplantation? Clin Chim Acta 2001; 310: 57–61.

Reff ME, Carner K, Chambers KS, et al. Depletion of B cells in vivo by a chimeric mouse human monoclonal antibody to CD20. Blood 1994; 83: 435–45.

Robson M, Coté I, Abbs I, et al. Thrombotic micro-angiopathy with sirolimus-based immunosuppression: potentiation of calcineurin-inhibitor-induced endothelial damage? Am J Transplant 2003; 3: 324–7.

Rojas E, Carlini RG, Clesca P, et al. The pathogenesis of osteodystrophy after renal transplantation as detected by early alterations in bone remodeling. Kidney Int 2003; 63: 1915–23.

Royer B, Zanetta G, Berard M, et al. A neutropenia suggesting an interaction between valacyclovir and mycophenolate mofetil. Clin Transplant 2003; 17: 158–61.

Ruggenenti P. Post-transplant hemolytic–uremic syndrome. Kidney Int 2002; 62: 1093–104.

Russ G, Segoloni G, Oberbauer R, et al. Superior outcomes in renal transplantation after early cyclosporine withdrawal and sirolimus maintenance therapy, regardless of baseline renal function. Transplantation 2005; 80: 1204–11.

Saikali JA, Truong LD, Suki WD. Sirolimus may promote thrombotic microangiopathy. Am J Transplant 2003; 3: 229–30.

Saurina A, Campistol JM, Piera C, et al. Conversion from calcineurin inhibitors to sirolimus in chronic allograft dysfunction: changes in glomerular haemodynamics and proteinuria. Nephrol Dial Transplant 2006; 2: 488–93.

Salvadori M, Holzer H, De Mattos A, et al. Enteric-coated mycophenolate sodium is therapeutically equivalent to mycophenolate mofetil in de novo renal transplant patients. Am J Transplant 2004; 4: 231–6.

Sartelet H, Toupance O, Lorenzato M, et al. Sirolimus-induced thrombotic microangiopathy is associated with decreased expression of vascular endothelial growth factor in kidneys. Am J Transplant 2005; 5: 2441–5.

Schaffellner S, Jakobi E, Kniepeiss D, et al. Center experience in liver transplantation (LTX): management of dermal side effects caused by sirolimus. Int Immunopharmaco 2005; 5: 137–40.

Schwimmer J, Nadasdy TA, Spitalnik PF, et al. De novo thrombotic microangiopathy in renal transplant recipients: a comparison of hemolytic uremic syndrome with localized renal thrombotic microangiopath. Am J Kidney Dis 2003; 41: 471–9.

Sennesael JJ, Bosmans JL, Bogers JP, et al. Conversion from cyclosporine to sirolimus in stable renal transplant recipients. Transplantation 2005; 80: 1578–85.

Serkova N, Jacobsen W, Niemann CU, et al. Sirolimus, but not the structurally related RAD (everolimus), enhances the negative effects of cyclosporine on mitochondrial metabolism in the rat brain. Br J Pharmacol 2001; 33: 875–85.

Shah OJ, Wang Z, Hunter T. Inappropriate activation of the TSC/Rheb/mTOR/S6K cassette induces IRS1/2 depletion, insulin resistance, and cell survival deficiencies. Curr Biol 2004; 14: 1650–6.

Sharma VK, Bologa RM, Xu GP, et al. Intragraft TGFβ$_1$ mRNA: a correlate of interstitial fibrosis and chronic allograft nephropathy. Kidney Int 1996; 49: 1297–303.

Shihab FS, Bennett WM, Andoh TF. Pirfenidone treatment decreases transforming growth factor-beta 1 and matrix protein and ameliorates fibrosis in chronic cyclosporine nephrotoxicity. Am J Transplant 2002; 2: 111–19.

Shihab FS, Bennett WM, Yi H, et al. Sirolimus increases transforming growth factor-beta1 expression and potentiates chronic cyclosporine nephrotoxicity. Kidney Int 2004; 65: 1262–71.

Sijpkens YW, Doxiadis II, Mallat MJ, et al. Early versus late acute rejection episodes in renal transplantation. Transplantation 2003; 75: 204–8.

Singh N. Invasive aspergillosis in organ transplant recipients: new issues in epidemiologic characteristics, diagnosis, and management. Med Mycol 2005; 43 (Suppl 1): S267–70.

Smak Gregoor PJH, van Gelder T, Van Besouw NM, et al. Randomized study on the conversion of treatment from cyclosporine to azathioprine or mycophenolate mofetil followed by dose reduction. Transplantation 2000; 70: 143–8.

Staatz CE, Willis C, Taylor PJ, Tett SE. Population pharmacokinetics of tacrolimus in adult kidney transplant recipients. Clin Pharmacol Ther 2002; 72: 660–9.

Stallone G, Infante B, Schena A, et al. Rapamycin for treatment of chronic allograft nephropathy in renal transplant patients. J Am Soc Nephrol 2005; 16: 3755–62.

Straathof-Galema L, Wetzels JF, Dijkman HB, et al. Sirolimus-associated heavy proteinuria in a renal transplant recipient: evidence for a tubular mechanism. Am J Transplant 2006; 2: 429–33.

Tamura K, Fujimura T, Tsutsumi T, et al. Transcriptional inhibition of insulin by FK506 and possible involvement of FK506 binding protein-12 in pancreatic β-cell. Transplantation 1995; 59: 1606–13.

Tan TC, Robinson PJ. Mechanisms of calcineurin-inhibitor induced neurotoxicity. Transplant Rev 2006; 20: 49–60.

Tang S, Chan TM, Lui SL, et al. Risk factors for avascular bone necrosis after transplantation. Transplant Proc 2000; 32: 1873–5.

Tauchi Y, Zushida L, Chono S, et al. Effect of dexamethasone palmitate–low density lipoprotein complex on cholesterol ester accumulation in aorta of atherogenic model mice. Biol Pharm Bull 2001; 24: 925–9.

Teutonico A, Schena PF, Di Paolo S. Glucose metabolism in renal transplant recipients: effect of calcineurin inhibitor withdrawal and conversion to sirolimus. J Am Soc Nephrol 2005; 16: 3128–35.

Thaunat O, Beaumont C, Chatenoud L, et al. Anemia after late introduction of sirolimus may correlate with biochemical evidence of a chronic inflammatory state. Transplantation 2005; 80: 1212–19.

Thorp M, DeMattos A, Bennett W, et al. The effect of conversion from cyclosporine to tacrolimus on gingival hyperplasia, hirsutism and cholesterol. Transplantation 2000; 69: 1218–20.

Tricot L, Lebbe C, Pillebout E, et al. Tacrolimus-induced alopecia in female kidney–pancreas transplant recipients. Transplantation 2005; 80: 1546–9.

Valente JF, Hricick D, Weigel K, et al. Comparison of sirolimus vs mycophenolate mofetil on surgical complications and wound healing in adult kidney transplantation. Am J Transplant 2003; 3: 1128–34.

Vanrenterghem Y, Ponticelli C, Morales J, et al. Prevalence and management of anemia in renal transplant recipients: a European Survey. Am J Transplant 2003; 3: 835–45.

Van Gelder T, Ter Meulen CG, Hené R, et al. Oral ulcers in kidney transplant recipients treated with sirolimus and mycophenolate mofetil. Transplantation 2003; 75: 788–91.

Vincenti F, Kirkman R, Light S, et al. Interleukin-2-receptor blockade with daclizumab to prevent acute rejection in renal transplantation. Daclizumab Triple Therapy Study Group. N Engl J Med 1998; 338: 161–5.

Vincenti F, de Andres A, Becker T, et al. Interleukin-2 receptor antagonist induction in modern immunosuppression regimens for renal transplant recipients. Transplant Int 2006; 19: 446–57.

Vitko S, Margreiter R, Weimar W, et al. Everolimus (Certican) 12-month safety and efficacy versus mycophenolate mofetil in de novo renal transplant recipients. Transplantation 2004; 78: 1532–40.

Weber LT, Shipkava M, Armstrong VW, et al. The pharmacokinetic–pharmacodynamic relationship for total and free mycophenolate mofetil therapy. A report of the German study group on mycophenolate mofetil therapy. J Am Soc Nephrol 2002; 13: 759–68.

Webster AC, Playford EG, Higgins G, et al. Interleukin 2 receptor anatagonists for renal transplant recipienta: a meta-analysis of randomized trials. Transplantation 2004; 77: 166–76.

Webster AC, Pankhurst T, Rinaldi F, et al. Monoclonal and polyclonal antibody therapy for treating acute rejection in kidney transplant recipients: a systematic review of randomized trial data. Transplantation 2006; 81: 953–65.

Weinstein RS, Jilka RL, Parfitt AM, Manolagas SC. Inhibition of osteoclastogenesis and promotion of apoptosis of osteoblasts and osteoclasts by glucocorticoids: potential mechanisms of their deleterious effects on bone. J Clin Invest 1998; 102: 274–82.

Weir MR, Ward MT, Blahut SA, et al. Long-term impact of discontinued or reduced calcineurin inhibitor in patients with chronic allograft nephropathy. Kidney Int 2001; 59: 1567–73.

Weir MR. Impact of immunosuppressive regimens on post-transplant diabetes mellitus. Transplant Proc 2001; 33 (Suppl 5A): 23S–6S.

Wever PC, Roest RW, Wolbink-Kamp AM, et al. OKT3-induced nephrotoxicity is associated with release of group II secretory phospholipase A2. Eur J Clin Invest 1996; 26: 873–8.

Wicke C, Halliday B, Allen D, et al. Effects of steroid and retinoids on wound healing. Arch Surg 2000; 135: 1265–70.

Williamson PM, Kohlhagen JL, Mangos GJ, et al. Acute effects of hydrocortisone on plasma nitrate/nitrite activity and forearm vasodilator responsiveness in normal human subjects. Clin Exp Pharmacol Physiol 2005; 32: 162–6.

Wong YT, Del-Rio-Martin J, Jaques B, et al. Audit of diabetes in a renal transplant population. Transplant Proc 2005; 37: 3283–5.

Wright S. Steroids and their mechanisms of action. Proc R Coll Physicians Edinb 1995; 25: 34–9.

Wu MJ, Wen MC, Chiu YT, et al. Rapamycin attenuates unilateral ureteral obstruction-induced renal fibrosis. Kidney Int 2006; 69: 2029–36.

Yang S, Zhang L. Glucocorticoids and vascular reactivity. Curr Vasc Pharmacol 2004; 2: 1–12.

Yango A, Morrissey P, Monaco A, et al. Successful treatment of tacrolimus-associated thrombotic microangiopathy with sirolimus conversion and plasma exchange. Clin Nephrol 2002; 5: 77–8.

Yorgin PD, Scandling JD, Belson A, et al. Late post-transplant anemia in adult renal transplant recipients. An underrecognized problem? Am J Transplant 2002; 2: 429–35.

7 RECURRENT PRIMARY DISEASE

Recurrence of the original disease following renal transplantation is a relatively frequent complication, which may contribute to the dysfunction and even loss of the kidney allograft. When compared with other transplant recipients, patients with post-transplant recurrent diseases have a significantly poorer graft survival in the long term (Hariharan et al., 1999). The incidence and severity of recurrence depend on the nature of the primary disease. Nevertheless, the risk of recurrence increases with time, and long exposure of the transplanted kidney to the recurrent disease increases the risk of graft function deterioration (Briganti et al., 2002).

Recurrence of primary disease

Primary glomerulonephritis (GN)

All forms of GN may recur on the kidney allograft, but the risk of recurrence is different for the various subtypes of GN (Table 7.1). However, even for a single subtype of GN, it is difficult to assess the risk of recurrence. In two large series, the recurrence of GN was the third most frequent cause of late graft failure after chronic allograft nephropathy and death, accounting for 8–12% of graft losses at 10 years after transplantation (Briganti et al., 2002; Ponticelli et al., 2002a). As the deleterious effect of recurrent GN may be diluted by the many other factors that interfere with long-term graft survival, there is no reason to discriminate against potential recipients with GN in selecting patients for renal transplantation. Nevertheless, for those patients who actually have recurrence, the relative risk of graft failure is almost doubled, the risk being particularly elevated for focal segmental glomerular sclerosis and for membranoproliferative GN.

Focal and segmental glomerulosclerosis (FSGS)

Patients with FSGS are at *high risk of recurrence* after renal transplantation. Approximately 20–40% of patients develop recurrence of FSGS in the first allograft (Abbott et al., 2001). There are two clinical presentations of FSGS after transplantation: an *early recurrence* with massive proteinuria within hours to days, and a *late*, more insidious recurrence several months or years after transplantation (Koushik and Matas, 2005).

Table 7.1   Risk of post-transplant recurrence for primary glomerular diseases

Disease	Estimated risk (%)	Predictive factors
Focal and segmental glomerular sclerosis	20–40	Permeability factors (?) Second graft after recurrence
Membranous GN	6–30	None
Membranoproliferative GN I	3–48	Low risk in Japanese population (?)
Membranoproliferative GN II	?	
IgA GN	9–60	Living donation (?) Young age
Anti-GBM GN antibodies	10–30	Circulating anti-GBM antibodies

The *pathogenesis* of recurrent FSGS is far from being established. The frequent occurrence of a rapid or even immediate relapse of proteinuria after transplantation suggests that at least some patients with FSGS have *circulating factor(s)* capable of altering glomerular permeability in normal grafts. Ten years ago, Savin *et al.* (1996) isolated a circulating factor with an apparent molecular mass of about 50 Da in patients with recurrent FSGS after transplantation, and hypothesized that it might initiate the renal injury. Dantal *et al.* (1998) reported that the albuminuric factor(s) are part of a complex with immunoglobulins. A few years later, Savin *et al.* (2003) found that the permeability activity is carried by small, highly glycosylated, hydrophobic protein(s) or peptide(s). Unfortunately, at present, the nature of circulating permeability factors is still unknown, and we still lack a reliable test for its presence and quantitation. More recently, the attention of investigators has focused on the *interpodocyte connection*. The slit diaphragm is structurally formed by extracellular proteins (such as nephrin, P-cadherin, etc.) anchored by a protein called podocin. It has been hypothesized that the permeability factor(s) may induce the redistribution and loss of nephrin as well as reduced expression of podocin (Doublier *et al.*, 2005). Recently, cases of FSGS associated with a *mutation of NPHS2* (encoding podocin) have been reported in both familial and sporadic forms of FSGS (Boute *et al.*, 2000). The risk of recurrence in patients with the NPHS2 mutation is low, around 8% (Bertelli *et al.*, 2003; Ruf *et al.*, 2004; Weber *et al.*, 2004). However, caution has been recommended in transplanting these patients with the kidneys of their parents who are carriers of the NPHS2 mutation, because it could increase the risk of recurrence (Vincenti and Ghiggeri, 2005). A role for *co-stimulatory molecule B7-1* in podocytes as an inducible modifier of glomerular permselectivity has been suggested. B7-1 in podocytes was found in genetic, drug-induced, immune-mediated, and bacterial toxin-induced experimental kidney diseases with nephrotic syndrome (Reiser *et al.*, 2004). It is also possible that a subset of patients with FSGS may produce anti-actin and anti-ATP synthase autoantibodies that may concur in altering glomerular permeability (Musante *et al.*, 2005).

It is difficult to predict the *risk of recurrence* in a single patient (Table 7.2). It seems, however, that in patients younger than 18 years, in recipients with better HLA matching, in patients with the collapsing variant of FSGS, and in those who have had a rapid progression of uremia, the risk of recurrence is higher (Tejani and Stablein, 1992; Dall'Amico *et al.*, 1999; Hariharan and Savin, 1999). Second grafts in those who have had recurrence in their first graft are generally accompanied by a further recurrence (Baum *et al.*, 2001), but sporadic cases of success have also been reported (Montagnino *et al.*, 2000). In an Italian study, 11 of 13 children who tested positive for the permeability factor versus four of 12 with a negative test had a recurrence of FSGS after renal transplantation (Dall'Amico *et al.*, 1999). As mentioned above, the familial form of FSGS associated with the NPHS2 mutation rarely recurs following transplantation (Weber *et al.*, 2004). Also, patients with the sporadic variety of FSGS who have homozygous or complex heterozygous podocin mutations have a low recurrence rate (Vincenti and Ghiggeri, 2005). In other patients with sporadic FSGS, a more complex and likely multifactorial etiology accounts for the recurrence of FSGS. There are conflicting results with living donation in FSGS. Baum *et al.* (2001) found that the results with living transplants in patients with FSGS were worse than in patients without FSGS, the graft survival being similar to that observed in cadaveric renal transplant recipients without FSGS. However, Cibrik *et al.* (2003), by reviewing the US Renal Data System database, found that the risk of death-censored graft loss was 1% per year in patients who received a zero HLA-mismatch from living donors versus a 4.4% loss per year for patients who received a zero HLA-mismatch from cadaveric donors. Abbott *et al.* (2001) reported a 10-year graft survival rate of 70% in patients with FSGS who received a living transplant. The risk of recurrence was higher in white than in non-white patients. Upon multivariate analysis, white recipient, younger age, acute rejection, and cadaveric transplant were associated with worse results.

In patients with early recurrence, proteinuria, usually in a nephrotic range, may precede the development of histologic lesions that develop a median 10–18 days after transplantation (Cochat *et al.*, 1996). Initial biopsies may show normal-appearing glomeruli with ultrastructural findings of diffuse podocyte effacement. Segmental lesions associated with endocapillary proliferation and foam cell accumulation (Figure 7.1) may occur later and progress to glomerular sclerosis and interstitial fibrosis (Stokes and De Palma, 2006). The spontaneous remission of proteinuria is exceptional. Patients with early recurrence of FSGS have a graft

Table 7.2 Factors that may influence the risk of recurrence of focal segmental glomerular sclerosis

Risk factors for recurrence	Low risk of recurrence
Age under 18 years	Familial form
Good HLA match	Sporadic form with NPHS2 mutation
Rapid progression to uremia	Slow progression to uremia
Positive circulating permeability factor (?)	Non-nephrotic proteinuria in the original disease
Second transplant after loss from recurrence	
White race	

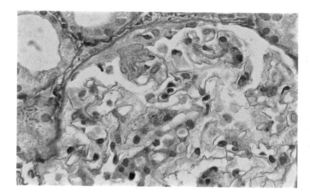

Figure 7.1 Recurrence of FSGS in a 16-year-old boy 15 days after transplantation, profuse proteinuria developed immediately. Graft biopsy showed the typical early features of FSGS: initial collapse of a small peripheral loop, adhering to the capsule through a crown of hypertrophic epithelial cells. (AFOG ×600)

failure rate of 30% at 3 years (Koushik and Matas, 2005), with a relative risk of graft failure of 2.25 when compared with patients without recurrence (Hariharan *et al.*, 1999).

The *management* of patients with recurrence of FSGS and nephrotic syndrome is difficult. The amelioration of proteinuria has been reported in a few children given very *high doses of cyclosporine* (Ingulli and Tejani, 1991). The aim of such an approach is to compensate the lipid binding of cyclosporine by elevated low-density lipoprotein (LDL) concentrations. After that report, some single-center experiences confirmed the possibility of reversing proteinuria by giving oral or intravenous cyclosporine at high doses in children with recurrence of FSGS (Cochat *et al.*, 1996; Salomon *et al.*, 2003; Raafat *et al.*, 2004). However, the long-term efficacy and tolerance of such a therapy remains to be established. Artero *et al.* (1992) treated nine patients with angiotensin-converting enzyme *(ACE) inhibitors*. Of them, five had lasting remission of proteinuria and stable renal function during treatment. An alternative approach is represented by the use of *plasmapheresis* or *immunoadsorption with protein A*. A review of the literature reported that in 58% of adults and in 74% of children treated with plasmapheresis because of the appearance of nephrotic syndrome, proteinuria improved and graft function stabilized, the response being better in patients treated earlier and more intensively (Bosch and Wendler, 2001). In a study, the response to plasmapheresis was similar in recurrent patients with podocin mutation and in those with idiopathic FSGS (Bertelli *et al.*, 2003). In some cases, prolonged plasmapheresis, up to 14 months, was needed to obtain complete remission (Haffner *et al.*, 2005). A protective role of *prophylactic plasmapheresis* (three sessions before transplantation) has been reported by Ohta *et al.* (2001). Of six patients who did not receive prophylactic treatment, four had recurrence of FSGS, while of 15 patients who were

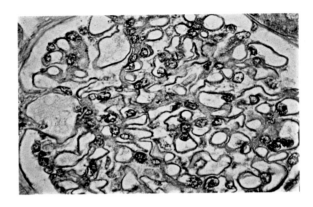

Figure 7.2 De novo membranous nephropathy in a patient transplanted because of polycystic kidney disease. Diffuse and regular thickening of capillary walls similar to that seen in idiopathic membranous nephropathy. (Jones silver ×480) (Courtesy of Dr G Banfi, Ospedale Maggiore, Milan, Italy)

given prophylactic plasmapheresis, only five had recurrence of FSGS. These data were confirmed by Gohh *et al.* (2005), who treated with pre-emptive plasmapheresis ten patients at high risk of recurrence; four of them had had a rapid course of recurrence and six had already lost their previous graft because of FSGS recurrence. Seven patients, including all four patients with first grafts and three of six with prior recurrence, were free of recurrence after 7–42 months. A long-term beneficial effect of *rituximab*, given weekly for 6 weeks, has been reported in a child with FSGS recurrence after transplantation who developed a large-cell lymphoma associated with Epstein–Barr virus infection (Pescovitz *et al.*, 2006).

In summary, the following patterns of response to plasmapheresis may be expected: (1) complete and sustained remission of proteinuria after a short course, (2) complete or partial remission with relapse of nephrotic proteinuria within weeks or months, (3) improvement of proteinuria with an early relapse after plasmapheresis is interrupted, and (4) no response. Unfortunately, it is impossible at present to predict what the response to plasmapheresis will be for the individual patient (Ponticelli *et al.*, 2002b). We suggest pre-emptive plamapheresis whenever possible, and particularly in patients receiving a kidney from a living donor and in those who lost a previous transplant from recurrence. After transplantation, patients with recurrent FSGS and severe nephrotic syndrome should be treated as soon as possible with an intensive course of plasmapheresis (an exchange a day for 3 days, then 2–3 exchanges per week for the first 2 weeks, followed by 1–2 exchanges per week). If complete disappearance of proteinuria is obtained, plasmapheresis treatment may be stopped. If proteinuria improves but remains over 2–3 g per day, we continue plasma exchanges at longer intervals. A further course of plasmapheresis may be attempted in the case of a relapse of nephrotic proteinuria. We also recommend the administration of high-dose ACE inhibitors or angiotensin receptor antagonists in order to exploit the antiproteinuric effect of these agents. The role of rituximab should be better elucidated by further studies.

Membranous nephropathy (MN)

Membranous nephropathy can develop in a transplanted kidney either as a recurrence of the original disease or as a *de novo* form. About one-third of allograft MN is caused by recurrence and two-thirds by *de novo* glomerulonephritis. The proportion of recurrence of MN is difficult to assess, as *de novo* form may develop even in transplant recipients with idiopathic MN as an original disease, with an indistinguishable histologic pattern (Figures 7.2–7.4). Recurrence is exceptional in children. In adults, the rate of recurrence averages 30% (Couser, 2005). No clinical or histologic factor may predict the risk of recurrence. In Caucasian patients, recurrence usually occurs within the second or third year after transplantation. In a series (Josephson *et al.*, 1994), post-transplant recurrence occurred earlier in recipients of a living-donor allograft (9.3±3 months after transplantation) than in cadaveric transplant recipients (18.2±7.5 months). However, a paper from Hong Kong reported that MN occurred later, at a mean of 45 months after transplantation (Chan *et al.*, 2005). Recurrence is not inhibited by cyclosporine (Montagnino *et al.*, 1989; Schwarz *et al.*, 1991).

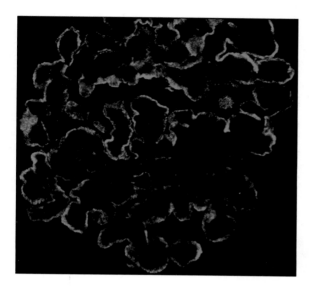

Figure 7.3 Immunofluorescence of the same case. Partial, fine granular deposits of IgG pathognomonic of membranous nephropathy. (×400)

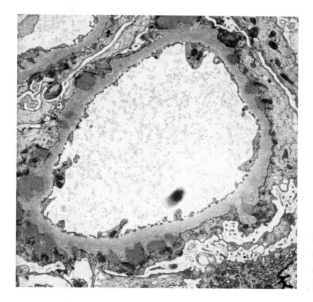

Figure 7.4 Membranous nephropathy, stage I–II: electron-dense globular deposits on the outer side of the glomerular basement membrane, separated by initial spikes. (×16 000)

Clinically, recurrence is heralded by the appearance of proteinuria, which is often in a nephrotic range (more than 3.5 g per day). Rarely, proteinuria may spontaneously improve or even disappear (Marcen *et al.*, 1996). With the exception of these cases, the nephrotic syndrome is usually resistant to treatment, and 60–65% patients progress to end-stage renal failure an average of 4 years after the diagnosis of recurrence (Josephson *et al.*, 1994; Cosyns *et al.*, 1998). The poor prognosis is not always attributable to MN, as many patients also show histologic evidence of rejection. There is no convincing evidence that corticosteroids, cytotoxic drugs, or other immunosuppressive agents may be of benefit in recurrent MN. Symptomatic treatment with diuretics, ACE inhibitors, AT1 receptor blockers, hypolipidemic drugs, and anticoagulants may help in reducing the signs and symptoms related to the nephrotic syndrome.

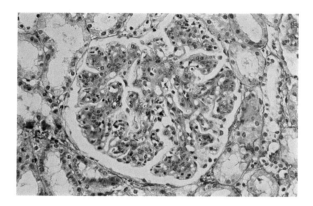

Figure 7.5 Recurrence of membranoproliferative glomerulonephritis type I. Diffuse hypercellularity, mainly due to mesangial cell proliferation, accompanied by mesangial matrix increase and diffuse, through irregular, thickening of the capillary walls. (AFOG ×300)

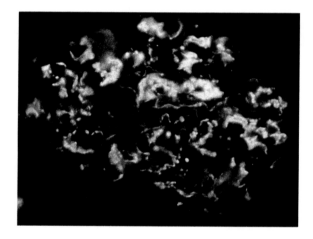

Figure 7.6 Immunostaining with C3 in coarse granular deposits in the mesangium and parietal position, corroborates the diagnosis of MPGN type I

Membranoproliferative glomerulonephritis (MPGN)

Type I MPGN accounts for approximately 80% of cases of idiopathic MPGN. It is characterized by electron-dense subendothelial deposits that contain immunoglobulins and complement under immunofluorescence. Clinically, the disease is characterized by hematuria, heavy proteinuria, hypertension, and impairment of renal function. The post-transplant recurrence rate is quite difficult to estimate because the characteristic lesions of type I MPGN on light microscopy (Figure 7.5) may mimic those seen in allograft glomerulopathy. However, under immunofluorescence, the recurrent type I MPGN shows greater intensity of C3 (Figure 7.6), while there is greater intensity of IgM in allograft glomerulopathy. On electron microscopy, type I MPGN shows subendothelial electron-dense deposits, while transplant glomerulopathy shows an electron-lucent zone in the subendothelial space (Andresdottir *et al.*, 1998; Figure 7.7).

The *recurrence rate* reached 48% at 4 years in a single-center report (Andresdottir *et al.*, 1997). The risk of recurrence is considerably lower in Japan, around 3%, suggesting a role for racial predisposition (Shimizu *et al.*, 1998). There are no clinical features prior to transplantation that can predict the risk of recurrence. Cyclosporine does not seem to be able to prevent recurrence, but may be protective against crescentic transformation (Ahsan *et al.*, 1997). The major clinical feature of recurrence is proteinuria, leading to the nephrotic syndrome and progression to renal insufficiency. The relative risk of *graft failure* is increased in patients with recurrence, ranging between 2.37 (Hariharan *et al.*, 1999) and 2.63 (Briganti *et al.*, 2002) in large surveys. Anedoctal cases of good response to long-term cyclophosphamide

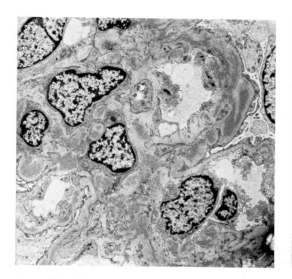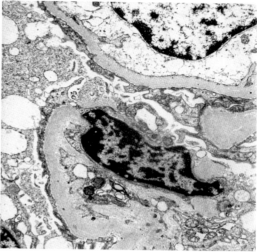

Figure 7.7 (a) Recurrence of MPGN type I. Together with the immunofluorescence pattern, electron microscopical investigation is mandatory to confirm the diagnosis of a recurrence of MPGN type I, disclosing the presence of deposits in the subendothelial and mesangial position (×16 000). (b) For diagnostic purposes the ultrastructural features of a case of 'chronic transplant glomerulopathy' are shown. There is a fairly homogeneous thickening of the 'lamina rara interna', in the absence of electron-dense deposits and cellular interposition. (×25 000) (Courtesy of Professor MJ Mihatsch, University of Basel)

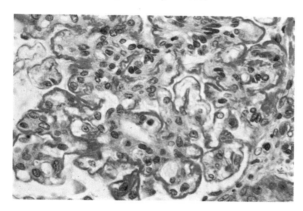

Figure 7.8 Recurrence of MPGN type II. Bright, continuous, ribbon-like deposits underline the capillary walls in this case of dense deposit disease (–), recurring 2 years after transplantation. (AFOG × 650) (Courtesy of Dr G Banfi, Ospedale Maggiore, Milan, Italy)

(Lien and Scott, 2000), high-dose mycophenolate mofetil (Wu *et al.*, 2004), or plasmapheresis (Saxena *et al.*, 2000) have been reported.

Type II MPGN, also called dense deposit disease, is characterized by intramembranous electron-dense deposits and is sometimes associated with partial lipodystrophy. C3 deposits can be found under immunofluorescence in the basal lamina surrounding the deposits and in the mesangium. The clinical expression of dense deposit disease is similar to that of MPGN type I. The histologic and ultrastructural features of *recurrent type II MPGN* may be similar to those seen in the original disease, but in early cases the typical alterations of the capillary wall are not seen under light microscopy (Figures 7.8 and 7.9), endocapillary proliferative glomerulonephritis being the earliest lesion of dense deposit disease (Aita *et al.*, 2006). However, dense deposits can be seen on electron microscopy. Under immunofluorescence, three patterns of glomerular C3 deposition have been described in recurrent type II MPGN (Andresdottir *et al.*, 1999): (1) globular deposition only in the mesangium, (2) mesangial deposits with linear deposits

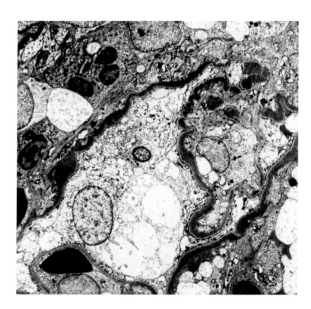

Figure 7.9 Recurrence of MPGN type II. Electron microscopy shows the characteristic dense transformation of the GBM (Courtesy of Professor MJ Mihatsch, University of Basel)

in the capillary walls, and (3) prominent linear deposits in the capillary walls. The histologic recurrence of dense deposits after renal transplantation is frequent, but in a number of patients with recurrence there are no clinical signs or symptoms. In one study, younger age at initial diagnosis and the presence of crescents on the original biopsy were independently associated with recurrence on multivariate analysis (Little et al., 2006). There is little information on the *long-term impact of recurrence*. In a European survey of pediatric transplant patients, 27 cases of MPGN type II were recorded. Ten grafts failed, but only in two patients was graft failure caused by recurrence (Broyer et al., 1992). More recently, Braum et al. (2005) reported the data collected by the North American Pediatric Renal Transplant Cooperative Study. In 75 children with type II MPGN, the 5-year patient survival was 50%, significantly lower than the 74% observed in other transplant patients of the registry. Living transplant recipients had a 5-year graft survival of 66%, significantly better than that of cadaveric transplant recipients. Recurrence was the main cause of graft loss in 15% of patients. In 18 children who underwent graft biopsy, recurrence was seen in 12 (67%). Patients with recurrence had higher serum creatinine levels and greater proteinuria than patients without recurrence. In adults, Andresdottir et al. (1999) reported 11 cases of recurrent type II MPGN. Eight patients with recurrence progressed to end-stage renal failure on average after 14 months. However, in only three patients, with crescents at biopsy, was recurrence the sole cause of graft failure.

Very rare cases of recurrence of *type III MPGN*, with electron-dense deposits in the mesangium as well as in subepithelial and subendothelial locations, have been reported. The patients progressed to dialysis within 3 months to 7 years after diagnosis (Morales et al., 1997; Ramesh Prasad et al., 2004). There is no effective therapy for recurrent type III MPGN.

IgA glomerulonephritis (IgA GN)

IgA GN is the most common recurrent GN after transplantation (Furness et al., 2002). *Histologic recurrence* (Figures 7.10 and 7.11) ranges between 9 and 61% (Table 7.3). These figures may be biased by the fact that not all recipients with microscopic hematuria and/or mild proteinuria are biopsied. Moreover, even asymptomatic patients may have histologic recurrence. Finally, it is likely that the incidence of IgA GN has different racial and geographical distributions. Recurrence may occur immediately after transplantation, but on average the diagnosis is made around 3 years after transplantation (Hariharan and Savin, 1999; Ponticelli et al., 2004). Some investigators reported a higher risk of recurrence for *living-related* transplants (Wang et al., 2001; Andresdottir et al., 2005), but others did not (Kim et al., 2001; Ponticelli

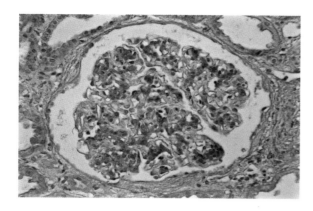

Figure 7.10 Recurrent IgAGN. Moderate mesangial enlargement due to mesangial cells proliferation and matrix increase. (PAS ×480)

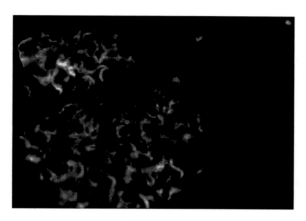

Figure 7.11 Recurrent IgAGN. The immunofluorescence shows the characteristic bright immunostaining for IgA, with parietal and mesangial pattern. (×400)

Table 7.3   Risk of biopsy-proven recurrence of IgA glomerulonephritis after transplantation

Author	Patients (*n*)	Recurrence (*n*)
Schwartz, 1991	8	1 (12%)
Odum, 1994	46	28 (61%)
Hartung, 1995	128	47 (37%)
Kim, 1996	75	36 (48%)
Frohnert, 1997	51	14 (27%)
Ohmacht, 1997	61	33 (54%)
Bumgardner, 1998a	61	18 (29%)
Freese, 1999	104	13 (12%)
Andresdottir, 2001	79	17 (21%)
Ponticelli, 2001	106	37 (35%)
Choy, 2003	75	14 (19%)
Chandrakantan, 2005	122	11 (9%)

et al., 2001). Recurrence tends to occur more frequently in *younger patients* (Ponticelli *et al.*, 2001). No other pre-transplant characteristics are predictive for recurrence. Nor is there evidence that the type of post-transplant immunosuppression may influence the risk of recurrence (Chandrakantan *et al.*, 2005). Hematuria and low-grade proteinuria represent the clinical expression of recurrence.

Lim *et al.* (1991) reported a more favorable *outcome* of the renal allograft in patients with IgA GN than in other transplant recipients, but others found that graft survival in an IgA group was similar to that of non-IgA renal transplant recipients (Bumgardner *et al.*, 1998a; Soler *et al.*, 2005). A retrospective analysis of the Eurotransplant data reported that 1207 patients with IgA GN had better death-censored graft survival at 1 year when compared with 7935 other renal transplant recipients, but the benefit was lost at 3 years, due to an accelerated decline in graft survival after the first year (Andresdottir *et al.*, 2005). The limit of this study rests on the large heterogeneity between patients with IgA GN and the control population. Better results were reported by a case–control study that compared the long-term outcome of 106 patients transplanted because of IgA GN with that of 212 non-IgA patients transplanted in the same period and in the same center (Ponticelli *et al.*, 2001). After censoring graft failures in the first 6 months, the 10-year graft survival probability was not significantly different between the two groups: 75% in patients with IgA GN and 82% in controls. The regression coefficient of the reciprocal of plasma creatinine was also similar in the two groups. In a Cox model analysis, IgA GN recurrence was not associated with an increased risk of graft failure. In the very long term, however, it is possible that recurrent IgA GN may represent a substantial risk factor for graft failure. Rarely, rapidly progressive renal failure caused by an underlying crescentic glomerulonephritis may occur (Benabdallah *et al.*, 2002; Kowalewska *et al.*, 2005).

There is no specific *therapy* for recurrent IgA GN. ACE inhibitors may be prescribed, as a controlled trial showed that their use could reduce proteinuria and preserve renal function in transplant recipients with IgA GN (Takahara *et al.*, 2002). Similar results were obtained with angiotensin II receptor antagonists in non-transplanted patients with IgA GN (Ohashi *et al.*, 2002). If recurrent crescentic IgA GN develops, a trial with high-dose corticosteroids, cyclophosphamide, and plasmapheresis may be attempted, although the results are usually poor.

Antiglomerular basement membrane glomerulonephritis (anti-GBM GN)

The recurrence of this disease is defined by linear deposits of IgG on glomerular capillary walls (Figure 7.12). Anti-GBM GN recurs in 10–30% of allografts particularly if *circulating anti-GBM antibodies* are present at the time of transplantation (Glassock, 1997). Conversely, in patients in whom antibodies cannot be detected, disease does not recur. In a series of ten patients with anti-GBM disease, no case of recurrence occurred (Deegens *et al.*, 2003). However, rare cases of recurrent anti-GBM GN accompanied by the reappearance of anti-GBM antibodies have been reported 7–8 years after transplantation in patients in whom anti-GBM antibodies had disappeared (Fonck *et al.*, 1998; Khandelwal *et al.*, 2004).

Clinical disease consequent to the glomerular deposits of anti-GBM antibodies occurs in less than 10% of cases, and only rarely leads to graft loss. In the past, bilateral nephrectomy of the native kidneys was performed in order to allow the disappearance of antibodies. This intervention is not recommended today. Most clinicians prefer to check the titer of circulating anti-GBM antibodies periodically and wait for 6–12 months before transplantation until the anti-GBM antibodies disappear. With such a policy, the recurrence of anti-GBM GN has virtually disappeared.

Necrotizing glomerulonephritis

The recurrence of necrotizing GN after transplantation is rare. Treatment with cyclophosphamide and corticosteroids is usually effective. Plasmapheresis and intravenous immunoglobulins may also be helpful in difficult cases (Lobbedez *et al.*, 2003).

Finnish type nephrotic syndrome

Congenital nephrotic syndrome of the Finnish type is caused by mutations in the NPHS1 gene which encodes nephrin, a cell adhesion protein located at the glomerular slit diaphragm. Renal transplantation is the only treatment. After transplantation the nephrotic syndrome recurs in 25% of cases, namely those

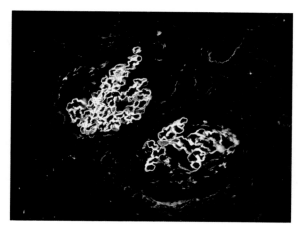

Figure 7.12 Early recurrence of antiGBM-GN in a patient with Goodpasture syndrome. Linear deposition of IgG along the GBM characterizes the reappearances of antiGBM disease in the graft. (×250)

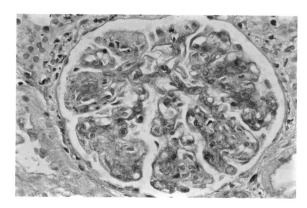

Figure 7.13 Diffuse proliferative lupus nephritis may recur in the graft with the same pattern, although sometimes with focal distribution. In this glomerulus hypercellularity is moderate; *mesangial expansion* with protein deposits, irregular but there is severe thickening of the capillary loops due to mesangial interposition and proteinaceous deposits. (AFOG ×400) (Courtesy of Dr G Banfi, Ospedale Maggiore, Milan, Italy)

with a genotype leading to the *absence of nephrin* (Patrakka *et al.*, 2002). On electron microscopy the fusion of foot processes and a decrease of slit diaphragms can be seen. High levels of *anti-nephrin antibodies* may be detected in the sera of children with recurrence, suggesting a pathogenic role for these antibodies (Wang *et al.*, 2001). Cyclophosphamide therapy may be effective, but most patients with recurrence lose their allografts.

Recurrence of systemic diseases

Lupus nephritis

The recurrence of lupus nephritis (Figure 7.13) is thought to be rare, ranging between 2 and 4% in some large series (Stone, 1998; Grimbert *et al.*, 1998). A higher level of histologic recurrence, up to 30%, was reported by Goral *et al.* (2003), even if the morphologic lesions were usually mild. It is possible that the recurrence of lupus nephritis may have been underestimated because of underreporting, insufficient follow-up, or failure to diagnose recurrence (Stone, 1998).

The *clinical outcome* is usually favorable. After transplantation many patients who were previously unresponsive to immunosuppression show little or no sign of active disease (Nossent *et al.*, 1991). A retrospective analysis of 100 renal transplants performed in young lupus patients found comparable patient and graft survival at 3 years to those seen in age-, race-, and gender-matched controls (Bartosh *et al.*, 2001). Another

Table 7.4   Graft survival in adult renal transplant patients with SLE and in well-matched controls

Author	Actuarial graft survival (years)	SLE transplant recipients (%)	Matched controls (%)
Stone, 1998	10	18.5	34.5
Bumgardner, 1998b	10	62	73
Grimbert, 1998	5	69	70
Azevedo, 1998	5	81	70
Ward, 2000	5	58	62
Deegens, 2003a	5	38	46
Moroni, 2005	15	69	67

study found that graft survival was similar in children with lupus and in those transplanted for other disease, but patient survival was lower in children with lupus (Gipson *et al.*, 2003). The prognosis has been reported to be good in adults (Haubitz *et al.*, 1997; Azevedo *et al.*, 1998; Alarcon-Segovia, 2000). However, only a few studies compared the results of renal transplantation in systemic lupus erythematosus (SLE) patients with those of well-matched controls (Table 7.4). The general impression is that the expectancies for patient and graft survival are similar in patients with SLE and in controls even in the long term. In our experience also, morbidity was similar in patients with lupus nephritis and in well-matched controls, with the exception of thrombotic events that were more frequent in SLE patients, particularly in those with antiphospholipid antibodies (Moroni *et al.*, 2005). Even in patients in whom recurrence has been clearly identified it is usually of little clinical relevance, and does not justify a reinforcement of immunosuppression, which should be reserved for exceptional cases showing a severe lupus flare-up. The introduction of cyclophosphamide and an increase in corticosteroid dosage are usually sufficient to obtain remission. Good results have also been achieved with the introduction of mycophenolate mofetil (Denton *et al.*, 2001).

The results are largely influenced by the clinical condition of the patient at transplantation. As patients who receive vigorous immunosuppression or long-term corticosteroid therapy are at higher risk of developing infection, cardiovascular disease, malignancy, and other severe complications after transplantation, it may be advisable to postpone transplantation by at least 1 year after entry to dialysis in these patients, to allow a 'wash-out' of previous corticosteroid and cytotoxic therapy (Ponticelli and Moroni, 2005).

Henoch–Schönlein purpura

A review of the literature reported a recurrence of IgA mesangial deposits in 53% of renal allografts performed in patients with Henoch–Schönlein purpura. Clinical recurrence with microscopic hematuria and proteinuria occurred in 18% of cases; graft loss from recurrence occurred in 11% of cases at 5 years (Meulders *et al.*, 1994).

Recurrence is frequent in children, while it is more rare in adults (Crown *et al.*, 1994). A few patients who have IgA ANCA (antineutrophil cytoplasmic antibodies) in the serum are particularly prone to recurrence of the disease after transplantation (Martin *et al.*, 1997). Recurrence can occur despite a delay of more than 1 year between the disappearance of proteinuria and transplantation. Clinical signs and symptoms may be absent. *Hematuria*, sometimes macroscopic, moderate proteinuria, and hypertension are common in patients with clinical evidence of recurrence. Histologic recurrence is characterized by focal and segmental necrotizing GN (Figure 7.14) with mesangial IgA deposits. The prognosis is more severe in adults than in children (Meulders *et al.*, 1994). In a European survey, graft survival in patients with recurrence was 57% at 2 years

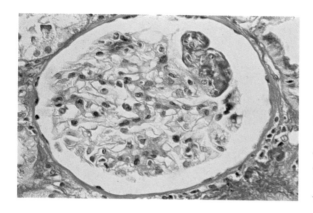

Figure 7.14 Recurrence of Henoch–Schönlein nephritis. Gross hematuria heralded the recurrence of focal and segmental necrotizing glomerulonephritis in this 35-year-old woman with Henoch–Schönlein purpura, 18 months after transplantation. (AFOG ×400)

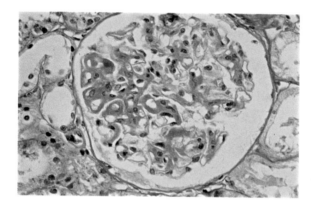

Figure 7.15 Recurrence of fibrillary/immunotactoid glomerulopathy. In the presence of an irregular 'membranoproliferative' pattern, as shown in this picture, one should also keep in mind the possibility of a recurrence of immunotactoid or fibrillary glomerulonephritis. (AFOG ×400) (Courtesy of Dr G Banfi, Ospedale Maggiore, Milan, Italy)

(Briggs and Jones, 1999a). Better results have been reported by Soler *et al.* (2005). In their small series the 5-year graft survival was 78%. The prognosis was more severe for cases with crescents at renal biopsy.

Fibrillary/immunotactoid glomerulopathy (FG)

This rare disease is characterized by the extracellular deposition of non-branching microfibrils or microtubules within the mesangium and capillary walls of renal glomeruli. Proteinuria, generally in a nephrotic range, hematuria, hypertension, and progressive course to renal failure are the main clinical features. There is limited information on the results of renal transplantation in FG because the diagnosis is difficult without electron microscopy (Figures 7.15 and 7.16). Of the 14 cases reported in the literature, fibril deposition recurred in six cases after 2 years or more. In spite of recurrence, the allografts functioned for 5–11 years (Samaniego *et al.*, 2001).

Amyloidosis

Primary amyloidosis may recur on the kidney allograft in about 25% of cases (Harrison *et al.*, 1993). Not all patients with recurrence of amyloid deposits show signs of renal disease. *Proteinuria*, usually causing a nephrotic syndrome, is the cardinal clinical sign. It often heralds progressive renal dysfunction. Unfortunately, many patients die from infections or cardiovascular complications even if the allograft function maintains stable. In a series of 105 renal transplants in patients with amyloidosis, graft survival was comparable to that seen in transplant patients with diabetes (Isoniemi *et al.*, 1994). Autologous stem cell and kidney transplantation may be proposed in cases with progressive primary amyloidosis (Merlini and Remuzzi, 2005).

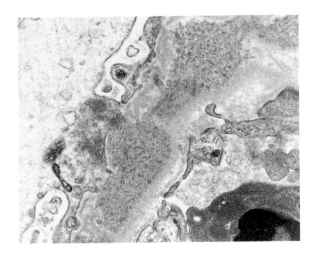

Figure 7.16 Electron microscopy shows the structured ('tactoid') deposits permeating the GBM. (Courtesy of Dr G Banfi, Ospedale Maggiore, Milan, Italy)

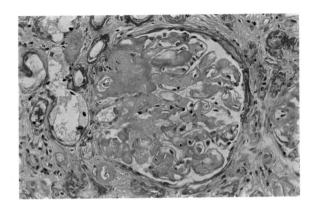

Figure 7.17 Recurrence of amyloidosis. The mesangial space is severely and irregularly dilated by the presence of a fluffy, cotton-like, slightly PAS-positve material in this patient with rheumatoid arthritis and recurrence of amyloidosis, 3.5 years after transplantation. (PAS ×300)

In *amyloidosis* secondary to *rheumatoid arthritis*, the risk of recurrence is correlated with the activity of the underlying primary disease (Figure 7.17). Good results have been reported in patients with *familial Mediterranean fever* (Sever et al., 2001). Recurrence is possible, but the early administration of colchicine, 1 mg/day indefinitely, can prevent the deposit of amyloid substance on the transplanted kidney. Moreover, transplanted patients with familial Mediterranean fever treated with colchicine showed a significantly lower amount of interstitial fibrosis in comparison with matched controls, suggesting a protective effect of this drug against interstitial fibrosis (Ozdemir et al., 2006). Renal transplantation is also indicated in patients with renal amyloidosis secondary to *Behcet's disease* (Ahuja et al., 2001; Akpolat et al., 2003), or in cases of *familial apolipoprotein II* amyloidosis (Magy et al., 2003). Successful liver and kidney transplantation has been reported in a case of *hereditary amyloidosis* caused by a mutation in fibrinogen A (Mousson et al., 2006).

In summary, the decision whether or not to transplant patients with amyloidosis should be based on the general condition of the patient rather than on the concern of recurrence.

Light-chain deposition disease (LCDD)

Light-chain deposition disease is characterized by the deposition of κ- or λ-immunoglobulin light chains in the kidneys and in other organs. About one-third of patients have no associated systemic illness, while in two-thirds, LCDD is associated with multiple myeloma or other lymphoplasmacytic disease (Figures 7.18

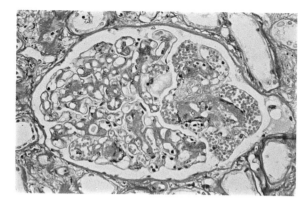

Figure 7.18 Recurrence of light-chain deposition disease. In this case, mesangial areas and capillary walls are markedly, although irregularly, widened by the presence of a homogeneous material that can mimic amyloid or glycosylated material of diabetes. (AFOG ×300)

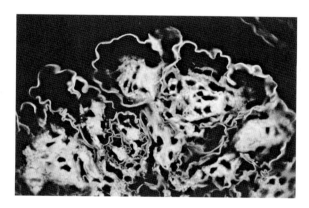

Figure 7.19 Recurrence of light-chain deposition disease. The immunofluorescence clarifies the nature of the disease showing linear parietal and homogeneous mesangial deposits of κ-chain (also present along TBM)

and 7.19). The indication for renal transplantation in these patients is controversial because of the risk of recurrence of LCDD on the graft, and the possibility of disease relapse in other organs (Short *et al.*, 2001). The prognosis is particularly poor when LCDD is associated with proliferative glomerulonephritis. Leung *et al.* (2004) reported their experience with renal transplantation in seven patients affected by LCDD. The disease recurred in five patients after a mean period of 33 months. Four of the five patients with recurrence died, and the fifth patient entered dialysis. Of the other two patients, one died from multiple myeloma and another one was still alive with graft functioning 13 years after transplantation.

Hemolytic–uremic syndrome (HUS)

HUS is a frequent cause of renal failure in children. Most cases are diarrhea-associated (D+HUS) and are usually related to exotoxins produced by *Escherichia coli* O157:H7. Other cases are not associated with diarrhea (D−HUS). Rarely, HUS may occur in several members of the same family (familial HUS). In about 30% of familial HUS, a mutation in the complement factor H gene may be detected. HUS may also occur in adults, and is frequently classified as thrombotic thrombocytopenic purpura (TTP). It may occur in pregnant women, as a complication of pneumonia, or after exposure to drugs such as oral contraceptives, mitomycin C, quinine, ticlopidine, clopidogrel, and calcineurin inhibitors (Ruggenenti *et al.*, 2001; Taylor and Neild, 2005). However, many cases do not demonstrate any etiological factors and are defined as idiopathic.

The possibility of *recurrence* of HUS after renal transplantation is well established, but the risk is variably estimated in different series. After renal transplantation, D+HUS usually does not recur (Ferraris *et al.*, 2002), while idiopathic D− or familial HUS may recur in 60–100% of children (Loirat and Niaudet,

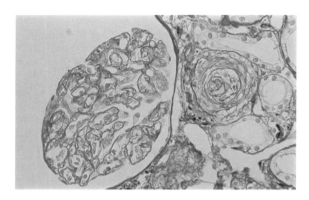

Figure 7.20 Recurrence of hemolytic–uremic syndrome. Acute graft deterioration developed 1 month after surgery in this woman who lost her native kidneys because of HUS. Graft biopsy revealed the recurrence of severe microangiopathy. The typical 'onion skin' aspect of a preglomerular arteriola is adjacent to the tributary glomerulus showing a moderate retraction of the tuft. (AFOG ×200) (Courtesy of Dr G Banfi, Ospedale Maggiore, Milan, Italy)

2003; Zimmerhackl et al., 2007). A high risk of recurrence ranging between 33 and 56% has been reported in adults, with an additional 16–20% of patients demonstrating thrombotic microangiopathy (TMA) in the absence of clinical manifestations (Conlon et al., 1996; Lahlou et al., 2000). Post-transplant recurrence seems to be particularly frequent in adults with autosomal recessive or autosomal dominant HUS (Kaplan and Leonard, 2000). In an analysis of the US Renal Data System, HUS recurred after transplantation in 29% of patients, with an incidence of 189/1000 person-years (Reynolds et al., 2003).

The *pathogenesis* of recurrent post-transplant TMA is still poorly defined. The human plasma protein factor H, which is a multifunctional multidomain protein, acts as a central regulator of the complement system. In addition to its complement regulatory activities, factor H interacts with a wide selection of ligands, such as the C-reactive protein, thrombospondin, bone sialoprotein, osteopontin, and heparin (Zipfel, 2001). In factor H-associated genetic HUS, the mutant factor H proteins can cause reduced binding to the central complement component C3b/C3d to endothelial cells, so favoring the progression of endothelial cell and microvascular damage (Manuelian et al., 2003). Therefore, uncontrolled complement activation and secondary endothelial injury may explain the high incidence of recurrent TMA in patients with factor H deficiency. The pathogenesis of idiopathic TTP has been linked to a deficiency of a metalloprotease referred as ADAMTS 13 (A Disintegrin And Metalloprotease with ThromboSpondin-1-like domains). This protease cleaves the large multimers of von Willebrand factor that can trigger platelet aggregation and microvascular thrombosis. A case report suggested that also patients with a congenital deficiency in the activity of von Willebrand factor-cleaving ADAMTS 13, or with acquired inhibition of ADAMTS 13, may be more susceptible to post-transplant recurrence (Pham et al., 2002), although the role of these abnormalities is still unclear (Nakazawa et al., 2003; Elliott et al., 2003). Apart from genetic predisposition, some factors such as calcineurin inhibitors, anti-mTOR agents, viral infection, and acute rejection may precipitate the recurrence of TMA after renal transplantation.

Clinically, the recurrence of HUS may be associated with hemolytic microangiopathy anemia, thrombocytopenia, hypertension, and progression to renal failure. Neurologic abnormalities and fever occur more rarely. In several cases, however, clinical signs and symptoms may be missing and the diagnosis rests on renal biopsy (Figure 7.20). Post-transplant TMA usually occurs in the early postoperative period, but sometimes occurs later, after some months (Olie et al., 2004). The *differential diagnosis* between recurrence and *de novo* HUS caused by calcineurin inhibitors, infections, or other factors can be difficult. Reversal after withdrawal of the offending drug or effective treatment of other factors implies *de novo* TMA. Also difficult is differential diagnosis from humoral rejection, although some clues, such as C4d deposits, are more frequent in humoral rejection (Mauiyyedi et al., 2002). Renal biopsy is needed in cases characterized by rapidly progressive graft dysfunction without systemic signs or symptoms of HUS.

The *prognosis* is poor in patients with recurrent HUS. In most cases the recurrence of HUS leads to loss of the allograft (Quan et al., 2001). The USRDS (United States Renal Data System) reported a patient survival at 3 years of 50% (Reynolds et al., 2003). In a review of 24 renal transplants in patients with diagnosis of

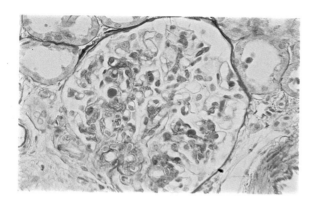

Figure 7.21 Recurrence of cryoglobulinemic nephritis. This case shows some highly characteristic features of cryoglobulinemic nephritis, which are irregularly and segmentally distributed. Pseudothrombi in some loops are associated with a segmental membranoproliferative pattern, without signs of monocyte inflammation. (AFOG ×400) (Courtesy of Dr G Banfi, Ospedale Maggiore, Milan, Italy)

HUS/TTP, the 2-year graft survival was 35%, but eventually all patients with recurrence lost their allograft (Conlon *et al.*, 1996). In another series, the 1-year graft survival in 17 adult patients with TMA recurrence was 29%, while survival in childhood-onset HUS was comparable to that in matched controls (Artz *et al.*, 2003).

Treatment is disappointing. Plasmapheresis or plasma infusion may obtain recovery from thrombocytopenia and microangiopathic anemia in some patients, but is generally ineffective on renal damage (Moake, 2002). In order to restore the defective factor H, combined liver and kidney transplantation has been performed in a few patients. In a child, no signs of hemolysis occurred after transplantation, but the liver was destroyed by a humoral rejection and the child died after a second uneventful liver transplantation. A 2-year-old girl with a recurrent form of D–HUS also received a combined liver and kidney transplantation. She died because of a never-functioning liver transplant (Remuzzi *et al.*, 2002, 2005). In another patient, liver transplantation led to a fatal outcome (Cheong *et al.*, 2004). These results suggest that liver transplantation should be cautiously applied to patients with HUS associated with factor H deficiency.

Mixed cryoglobulinemic nephritis (MCN)

Mixed cryoglobulinemic nephritis is a rare disease usually associated with hepatitis C virus, characterized by vasculitis and by glomerular changes resembling membranoproliferative glomerulonephritis. Only a few patients with MCN have been submitted to renal transplantation. By reviewing the literature, Tarantino *et al.* (1994) found a recurrence of MCN in 70% of cases. However, it is still unclear whether the recurrence of MCN may interfere with the evolution of the transplanted kidney. In our own experience of two patients with MCN submitted to transplantation, one lost his kidney because of acute rejection and the other still has his kidney allograft functioning 8 years after transplantation in spite of histologic recurrence (Figure 7.21).

Vasculitis

Wegener's granulomatosis (WG)

WG recurs in about 17% of cases after transplantation (Nachman *et al.*, 1999). Post-transplant immunosuppression does not influence the probability of recurrence. However, rarely, a few patients may show a recurrence many years after transplantation (Fan *et al.*, 2001). In spite of the risk of recurrence the patient and graft survival rates are similar in patients with WG and in other kidney transplant recipients (Briggs and Jones, 1999b; Deegens *et al.*, 2003a, 2003b).

The optimal timing for transplantation is not clear. A successful outcome was obtained even in patients with a short interval between clinical onset and transplantation. The presence in the serum of ANCA may increase the risk of recurrence, but not significantly (Nachman *et al.*, 1999). Cyclophosphamide and corticosteroids may stabilize renal function in most patients with recurrence (Nyberg *et al.*, 1997; Oka *et al.*, 2000), but this additional treatment can expose the patient to the risk of over-immunosuppression.

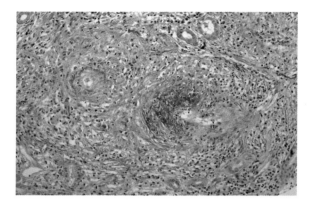

Figure 7.22 Recurrence of microscopic polyarteritis 8 years renal transplantation. Segmental but complete necrosis of a branch of interlobular artery, with severe parietal inflammation is pathognomonic of ANCA-associated micropolyarteritis. (AFOG ×250)

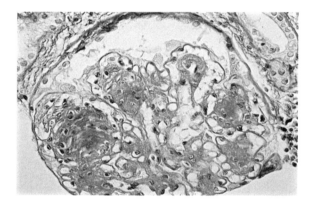

Figure 7.23 Recurrence of diabetic glomerulosclerosis. In its full pattern, as in this case, diabetic glomerulosclerosis usually recurs in the graft only after years of ill-controlled disease. (AFOG ×480) (Courtesy of Dr G Banfi, Ospedale Maggiore, Milan, Italy)

Microscopic polyarteritis

The risk of recurrence was lower than 3% in a European survey. However, the graft survival was lower than that seen in patients with other renal diseases due to the high rate of death caused by cardiovascular complications (Briggs and Jones, 1999b). Cases with lung or kidney involvement can be successfully treated with intravenous high-dose methylprednisolone pulses (Rostaing *et al.*, 1997) (Figure 7.22).

Recurrence of metabolic disease

Diabetic nephropathy

Histologic recurrence of diabetic nephropathy has been reported to occur in almost 40% of diabetic patients, on average 6.7 years after transplantation (Bhalla *et al.*, 2003). In patients with proteinuria and renal insufficiency the typical nodular intercapillary glomerulosclerosis (Figure 7.23) is seen infrequently, while vascular changes are predominant (Hariharan *et al.*, 1996).

The *progression* of histologic lesions in the transplanted kidney is usually slow, but more rapid than in the original disease, perhaps because of the lower nephron mass, the use of nephrotoxic agents such as cyclosporine or tacrolimus, and the frequent hypertension. Microalbuminuria heralds the presence of renal morphologic abnormalities. Overt proteinuria and nephrotic syndrome develop later, preceding the onset of progressive renal failure. Frequent recurrence accounted for only 1.8% of graft losses in the

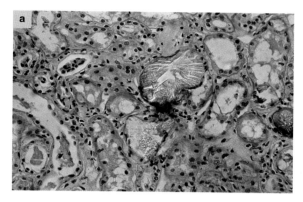

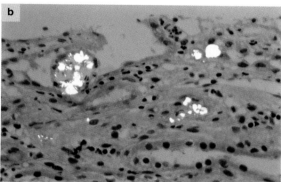

Figure 7.24 (a) Diffuse tubular damage with focal epithelial necrosis and diffuse interstitial inflammation. Some dilated tubular segments are filled with cellular debris and protein cast, but the central and largest segment is filled by needles of crystals, laying circumferentially on the luminal side of the tubular basement membrane, which shows partial disruption. (b) At polarized light the intraluminal crystals show birefringence. Such morphologic features are characteristic of crystals made of oxalic acid which, in this woman affected by primary oxaluria, massively precipitated destroying the graft 6 months after transplantation. (Courtesy of Dr G Banfi, Ospedale Maggiore, Milan, Italy)

largest series of renal transplants in diabetic recipients (Basadonna *et al.*, 1992). This is probably due to the fact that the mean interval between the onset of insulin-dependent diabetes and the development of overt nephropathy in renal transplant recipients is several years (Hariharan *et al.*, 1996).

To prevent the development of diabetic transplant nephropathy, strict glycemic control should be recommended. ACE inhibitors and/or angiotensin receptor antagonists may be helpful in slowing the progression of renal disease, and should be started as early as possible.

Oxalosis (primary hyperoxaluria)

Primary hyperoxaluria (PH) is a term to indicate two genetic disorders of glyoxylate metabolism leading to an excessive synthesis and urine excretion of oxalic acid. PH type I is caused by a defect of α-ketoglutarate: glyoxylate carboxylase. PH type II is caused by a defect of the enzyme D-glyceric dehydrogenase. In infancy, the disease is characterized by nephrocalcinosis and widespread oxalate deposition, particularly in blood vessel walls and in bone. Most commonly the disease is characterized by severely recurrent nephrolithiasis. Large amounts of pyridoxine (200–400 mg per day) may decrease the oxalate excretion in some patients with PH type I (pyridoxine responders).

After renal transplantation, patients with PH may show a *rapid recurrence* with deposition of oxalate in the allograft that results in allograft loss (Figure 7.24). Thus, for most patients a double liver and kidney transplant is necessary. The transplanted liver may restore the missing enzyme and prevent cardiovascular complications which represent the major cause of death (Detry *et al.*, 2002). It is advisable to perform the liver and kidney transplantation before dialysis in order to prevent the consequences of the oxalate burden on target organs.

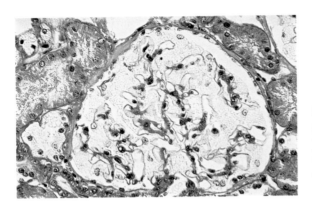

Figure 7.25 Recurrence of Fabry's disease. The glomerulus shows the characteristic fine web of foamy, enlarged visceral podocytes, wrapping up the loops, which appear well preserved. (AFOG ×250) (Courtesy of Dr G Banfi, Ospedale Maggiore, Milan, Italy)

In patients with PH type I who respond to pyridoxine and in patients with type II, which is less severe than type I, isolated renal transplantation may be done successfully (Monico and Milliner, 2001). *Forced diuresis* and *administration of high-dose pyridoxine* after transplantation are mandatory in these cases. A survey of 190 adult renal transplant recipients who had PH showed that the death-censored graft survival was superior in patients who received a combined liver and kidney transplant than in the recipients of a kidney alone (Cibrik *et al.*, 2002).

Cystinosis

This is a rare metabolic disease inherited as an autosomal recessive trait and characterized by the intracellular accumulation of free cystine in many organs, including the kidney. Renal transplantation in children with cystinosis gives results comparable to those in children with other renal diseases (Ehrich *et al.*, 1991). *Cystinosis does not recur*, even if some accumulation of cystine may be seen in the renal interstitium. These cystine deposits are thought to derive from macrophage invasion of host origin, and have no clinical consequences on the graft. Despite successful transplantation, accumulation of *cystine in other organs* continues and can lead to disabling consequences, such as ophthalmological problems, distal myopathy with muscle wasting, swallowing difficulties, pulmonary dysfunction, diabetes, and central nervous system deterioration (Gahl *et al.*, 2002). The early and continuous administration of cysteamine, 60–90 mg/kg/day q.i.d. every 6 hours, may lower by 90% the content of cysteamine in leukocytes, improve the annual growth rate, and allow a nearly normal life (Kleta and Gahl, 2004). Cysteamine in the form of eye-drops may prevent corneal accumulation.

Fabry's disease

This disease is caused by a deficiency of the enzyme α-galactosidase with the consequent accumulation of glycosphyngolipids in most tissues, including the kidney. Angiokeratomata, corneal dystrophy, acroparesthesias, mitral valve defect, and cardiovascular disease are frequent clinical features. Renal failure is the most common cause of death. Enzyme replacement therapy with high-dose α-galactosidase is now available (Caplan *et al.*, 2001). Two different agalsidase formulations have been obtained, one from human fibroblast and one from Chinese hamster ovary cells. Both products have proved to be effective and safe.

Results with renal transplantation were poor in the past, mostly because of premature cardiovascular and cerebrovascular deaths. Recurrence of the disease on kidney allograft may occur (Figure 7.25), but the impact in the long-term is still unclear (Sessa *et al.*, 2002). More recent data showed that the short-term and long-term graft survival is comparable to that in kidney transplant recipients with other primary diseases (Obrador *et al.*, 2002). *Enzyme replacement therapy* in renal transplant patients was well tolerated and preserved renal graft function, improved extra-renal symptoms, and preserved cardiomyopathy progression at least in the short term (Mignani *et al.*, 2004).

Lipoprotein glomerulopathy (LG)

This rare disease is characterized by intracapillary lipoprotein deposits associated with proteinuria often in a nephrotic range, and qualitative changes in plasma apolipoprotein E. Cases of recurrence have been reported in both living kidney and cadaveric kidney recipients, suggesting a role for humoral components resulting from abnormal lipoprotein metabolism, probably linked to apolipoprotein E (Miyata et al., 1999). Although the majority of patients lost their graft after recurrence, one case with stable graft function 4 years after recurrence has been described (Mourad et al., 1998).

References

Abbott KC, Sawyers ES, Oliver JD III, et al. Graft loss due to recurrent focal segmental glomerulosclerosis in renal transplant recipients in the United States. Am J Kidney Dis 2001; 37: 366–73.

Ahsan N, Manning EC, Dabbs DJ, et al. Recurrent type I membranoproliferative glomerulonephritis after renal transplantation and protective role of cyclosporine in acute crescentic transformation. Clin Transplant 1997; 11: 9–14.

Ahuja TS, Boughton J, Weiss V, et al. Renal Behcet's disease: a cumulative analysis. Semin Arthritis Rheum 2001; 31: 317–37.

Akpolat T, Diri B, Oguz Y, et al. Behcet's disease and renal failure. Nephrol Dial Transplant 2003; 18: 888–9.

Alarcon-Segovia D. Kidney transplantation is a safe therapeutic tool in systemic lupus erythematosus. Clin Exp Rheumatol 2000; 18: 185–6.

Aita K, Ito S, Tanabe K, et al. Early recurrence of dense deposit disease with marked endocapillary proliferation after renal transplantation. Pathol Int 2006; 56: 101–9.

Andresdottir MB, Assmann KJ, Hojitsma AJ, et al. Recurrence of type I membranoproliferative glomerulonephritis after renal transplantation: analysis of the incidence, risk factors and impact on graft survival. Transplantation 1997; 63: 1628–33.

Andresdottir MB, Assmann KJ, Koene RA, Wetzels JF. Immunohistological and ultrastructural differences between recurrent type I membranoproliferative glomerulonephritis and chronic transplant glomerulopathy. Am J Kidney Dis 1998; 32: 582–8.

Andresdottir MB, Assman KJ, Hojistma AJ, et al. Renal transplantation in patients with dense deposit disease: morphological characteristics of recurrent disease and clinical outcome. Nephrol Dial Transplant 1999; 14: 1723–31.

Andresdottir MB, Haasnot GW, Doxiadis II, et al. Exclusive characteristics of graft survival and risk factors in recipients of immunoglobulin A nephropathy: a retrospective analysis of registry data. Transplantation 2005; 80: 1012–18.

Artero M, Biava C, Amend W. Recurrent focal glomerulosclerosis. Natural history and response to therapy. Am J Med 1992; 92: 375–83.

Artz MA, Steenbergen EJ, Hoitsma AJ, et al. Renal transplantation in patients with hemolytic uremic syndrome: high rate of recurrence and increased incidence of acute rejection. Transplantation 2003; 15: 821–6.

Azevedo LS, Romao JE, Malheiros D, et al. Renal transplantation in systemic lupus erythematosus. A case control study of 45 patients. Nephrol Dial Transplant 1998; 13: 2894–8.

Bartosh SM, Fine RN, Sullivan EK. Outcome after transplantation of young patients with systemic lupus erythematosus: a report of the North America pediatric renal transplant cooperative group. Transplantation 2001; 72: 973–8.

Basadonna G, Matas AJ, Najarian JS, et al. Transplantation in diabetic patients: the University of Minnesota experience. Kidney Int 1992; 42: S193–8.

Baum MA, Stablein DM, Panzarino VM, et al. Loss of living donor renal allograft advantage in children with focal segmental glomerulosclerosis. Kidney Int 2001; 59: 328–33.

Benabdallah L, Rerolle JP, Peraldi MN, et al. An unusual recurrence of crescentic nephritis after renal transplantation for IgA nephropathy. Am J Kidney Dis 2002; 40: E20.

Bertelli R, Ginevri F, Caridi G, et al. Recurrence of focal segmental glomerulosclerosis in patients with mutations of podocin. Am J Kidney Dis 2003; 41: 1314–21.

Bhalla V, Nast CC, Stollenwerk N, et al. Recurrent and de novo diabetic nephropathy in renal allografts. Transplantation 2003; 75: 66–71.

Bosch T, Wendler T. Extracorporeal plasma treatment in primary and recurrent focal segmental glomerular sclerosis. Ther Apher 2001; 5: 155–60.

Boute N, Gribouval O, Roselli S, et al. NPHS2 encoding the glomerular protein is mutated in autosomal recessive steroid-resistant nephritic syndrome. Nat Genet 2000; 24: 349–54.

Braum MC, Stablein DM, Hamiwka LA, et al. Recurrence of membranoproliferative glomerulonephritis type II in renal allografts: the North American Pediatric Renal Transplant Cooperative Study experience. J Am Soc Nephrol 2005; 16: 2225–33.

Briganti EM, Russ GR, McNeil JJ, et al. Risk of renal allograft loss from recurrent glomerulonephritis. N Engl J Med 2002; 347: 103–9.

Briggs JD, Jones E. Recurrence of glomerulonephritis following renal transplantation. Nephrol Dial Transplant 1999a; 14: 564–5.

Briggs JD, Jones E. Renal transplantation for uncommon diseases. Nephrol Dial Transplant 1999b; 14: 570–5.

Broyer M, Selwood N, Brunner F. Recurrence of primary renal disease on kidney graft. A European experience. J Am Soc Nephrol 1992; 2: 5255–7.

Bumgardner GL, Amend WC, Ascher NL, Vincenti EG. Single-center long-term results of renal transplantation for IgA nephropathy. Transplantation 1998a; 65: 1053–60.

Bumgardner GL, Mauer SM, Payne W, et al. Single-center 1–15 years results of renal transplantation in patients with systemic lupus erythematosus. Transplantation 1998b; 46: 703–9.

Caplan L, Linthorst GE, Desnick RJ. Safety and efficacy of recombinant human α-galactosidase A-replacement therapy in Fabry's disease. N Engl J Med 2001; 345: 9–16.

Chan KW, Chan GS, Tang S. Glomerular pathology of allograft kidneys in Hong Kong. Transplant Proc 2005; 37: 4293–6.

Chandrakantan A, Ratanapanichkich P, Said P, et al. Recurrent IgA nephropathy after renal transplantation despite immunosuppressive regimen with mycophenolate mofetil. Nephrol Dial Transplant 2005; 20: 1214–21.

Cheong HI, Lee BS, Kang HG, et al. Attempted treatment of factor H deficiency by liver transplantation. Pediatr Nephrol 2004; 19: 454–8.

Choy BY, Chan TM, Lo SK, Lai KN. Renal transplantation in patients with primary immunoglobulin A nephropathy. Nephrol Dial Transplant 2003; 18: 2399–404.

Cibrik DM, Kaplan B, Arnorfer JA, Meier-Kriesche HU. Renal allograft survival in patients with oxalosis. Transplantation 2002; 74: 707–10.

Cibrik DM, Kaplan B, Campbell DA, Meier-Kriesche HU. Renal allograft survival in transplant recipients with focal segmental glomerulosclerosis. Am J Transplant 2003; 3: 64–7.

Cochat P, Schell M, Ranchin B, et al. Management of recurrent nephrotic syndrome after kidney transplantation in children. Clin Nephrol 1996; 46: 17–20.

Conlon PJ, Brennan DC, Pfaf WW, et al. Renal transplantation in adults with thombotic thrombocytopenic purpura/haemolytic–uraemic syndrome. Nephrol Dial Transplant 1996; 11: 1810–14.

Cosyns JP, Couchoud C, Pouteil-Noble C, et al. Recurrence of membranous nephropathy after renal transplantation: probability, outcome and risk factors. Clin Nephrol 1998; 50: 144–53.

Couser W. Recurrent glomerulonephritis in the renal allograft: an update of selected areas. Exp Clin Transplant 2005; 1: 283–8.

Crown AL, Woolfson RG, Griffiths MH, et al. Recurrent systemic Henoch–Schönlein purpura in an adult following renal transplantation. Nephrol Dial Transplant 1994; 9: 423–5.

Dall'Amico R, Ghiggeri G, Carraro M, et al. Prediction and treatment of recurrent focal segmental glomerulosclerosis after renal transplantation in children. Am J Kidney Dis 1999; 34: 1048–55.

Dantal J, Godfrin Y, Koll R, et al. Antihuman immunoglobulin affinity immunoadsorption strongly decreases proteinuria in patients with relapsing nephrotic syndrome. J Am Soc Nephrol 1998; 9: 1709–15.

Deegens JK, Artz MA, Hoijtsma AJ, Wetzels JF. Outcome of renal transplantation in patients with systemic lupus erythematosus. Transpl Int 2003a; 16: 411–18.

Deegens JK, Artz MA, Hoitsma AJ, Wetzels JF. Outcome of renal transplantation in patients with pauci-immune small vessel vasculitis or anti-GBM disease. Clin Nephrol 2003b; 59: 1–9.

Denton MD, Galvanek EG, Singh A, Sayegh MH. Membranous nephritis in a renal allograft: response to mycophenolate mofetil. Am J Transplant 2001; 1: 288–92.

Detry O, Honore P, DeRoover A, et al. Reversal of oxalosis cardiomyopathy after combined liver and kidney transplantation. Transpl Int 2002; 15: 50–2.

Doublier S, Musante G, Lupia E, et al. Direct effects of plasma protein factors from patients with idiopathic FSGS on nephrin and podocyte expression in human podocytes. Int J Mol Med 2005; 16: 49–58.

Ducloux D, Rebibou JM, Smhoun-Ducloux S, et al. Recurrence of hemolytic–uremic syndrome in renal transplant recipients: a meta-analysis. Transplantation 1988; 65: 1405–7.

Ehrich JHH, Brodehl J, Byrd DY, et al. Renal transplantation in 22 children with nephropatic cystinosis. Pediatr Nephrol 1991; 5: 708–14.

Elliott MA, Nichols WL Jr, Plumhoff EA, et al. Posttransplantation thrombotic thrombocytopenic purpura: a single-center experience and a contemporary review. Mayo Clin Proc 2003; 78: 421–30.

Fan SL, Lewis KE, Ball E, et al. Recurrence of Wegener's granulomatosis 13 years after renal transplantation. Am J Kidney Dis 2001; 38: E32.

Ferraris JR, Ramirez JA, Ruiz S, et al. Shiga-toxin-associated hemolytic uremic syndrome: absence of recurrence after renal transplantation. Pediatr Nephrol 2002; 17: 809–14.

Fonck C, Loute G, Cosyns JP, Pirson Y. Recurrent fulminant anti-glomerular basement membrane nephritis at 7-year interval. Am J Kidney Dis 1998; 32: 323–7.

Freese P, Svalander C, Norden G, Nyberg G. Clinical risk factors for recurrence of IgA nephritis. Clin Transplant 1999; 13: 313–17.

Frohnert PP, Donadio JV, Velosa JA, et al. Recurrent immunoglobulin A nephropathy after renal transplantation. Clin Transplant 1997; 11: 127–33.

Furness PN, Roberts ISD, Briggs JD. Recurrent glomerular disease in transplants. Transplant Proc 2002; 34: 242.

Gahl WA, Thoene JG, Schneider JA. Cystinosis. N Engl J Med 2002; 347: 111–21.

Gipson DS, Ferris ME, Dooley MA, et al. Renal transplantation in children with lupus nephritis. Am J Kidney Dis 2003; 41: 455–63.

Glassock RJ. Crescentic glomerulonephritis. In Ponticelli C, Glassock RJ, eds. Treatment of Primary Glomerulonephritis. Oxford: Oxford University Press, 1997: 234–54.

Gohh RY, Yango AF, Morrissey PE, et al. Preemptive plasmapheresis and recurrence of FSGS in high-risk renal transplant recipients. Am J Transplant 2005; 5: 2907–12.

Goral S, Ynares C, Shappell SB, et al. Recurrent lupus nephritis in renal transplant recipients revisited: it is not rare. Transplantation 2003; 75: 651–6.

Grimbert P, Frappier J, Bedrossian J, et al. Long-term outcome of kidney transplantation in patients with systemic lupus erythematosus: a multicenter study. Groupe Cooperatif de Transplantation d'Ile de France. Transplantation 1998; 66: 1000–3.

Haffner K, Zimmerhackl LB, von Schnakenburg C, et al. Complete remission of post-transplant FSGS recurrence by long-term plasmapheresis. Pediatr Nephrol 2005; 20: 994–7.

Hariharan S, Smith RD, Viero R, et al. Diabetic nephropathy after renal transplantation. Transplantation 1996; 62: 632–5.

Hariharan S, Savin V. Recurrent and de novo glomerular diseases after renal transplantation. Graft 1999; 2 (Suppl 2): S113–18.

Hariharan S, Adams MB, Brennan DC, et al. Recurrent and de novo glomerular disease after renal transplantation. A report from the Renal Allograft Disease Registry (RADR). Transplantation 1999; 68: 635–41.

Harrison KL, Alpers CE, Davis CL. De novo amyloidosis in a renal allograft: a case report and review of the literature. Am J Kidney Dis 1993; 22: 468–76.

Hartung R, Livingston B, Excell L, et al. Recurrence of IgA deposits/disease in grafts. Contrib Nephrol 1995; 111: 13–16.

Haubitz M, Kliem V, Koch KM, et al. Renal transplantation for patients with autoimmune disease: single-center experience with 42 patients. Transplantation 1997; 15: 1251–7.

Heidet L, Gagnadoux MF, Beziau A, et al. Recurrence of de novo membranous glomerulonephritis on renal grafts. Clin Nephrol 1994; 41: 314–18.

Ingulli E, Tejani A. Incidence, treatment and outcome of recurrent focal segmental glomerulosclerosis posttransplantation in 42 allografts in children: a single center experience. Transplantation 1991; 51: 401–5.

Isoniemi H, Kyllunen L, Ahonen J, et al. Improved outcome of transplantation in amyloidosis. Transpl Int 1994; 7 (Suppl 1): S298–300.

Josephson MA, Spargo B, Hollandsworth DO, Thistlewait MD. The recurrence of membranous glomerulopathy in a renal transplant recipient: case report and literature review. Am J Kidney Dis 1994; 24: 873–8.

Kaplan BS, Leonard MB. Autosomal dominant hemolytic uremic syndrome: variable phenotypes and transplant results. Pediatr Nephrol 2000; 14: 464–8.

Khandelwal M, McCormick BB, Lajoie G, et al. Recurrence of anti-GBM disease 8 years after renal transplantation. Nephrol Dial Transplant 2004; 19: 491–4.

Kim YS, Jeong HJ, Choi HK, et al. Renal transplantation in patients with I$_g$A nephropathy. Transplant Proc 1996; 28: 1543.

Kim YS, Moon JI, Jeong HJ, et al. Live donor renal allograft in end-stage renal failure patients from immunoglobulin A nephropathy. Transplantation 2001; 71: 233–8.

Kleta R, Gahl WA. Pharmacological treatment of nephropathic cystinosis with cysteamine. Expert Opin Pharmacother 2004; 5: 2255–62.

Koushik R, Matas AJ. Focal segmental glomerular sclerosis in kidney allograft recipients: an evidence-based approach. Transplant Rev 2005; 19: 78–87.

Kowalewska J, Juan S, Sustento-Reodica N, et al. IgA nephropathy with crescents in kidney transplant recipients. Am J Kidney Dis 2005; 45: 167–75.

Lahlou A, Lang P, Charpentier B, et al. Hemolytic uremic syndrome. Recurrence after renal transplantation. Groupe Cooperatif de l'Ile de France (GCIF). Medicine (Baltimore) 2000; 79: 90–102.

Leung N, Lager DJ, Gertz MA, et al. Long-term outcome of renal transplantation in light-chain deposition disease. Am J Kidney Dis 2004; 43: 147–53.

Lien YH, Scott K. Long-term cyclophosphamide treatment for recurrent type I membranoproliferative glomerulonephritis after transplantation. Am J Kidney Transplant 2000; 35: 539–43.

Lim EC, Chia D, Terasaki PI. Studies of sera from IgA nephropathy patients to explain high kidney graft survival. Hum Immunol 1991; 32: 81–6.

Little MA, Dupont P, Campbell E, et al. Severity of primary MPGN, rather than MPGN type, determines renal survival and post-transplantation recurrence risk. Kidney Int 2006; 69: 504–5.

Lobbedez T, Comoz F, Renaudineau E, et al. Recurrence of ANCA-positive glomerulonephritis immediately after renal transplantation. Am J Kidney Dis 2003; 42: 52–6.

Loirat C, Niaudet P. The risk of recurrence of hemolytic uremic syndrome after renal transplantation in children. Pediatr Nephrol 2003; 18: 1095–101.

Magy N, Liepnieks JJ, Yazaki M, et al. Renal transplantation for apolipoprotein AII amyloidosis. Amyloid 2003; 10: 224–8.

Manuelian T, Hellwage J, Meri S. Mutations in factor H reduce binding affinity to C3b and heparin and surface attachment to endothelial cells in hemolytic uremic syndrome. J Clin Invest 2003; 111: 1181–90.

Marcen R, Mampso F, Tervel JL, et al. Membranous nephropathy: recurrence after kidney transplantation. Nephrol Dial Transplant 1996; 11: 1129–33.

Martin SJ, Audrain MA, Baranger T, et al. Recurrence of immunoglobulin A nephropathy with immunoglobulin A antineutrophil cytoplasmic antibodies following renal transplantation. Am J Kidney Dis 1997; 29: 125–31.

Mauiyyedi S, Crespo M, Collins AB, et al. Acute humoral rejection in kidney transplantation II. Morphology, immunopathology, and pathologic classification. J Am Soc Nephrol 2002; 13: 779–87.

Merlini G, Remuzzi G, Autologous stem cell and kidney transplantation for primary amyloidosis associated with ESRD: which should come first? Am J Transplant 2005; 5: 1585–6.

Meulders Q, Pirson Y, Cosyns JP, et al. Course of Henoch–Schönlein nephritis after renal transplantation. Transplantation 1994; 58: 1172–86.

Mignani R, Panichi V, Giudicissi A, et al. Enzyme replacement therapy with algasidase beta in kidney transplant patients with Fabry's disease: a pilot study. Kidney Int 2004; 65: 1381–5.

Miyata T, Sugiyama S, Nangaku M, et al. Apolipoprotein E2/E5 variants in lipoprotein glomerulopathy recurred in renal transplanted kidney. J Am Soc Nephrol 1999; 10: 1590–5.

Moake JL. Thrombotic microangiopathies. N Engl J Med 2002; 347: 589–600.

Monico CG, Milliner DS. Combined liver–kidney and kidney-alone transplantation in primary hyperoxaluria. Liver Transpl 2001; 7: 954–63.

Montagnino G, Colturi C, Banfi G, et al. Membranous nephropathy in cyclosporine-treated renal transplant patients. Transplantation 1989; 47: 725–7.

Montagnino G, Tarantino A, Banfi G, et al. Double recurrence of FSGS after two renal transplants with complete regression after plasmapheresis and ACE inhibitors. Transpl Int 2000; 13: 166–8.

Morales JM, Martinez MA, Munoz de Bustillo E, et al. Recurrent type III membranoproliferative glomerulonephritis after kidney transplantation. Transplantation 1997; 63: 1186–8.

Moroni G, Tantardini F, Galleli B, et al. The long-term prognosis of renal transplantation in patients with lupus nephritis. Am J Kidney Dis 2005; 45: 903–11.

Mourad G, Djamali A, Turc-Baron C, Cristol JP. Lipoprotein glomerulopathy: a new cause of nephrotic syndrome after renal transplantation. Nephrol Dial Transplant 1998; 13: 1292–4.

Mousson C, Heyd B, Justrabo E, et al. Successful hepatorenal transplantation in hereditary amyloidosis caused by a frame-shift mutation in fibrinogen A alpha-chain gene. Am J Transplant 2006; 6: 632–5.

Musante L, Candiano G, Bruschi M, et al. Circulating anti-actin and anti-ATP synthase antibodies identify a sub-set of patients with idiopathic nephrotic syndome. Clin Exp Immunol 2005; 141: 491–9.

Nachman PH, Segelmark M, Westman K, et al. Recurrent ANCA-associated small vessel vasculitis after transplantation: a pooled analysis. Kidney Int 1999; 56: 1544–50.

Nakazawa Y, Hashikura Y, Urata K, et al. Von Willebrand factor-cleaving protease activity in thrombotic microangiopathy after living donor liver transplantation: a case report. Liver Transpl 2003; 9: 1328–33.

Nossent HC, Swaak TJG, Berden JHM. Systemic lupus erythematosus after renal transplantation: patient and graft survival and disease activity. Ann Intern Med 1991; 114: 183–8.

Nyberg G, Akensson P, Norden G, Wieslander J. Systemic vasculitis in a kidney transplant population. Transplantation 1997; 63: 1273–7.

Obrador GT, Ojo A, Thadhani R. End-stage renal disease in patients with Fabry disease. J Am Soc Nephrol 2002; 6 (Suppl 2): S144–7.

Odum J, Peh C, Clarkson A, et al. Recurrence of mesangial IgA nephritis following renal transplantation. Nephrol Dial Transplant 1994; 9: 309–12.

Ohmacht Ch, Kliem V, Burg M, et al. Recurrent Immunoglobulin A nephropathy after renal transplantation. transplantation 1997; 64: 1493–6.

Ohta K, Kawaguchi H, Hattori M, et al. Effect of pre- and postoperative plasmapheresis on posttransplant recurrence of focal segmental glomerulosclerosis in children. Transplantation 2001; 71: 628–33.

Ohashi H, Oda H, Ohno M, et al. Losartan reduces proteinuria and preserves renal function in hypertensive patients with IgA nephropathy. Clin Exp Nephrol 2002; 6: 224–8.

Oka K, Moriyama T, Izumi M, et al. A case of relapse of C-ANCA-associated glomerulonephritis in post-transplant patients. Clin Transplant 2000; 14 (Suppl 3): 33–6.

Olie KH, Florquin S, Groothoff JW, et al. Atypical relapse of haemolytic uremic syndrome after transplantation. Pediatr Nephrol 2004; 19: 1173–6.

Ozdemir BH, Ozdemir FN, Sezer S, et al. Does colchicine have an antifibrotic effect on development of interstitial fibrosis in renal allografts of recipients with familial mediterranean fever? Transplant Proc 2006; 38: 473–6.

Patrakka J, Ruotsalainen V, Reponen P, et al. Recurrence of nephrotic syndrome in kidney grafts of patients with congenital nephrotic syndrome of the Finnish type: role of nephrin. Transplantation 2002; 73: 394–403.

Pescovitz MD, Book BK, Sidner RA. Resolution of recurrent focal segmental glomerulosclerosis proteinuria after rituximab treatment. N Engl J Med 2006; 354: 1961–3.

Pham P, Danovitch G, Wilkinson A, et al. Inhibitors of ADAMTS 13: a potential factor in the cause of thrombotic microangiopathy in a renal allograft recipient. Transplantation 2002; 74: 1077–80.

Ponticelli C, Traversi L, Feliciani A, et al. Kidney transplantation in patients with IgA mesangial glomerulonephritis. Kidney Int 2001; 60: 1948–54.

Ponticelli C, Villa M, Cesana B, et al. Risk factors for late kidney allograft failure. Kidney Int 2002a; 62: 1848–54.

Ponticelli C, Campise M, Tarantino A. The different patterns of response to plasmapheresis of recurrent focal and segmental glomerulosclerosis. Transplant Proc 2002b; 34: 3069–71.

Ponticelli C, Traversi L, Banfi G. Renal transplantation in patients with IgA mesangial glomerulonephritis Pediatr. Transplant 2004; 8: 334–8.

Ponticelli C, Moroni G. Renal transplantation in lupus nephritis. Lupus 2005; 14: 95–8.

Quan A, Sullivan EK, Alexander SR. Recurrence of hemolytic uremic syndrome after renal transplantation in children: a report of the North American Pediatric Renal Transplant Cooperative Study. Transplantation 2001; 72: 742–5.

Raafat RH, Kalia A, Travis LB, Diven SC. High-dose cyclosporine therapy for recurrent focal segmental glomerulosclerosis in children. Am J Kidney Dis 2004; 44: 50–6.

Ramesh-Prasad GV, Shamy F, Zaltzman JS. Recurrence of type III membranoproliferative glomerulonephritis after renal transplantation. Clin Nephrol 2004; 61: 80–1.

Reiser J, von Gersdorff G, Loos M, et al. Induction of B7-1 in podocytes is associated with nephrotic syndrome. J Clin Invest 2004; 113: 1390–7.

Reynolds JC, Agodoa LY, Yuan CM, Abbott KC. Thrombotic microangiopathy after renal transplantation in the United States. Am J Kidney Dis 2003; 42: 1058–68.

Remuzzi G, Ruggenenti P, Codazzi D, et al. Combined kidney and liver transplantation for familial haemolytic uraemic syndrome. Lancet 2002; 359: 1671–2.

Remuzzi G, Ruggenenti P, Colledan M, et al. Hemolytic uremic syndrome: a fatal outcome after kidney and liver transplantation performed to correct factor H gene mutation. Am J Transplant 2005; 5: 1146–50.

Rostaing L, Modesto A, Oksman F, et al. Outcome of patients with antineutrophilic cytoplasmic auto-antibodies associated vasculitis after cadaveric renal transplantation. Am J Kidney Dis 1997; 29: 96–102.

Ruf RG, Lichtenberger A, Karle SM, et al. Patients with mutation in NPSH2 (podocin) do not respond to standard steroid treatment of nephritic syndrome. J Am Soc Nephrol 2004; 15: 722–32.

Ruggenenti P, Noris M, Remuzzi G. Thrombotic microangiopathy, hemolytic uremic syndrome, and thrombotic thrombocytopenic purpura. Kidney Int 2001; 60: 831–46.

Salomon R, Gagnadoux MF, Niaudet P. Intravenous cyclosporine therapy in recurrent nephrotic syndrome after transplantation in children. Transplantation 2003; 75: 810–14.

Samaniego M, Nadasdy GM, Laszik Z, Nadasdy T. Outcome of renal transplantation in fibrillary glomerulonephritis. Clin Nephrol 2001; 55: 159–66.

Savin VJ, Sharma R, Sharma M, et al. Circulating factor associated with increased glomerular permeability to albumin in recurrent focal segmental glomerulosclerosis. N Engl J Med 1996; 334: 878–83.

Savin VJ, McCarthy ET, Sharma M. Permeability factors in focal segmental glomerulosclerosis. Semin Nephrol 2003; 23: 147–60.

Saxena R, Frankel WL, Sedmark DD, et al. Recurrent type I membranoproliferative glomerulonephritis in a renal allograft: successful treatment with plasmapheresis. Am J Kidney Dis 2000; 35: 749–52.

Schwartz A, Krause PH, Offermann G, Keller F. Recurrent and de novo renal disease after kidney transplantation with or without cyclosporine A. Am J Kidney Dis 1991; 5: 524–31.

Sessa A, Meroni M, Battini G. Renal transplantation in patients with Fabry's disease. Nephron 2002; 91: 348–51.

Sever MS, Turkmen A, Sahin S, et al. Renal transplantation in amyloidosis secondary to familial Mediterranean fever. Transplant Proc 2001; 33: 3392–3.

Shimizu T, Tanabe K, Oshima T, et al. Recurrence of membranoproliferative glomerulonephritis in renal allografts. Transplant Proc 1998; 30: 3910–13.

Short AK, O'Donoghue DJ, Riad HN, et al. Recurrence of light chain nephropathy in a renal allograft. A case report and review of the literature. Am J Nephrol 2001; 21: 237–41.

Soler MJ, Mir M, Rodriguez E, et al. Recurrence of IgA nephropathy and Henoch–Schoenlein purpura after kidney transplantation: risk factors and graft survival. Transplant Proc 2005; 37: 3705–9.

Stokes MB, De Palma J. Post-transplantation nephrotic syndrome. Kidney Int 2006; 69: 1088–91.

Stone JH. End-stage renal disease in lupus: disease activity, dialysis, and the outcome of transplantation. Lupus 1998; 7: 654–9.

Takahara S, Moriyama T, Kokado Y, et al. Randomized prospective study of effects of benazepril in renal transplantation: an analysis of safety and efficacy. Clin Exp Nephrol 2002; 6: 242–7.

Tarantino A, Moroni G, Banfi G, et al. Renal replacement therapy in cryoglobulinemic nephritis. Nephrol Dial Transplant 1994; 9: 1426–30.

Taylor CM, Neild G. Acute renal failure associated with microangiopathy (haemolytic–uraemic syndrome and thrmbotic thrombocytopenic purpura). In Davison A, Cameron JS, Grunfeld JP, et al., eds. Oxford Textbook of Clinical Nephrology. Oxford: Oxford University Press, 2005: 1545–64.

Tejani A, Stablein DH. Recurrence of focal segmental glomerulosclerosis posttransplantation: a special report of the North American Pediatric Renal Transplant Cooperative Study. J Am Soc Nephrol 1992; 2 (Suppl): S258–63.

Vincenti F, Ghiggeri GM. New insights into the pathogenesis and the therapy of recurrent focal glomerulosclerosis. Am J Transplant 2005; 5: 1179–85.

Wang AYM, Mac-Moune Lai F, Yu AWY, et al. Recurrent IgA nephropathy in renal transplant allografts. Am J Kidney Dis 2001; 38: 588–96.

Wang SX, Ahola H, Palmen T, et al. Recurrence of nephrotic syndrome after transplantation in CNF is due to autoantibodies in nephrin. Exp Nephrol 2001; 9: 327–31.

Ward MM. Outcomes of renal transplantation among patients with end-stage renal disease caused by lupus nephritis. Kidney Int 2000; 57: 2136–43.

Weber S, Gribouval O, Esquivel EL, et al. NPHS2 mutation analysis shows genetic heterogeneity of steroid-resistant nephrotic syndrome and low post-transplant recurrence. Kidney Int 2004; 66: 571–9.

Wu J, Jaar BG, Briggs WA, et al. High-dose mycophenolate mofetil in the treatment of posttransplant glomerular disease in the allograft: a case series. Nephron Clin Pract 2004; 98: c61–6.

Zipfel PF. Complement factor H: physiology and pathophysiology. Semin Thromb Hemost 2001; 27: 191–9.

Zimmerhackl LB, Scheiring J, Profer F, et al. Renal transplantation in HUS patients with disorders of complement regulation. Pediatr Nephrol 2007; 22: 10–60.

DE NOVO RENAL DISEASE

De novo glomerular disease

Glomerular diseases in the Kidney allograft are more often caused by the recurrence of the original disease. However, in a number of cases different types of de novo glomerlar diseases may develop in the transplanted kidney, triggered by autoimmune processes, diabetes, drug toxicity or infections.

Minimal change nephropathy

Occasional cases of *de novo* minimal change nephropathy meeting strict clinical–pathologic criteria for diagnosis have been reported. Nephrotic syndrome is the usual presentation (Zafarmand et al., 2002; Newstead, 2003; Audard et al., 2005b), but reversible acute renal failure may also occur (Marcowitz et al., 1998). The disease develops early after transplantation, usually within 4 months. Steroids, ACE inhibitors, and angiotensin receptor blockers have been used. Sustained remission of proteinuria can be achieved in most cases within a year, but some patients may enter remission after 3 or more years (Zafarmand et al., 2002).

Membranous nephropathy

De novo MN is the second cause of nephrotic syndrome after renal transplantation (Davison and Johnston, 1992). A pediatric series, in which control allograft biopsy was performed even in the absence of signs of nephropathy, reported *de novo* MN in 9% of cases. Of these, however, a quarter showed no sign of renal disease and another quarter had only mild proteinuria (Antignac et al., 1988). A large number of cases of *de novo* MN were reported in retransplanted patients (Heidet et al., 1994). MN usually occurs months or years after transplantation, but rare cases of *de novo* MN have been described 3 months after engrafment (Gough et al., 2005).

In a number of cases, the etiological agent of *de novo* MN may be identified. *De novo* MN is often associated with *hepatitis B (HBV) infection* (Lai et al., 1991). Cases of *de novo* MN have also been described in *HCV-positive* patients (Cruzado et al., 2001). In some cases the HCV core protein was found in the glomeruli, suggesting that HCV infection may cause MN through immune complex deposition (Okada et al., 1996). A case of *de novo* MN developed in a patient converted from cyclosporine to *sirolimus*; glomerulonephritis reversed after the patient stopped sirolimus and was reconverted to cyclosporine (Dittrich et al., 2004).

The *pathogenesis* is unclear. The disease has been considered an expression of chronic rejection, as lesions of rejection may be associated with MN or may even antedate it (Truong et al., 1989). However, this hypothesis is challenged by the observation that *de novo* MN may also occur following transplantation between identical twins (Bansal et al., 1986). It is possible that MN is caused by an autoimmune response to unknown antigens of glomerular or tubular origin, with consequent *in situ* deposition of immune complexes in a subepithelial position.

The *histopathological* findings in some cases may either be similar to those of classical membranous nephropathy, or be more subtle, showing focal segmental variation in severity, often in conjuction with the features of chronic allograft nephropathy (Sebire and Bockenhauer, 2005).

The *prognosis* as well as the risk factors that may predict a poor outcome are not well established. Truong *et al.* (1989) found that 42% of adults lost their allograft on average 3 years after the diagnosis. In children, 60% lost their graft on average 6 years after the diagnosis (Heidet *et al.*, 1994). On the other hand, Antignac *et al.* (1988) did not observe a progressive course in patients with mild or absent proteinuria, and Schwarz *et al.* (1994) reported that the 5-year graft survival rate was similar in 21 patients with *de novo* MN and in 851 other renal transplant recipients.

The *treatment* of 'idiopathic' *de novo* MN is elusive. There is no evidence that reinforcement of immunosuppressive treatment or the introduction of cytotoxic agents is of any benefit (Poduval *et al.*, 2003). However, in a few patients, remission of the nephrotic syndrome and stabilization of renal function were obtained by reinforcing the doses of oral prednisone (Schwarz *et al.*, 1994). Antiviral therapy may be effective in cases associated with HBV infection (Farrell and Teoh, 2006).

Membranoproliferative glomerulonephritis

De novo membranoproliferative GN may develop after transplantation in patients infected with hepatitis C virus. Both type I and type III MPGN can occur in HCV-positive renal transplant patients (Cruzado *et al.*, 2001). Some cases may be associated with cryoglobulinemia (Morales, 2004), but in a number of patients with *de novo* MPGN the search for circulating cryoglobulins proved negative (Roth *et al.*, 1995). The development of MPGN usually results in an accelerated loss of the graft (Hammoud *et al.*, 1996; Cruzado *et al.*, 2001). A case of type I MPGN developed 7 years after transplantation has been reported in a *HGV*-positive patient who proved to be HCV- and HBV-negative. The presence of the HGV genome was detected in glomeruli and tubules (Berthoux *et al.*, 1999). A case of MPGN developed after conversion from cyclosporine to sirolimus has been reported. The disease disappeared after the patient stopped sirolimus and reintroduced cyclosporine (Dittrich *et al.*, 2004).

Collapsing glomerulopathy

Collapsing glomerulopathy is a variant of focal segmental glomerular sclerosis characterized by severe proteinuria and rapidly progressive renal failure. A *de novo* collapsing glomerulopathy may occur in about 0.6% of renal transplants (Meehan *et al.*, 1998). The *etiopathogenesis* is unknown. The morphologic pattern and clinical features in renal allografts suggest that post-transplant collapsing glomerulopathy may not represent the same disease process affecting native kidneys, but rather represents a pattern of renal injury (Nadasdy *et al.*, 2002). Among other factors, hemodynamic disturbance may play a role in the development of the pattern of collapsing glomerulopathy in renal allografts. Viral etiology may also be involved. A case of *de novo* collapsing glomerulopathy and red cell aplasia has been reported in a renal transplant patient with persistent parvovirus B19 infection (Moudgil *et al.*, 1997). Further studies demonstrated a specific association between parvovirus infection and collapsing glomerulopathy in non-transplant patients (Moudgil *et al.*, 2001).

The characteristic *glomerular lesions* are capillary loop collapse with prominent podocytes filling Bowman's space, often associated with severe tubulointerstitial injury and obliterative vascular changes (Nadasdy *et al.*, 2002). However, these histologic findings are often associated with acute rejection, diabetic nephropathy, and/or immune complex glomerulonephritis (Stokes *et al.*, 1999). Contrary to what is observed in non-transplanted kidneys, post-transplant collapsing glomerulopathy is not always associated with severe proteinuria. The *prognosis* is severe, with a high rate of graft loss (Meehan *et al.*, 1998; Stokes *et al.*, 1999).

Diabetic nephropathy

After renal transplantation some 45% of patients may show abnormal glucose tolerance and 20–25% may develop diabetes (Cosio *et al.*, 2002; Mathew *et al.*, 2003; Kasiske *et al.*, 2003). A number of risk factors have been identified (Table 8.1). An Australian survey showed that older age, abnormal glucose tolerance before transplantation, rapid gain in dry weight on dialysis, and high-dose prednisone or calcineurin inhibitors are factors associated with the development of post-transplant diabetes (Mathew *et al.*, 2003).

Table 8.1   Main risk factors for post-transplant diabetes mellitus

Family history of diabetes
Older recipient age
HCV-seropositive status
High body mass index
High dose of CNI (tacrolimus > cyclosporine)
High doses of concomitant corticosteroids
Afro-American race
Hispanic ethnicity

By reviewing USRDS (United States Renal Data System) data, Kasiske et al. (2003) found that African-American race, Hispanic ethnicity, elevated body mass index, and tacrolimus were the strongest risk factors for post-transplant diabetes. An association between diabetes and HCV positivity has also been noted (Yildiz et al., 2002; Fabrizi et al., 2005).

Nephropathy due to *de novo* diabetes seems to occur as frequently as recurrent diabetic nephropathy. The mean time of histologic diabetic nephropathy occurrence ranges around 6.7 years for recurrent diabetes and 5.9 years for *de novo* post-transplant diabetes (Bhalla et al., 2003). However, the longer is the duration of post-transplant diabetes the higher is the risk of developing diabetic nephropathy.

Post-transplantation diabetes may aggravate the patient and graft *prognosis*. De novo diabetes is associated with an increased mortality (Cosio et al., 2002; Kasiske et al., 2003). The development of diabetes has a deleterious impact on long-term graft outcome. Plasma creatinine levels and 12-year graft survival (48% vs. 72%) were significantly worse in transplant patients who developed diabetes than in controls (Miles et al., 1998). The long-term graft survival is poorer in patients with post-transplant diabetes than in non-diabetic transplant recipients (Miles et al., 1998; Cosio et al., 2002).

Efforts should be made to *prevent* the possible development of post-transplant diabetes. Diet, physical activity, and reducing the doses of corticosteroids and calcineurin inhibitors whenever possible are effective measures for minimizing glucose intolerance in renal transplant recipients. In patients with diabetes, an improvement in glucose control is the most important therapeutic approach in primary prevention. A target of glycated hemoglobin levels < 7% should be recommended in all patients with diabetes (Fioretto et al., 2006). ACE inhibitors and/or angiotensin receptor blockers (Brenner et al., 2001; Remuzzi et al., 2006) may be useful to retard the onset of microalbuminuria and to slow the progression of renal disease in patients with diabetic nephropathy.

Antiglomerular basement membrane nephritis in Alport's syndrome

Approximately 15% of Alport's patients who have undergone kidney transplantation develop transient IgG linear deposition along the glomerular basement membrane (GBM) without anti-GBM antibodies, and about 3% develop anti-GBM disease (Byrne et al., 2002). The immunization of Alport's patients is caused by the presence in the transplanted kidney of *antigenic epitopes* that are lacking in the native kidneys. These antibodies, which are directed against the α_3, α_4, and α_5 chains of type IV collagen can be detected in the serum (Hudson et al., 2003).

IgG deposition along the GBM does not usually have any relevant effect on allograft function. However, some 3–5% of Alport's patients, mainly those with a juvenile type, develop immunization against graft GBM. In these patients, anti-GBM antibodies remain tightly bound to the GBM, producing continuing inflammation and eventually leading to severe *crescentic glomerulonephritis* (Rutgers et al., 2000). This complication manifests within the first year. The diagnosis is based on the detection of circulating anti-GBM antibodies and renal biopsy. The prognosis is poor. Intensive plasma exchange therapy may be attempted in order to remove the anti-GBM antibodies, but only a few patients respond to treatment. Retransplantation also carries a poor prognosis (Browne et al., 2004).

mTOR inhibitor-induced glomerulonephritis (?)

Experimental studies showed that in a 'full-dose' anti-Thy1 model, everolimus caused adverse effects with a high mortality rate, progressive apoptosis, crescent formation, and glomerulosclerosis (Daniel et al., 2005). In clinical renal transplantation, Dittrich et al. (2004) described four patients who developed post-transplantation glomerulonephritis after conversion from calcineurin inhibitor-based immunosuppression to sirolimus. In all four patients, nephrotic-range proteinuria occurred 2–9 months after conversion from cyclosporine to sirolimus. Renal biopsy showed membranoproliferative GN type I in one case, membranous nephropathy in another, and IgA GN in two cases. Cyclosporine was reintroduced, and resulted in complete remission of proteinuria and stabilized renal function in all patients. Mainra et al. (2005) reported a further case of minimal change nephropathy in a sirolimus-treated patient that reversed after switching to cyclosporine. However, the large variety of glomerular diseases and the prompt reversal after the reintroduction of cyclosporine make the etiological role of sirolimus doubtful. A possible alternative explanation could be that, even before the administration of sirolimus, these patients were already carriers of glomerulonephritis, but proteinuria was masked by the anti-proteinuric effect of cyclosporine.

Acute post-bacterial glomerulonephritis

Only few cases of post-infectious glomerulonephritis have been reported in renal transplant recipients. In contrast with the typical post-streptococcal GN, the etiology of infections may be variable. Most cases have graft dysfunction at presentation. The outcome may be severe in the long term. The role of therapy, if any, is still undefined (Moroni et al., 2004).

Necrotizing glomerulonephritis

The occurrence of rapidly progressive necrotizing glomerulonephritis after kidney transplantation is rare, and usually leads to graft failure. Reinforcement of corticosteroid therapy and the introduction of cyclophosphamide were able to induce recovery in a transplant patient with necrotizing GN (Campise et al., 2003).

Immunotactoid glomerulopathy

The association of immunotactoid glomerulopathy with cytomegalovirus infection in a renal transplant recipient has been reported (Rao et al., 1994). In the patient described, the morphologic lesions of immunotactoid glomerulopathy and clinical renal disease reversed after recovery from the viral infection.

Light-chain deposition disease (LCDD)

Rare cases of de novo LCDD have been reported in renal transplant recipients without previous history of multiple myeloma. κ Light chain deposition (Ecder et al., 1996) is more frequent, but also cases of λ chain deposition (Tanenbaum et al., 2005) in renal allograft have been reported.

Interstitial nephritis

Acute interstitial nephritis is a rare complication which can pose problems of differential diagnosis in renal transplantation, as the lesions resemble those of acute cellular rejection. Viral infection and drugs are the most frequent causes of acute interstitial nephritis.

Virus-associated interstitial nephritis

Several viruses may trigger interstitial nephritis. Early diagnosis and appropriate treatment are important in order to avoid potentially dangerous anti-rejection therapy and to obtain reversibility of interstitial lesions.

Cytomegalovirus

Cytomegalovirus (CMV) rarely causes mild interstitial nephritis. The diagnosis may be suspected when the renal function deteriorates during a CMV infection. At renal biopsy, cytopathic changes can be recognized easily. Viral inclusions may be seen in tubular and glomerular cells. The use of monoclonal antibodies against CMV should be employed for a correct diagnosis. The presence of viruria may facilitate the diagnosis.

After diagnosis, a course of *treatment* with ganciclovir or foscarnet (Wong *et al.*, 2002) is usually effective in eradicating viruses from kidney tissue. There are contrasting opinions about the effect of CMV interstitial nephritis on long-term graft function. In a series of ten cases with CMV inclusions in the allograft and florid interstitial nephritis in seven, no graft loss attributable primarily to CMV was observed (Kashyap *et al.*, 1999), but in a case report, CMV nephritis eventually caused irreversible graft failure in the long term (Trimarchi *et al.*, 2001).

Herpesvirus 1 or 2

Herpesvirus 1 or 2 rarely causes interstitial nephritis. Usually this occurs in the first weeks after transplantation, and may be concomitant with mucocutaneous lesions. At renal biopsy, nuclear clearing, necrosis, and inclusions in tubular cells may be seen. Acyclovir and a reduction of immunosuppressive therapy may be helpful in reversing this type of interstitial nephritis, although there is little information about the clinical outcome of these cases.

Adenovirus

Adenovirus infections affecting renal allografts are extremely rare. These cases bear some similarities to polyomavirus nephritis, as they present with allograft dysfunction and demonstrate, in urine sediment, the so-called decoy cells, i.e. tubular cells showing intranuclear inclusions with a halo surrounded by a ring of marginated chromatin and smudged nuclei (Asim *et al.*, 2003). Glassy-appearing nuclear smudging and extensive tubular necrosis with granulomatous interstitial nephritis may allow a differential diagnosis from rejection (Colvin, 1996). Immunoperoxidase stains for viral antigen can establish the etiology. The renal impairment is severe. Hemorrhagic cystitis may also occur. There is no specific antiviral therapy available for adenovirus infection. A reduction in the intensity of immunosuppression may result in an improvement of graft function (Asim *et al.*, 2003).

BK polyomavirus

The human polyomavirus family contains two viruses, the JC virus and the BK virus. These viruses are usually acquired in childhood, probably through the oral route. While the JC virus is usually located in the central nervous system, the BK virus remains latent in the urinary tract. Intense immunosuppression can favor the *reactivation* of BK virus in transplanted kidneys. Reactivation of BK virus may cause an interstitial nephritis that slowly progresses to graft loss in more than half of cases (Hirsch, 2002). BK virus infection transcribes proinflammatory genes equal in character to and larger in magnitude than those seen with acute rejection, and creates a microenvinronment that promotes graft fibrosis (Mannon *et al.*, 2005).

The *incidence* of interstitial nephritis caused by BK virus is more frequent in patients treated with tacrolimus and mycophenolate mofetil (Ramos *et al.*, 2002; Nickeleit *et al.*, 2003). However, cases who have never received calcineurin inhibitors have also been reported (Lipshutz *et al.*, 2004). The development of BK virus nephritis is often (Hirsch *et al.*, 2002), but not invariably (Elli *et al.*, 2002), associated with anti-rejection treatment. There are no clinical signs or symptoms of BK virus nephropathy, except for a progressive deterioration of graft function.

The *diagnosis* is based on a combination of urine cytology, viral load in plasma, and cytopathic changes in graft biopsy. Cells in the urine that have viral inclusions, so-called 'decoy cells' (Figure 8.1), may be seen frequently in patients with replicating BK virus (Binet *et al.*, 1999), but are not specific. BK virus replication in the allograft has been correlated with the detection of virus DNA in the plasma by polymerase chain reaction (PCR) (Limaye *et al.*, 2001), which may be useful for monitoring the course of infection and related nephropathy (Hirsch *et al.*, 2002). At renal biopsy, BK virus nephritis is characterized by an interstitial

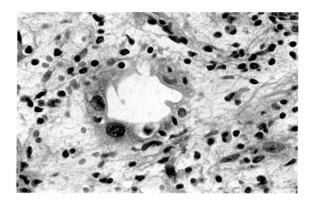

Figure 8.1 Viral cytopathy. Enlarged nuclei of epithelial tubular cells containing multiple vacuoles, in a patient with polyoma BK virus nephritis (H.E. ×480)

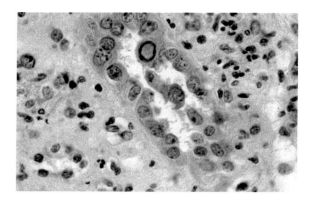

Figure 8.2 Viral cytopathy. Enlarged nuclei resembling a glass watch with peripheral distribution of chromatin in a case of BK virus nephritis (H.E. ×480)

infiltrate rich in plasma cells and by cytopathic changes caused by virus infiltration (Figure 8.2). On electron microscopy it is possible to see intranuclear viral inclusions in clusters. Detection in the kidney tissue of simian virus SV40T antigen by specific monoclonal antobodies and/or histologic demonstration of viral alterations on graft biopsy are the most important clues to BK virus nephritis.

The *prognosis* is severe. In many patients there is progressive deterioration of renal function, with ultimate graft loss. However, recent advances in management strategies have improved graft survival. Graft loss within 2 years from clinical diagnosis, which was almost the rule until recently, is uncommon today, although functional decline still occurs frequently (Wadei *et al.*, 2006).

Treatment is mainly based on a reduction of immunosuppression, which may stabilize graft function in some cases (Randhawa *et al.*, 1999) but may render patients more susceptible to acute rejection (Ramos *et al.*, 2002). The antiviral cidofovir (Bjorang *et al.*, 2002; Kadambi *et al.*, 2003) or leflunomide (Nickeleit *et al.*, 2003) may also be useful. A possible strategy may consist of withdrawing mycophenolate mofetil (MMF) while progressively halving the dose of tacrolimus. In the mean time, leflunomide may be introduced at an initial dose of 100 mg per day for 3 days followed by 20 mg in a single daily administration. In the case of no response, cidofovir, 2.5–3.3 mg/kg, may be added every 2 weeks for 4 weeks. As this agent is nephrotoxic, probenecid should also be given together with generous hydration, if there are no contraindications. Whether and when to retransplant patients who have lost their graft because of polyoma virus infection are still open questions. Cases of successful retransplantation after a first graft failure due to polyoma virus have also been reported (Poduval *et al.*, 2002; Ginevri *et al.*, 2003, Hirsch and Ramos, 2006). Judicious retransplantation may be considered in patients with negative PCR in the blood and urine.

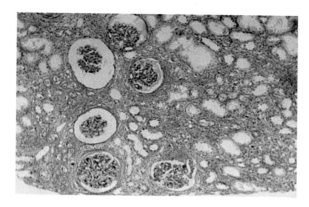

Figure 8.3 Interstitial fibrosis and tubular atrophy in a renal transplant recipient with interstitial nephritis probably caused by allopurinol (AFOG ×120)

Drug-induced interstitial nephritis

A number of drugs may be responsible for interstitial nephritis. These include antibiotics, sulfonamides, allopurinol, diuretics, non-steroidal anti-inflammatory drugs, etc. The clinical diagnosis may be difficult. Fever, skin rash, and eosinophilia may be lacking or mild, because basic immunosuppression may mask the typical signs and symptoms of interstitial nephritis. A superimposed interstitial nephritis may be suspected when a sudden increase in plasma creatinine occurs in a transplant patient who took even a single dose of a potential allergen.

As drug-associated interstitial nephritis may show histologic features identical to those of acute rejection, namely tubulitis, mononuclear interstitial infiltrate, and eosinophilia, differential diagnosis from renal biopsy can also be difficult. However, endothelialitis is typical of acute rejection, and, when present, allows a correct diagnosis.

While in some cases the removal of the offending drug may be sufficient to reverse renal dysfunction, in other instances a course of high-dose corticosteroids may be necessary. A delay in diagnosis and treatment may lead to progressive interstitial fibrosis and tubular atrophy (Figure 8.3), eventually resulting in chronic allograft dysfunction.

Pyelonephritis

Infection of the urinary tract is frequent in renal transplant recipients. Most infections are localized in the lower urinary tract and are often asymptomatic. More rare are infections of the upper urinary tract that may be responsible for acute or chronic pyelonephritis. Urological complications, vesicoureteral reflux, and diabetes mellitus may predispose to the development of pyelonephritis.

Acute pyelonephritis

Although acute pyelonephritis may occur at any time, it is more frequent in the early post-transplant period because of catheterization, stenting, vesicoureteral reflux, and/or anti-rejection treatment. Even in patients who received anti-reflux surgery before transplantation, the risk of pyelonephritis is more elevated than in other transplant recipients (Basiri et al., 2006).

Clinical and laboratory features

This form of acute interstitial nephritis, due to bacterial invasion of the kidney, usually produces a *septic picture*. Symptoms develop rapidly and include high fever, shaking chills, tachycardia, muscular tenderness, nausea, vomiting, and diarrhea. Cystitis and/or macroscopic hematuria may or may not be present. Severe hypotension and oliguria may develop in the most severe cases.

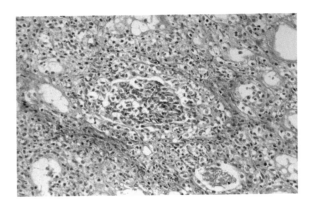

Figure 8.4 Acute pyelonephritis: tubuli display severe disruption by inflammatory cells constituted mainly by neutrophils which fill, together with necrotic tubular cells, the lumina. (AFOG ×250)

Laboratory investigations show elevated levels of C-reactive protein and leukocytosis in most patients. However, transplant recipients under treatment with azathioprine, MMF, or antilymphocyte antibodies may show neutropenia. Leukocytes, erythrocytes, and leukocyte casts are usually seen in the urine sediment. However, if the infective focus does not communicate with urine, both the urinary sediment and the urine culture may be negative. In case of sepsis, bacteria can be isolated from the blood culture. Most cases of acute pyelonephritis are due to *Gram-negative* bacteria such as *Escherichia coli, Proteus* species, and *Pseudomonas* species. *Enterobacter* is the predominant Gram-positive bacterium. Opportunistic micro-organisms and fungi may also be responsible for acute pyelonephritis. Particularly severe are the few cases of emphysematous pyelonephritis.

An increase in plasma creatinine is frequent and sometimes severe, often favored by profuse sweating, vomiting, and/or diarrhea. This may raise some problems of *differential diagnosis* from acute rejection, particularly in the early post-transplant period. Prior complications and/or instrumentation of the urinary tract orientate toward acute pyelonephritis. Ultrasonography may be helpful if urinary obstruction, fistula, or stones are present. Renal biopsy may show a massive interstitial infiltrate rich in polymorphonuclear cells, with focal disruption of the tubular structure (Figure 8.4). However, if the infiltrates are striped (or patchy), not uniform, the renal biopsy can also be unrepresentative.

Prognosis

Usually, acute pyelonephritis responds favorably to antibiotics, but those cases caused by acute urinary obstruction or urine fistula require urine diversion or surgery. Many patients with emphysematous pyelonephritis had to be transplantectomized, but in some cases percutaneous drainage and nephrostomy were able to preserve graft function (Cheng *et al.*, 2001).

There is little informaton on the *long-term consequences* of acute pyelonephritis. A retrospective study reported that, taken as a whole, acute pyelonephritis was not associated with a poor long-term outcome. However, early pyelonephritis (within the first 3 months) was significantly detrimental for late graft function (Giral *et al.*, 2002). There is also evidence that acute pyelonephritis may activate the immune system and trigger acute or chronic rejection (Audard *et al.*, 2005a).

Treatment

Pending urine culture and sensitivity, parenteral antimicrobial therapy should be promptly instituted together with electrolyte and fluid replacement. Immunosuppressive treatment should be reduced if signs of sepsis are present. Third-generation cephalosporins, ampicillin sulbactam, imipenem, aztreonam, and fluoroquinolones are active against the bacteria most frequently involved. Aminoglycosides are very useful, but should be handled with caution because of their potential nephrotoxicity. Intravenous therapy should be continued for at least 48 hours after fever disappears. Then, oral antimicrobial agents should be given for at least 4 weeks in order to prevent relapses.

Chronic pyelonephritis

Chronic pyelonephritis due to bacterial infection of the allograft is a rare cause of progressive chronic allograft dysfunction. The few cases are usually caused by recurrent stones, ureteral stenosis, or massive vesicoureteral reflux. On the other hand, some studies reported that vesicoureteral reflux in the transplanted kidney does not influence the long-term graft function and survival (Fontana et al., 1999), but is associated with an increased risk of acute pyelonephritis (Ranchin et al., 2000).

Clinically, chronic pyelonephritis may be asymptomatic. Some patients with stones may have renal colic, and others may complain of cystitis. Usually, the *diagnosis* is established because a patient with a persistently positive urine culture and/or progressive increase in plasma creatinine is submitted to ultrasonography. This reveals changes of decreased renal size and segmental cortical scarring. Intravenous pyelography confirms these findings and also shows blunting and dilatation of the calyces, and ureteral dilatation in cases of vesicoureteral reflux. Urinary tuberculosis can give similar changes, but ureteral strictures and a contracted bladder can also be frequently found. Renal biopsy may show neutrophilic interstitial nephritis, a progressive disease, not always caused by a clear infectious etiology, which may be seen in up to 5% of transplant patients (de Castro et al., 1998). Surgical *treatment* is indicated in patients with urinary obstruction or stones resistant to lithotripsy. Continuous prophylaxis with low-dose sulfamethoxazole–trimethoprim, nitrofurantoin, or other antimicrobial agents may be indicated to reduce the risk of acute infections.

Renal vascular disease

Cholesterol embolization

Cholesterol crystal embolism is an increasingly frequent complication of atherosclerosis or its treatment, which may lead to multiorgan distal ischemia. When the disease affects the kidney, rapidly progressive renal failure and/or malignant hypertension may develop. The occurrence of *acute renal failure* in an atherosclerotic patient who has recently been treated with a stent, bypass, or anticoagulaton should raise the suspicion of atheroembolism, particularly in the presence of livedo reticularis, eosinophilia, and/or hypocomplementemia.

Renal cholesterol embolization may rarely occur in renal transplant recipients. A score of cases have been reported in the literature (Ripple et al., 2000). The origin of the graft atheroembolism was the recipient in about half the cases and the donor in the remaining cases. The *prognosis* was good when cholesterol emboli originated in the recipient, while most cases of donor origin developed progressive graft dysfunction. The reason for the difference could be attributed to more extensive cholesterol embolism from atherosclerotic cadaveric donors during organ procurement. There is no recommended treatment for patients with evolving renal failure. The prompt institution of *corticosteroid* therapy (Mann and Sos, 2001) or *statins* (Scolari et al., 2003) has been reported to be of benefit in some non-transplanted patients with renal atheroembolism.

De novo thrombotic microangiopathy (TMA)

The incidence of *de novo* post-transplant TMA has been differently estimated. In the analysis of USRDS data, *de novo* TMA was reported in only 0.8% of cases (Reynolds et al., 2003), while in a large series, 26 of 188 (14%) kidney and pancreas–kidney transplant recipients treated with cyclosporine developed *de novo* hemolytic–uremic syndrome (Zarifian et al., 1999).

Etiopathogenesis

A number of factors may increase the risk of developing a TMA in transplanted kidneys (Table 8.2). They include marginal kidneys (Pelle et al., 2005), cytomegalovirus infection (Waiser et al., 1999), parvovirus B19 infection (Murer et al., 2000), BK polyoma virus nephritis (Petrogiannis-Haliotis et al., 2001), antiphospholipid antibodies (Jumani et al., 2004), anticardiolipin antibodies in HCV-positive patients (Baid et al., 1999), or malignancy (Gohh et al., 1997). However, the most important risk factors are by far represented by the calcineurin inhibitors (CNI), cyclosporine (Zarifian et al., 1999) and tacrolimus (Lin et al., 2003), as well as

Table 8.2   Etiological factors for post-transplant thrombotic microangiopathy

Drugs	Virus	Miscellaneous
Cyclosporine	Cytomegalovirus	Marginal kidneys
Tacrolimus	Parvovirus B19	Antiphospholipid antibodies
Sirolimus	Polyoma BK virus	Malignancy
Everolimus	Hepatitis C	Severe hypertension
OKT3		

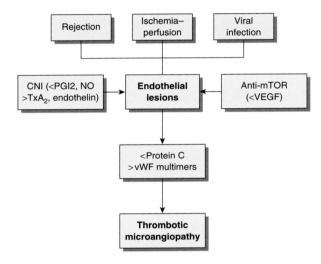

Figure 8.5 Pathogenetic mechanisms leading to *de novo* thrombotic microangiopathy. CNI, calcineurin inhibitors; PGI2, prostacyclin; TxA$_2$, thromboxane A$_2$; VEGF, vascular endothelial growth factor; vWF, von Willebrand factor

the anti-mTOR (mammalian target of rapamycin) drugs, sirolimus and everolimus (Saikali *et al.*, 2003; Sartelet *et al.*, 2005). The risk of *de novo* TMA is particularly increased when CNI and anti-mTOR agents are used in association (Langer *et al.*, 2002; Robson *et al.*, 2003). Cases of TMA have also been reported in transplant patients during treatment with OKT3 (Abramowicz *et al.*, 1992).

The *pathogenesis* of *de novo* post-transplant TMA is still poorly understood (Figure 8.5). It is possible to speculate that the endothelial lesions caused by ischemia–reperfusion injury (Land, 2005), viral infection (Maslo *et al.*, 1997; Guetta *et al.*, 2001), and/or rejection may be amplified by the endothelial injury caused by immunosuppressive drugs. CNI activate the renin–angiotensin system, increase the synthesis of vasoconstrictor agents such as endothelin and thromboxane A$_2$, and have a direct effect on renal vessels, while decreasing the vasodilators nitric oxide and prostacyclin (Burdmann *et al.*, 2003). As a consequence, arteriolar lesions characterized by mucinoid thickening of the intima or nodular hyalinosis (Mihatsch *et al.*, 1998) may develop. The concomitant increased platelet aggregation caused by the above-mentioned abnormalities and a pro-necrotic activity of cyclosporine in endothelial cells (Raymond *et al.*, 2003), together with reduced production of protein C, enhanced production of plasminogen activator inhibitor, and increased production of von Willebrand factor multimers, may eventually lead to TMA. The combination of CNI with mTOR may concomitantly exert pro-necrotic and antiangiogenic effects on endothelial cells (Fortin *et al.*, 2004). In fact, mTOR inhibitors may act as a subsequent aggressor, as it has been demonstrated that sirolimus may induce downregulation of vascular endothelial growth factor (Schrijvers *et al.*, 2004; Sartelet *et al.*, 2005), which is required for endothelial repair from CNI nephrotoxicity and TMA (Figure 8.6).

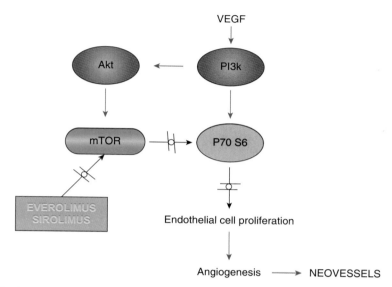

Figure 8.6 After immunological or non-immunological insults, endothelial cells slough into the circulation. Replacement occurs via the induced proliferation of neighboring endothelial cells and by neoformation of capillaries. These processes are under the control of vascular endothelial growth factor (VEGF) that activates the cascade of kinases governed by phosphatidylinositol 3 kinase (PI3k). A key role is played by the downstream effector of PI3k, a serine–threonine kinase called mTOR. This kinase can be inhibited by sirolimus or everolimus, thus impeding the proliferation of endothelial cells and angiogenesis.

Clinical and histologic features

Usually, *de novo* TMA occurs in the early post-transplant days, but it may also develop 2–6 years after transplantation (Katafuchi *et al.*, 1999; Zarifian *et al.*, 1999; Karthikeyan *et al.*, 2003). The clinical presentation of *de novo* post-transplant TMA may be variable. Some patients may show the clinical and laboratory features of HUS/TTP (hemolytic–uremic syndrome/thrombotic thrombocytopenic purpura), although milder than seen in non-transplant patients. Other patients show only progressive graft dysfunction, often associated with arterial hypertension.

Histologically, TMA is characterized by arterial and glomerular changes. Arterial TMA may involve preglomerular arterioles (Figure 8.7) and interlobular arteries, but not interlobar arteries. There is an initial deposition of fibrin in the subendothelial space and lumen, followed by intimal proliferation, stenosis of the lumen, and thrombosis. Glomerular changes may consist of glomerular lobulation with images of double contour and destruction of the mesangial matrix (mesangiolysis). Often there is patchy glomerular thrombosis of the glomeruli (Figure 8.8). In cases without extra-renal signs or symptoms, differential diagnosis between TMA and vascular rejection may be difficult, even with graft biopsy. It has been pointed out that intimal expansion with mononuclear cells and neutrophilic infiltration of the subendothelial layer favors humoral rejection (Mor *et al.*, 2000). The positive staining of peritubular capillaries with C4d is another feature of humoral rejection (Mauiyyedi *et al.*, 2002). However, cases of recurrent TMA with positive C4d staining have been reported (Karthikeyan *et al.*, 2003).

Prognosis

The prognosis is less severe than with recurrent TMA. It may depend on the severity of histologic lesions and clinical features. Patients with isolated glomerular TMA usually have a good outcome (Bren *et al.*, 2005). Prognosis is more favorable when TMA occurs later in the post-transplant course or when it affects recipients of allografts from living donors (Wiener *et al.*, 1997). Graft loss is rare in patients with TMA

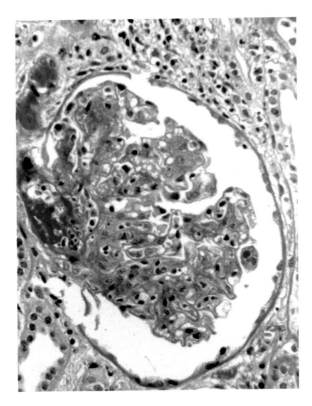

Figure 8.7 Post-transplant thrombotic microangiopathy. Preglomerular and hilar thrombosis of the glomerulus in a patient with recurrent post-transplant thrombotic microangiopathy (AFOG ×240)

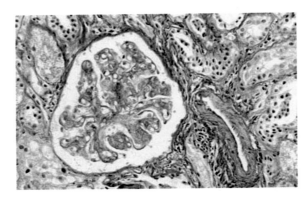

Figure 8.8 Post-transplant thrombotic microangiopathy. Patchy thrombosis of some loops of one glomerulus in a patient with de novo thrombotic microangiopathy. (AFOG ×240)

localized only to the kidney, while patients with systemic signs and symptoms of HUS are more likely to need dialysis treatment and to lose allograft function (Schwimmer *et al.*, 2003).

Treatment

Therapeutic guidelines for *de novo* TMA are not well defined. Complete withdrawal of the *offending drug* is essential (Oyen *et al.*, 2006), although not all patients respond (Manzoor *et al.*, 2006). In a few cases, reversal of TMA was obtained by switching from cyclosporine to tacrolimus (Franz *et al.*, 1998) or from tacrolimus to sirolimus (Yango *et al.*, 2002). However, it should be kept in mind that all CNI and mTOR inhibitors may potentially lead to TMA. Therefore, these changes of therapy should be made with great caution. *Plasma exchange* in addition to CNI withdrawal resulted in a graft salvage rate of 80% in two series (Mor *et al.*, 2000; Karthikeyan *et al.*, 2003) and in other single cases (Trimarchi *et al.*, 2001; Pham *et al.*, 2002). In cases with cytomegalovirus infection, ganciclovir may resolve TMA in cases resistant to plasmapheresis and CNI withdrawal (Jeejeebhoi *et al.*, 1998). Reinstitution of the offending CNI has been successfully made in a number of patients after recovery of graft function (Young *et al.*, 1996; Wiener *et al.*, 1997; Karthikeyan and Zaltzman, 2003). However, it should be recommended that the offending drug be reintroduced with extreme caution.

References

Abramowicz D, Pradier O, Marchant A, et al. Induction of thrombosis within renal grafts by high-dose prophylactic OKT3. Lancet 1992; 339: 777–8.

Antignac C, Hinglais N, Gubler MC, et al. De novo membranous glomerulonephritis in renal allografts in children. Clin Nephrol 1988; 30: 1–6.

Asim M, Chong-lopez A, Nickeleit V. Adenovirus infection of a renal allograft. Am J Kidney Dis 2003; 41: 696–701.

Audard V, Amor M, Desvaux D, et al. Acute graft pyelonephritis: a potential cause of acute rejection in renal transplant. Transplantation 2005a; 80: 1128–30.

Audard V, Pardon A, Claude O, et al. Necrotizing fasciitis during de novo minimal change nephrotic syndrome in a kidney transplant recipient. Transpl Infect Dis 2005b; 7: 89–92.

Baid S, Pascual M, Williams WW Jr, et al. Renal thrombotic microangiopathy associated with anticardiolipin antibodies in hepatitis C positive renal allograft recipients. J Am Soc Nephrol 1999; 10: 146–53.

Bansal VK, Koseny GA, Fresco R, et al. De novo membranous nephropathy following transplantation between conjoint twins. Transplantation 1986; 41: 404–8.

Basiri A, Otookesh H, Simforoosh N, et al. Does pre-transplantation antireflux surgery eliminate post-renal transplantation pyelonephritis in children? J Urol 2006; 175: 1490–2.

Berthoux P, Laurent B, Cecillon S, Berthoux F. Membranoproliferative glomerulonephritis with subendothelial deposits (type 1) associated with hepatitis G virus infection in a renal transplant patient. Am J Nephrol 1999; 19: 513–18.

Bhalla V, Nast CC, Stollenwerk N, et al. Recurrent and de novo diabetic nephropathy in renal allografts. Transplantation 2003; 75: 66–71.

Binet L, Nickeleit V, Hirsch HH, et al. Polyoma virus disease under immunosuppressive drugs. Transplantation 1999; 67: 918–22.

Bjorang O, Tveitan I, Midvedt K, et al. Treatment of polyomavirus infection with cidofovir in a renal transplant recipient. Nephrol Dial Transplant 2002; 17: 2023–5.

Bren A, Pajek J, Grego K, et al. Follow-up of kidney graft recipients with cyclosporine-associated hemolytic–uremic syndrome and thrombotic microangiiopathy. Transplant Proc 2005; 37: 1889–91.

Brenner BM, Cooper ME, de Zeeuw D, et al. Effects of losartan on renal and cardiovascular outcomes in patients with type 2 diabetes and nephropathy. N Engl J Med 2001; 345: 861–9.

Browne G, Brown PA, Tomson CR, et al. Retransplantation in Alport post-transplant anti-GBM disease. Kidney Int 2004; 65: 675–81.

Burdmann EA, Andoh TF, Yu L, Bennett WM. Cyclosporine nephrotoxicity. Semin Nephrol 2003; 23: 465–76.

Byrne MC, Budisavljevic MN, Fanz Z, et al. Renal transplant in patients with Alport's syndrome. Am J Kidney Dis 2002; 39: 769–75.

Campise M, Tarantino A, Banfi G, Ponticelli C. Necrotizing glomerulonephritis in a living donor kidney transplant recipient. Transplant Proc 2003; 35: 1368–9.

Cheng YT, Wang HP, Hsieh HH. Emphysematous pyelonephritis in a renal allograft: successful treatment with percutaneous drainage and nephrostomy. Clin Transplant. 2001; 15: 364–7.

Cosio FG, Pesavento TE, Kim S, et al. Patient survival after renal transplantation: IV. Impact of post-transplant diabetes. Kidney Int 2002; 62: 1440–6.

Cruzado JM, Carrera M, Torras J, Grinyo JM. Hepatitis C virus infection and de novo glomerular lesions in renal allografts. Am J Transplant 2001; 1: 171–8.

Daniel C, Renders L, Amann K, et al. Mechanisms of everolimus-induced glomerulosclerosis after glomerular injury in the rat. Am J Transplant 2005; 5: 2849–61.

Davison AM, Johnston PA. Allograft membranous nephropathy. Nephrol Dial Transplant 1992; 7 (Suppl 1): 114–18.

de Castro MC, Saldanha LB, Nahas W. Post-transplant neutrophilic interstitial nephritis, an important cause of graft dysfunction. Transpl Int 1998; 11 (Suppl 1) : S144–6.

Dittrich F, Schumaldienst S, Soleiman A, et al. Rapamycin-associated posttransplantation glomerulonephritis and its remission after reintroduction of calcineurin inhibitor therapy. Transpl Int 2004; 17: 215–20.

Ecder T, Tbakhi A, Braun WE, et al. De novo light-chain deposition disease in a cadaver renal allograft. Am J Kidney Dis 1996; 28: 461–5.

Elli A, Banfi G, Fogazzi G, et al. BK polyoma virus interstitial nephritis in a renal transplant patient with no previous acute rejection episodes. J Nephrol 2002; 15: 313–16.

Fabrizi F, Martin P, Dixit V, et al. Post-transplant diabetes mellitus and HCV seropositive status after renal transplantation: meta-analysis of clinical studies. Am J Transplant 2005; 5: 2433–40.

Farrell GC, Teoh NC, Management of chronic hepatitis B virus infection: a new era of disease control. Intern Med J 2006; 36: 100–13.

Fioretto P, Bruseghin M, Berto I, et al. Renal protection in diabetes: role of glycemic control. J Am Soc Nephrol 2006; 17 (Suppl 2): S86–9.

Fontana I, Ginevri F, Arcuri V, et al. Vesico-ureteral reflux in pediatric kidney transplants: clinical relevance to graft and patient outcome. Pediatr Transplant 1999; 3: 206–9.

Fortin MC, Raymond MA, Madore F, et al. Increased risk of thrombotic microangiopathy in patients receiving a cyclosporine–sirolimus combination. Am J Transplant 2004; 4: 946–52.

Franz M, Regele H, Schmaldienst S, et al. Posttransplant haemolytic uremic syndrome in adult retransplanted kidney graft recipients: advantage of FK506 therapy? Transplantation 1998; 1: 1258–62.

Ginevri F, Pastorino N, de Santis R, et al. Retransplantation after kidney graft loss due to polyoma BK virus nephropathy: successful outcome without original allograft nephrectomy. Am J Kidney Dis 2003; 42: 821–5.

Giral M, Pascuariello G, Karam G, et al. Acute graft pyelonephritis and long-term kidney allograft outcome. Kidney Int 2002; 61: 1880–6.

Gohh RY, Williams ME, Crosson AW, et al. Late renal allograft failure secondary to thrombotic microangiopathy associated with disseminated malignancy. Am J Nephrol 1997; 17: 176–80.

Gough J, Yilmaz A, Yilmaz S, Benediktsson H. Recurrent and de novo glomerular immune-complex deposits in renal transplant biopsies. Arch Pathol Lab Med 2005; 129: 231–3.

Guetta E, Scarpati EM, DiCorleto PE. Effect of cytomegalovirus immediate early gene products on endothelial cell gene activity. Cardiovasc Res 2001; 50: 538–46.

Hammoud H, Haem J, Laurent B, et al. Glomerular disease during HCV infection in renal transplantation. Nephrol Dial Transplant 1996; 11 (Suppl 4): 54–5.

Heidet L, Gagnadoux MF, Beziau A, et al. Recurrence of de novo membranous glomerulonephritis on renal grafts. Clin Nephrol 1994; 41: 314–18.

Hirsch HH. Polyomavirus BK nephropathy: a (re)emerging complication in renal transplantation. Am J Transplant 2002; 2: 25–30.

Hirsch HH, Knowles W, Dickenmann M, et al. Prospective study of polyomavirus type BK replication and nephropathy in renal-transplant-recipients. N Engl J Med 2002; 347: 488–96.

Hirsch HH, Ramos E. Retransplantation after polyomavirus-associated nephropathy: just do it? Am J Transplant 2006; 6: 7–9.

Hudson BG, Tryggvason K, Sundaramoorthy M, Neilson EG. Alport's syndrome, Goodpasture's syndrome, and type I collagen. N Engl J Med 2003; 348: 2543–56.

Jeejeebhoy FM, Zaltzman JS. Thrombotic microangiopathy in association with cytomegalovirus infection in a renal transplant patient: a new treatment strategy. Transplantation 1998; 65: 1645–8.

Jumani A, Hala K, Tahir S, et al. Causes of acute thrombotic microangiopathy in patients receiving kidney transplantation. Exp Clin Transplant 2004; 2: 268–72.

Kadambi P, Josephson MA, Williams J, et al. Treatment of refractory BK virus-associated nephropathy with cidofovir. Am J Transplant 2003; 3: 186.

Karthikeyan V, Parasuraman R, Shah V, et al. Outcome of plasma exchange therapy in thrombotic microangiopathy after renal transplantation. Am J Transplant 2003; 3: 1289–94.

Katafuchi R, Saito S, Ikeda K, et al. A case of late onset cyclosporine-induced haemolytic uremic syndrome resulting in renal graft loss. Clin Transplant 1999; 13 (Suppl 1): 54–8.

Kashyap R, Shapiro R, Jordan M, Randhawa PS. The clinical significance of cytomegaloviral inclusions in the allograft kidney. Transplantation 1999; 67: 98–103.

Kasiske B, Snyder JJ, Gilbert D, Matas AJ. Diabetes mellitus after kidney transplantation in the United States. Am J Transplant 2003; 3: 178–85.

Lai KN, Li PKT, Lui SF, et al. Membranous nephropathy related to hepatitis B virus. N Engl J Med 1991; 324: 1457–63.

Land WG. The role of postischemic reperfusion injury and other nonantigen-dependent inflammatory pathways in transplantation. Transplantation 2005; 79: 505–14.

Langer RM, Van Buren CT, Katz SM, Kahan BD. De novo haemolytic uremic syndrome after kidney transplantation patients treated with cyclosporine–sirolimus combination. Transplantation 2002; 73: 756–60.

Limaye AP, Jerome KR, Kuhr CS, et al. Quantitation of BKV load in serum for the diagnosis of BK virus-associated nephropathy in renal transplant recipients. J Infect Dis 2001; 183: 1669–72.

Lin CC, King KL, Chao YW, et al. Tacrolimus-associated hemolytic uremic syndrome: a case analysis. J Nephrol 2003; 16: 580–5.

Lipshutz GS, Flechner SM, Govani MV, Vincenti F. BK nephropathy in kidney transplant recipients treated with a calcineurin inhibitor-free immunosuppression regimen. Am J Transplant 2004; 4: 2132–4.

Mainra R, Mulay A, Bell R, et al. Sirolimus use and de novo minimal change nephropathy following renal transplantation [Letter]. Transplantation 2005; 80: 1816.

Mann SJ, Sos TA. Treatment of atheroembolism with corticosteroids. Am J Hypertens 2001; 8: 831–4.

Mannon RB, Hoffmann SC, Kampen RL, et al. Molecular evaluation of BK polyomavirus nephropathy. Am J Transplant 2005; 5: 2883–93.

Manzoor K, Ahmed E, Akhtar F, et al. Cyclosporine withdrawal in post-renal transplant microangiopathy. Clin Transplant 2006; 20: 43–7.

Markowitz GS, Stemmer CL, Croker BP, D'Agati VD. De novo minimal change disease. Am J Kidney Dis 1998; 32: 508–13.

Maslo C, Peraldi MN, Desenclos JC, et al. Thrombotic microangiopathy and cytomegalovirus disease in patients infected with human immunodeficiency virus. Clin Infect Dis 1997; 24: 350–5.

Mathew TH, Rao M, Job V, et al. Post-transplant hyperglycemia: a study of risk factors. Nephrol Dial Transplant 2003; 18: 164–71.

Mauiyyedi S, Crespo M, Collins AB, et al. Acute humoral rejection in kidney transplantation: II. Morphology, immunopathology, and pathologic classification. J Am Soc Nephrol 2002; 13: 779–87.

Meehan SM, Pascual M, Williams WW, et al. De novo collapsing glomerulopathy in renal allografts. Transplantation 1998; 65: 1192–7.

Mihatsch MJ, Kyo M, Morozumi K, et al. The side-effects of ciclosporine-A and tacrolimus. Clin Nephrol 1998; 49: 356–63.

Miles AM, Sumrani N, Horowitz R. Diabetes mellitus after renal transplantation: as deleterious as non-transplant-associated diabetes? Transplantation 1998; 65: 380–4.

Mor E, Lustig A, Tovar N, et al. Thrombotic microangiopathy early after kidney transplantation: hemolytic uremic syndrome or vascular rejection? Transplant Proc 2000; 32: 686–7.

Morales JM. Hepatitis C virus infection and renal disease after renal transplantation. Transplant Proc 2004; 36: 760–2.

Moroni G, Papaccioli D, Banfi G, et al. Acute post-bacterial glomerulonephritis in renal transplant patients: description of three cases and review of the literature. Am J Transplant 2004; 4: 132–6.

Moudgil A, Shidban H, Nast CC, et al. Parvovirus B19 infection-related complications in renal transplant recipients: treatment with intravenous immunoglobulin. Transplantation 1997; 64: 1847–50.

Moudgil A, Nast CC, Bagga A, et al. Association of parvovirus B19 infection with idiopathic collapsing glomerulopathy. Kidney Int 2001; 59: 2126–33.

Murer L, Zacchello G, Bianchi D, et al. Thrombotic microangiopathy associated with parvovirus B19 infection after renal transplantation. J Am Soc Nephrol 2000; 11: 1132–7.

Nadasdy T, Allen C, Zand MS. Zonal distribution of glomerular collapse in renal allografts: possible role of vascular changes. Hum Pathol 2002; 33: 437–41.

Newstead CG. Recurrent disease in renal transplants. Nephrol Dial Transplant 2003; 18 (Suppl 6): 68–74.

Nickeleit V, Singh HK, Mihatsch MJ. Polyomavirus nephropathy: morphology, pathophysiology, and clinical management. Curr Opin Nephrol Hypertens 2003; 12: 599–605.

Okada K, Takishita Y, Shimomura H, et al. Detection of hepatitis C virus core protein in the glomeruli of patients with membranous glomerulonephritis. Clin Nephrol 1996; 45: 71–6.

Oyen O, Strom EH, Midtvet K, et al. Calcineurin inhibitor-free immunosuppression in renal allograft recipients with thrombotic microangiopathy/hemolytic uremic syndrome. Am J Transplant 2006; 6: 412–18.

Pelle G, Xu Y, Khoury N, et al. Thrombotic microangiopathy in marginal kidney after sirolimus use. Am J Kidney Dis 2005; 46: 1124–8.

Petrogiannis-Haliotis T, Sakoulas G, Kirby J. BK-related polyomavirus vasculopathy in a renal-transplant recipient. N Engl J Med 2001; 345: 1250–5.

Pham P, Danovitch G, Wilkinson A, et al. Inhibitors of ADAMTS 13: a potential factor in the cause of thrombotic microangiopathy in a renal allograft recipient. Transplantation 2002; 74: 1077–80.

Poduval RD, Meehan SM, Woodle ES, et al. Successful retransplantation after renal allograft loss to polyoma virus interstitial nephritis. Transplantation 2002; 73: 1166–9.

Poduval RD, Josephson MA, Javaid B. Treatment of de novo and recurrent membranous nephropathy in renal transplant patients. Semin Nephrol 2003; 23: 392–9.

Ramos E, Drachenberg CB, Papadimitriou JC, et al. Clinical course of polyoma virus nephropathy in 67 renal transplant patients. J Am Soc Nephrol 2002; 13: 2145–51.

Ranchin B, Chapuis F, Dawhara M, et al. Vesico-ureteral reflux after kidney transplantation in children. Nephrol Dial Transplant 2000; 15: 1852–8.

Randhawa PS, Finkelstein S, Scantlebury V, et al. Human polyoma virus-associated interstitial nephritis in the allograft kidney. Transplantation 1999; 67: 103–9.

Rao KV, Hafner GP, Crary GS. De novo immunotactoid glomerulopathy of the renal allograft: possible association with cytomegalovirus infection. Am J Kidney Dis 1994; 24: 97–103.

Raymond MA, Mollica L, Vigneault N, et al. Blockade of apoptotic machinery by cyclosporine A redirects cell death towards necrosis in arterial endothelial cells: regulation by reactive oxygen species and cathepsin D. FASEB J 2003; 17: 515–17.

Remuzzi G, Macia M, Ruggenenti P. Prevention and treatment of diabetic renal disease in type 2 diabetes: the BENEDICT study. J Am Soc Nephrol 2006; 17 (Suppl 2): S90–7.

Reynolds JC, Agodoa LY, Yuan CM, Abbott KC. Thrombotic microangiopathy after renal transplantation in the United States. Am J Kidney Dis 2003; 42: 1058–68.

Ripple MG, Charney D, Nadasdy T. Cholesterol embolization in renal allografts. Transplantation 2000; 69: 2221–5.

Robson M, Coté I, Abbs I, et al. Thrombotic micro-angiopathy with sirolimus-based immunosuppression: potentiation of calcineurin-inhibitor-induced endothelial damage? Am J Transplant 2003; 3: 324–7.

Roth D, Cirocco R, Zucker K, et al. De novo membranoproliferative glomerulonephritis in hepatitis C virus-infected renal allograft recipients. Transplantation 1995; 59: 1676–82.

Rutgers A, Meyers KE, Canziani G, et al. High affinity of anti-GBM antibodies from Goodpasture and transplanted Alport patients to alpha 3 (IV) NC1 collagen. Kidney Int 2000; 58: 115–22.

Saikali J, Truong L, Suki W. Sirolimus may promote thrombotic microangiopathy. Am J Transplant 2003; 3: 229–30.

Sartelet H, Toupance O, Lorenzato M, et al. Sirolimus-induced thrombotic microangiopathy is associated with decreased expression of vascular endothelial growth factor in kidneys. Am J Transplant 2005; 5: 2441–7.

Schrijvers BF, Flyvbjerg A, De Vries AS. The role of vascular endothelial growth factor (VEGF) in renal pathophysiology. Kidney Int 2004; 65: 2003–17.

Schwarz A, Krause PH, Offermann G, Keller F. Impact of de novo membranous glomerulonephritis on the clinical course after kidney transplantation. Transplantation 1994; 58: 650–4.

Schwimmer J, Nadasdy TA, Spitalnik PF, et al. De novo thrombotic microangiopathy in renal transplant recipients: a comparison of hemolytic uremic syndrome with localized renal thrombotic microangiopathy. Am J Kidney Dis 2003; 41: 471–9.

Scolari F, Ravani P, Pola A, et al. Predictors of renal and patient outcomes in atheroembolic renal disease: a prospective study. J Am Soc Nephrol 2003; 14: 1584–90.

Sebire NJ, Bockenhauer D. Posttransplant de novo membranous nephropathy in childhood. Fetal Pediatr Pathol 2005; 24: 95–103.

Stokes MB, Davis CL, Alpers CE. Collapsing glomerulopathy in renal allografts: a morphological pattern with diverse clinicopathologic associations. Am J Kidney Dis 33: 658–66.

Tanenbaum ND, Howell DN, Middleton JP, Spurney RF. Lambda light chain deposition disease in a renal allograft. Transplant Proc 2005; 37: 4289–92.

Trimarchi H, Freixas E, Rabinovich O, et al. Cyclosporine-associated thrombotic microangiopathy during daclizumab induction: a suggested therapeutic approach. Nephron 2001; 87: 361–4.

Truong L, Gelfand J, D'Agati V, et al. De novo membranous glomerulonephropathy in renal allografts: a report of 10 cases and review of the literature. Am J Kidney Dis 1989; 14: 131–44.

Wadei HM, Rule AD, Lewin M, et al. Kidney transplant function and histological clearance of virus following diagnosis of polyomavirus-associated nephropathy (PVAN). Am J Transplant 2006; 6: 1025–32.

Waiser J, Budde K, Rudolph B, Ortner MA, Neumayer HH. De novo haemolytic uremic syndrome postrenal transplant after cytomegalovirus infection. Am J Kidney Dis 1999; 34: 556–9.

Wiener Y, Nakhleh RE, Lee MW, et al. Prognostic factors and early resumption of cyclosporine A in renal allograft recipients with thrombotic microangiopathy and haemolytic uremic syndrome. Clin Transplant 1997; 11: 157–62.

Wong KM, Chan YH, Chan SK, et al. Cytomegalovirus-induced tubulointerstitial nephritis in a renal allograft treated by foscarnet therapy. Am J Nephrol 2002; 20: 222–4.

Yango A, Morrissey P, Monaco A, et al. Successful treatment of tacrolimus-associated thrombotic microangiopathy with sirolimus conversion and plasma exchange. Clin Nephrol 2002; 5: 77–8.

Yildiz A, Tutuncu Y, Yazici H, et al. Association between hepatitis C virus infection and development of posttransplantation diabetes mellitus in renal transplant recipients. Transplantation 2002; 74: 1109–13.

Young BA, Marsh CL, Alpers CE, Davis CL. Cyclosporine-associated thrombotic microangiopathy/haemolytic uremic syndrome following kidney and kidney–pancreas transplantation. Am J Kidney Dis 1996; 28: 561–71.

Zafarmand AA, Baranowska-Daca E, Ly PC, et al. De novo minimal change disease associated with reversible post-transplant nephrotic syndrome. A report of five cases and review of the literature. Clin Transplant 2002; 16: 350–61.

Zarifian A, Meleg-Smith S, O'Donovan R, et al. Cyclosporine-associated thrombotic microangiopathy in renal allografts. Kidney Int 1999; 55: 2457–66.

For many years infections have been the most frequent cause of death in kidney transplant recipients. More recently, improved methods of immunosuppression and progress in the diagnosis and treatment of infection have led to a consistent decline in the incidence of fatal infections. However, even today, infection still occurs in most transplant recipients and accounts for 15–20% of deaths after transplantation (Briggs, 2001). The transplant physician has to face many challenges with transplant infections, and among them it should be noted that: (1) signs and symptoms of the infection may be attenuated by immunosuppressive therapy, with possible delays in diagnosis and treatment (Rubin, 2004); (2) the range of micro-organisms is far broader than in the general population; (3) the novel immunosuppressive agents have led to continuous changes of infectious complications (Humar and Michaels, 2006); and (4) simultaneous and sequential infections are common in transplant recipients.

Since the consequences of infection in immunosuppressed patients can be devastating, all efforts should be made to prevent infection. If an infection develops, it is important to establish the etiological diagnosis as quickly as possible and to institute an effective therapeutic regimen rapidly.

Prophylaxis

Prevention of infections is one of the primary goals in the management of renal transplant recipients. Theoretically, the best chance of prevention is represented by low immunosuppression; however, avoiding rejection remains a difficult task even with modern immunosuppressive therapy.

General measures

A number of *general measures* may be taken to prevent infections (Table 9.1). To lower the risk of postoperative infections, the use of drainage catheters, indwelling stents, vein catheters, and other foreign bodies should be reduced to a minimum. Apart from the recommendation of hand-washing, which removes most Gram-negative rods in a few seconds (Larson, 1995), some general measures should be taken during hospitalization. These include the removal of plants and fresh flowers, which carry pathogenic micro-organisms (Risi and Tomascak, 1998), from around the patient, hot water supply decontamination, and protection from other potentially infected patients. There should be regular inspection of air conditioning, showers, and water reservoirs to prevent the risk of Legionnaires' disease (Fields *et al.*, 2002).

Many transplant centers use a cephalosporin for 1–3 days to prevent wound infection. Oral washing with nystatin to prevent oral or gastrointestinal fungal infections is often used, but the administration of fluconazole at a dose of 100 mg per day is superior and does not interfere with the pharmacokinetis of cyclosporine (Paya, 2002). It is current practice to administer one tablet of trimethoprim 160 mg and sulfamethoxazole 800 mg every 24 or 48 hours, for 6–12 months after transplantation, in order to reduce the risk of urinary infections, and of infections caused by *Pneumocystis carinii* (Centers for Disease Control 1995), *Listeria*, *Nocardia*, and *Toxoplasma* (Rubin, 2004). At these doses, nephrotoxicity of trimethoprim–sulfamethoxazole is rare, but a mild increase in serum creatinine is possible.

Prevention of viral infection

Viral infections are particularly frequent and severe in renal transplant recipients (Table 9.2). As many as 70–80% of kidney transplant recipients may show laboratory evidence of *cytomegalovirus* (CMV) infection

Table 9.1 General measures for infection prophylaxis

Regular inspection of air-conditioning and water reservoirs
Minimal use of catheters, stents, and other foreign bodies
Protection from other infected patients
Oral washing with nystatin and/or fluconazole 100 mg per day
Trimethoprim–sulfamethoxazole 1 tablet every 24–48 hours
Cephalosporin for 1–3 days

after transplant, and a significant number of patients develop tissue-invasive disease with considerable morbidity and occasional mortality. It is highly recommended that donor and recipient are screened by CMV serology before transplantation. Monitoring once a month using a quantitative viral load assay for the first year is also recommended (Humar and Michaels, 2006). Many transplant centers recommend anti-CMV *prophylaxi*s in high-risk patients such as seronegative recipients who receive the graft from seropositive donors, or patients treated with monoclonal or polyclonal antilymphocyte antibodies. Prophylaxis with intravenous immunoglobulins or oral ganciclovir may significantly reduce CMV infection and disease in seronegative renal transplant patients receiving their kidneys from seropositive donors. However, there are three main drawbacks with prophylaxis (Singh and Yu, 2005): (1) the duration of prophylaxis is very long, about 100 days; (2) between 3 and 18% of patients may develop a late onset CMV disease; and (3) there is a high potential for resistance. The risk of resistance is higher with oral ganciclovir that has a low bioavailability (Varga et al., 2005), while resistance is rare after prophylaxis with valganciclovir (Boivin et al., 2004). Other centers prefer to start *pre-emptive* treatment when elevated levels of pp65 antigenemia or virus replication signs are found before CMV disease develops. The value of these approaches is still controversial, in view of the possible risk of inducing virus resistance (Ketteler et al., 2003). On the other hand, deferred strategies may have a deleterious effect on long-term graft function (Geddes et al., 2003). A recent meta-analysis of the randomized trials with pre-emptive therapy in organ transplant recipients did not resolve the problem. Pre-emptive therapy was effective in preventing CMV disease, but further trials were advocated to determine better the relative risks and harms (Strippoli et al., 2006). The risk of viral resistance is largely associated with the type of antiviral agent used for prophylaxis or pre-emptive therapy. Intravenous ganciclovir is quite effective, but its administration twice a day may cause logistical problems in non-hospitalized patients. Oral ganciclovir or valganciclovir has also been used for prevention of CMV infection. Oral ganciclovir has a poor absorption (6%), requires the administration of many pills per day, and can give resistance. Valganciclovir is an oral prodrug of ganciclovir with a ten-fold greater bioavailability (60%) and is as effective as oral ganciclovir for prevention, but two pills per day are sufficient, and, of much importance, it does not confer viral resistance (Reusser, 2001). Cidofovir has been used with good results as primary pre-emptive therapy (Chakrabarti et al., 2001), but it should be reserved for the treatment of severe ganciclovir-resistant cases as it may cause acute graft failure in renal transplant patients (Bienvenu et al., 2002).

Valacyclovir has demonstrated efficacy for other *herpes virus* prophylaxis (Squifflet and Legendre, 2002). Most transplant recipients have preformed antibodies against the *Epstein–Barr virus* (EBV). The few seronegative patients carry a high risk of receiving an EBV-positive kidney with the consequent risk of infection. While in some patients EBV infection causes benign polyclonal hyperplasia, in other transplant recipients it may cause a B-cell monoclonal lymphoproliferative reaction. Thus, EBV-seronegative patients should not be treated with antilymphocyte antibodies that render them more susceptible to an increased risk of viral infection. Seronegative transplant recipients and those receiving antilymphocyte antibodies should be given prophylaxis with valacyclovir or valgancyclovir for the first 3 months after transplantation. In addition, EBV viremia should be carefully monitored to reduce immunosuppression, or in order to give a quick antiviral treatment in the case of EBV infection (Shroff et al., 2002). Real-time polymerase chain reaction is superior to serology for measuring the viral load (Wagner et al., 2002).

Table 9.2 Preventive measures against viral infection

Cytomegalovirus

Prophylaxis: In CMV-seronegative recipients of CMV-seropositive kidneys and/or in patients receiving antilymphocyte antibodies, intravenous ganciclovir or oral valganciclovir for up to 3 months (risk of viral resistance)
Pre-emptive therapy: Monitor regularly viral load and/or pp65 antigenemia. Start intravenous ganciclovir whenever CMV DNA or pp65 antigenemia positive

Herpes virus

In patients with a history of recurrent infection, acyclovir or valacyclovir

Epstein–Barr virus

In EBV-negative recipients of EBV-positive kidneys and/or in patients receiving antilymphocyte antibodies, oral valacyclovir, or valganciclovir for 3 months

Varicella

Vaccination

Influenza

Vaccination

Vaccination against *varicella* is recommended in transplant candidates without humoral immunity (Olson *et al.*, 2001). Zoster immune globulins and antiviral prophylaxis should be administered to the recipient if some relative is infected with varicella. Yearly influenza vaccine has also been recommended in circumstances such as influenza epidemics and nosocomial outbreaks (Slifkin *et al.*, 2004). In a study in 49 renal transplant recipients, no negative effects on graft outcome were seen after vaccination. However, only 46% of patients developed antibodies to influenza A and 20% to influenza B (Sanchez-Fructuoso *et al.*, 2000).

Positive tuberculin test

Whether transplant recipients with a positive *tuberculin* test should receive anti-tuberculous prophylaxis or not is still a matter of discussion. The European Best Practice Guidelines for Renal Transplantation (Berhoux *et al.*, 2002) suggested prophylaxis with isoniazide (INH), 300 mg a day for 9 months, for patients with a history of inadequately treated tuberculosis or in patients who are positive for tuberculin. As an alternative approach, 2 months of rifampin plus pyrazinamide may be suggested. However, a number of uremic patients have tuberculin anergy (Woeltje *et al.*, 1998). Moreover, these drugs may cause hepatotoxicity and can interfere with the metabolism of calcineurin inhibitors and anti-mTOR (mammalian target of rapamycin) agents. Finally, it must be pointed out that there are more and more forms of isoniazid-resistant tuberculosis. Therefore, in patients with positive tuberculin tests and no other risk factors for tuberculosis (such as recent tuberculin conversion, protein calorie malnutrition, history of active tuberculosis), it has been suggested that active surveillance is preferred to prophylactic therapy (Rubin, 2005).

Bacteremic donors

A special problem is represented by kidneys coming from bacteremic donors. In the case of bacteremia caused by bland organisms, such as Enterobacteriaceae, *Streptococcus viridans*, or penicillin-sensitive

Table 9.3   Timetable of infections in renal transplant recipients

0–1 month

Bacterial:	wound infection, pneumonia, urinary tract infection, pyelitis, bacteremia
Viral:	herpes simplex, hepatitis

1–6 months

Viral:	CMV, Epstein–Barr, varicella zoster
Fungal:	*Candida, Aspergillus, Cryptococcus*
Bacterial:	*Listeria, Legionella, Nocardia*
Prortozoa:	*Pneumocystis carinii*

>6 months

Bacterial:	community micro-organism, mycobacteriosis
Viral:	hepatitis B or C, CMV chorioretinitis

pneumococci and meningococci, a short course of bactericidal antibiotics may be sufficient to eradicate the micro-organism. In the case of infections caused by *Staphylococcus aureus, Pseudomonas aeruginosa, Acinetobacter baumannii*, or penicillin-resistant streptococci, a minimum of 2 weeks of bactericidal therapy is required. Blood cultures should remain negative over a period of a week after antibiotic therapy. Donors with infections caused by vancomycin-resistant enterococcal infections or salmonella, fungal, nocardial, or active mycobacterial infection should be excluded (Rubin and Fishman, 1998).

Timetable for infection

In the transplant recipient, infections can be caused by nosocomial micro-organisms, opportunistic micro-organisms, or micro-organisms of the community. The type, frequency, and severity of the infection are roughly related to the level of immunosuppression, and the duration of immunosuppressive therapy. According to Rubin (1993), there is a relatively stereotypical pattern in the timetable of post-transplant infections. In the first month following transplantation, most infections are accounted for by nosocomial micro-organisms. In the period between the first and the sixth months, opportunistic infections derived from endogenous flora are frequent. After the sixth month, the type of infection is similar to that observed in the general population. However, patients with poor allograft function or vigorous immunosuppression are still exposed to an increased risk of viral and opportunistic infections (Table 9.3).

Infection in the first month

During the first month after transplantation, opportunistic infections are rare. Some patients have a recurrence of infection that was present in the donor or the recipient but was unrecognized or insufficiently treated (Fishman, 2002). Most infections occurring in this period are nosocomial bacterial or candidal infections of the surgical wound, lungs, urinary tract, or vascular devices. These infections are similar to those seen in non-transplanted patients who received a comparable amount of surgery (Rubin, 2002). Active infection is rarely transmitted when the allograft comes from a donor with bacteremia or fungemia. Such infections can seed at the vascular suture lines, leading to the formation of mycotic aneurysms causing arterial disruption (Rubin and Fishman, 1998).

Infections at 1–6 months

After the first month, the combination of sustained immunosuppression and infections with immuno-modulating viruses (particularly CMV, but also EBV, other herpes viruses, and hepatitis viruses) opens the possibility for opportunistic infections due to *Pneumocystis carinii*, *Aspergillus*, *Listeria monocytogenes*, and *Candida*. Particularly frequent in this period are infections caused by CMV, which account for 67% of cases of fever (Rubin, 2002). The lung, central nervous system, retina, urinary tract, and gastrointestinal tract are the most frequent sites of infection.

Infections after the sixth month

After the first 6 months from transplantation, kidney transplant function becomes the main predictor of risk for infection (Schmidt and Oberbaum, 1999). For patients with good renal function the incidence and type of infections are similar to those of the general community and are primarily respiratory. Urinary tract infections are frequent but are usually benign. In cases with chronic rejection, a more intensive immunosuppressive therapy can expose the patient to opportunistic infections. Lifelong prophylaxis with trimethoprim–sulfamethoxazole and/or antifungal prophylaxis has been recommended for these patients (Fishman and Rubin, 1998). Another subset of renal transplant recipients have chronic infection with CMV, EBV, hepatitis B or C virus, or papillomavirus. These infections may be progressive and lead to chorioretinitis, lymphoma, liver failure, or squamous-cell cancer. Leishmaniasis, ehrlichiosis, and other rare infectious diseases may also occur.

Approach to the febrile transplant patient

Although fever is not always present in an infected immunosuppressed patient, it remains the most common manifestation of an infection in a transplant patient. A number of clinical, laboratory, and radiological investigations are recommended in the febrile transplant patient. The first *differential diagnosis* should be between infection and rejection (Table 9.4). Usually an acute rejection causing fever is easy to detect because it is associated with typical signs and symptoms, such as a rapid increase in plasma creatinine, oliguria, proteinuria, and tenderness of the allograft. However, a similar clinical picture can be present in the case of pyelitis, perirenal hematoma, lymphocele, urinary fistula, or stenosis. Ultrasonography of the kidney, ureter, and bladder is usually sufficient for a correct diagnosis, but in the most difficult cases intravenous urography, computed tomography, or renal biopsy may be required.

A vigorous search for the *focus of infection* is imperative. Although localized sites of infection can be identified in many cases, some infections manifest themselves with signs and symptoms of a systemic disease without findings of a focal infection. This is particularly frequent in the case of CMV infection, but may also occur in febrile patients with bacteremia or fungemia.

While waiting for the results of blood culture, the history, the site of infection, and the time of infection can orientate the *empiric antibacterial therapy*. Septicemia in renal transplant patients is usually due to a Gram-negative organism, particularly in the setting of neutropenia; more rarely it may be sustained by *Staphylococcus aureus* and *Listeria monocytogenes*. Today, empiric therapy is usually based on the administration of a single drug active on Gram-negative bacteria, i.e. imipenem, ceftazidime, or piperacillin–tazobactam. If the patient is continuing to have signs and symptoms, an additional Gram-positive and anti-fungal empiric therapy is recommended (Marty and Rubin, 2006). In all patients with severe infection, exogenous immunosuppression must be reduced as much as possible.

Viral infections

Cytomegalovirus (HHV-5)

Human cytomegalovirus is a double-stranded DNA virus belonging to the family of β-herpesviridae. It is also called human herpes virus 5. The replication of CMV involves three types of genes: immediate early

Table 9.4 Investigations in a renal transplant recipient with fever

Rejection	Infection
PI, creatinine	Hemocrome (differential count)
Urinalysis (sodium, protein, sediment)	Mucosal plugging
Graft ultrasonography	Cultures (blood, urine, secretions)
Fine needle aspiration	CMV antigenemia
Renal biopsy	Anti-*Legionella*, *Candida*, *Mycoplasma* antibodies
	Pulmonary
	Chest X-ray (bronchial iavage)
	Cardiac
	Echocardiogram
	Urinary
	Graft, native kidney, bladder, and prostate ultrasonography
	Neurologic
	Liquor
	Cerebral CT
	Intestinal–hepatic
	Stool culture
	Liver and pancreas ultrasonography
	Serodiagnosis

genes encoding IE proteins; early genes encoding E antigens; and late genes encoding L antigens. The H65 matrix is a late antigen. CMV is the most frequent virus infecting renal transplant recipients. There are three forms of CMV infection in transplant patients: primary infection, secondary or reactivated infection, and superinfection.

The *primary infection* is the most severe form. Some 30–50% of adults are seropositive for CMV. The virus can reside in the kidney, and it is through the allograft that seronegative transplant recipients become infected. It has been estimated that seropositive patients may develop CMV disease in about 10% of cases (Brennan, 2001), while seronegative recipients from seropositive donors have a greater than 50% risk of symptomatic disease (Rubin, 1993). *Reactivation* occurs in a patient who is already a carrier of the virus. Activation from latency can be induced by several factors: therapy with antilymphocyte antibodies or other immunosuppressive agents; allogeneic reactions; and systemic infections. Systemic inflammation can reactivate CMV from latency through intracellular messengers stimulated by proinflammatory cytokines (Fietze *et al.*, 1994). *Superinfection* occurs when the donor and the recipient are both seropositive and the virus of donor origin reactivates. For clinical aims it has been proposed to differentiate between CMV active infection and CMV disease (Humar and Michaels, 2006). *CMV active infection* can be diagnosed by growing the virus *in vitro* or finding evidence of replication using nucleic acid-based assays or antigenemia. *CMV disease* is defined by evidence of CMV infection with attributable symptoms.

Clinical presentation and complications

The typical CMV disease manifests itself with fever, anorexia, myalgias, headache, and malaise, which usually occur between 1 and 4 months after transplantation; however, the onset of CMV disease may occur

Table 9.5 Clinical characteristics of CMV disease

Time of onset
More frequent 1–4 months after transplantation, later onset in case of prophylaxis

Predisposing factors
CMV– recipient/CMV+ donor
Previous therapy with antilymphocyte antibodies, OKT3, high-dose steroid
Retransplantation
Concurrent infection with HHV-6/HHV-7

Symptoms
Fever, anorexia, myalgias, headache, malaise

Signs
Anemia, leukopenia, lymphocytosis, thrombocytopenia, increase in transaminases

Specific tests
Antigenemia (pp65) > 100/200 0000 PBL, CMV DNA > 25 000 copies/ml

Direct consequences
Pneumonitis, gastrointestinal complications, hepatitis, encephalitis, myocarditis

Indirect consequences
Opportunistic infections, acute rejection, chronic rejection, lymphoproliferative disorders

later if the patient received a prophylactic treatment with IV ganciclovir or valganciclovir (Table 9.5). It may be associated with anemia, leukopenia, thrombocytopenia, mild lymphocytosis with atypical lymphocytes, and mild hepatitis. Some patients, particularly those affected by primary infection, may develop pneumonitis, gastrointestinal complications, hepatitis, encephalitis, or myocarditis. On the other hand, it must be noted that a reactivated and, less frequently, a primary infection may be asymptomatic, but may render the patient more susceptible to opportunistic infections, such as *P. carinii* pneumonia or invasive aspergillosis (Paya, 1999). While powerful anti-rejection therapy increases viral replication, CMV infection may, in turn, favor the development of acute rejection (Sagedal *et al.*, 2002), particularly in CMV mismatched (donor +/recipient–) patients (McLaughlin *et al.*, 2002). CMV infection may also expose patients to an increased risk of chronic allograft nephropathy (Tong *et al.*, 2002) through overproduction of mediators, cytokines, chemokines, and growth factors. An association has also been shown between CMV infection and atherosclerosis (Blum *et al.*, 2003; Vliegen *et al.*, 2004). Finally, CMV infection may favor the occurrence of lymphoproliferative disorders both directly, because CMV may exert an oncogenic effect (Rubin, 2002), and by favoring the development of EBV infection (Fishman and Rubin, 1998).

Diagnosis

The diagnosis of CMV infection is based on the demonstration of virus in the blood and the quantification of viral load. Blood viral culture, detection of viral genetic material by real-time polymerase chain reaction (PCR), and detection of CMV antigenemia have been employed to obtain an early and correct diagnosis of CMV infection in order to guide prophylactic and therapeutic strategies. Each technique has a different diagnostic meaning and clinical impact.

Viral culture of peripheral blood leukocytes (PBL) provides a direct demonstration of the presence of CMV. However, this technique takes a long time to obtain the final results, and cannot be used for early

Table 9.6   Dose adjustment for the principal antiviral agents according to creatinine clearance. For cidofovir, see text

Creatinine clearance (ml/min)	Acyclovir	Intravenous ganciclovir	Foscarnet	Valacyclovir	Valganciclovir
>70	5–15 mg/kg/8 h	5.0 mg/kg/12 h	100 mg/kg/12 h	500 mg/kg/6 h	450 mg/12 h
50–69	5–15 mg/kg/12 h	2.5 mg/kg/12 h	50 mg/kg/12 h	500 mg/kg/8 h	450 mg/24 h
25–49	5–15 mg/kg/12 h	2.5 mg/kg/24 h	25 mg/kg/12 h	500 mg/kg/12 h	450 mg/48 h
10–24	5–15 mg/kg/24 h	1.5 mg/kg/24 h	12.5 mg/kg/12 h	500 mg/kg/24 h	450 mg/72 h
<10	2.5–5 mg/kg/24 h	1.25 mg/kg/48 h	Avoid or 5 mg/kg after dialysis	500 mg/kg/24 h	450 mg once a week. Doses can be doubled for induction

diagnosis. The *shell vial* modification of the conventional buffy-coat culture technique, which shortens the time of viral culture, was developed a few years ago. However, it is not useful for early diagnosis (Murray *et al.*, 1997), and is not correlated with the clinical course of the infection (Tanabe *et al.*, 1997).

The CMV antigen test is an immunocytochemical method that, by using a monoclonal antibody specific for the *pp65 CMV* matrix protein, allows detection and quantification of positive PBL directly on a buffy-coat preparation. This protein is abundantly produced in excess during viral replication at different body sites, and is picked up by PBL. High levels of CMV antigenemia have been found in patients with overt disease, whereas low levels correlate with asymptomatic infections (Van der Berg *et al.*, 1989). In order to identify patients at higher risk of overt disease as early as possible, and to define pre-emptive strategies, threshold values of antigenemia have been determined. In one study, a threshold of 100 pp65-positive/200 000 PBL was chosen in solid-organ recipients (Grossi *et al.*, 1995). Slightly different thresholds have been suggested in other studies (Murray *et al.*, 1997), likely due to technical reasons and to underlying clinical circumstances, such as the level of immunosuppression.

PCR can also be used to detect CMV DNA. Whole blood in comparison with plasma is the optimal blood compartment for detection of CMV DNA in transplant patients (Tong *et al.*, 2000a; Razonable *et al.*, 2002). This test has a good sensitivity and specificity and can detect the presence of viremia even before the onset of symptoms. The quantitative determination of viral DNA in blood has been proposed as the assay of choice in monitoring solid organ recipients at high risk (Gerna *et al.*, 2001). It proved to correlate more closely with clinical symptoms in a high-risk population than antigenemia. This could be due to the fact that CMV DNA in leukocytes is the only genuine expression of viral replication occurring at different sites, while the pp65 matrix protein is produced in excess during viral replication and assembly. A threshold of 25 000 copies/ml has been proposed to distinguish between symptomatic and asymptomatic patients.

Treatment

The treatment of clinical CMV disease requires the administration of intravenous *ganciclovir* for a minimum of 2–4 weeks. However, many investigators are in favor of more prolonged treatments. Ganciclovir is a guanosine analog that, after intracellular phosphorylation, inhibits DNA polymerase activity and is incorporated in the viral DNA with consequent inhibition of synthesis of the chain. Ganciclovir should be administered at dose of 5 mg/kg every 12 hours with adjustment in the case of renal dysfunction (Table 9.6). In order to prevent relapses or resistance, treatment should be continued until the clearance of viremia before intravenous administration is documented. While the efficacy of oral ganciclovir in preventing relapses is questionable (Fishman and Rubin, 1998), oral *valganciclovir*, a prodrug largely and rapidly metabolized to ganciclovir, shows an efficacy comparable to that of intravenous ganciclovir (Kalpoe *et al.*, 2005). Serious side-effects of ganciclovir are infrequent, and include reversible neutropenia in 25–40% of patients, thrombocytopenia in about 20% of patients, irritation at the infusion site, and rarely a dose-dependent deterioration of renal function, probably due to crystallization of the drug in renal tubules (Dunn *et al.*, 1991). Generalized seizures have been reported (Barton *et al.*, 1992). Occasionally, allergic reactions may also occur. In cases of overt CMV infection, a decrease of immunosuppressive therapy and trimethoprim–sulfamethoxazole administration to prevent *P. carinii* infection are also recommended.

Some patients, particularly CMV-negative recipients of organs from seropositive donors (Limaye, 2002), may develop *resistance* to ganciclovir, which is manifested by a progression of CMV disease and persistence of viremia in spite of therapy. Ganciclovir-resistant CMV usually responds to foscarnet or to cidofovir. *Foscarnet* is an analog of pyrophosphate that inhibits the viral DNA polymerase and interferes with the exchange of pyrophosphate from phosphorylated deoxynucleotides. Foscarnet must be given intravenously for 14–21 days. The initial dose is 60 mg/kg every 8 hours, but the dose should be adjusted according to the renal function, as the drug is eliminated by glomerular filtration and tubular secretion. The maintenance dose is 120 mg/kg per day. Again, the dosage should be modified according to the creatinine clearance (Table 9.6). Foscarnet may be responsible for several side-effects: fever, nausea, anemia, diarrhea, vomiting, headache, and seizures. The most severe side-effect is renal toxicity. The drug may cause a substantial increase in plasma creatinine values and may be responsible for acute tubular necrosis (Deray *et al.*, 1989) or crystalline glomerulonephritis with nephrotic syndrome (Zanetta *et al.*, 1999). The administration of a saline infusion, 2.5 l/day throughout treatment with foscarnet, reduces the risk of nephrotoxicity. Other nephrotoxic drugs, such as cyclosporine, tacrolimus, amphotericin B, and aminoglycosides should be stopped, or their dosage reduced, during foscarnet administration. Electrolyte imbalance, especially hypocalcemia, is also common under foscarnet therapy (Balfour, 1999). *Cidofovir* is an acyclic nucleoside phosphonate derivative which inhibits the viral DNA polymerase. The drug may exert severe renal toxicity (Ljungman, 2001) and is contraindicated in patients with renal insufficiency. Cidofovir should be used with probenecid (2 g, 3 hours before cidofovir administration) and previous hydration with saline solution. In patients with normal renal function, the dose is 5 mg/kg once a week for the first week and then every 2 weeks for a maximum of 4 weeks. Because of its renal toxicity profile (Bienvenu *et al.*, 2002), its administration to renal transplant recipients requires the regular monitoring of serum creatinine. The dose should be halved in the case of an increase of 0.2–0.3 mg/dl; the drug should be stopped if serum creatinine increases to ≥0.5 mg/dl. New inhibitors of CMV replication, inhibitors of the terminase complex, and inhibitors of the viral protein kinase UL97 are under investigation (Emery and Hassan-Walker, 2002).

Influenza A and B

There is little information about the incidence and consequences of influenza in renal transplant patients. It is reasonable to assume that the incidence should be similar or, more probably, higher than in the general population. In a series of 30 organ transplant recipients with influenza, five (17%) developed bacterial pneumonia and three other patients developed myocarditis, myositis, and bronchiolitis obliterans, respectively. Variable degrees of acute rejection were seen in 18 of the patients (Vilchez *et al.*, 2002a). It is still uncertain whether the available anti-influenza virus agents (zanamir, amantadine, rimantadine, oseltamivir) may prevent the serious complications of influenza in renal transplant patients.

Epstein–Barr virus (HHV-4)

EBV infection may cause a self-limited mononucleosis syndrome in the general population, which is particularly frequent in adolescents. Organ transplant patients may suffer from either an asymptomatic *EBV infection*, defined by the presence of a detectable EBV viral load, or by *EBV disease*, defined by the presence of active infection associated with signs and symptoms. The most worrying effect of EBV infection in

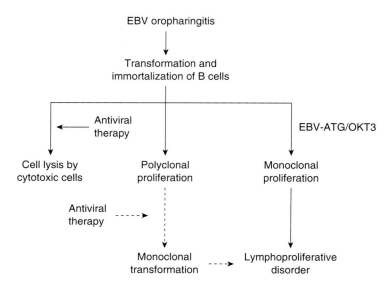

Figure 9.1 Possible evolutions of Epstein–Barr virus (EBV) infection

renal transplant recipients is represented by its oncogenic potential. EBV replication in the oropharynx results in infection, transformation, and immortalization of B cells. In the normal subject these transformed B cells are eliminated by specific cytotoxic cells. In the immunosuppressed renal transplant recipient, this surveillance mechanism may be impaired, thus making possible the development of uncontrolled proliferation resulting in malignant *lymphoproliferative disorders* (Figure 9.1).

It is recommended that serology be obtained for both donor and recipient before transplantation. Patients at risk, i.e. seronegative transplant patients who receive a kidney from a seropositive donor and those treated with antilymphocyte antibodies, may benefit from *antiviral prophylaxis* with valacyclovir or valganciclovir for the first 3 months after transplantation. Although a number of patients may develop EBV disease, the risk of post-transplant lymphoproliferative disorders is lowered in patients who received antiviral prophylaxis (Funch *et al.*, 2005). Of clinical interest, the mTOR inhibitors everolimus and sirolimus have been shown to inhibit the growth of EBV-infected lymphoma cells (Majewski *et al.*, 2003; Nepomuceno *et al.*, 2003).

The role of antiviral agents for the *treatment* of EBV infection is still under discussion. The combination of reducing immunosuppression, antiviral agents, and CMV immunoglobulins obtained a significant reduction of EBV DNA levels in a consistent number of organ transplant recipients in one study (Holmes *et al.*, 2002), while it was ineffective in another (Humar *et al.*, 2006b). A different approach consists of the infusion of autologous EBV-specific cytotoxic T lymphocytes prepared from peripheral blood mononuclear cells recovered at the time of virus reactivation. An increased virus-specific immune response and reduced viral load can be obtained with such a strategy, which can be proposed, therefore, for the prevention of lymphoproliferative disorders (Comoli *et al.*, 2002).

Varicella zoster virus (HHV-3)

The dermatosomal zoster is about ten times more common in renal transplant recipients than in healthy individuals.

Herpes zoster

Herpes zoster occurred in 7.4% of renal transplant recipients in a series, being more frequent in patients who received antilymphocyte antibodies (Gourishankar *et al.*, 2004). The infection tends to follow a more protracted course in the immunosuppressed patient, but visceral dissemination rarely occurs. Oral acyclovir (800 mg four times a day for 7 days) or intravenous acyclovir in the most severe cases (250–500 mg/m^2

every 8 hours for 7 days) may halt the progression of herpes zoster in an immunocompromised host. High-dose acyclovir may rarely cause renal dysfunction because of crystallization of the drug in renal tubules (Balfour, 1999). Valacyclovir, an L-valine ester of acyclovir, exhibits better oral biovailability. Controlled trials in immunocompetent patients with herpes zoster showed that valacyclovir, at a dose of 1000 mg three times a day for 7 days, significantly reduced the median pain duration when compared with acyclovir 800 mg five times a day for 7 days (Lin et al., 2001). A rare, severe, and still unexplained complication of valacyclovir is represented by thrombotic microangiopathy (Balfour, 1999).

Varicella (chicken-pox)

A much more serious occurrence is chicken-pox. This complication is more frequent and severe in children (Lynfield et al., 1992), but may also occur in adults (Fehr et al., 2002). In renal transplant patients, varicella may be a devastating disease, causing encephalitis, pneumonia, hepatitis, pancreatitis, disseminated intravascular coagulation, and gastrointestinal ulcerations. Pre-transplant *vaccination* with a two-dose regimen of varicella vaccine is recommended in seronegative transplant candidates (Geel et al., 2005), and can be done successfully also after transplantation (Furth et al., 2003; Chaves Tdo et al., 2005). If a patient without antibodies to varicella zoster is exposed to chicken-pox, then varicella zoster *immune globulins* should be given within 72 hours of exposure. The usual dose for intramuscular administration is 125 U/10 kg body weight in children, up to a maximum of 625 U. Post-exposure acyclovir prophylaxis is also useful (Goldstein et al., 2000). If chicken-pox develops, *intravenous acyclovir* should be promptly instituted (10 mg/kg every 8 hours for 7–10 days, with dosage decreases for renal dysfunction); in the case of combined varicella zoster and CMV infection, ganciclovir can be used (Aitken et al., 1999).

Herpes simplex virus (HHV-1 and -2)

Reactivation of herpes simplex virus (HSV) infection is common in renal transplant recipients. Infection usually involves the orolabial region, and less commonly the anogenital area. The diagnosis rests on the typical vesicular lesions. More rarely the HSV infection may affect the conjunctiva, or the cornea. Occasionally, life-threatening hepatitis, pneumonitis, or encephalitis occurs. In the latter cases, diagnosis is difficult. It may be confirmed by biopsy tissue, by culture, or by DNA/RNA-based assay. Topical acyclovir is ineffective and is not recommended. Most patients respond well to oral acyclovir (200–400 mg five times per day for 7 days) or valacyclovir (500 mg twice a day for 3 days). In the case of encephalitis or other visceral localization, high-dose intravenous acyclovir (10 mg/kg every 8 hours for 10–14 days) is the treatment of choice.

Human herpes virus 6 (HHV-6)

Human herpes virus 6 infection occurs in 31–55% of organ transplant recipients, usually 2–4 weeks after transplantation as a result of reactivation caused by intense immunosuppression. In many cases there is a co-infection or a reactivation of HHV-6, HHV-7, and CMV together (Tong et al., 2000b). Two variants have been identified: A and B. Renal transplant patients are infected almost exclusively with variant B. The *clinical sequelae* of HHV-6 may range from a self-limited febrile viral syndrome to tissue-invasive disseminated disease. Bone marrow suppression, meningoencephalitis, interstitial pneumonitis, and a mononucleosis syndrome are the most commonly reported types of clinical disease. An increased risk of acute rejection has also been reported (Clark, 2002). Apart from direct morbidity, the immune dysregulation triggered by HHV-6 may facilitate superinfections with other opportunistic pathogens. Human HHV-6 responds to ganciclovir and foscarnet, but is resistant to acyclovir (Singh and Carrigan, 1996).

Human herpes virus 7 (HHV-7)

HHV-7 is another recently identified β-herpes virus genetically related to human cytomegalovirus. The infection usually occurs in children, and may be reactivated after organ transplantation. The infection causes an aspecific febrile illness, including exanthema subitum. A tissue-invasive disease is extremely rare. The diagnosis can be made by PCR. There is growing evidence that the HHV-7 infection may be linked to an increased risk of CMV disease (Tong et al., 2000b; Clark, 2002).

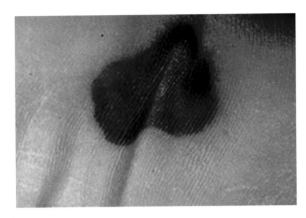

Figure 9.2 Kaposi's sarcoma

Human herpes virus 8 (HHV-8) (see also Chapters 11 and 14)

Human herpes virus 8 is a virus sharing biochemical and biological properties with the herpesviridae family, namely the ability to establish a latent infection that may reactivate with immunosuppression. There is now solid evidence linking Kaposi's sarcoma (both in endemic and in non-endemic form, in HIV, and in transplant-associated forms) to HHV-8 infection (Cathomas et al., 1997).

Kaposi's sarcoma is an angioproliferative disease. It generally starts as a hyperplastic reactive-inflammatory and angiogenic process which may evolve into monomorphic nodules that can be clonal and resemble a sarcoma (Figure 9.2). The prevalence of Kaposi's sarcoma in organ transplant recipients varies between 0.5 and 5%, depending on the patient's country of origin (Tan and Goh, 2006). Kaposi's sarcoma may develop in transplant recipients either as a consequence of a reactivated infection in a seropositive patient or as a primary infection in a patient without HHV-8-specific antibodies. In the latter case, a primary infection may be transmitted from the donor through the graft (Regamey et al., 1998). It is likely that factors other than immunosuppression are required for Kaposi's sarcoma to develop. The first therapeutic approach in transplant recipients is reduction or even withdrawal of immunosuppression. A response to treatment with an antiviral agent, cidofovir (Hammoud et al., 1998) or foscarnet (Luppi et al., 2002), has been reported. Preclinical studies indicate that protease inhibitors, which have antiangiogenic activity, are associated with the regression of Kaposi's sarcoma in treated patients (Toschi et al., 2002). In a number of cases the conversion from calcineurin inhibitors to sirolimus led to the cure of cutaneous (Campistol et al., 2004; Stallone et al., 2005) and even visceral (Mohsin et al., 2005) Kaposi's sarcoma. In some patients, however, no effect of sirolimus on the outcome of Kaposi's sarcoma was noted (Descoeudres et al., 2006).

Polyoma virus (see also Chapter 8)

The human polyoma virus family contains the BK virus (BKV), the JC virus, and the simain virus 40 (SV40), which are classified as 'slow' viruses. Polyoma viruses are usually acquired in childhood and remain latent in the kidney, liver, brain, lymphocytes, and perhaps lung. BK virus may be found, by cytology, in the urine of about 20–40% of renal transplant recipients. The clinical significance of this finding remains unclear, as in many patients BK virus does not cause significant morbidity. However, in renal transplant recipients, reactivation of *JC virus* may result in the development of progressive multifocal leukoencephalopathy, while *reactivation of BKV* latent in renal tubuli may lead to graft dysfunction and even graft loss.

JC virus infection

JC virus reactivation may lead to the development of progressive multifocal *leukoencephalopathy*. Seroepidemiological studies indicate that infection with this virus typically occurs before the age of 20 years. No primary illness owing to JC virus infection has been recognized, and the means of spread from

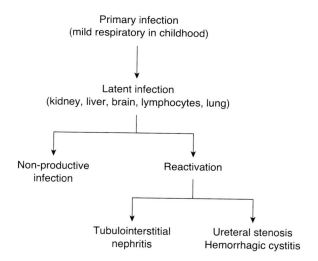

Primary infection
(mild respiratory in childhood)

↓

Latent infection
(kidney, liver, brain, lymphocytes, lung)

Non-productive infection   Reactivation

Tubulointerstitial   Ureteral stenosis
nephritis   Hemorrhagic cystitis

Figure 9.3   Possible evolution of BK virus infection

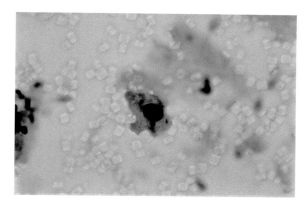

Figure 9.4   Polyoma virus in the urinary sediment. Light micrograph of urine cytology showing a tubular epithelial cell with characteristic intranuclear inclusion. (Courtesy of Dr F Egidi, University of Tennessee.)

person to person remains obscure. Following infection, the virus becomes latent in bone marrow, spleen, tonsils, and other tissues (Berger and Houff, 2006). Although JC virus is widely latent in patients accepted for transplantation, reactivation is infrequent (Randhawa *et al.*, 2005), and JC virus-related leukoencephalopathy remains a rare disease. The differential diagnosis between JC virus- and cyclosporine-induced leukoencephalopathy may be difficult (Koralnik, 2002).

BK virus nephropathy

The reactivation of BK virus occurs more often after the treatment of rejection, and in patients given tacrolimus and mycophenolate mofetil (Binet *et al.*, 1999; Ramos *et al.*, 2002) (Figure 9.3). *Primary infection* with BKV may also occur in children (Vats, 2004). The prevalence of polyomavirus BK nephropathy in renal transplant recipients ranges between 3 and 8% (Nickeleit *et al.*, 2003; Kiberd, 2005). The *diagnosis* is made on average between 6 and 12 months post-transplantation. BK virus infection may cause ureteral stenosis, hemorrhagic cystitis, and more often interstitial nephritis with a large number of plasma cells that leads to progressive graft loss. The presence of viral inclusions, known as 'decoy cells', in the urine (Figure 9.4), and the presence of BK virus DNA in plasma and urine, have been proposed as markers for the replication of BK virus infection (Nickeleit *et al.*, 2002; Hirsch *et al.*, 2002). The sensitivity of

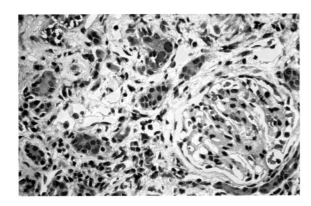

Figure 9.5 Renal biopsy. Interstitial nephritis caused by polyoma virus. The infiltrate is mainly composed of plasma cells and lymphocytes with interstitial fibrosis. (Courtesy of Dr F Egidi, University of Tennessee.)

decoy cells is 100% but the predictive value is low, only 27%. The diagnosis may be confirmed by the demonstration of viremia or viruria, which has a sensitivity of 100%, a specificity of 92%, and a predictive value of 74% (Randhawa et al., 2002). The final diagnosis may be made by renal biopsy, which shows an *interstitial nephritis* with an infiltrate rich in plasma cells (Figure 9.5), and atypical intranuclear viral inclusion bodies. It is important, however, to make an early diagnosis before severe histologic lesions develop. BKV replication in the urine should be screened every 3 months during the first 2 years post-transplant, and whenever allograft dysfunction is noted. A positive screening result should be confirmed in <4 weeks and assessed by quantitative assays (Hirsch et al., 2005).

The *prognosis* depends on the timelines of diagnosis. When diffuse interstitial nephritis associated with graft dysfunction is present, the prognosis is severe, with graft loss as high as 50% which may progress to 90% if interstitial nephritis is advanced (Drachenberg et al., 2004). Fibrosis at the time of diagnosis predicts subsequent functional decline (Wadei et al., 2006). The progression may be due to the fact that renal allografts with polyoma BKV nephritis transcribe proinflammatory genes equal in character and larger in magnitude to those seen during acute cellular rejection, thus creating a transcriptional microenvironment that promotes graft fibrosis (Mannon et al., 2005).

There is no specific *treatment* for BK virus infection (Figure 9.6). A reduction of immunosuppression may stabilize renal function in a few cases, but may expose the patient to the risk of acute rejection (Ramos et al., 2002). Once again, the success of this intervention depends on the time of diagnosis. The addition of cidofovir has been found to be helpful in a few cases (Bjorang et al., 2002; Vats et al., 2003). The standard dose is 5 mg/kg weekly for 2 weeks followed by one administration every 2 weeks. However, this drug is nephrotoxic, and its administration in patients with impaired graft function may further worsen renal insufficiency. In renal transplant patients the dose may range between 2.5 and 3.3 mg/kg intravenously biweekly (Hirsch et al., 2005), but may be further reduced in the presence of renal insufficiency. Pretreatment with probenecid and weekly adjuvant low-dose cidofovir, together with lowering immunosuppression, proved able to halt the progression of renal disease without causing nephrotoxicity in eight patients with polyoma virus nephropathy (Kuypers et al., 2005). Another approach may consist of withdrawing micophenolic acid and replacing, completely or partially, tacrolimus with leflunomide, an immunomodulant agent with antiviral properties. The recommended dose is 100 mg per day for 3 days followed by maintenance of 10–20 mg per day. Leflunomide may be given alone or in combination with cidofovir (Hariharan, 2006).

Parvovirus B19 (PVB-19)

Human PVB-19 is a small single-stranded DNA virus of the family parvoviridae. PVB-19 gains access to the human host by inhalation, but may also be transmitted by blood or by transplanted organs. Clinically, the acute infection is characterized by rash, fever, arthralgias, and anemia. In renal transplant recipients the presentation may be variable, with possible renal involvement. Hypertension, nephrotic syndrome, hematuria, and progressive deterioration of renal function may occur. Occasionally, in immunosuppressed

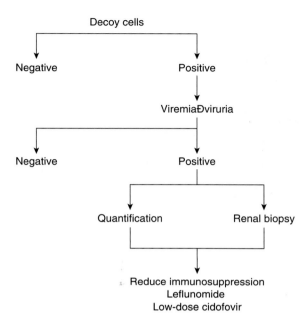

Figure 9.6 Diagnostic and therapeutic approach for BK interstitial nephritis

patients, a lack of protective antibodies allows PVB-19 to persist. In these cases PVB-19 can cause an abrupt cessation of red cell production, which provokes severe anemia. White cell and platelet count may also fall. Usually aplastic crisis is self-limited, but, in rare cases, anemia causes fatal cerebrovascular or cardiovascular events (Young and Brown, 2004). The diagnosis is based on an increase in specific IgM that can be seen in many but not all cases. The eradication of PVB-19 in immunosuppressed patients is difficult, but the use of intravenous immunoglobulins (0.4 g/kg for 5–10 days) can obtain recovery in some cases (Barsoum et al., 2002; Kumar et al., 2005).

Sepsis

Incidence

Sepsis is a syndrome defined by the presence of two or more features of systemic inflammation such as: fever or hypothermia, leukocytosis or leukopenia, tachycardia and tachypnea, or supranormal minute ventilation (Bone et al., 1992). Renal transplant patients have an adjusted incidence ratio of hospitalization for septicemia of 41.5 when compared with the general population (Abbott et al., 2001). Most cases occur within 6 months after transplantation. The lung and the urinary tract are the most common sites of infection, followed by the abdomen, but in several cases a definite site of infection cannot be recognized. Pleural, peritoneal, and paranasal sinus infections can easily be overlooked, even with the use of computed tomography (Wheeler and Bernard, 1999). In about 20–30% of patients, cultures are sterile. A useful marker for differential diagnosis may be the serum level of lipopolysaccharide-binding protein, which is elevated in a case of bacterial infection while being normal in a case of viral infection or acute rejection (Kaden et al., 2002).

Metabolic consequences

At the onset, sepsis is characterized by an increase in anti-inflammatory mediators. However, as sepsis persists, there is a shift to an anti-inflammatory immunosuppressive state even in non-transplanted

Table 9.7   Main therapeutic measures in patients with sepsis

Antimicrobial therapy	Hemodynamic stability	Microperfusion
Waiting for micro-organism isolation	Adequate hydration	Oxygen supply (usually inadequate)
Broad-spectrum antibiosis		
Specific antimicrobial agent after isolation	Low-dose corticosteroids	Control of glycemia
	Dopamine	Activated protein C

patients. The potential mechanisms leading to immunosuppression and failure to eradicate pathogens may consist of a shift from Th1 to Th2 cell response, anergy, apoptotic loss of CD4 T cells and B cells, loss of macrophage expression of HLA class II and co-stimulatory molecules, and an immunosuppressive effect of apoptotic cells (Hotchkiss and Karl, 2002). The most important consequences of sepsis are represented by insufficient microperfusion and defective oxygenation of tissue cells, in spite of the correction of systemic oxygen delivery variables (Ince, 2005). One mechanism leading to inadequate oxygen supply is represented by hyperglycemia, a frequent complication of sepsis caused by the overproduction of the proinflammatory mediator TNFα. In turn, hyperglycemia modifies inflammatory and immune reactions and enhances the production of reactive oxygen species.

Prognosis

The prognosis of sepsis largely depends on organ involvement. The average risk of death increases by 15–20% with the failure of each organ. In addition to the number of organ failures, the severity of each failure worsens the prognosis (Wheeler and Bernard, 1999). Other poor prognostic factors are granulocytopenia and persisting septicemia. In renal transplant recipients hospitalized for septicemia, the mean patient survival is 9.0 years, compared with 15.7 years for all other recipients (Abbott et al., 2001).

Treatment

Treatment relies on antimicrobial therapy that should be guided by isolation of the etiologic micro-organism. When the pathogen is not identified, broad antibiotic coverage is usually started, narrowing the therapy when microbiological data are available. In some cases, antimicrobial therapy may paradoxically precipitate sepsis syndrome by liberating microbial products. Supportive therapy is also of critical importance (Table 9.7). Adequate fluid and electrolyte administration are the first measures to maintain hemodynamic stability and prevent dysfunction of the kidney and other organs. The use of low-dose corticosteroids in patients with septic shock is useful not only in the case of corticosteroid insufficiency. These agents may improve survival because of their anti-inflammatory properties and their profound effects on the cardiovascular system (Annane and Cavaillon, 2003). In the case of hypotension sustained by low systemic vascular resistance, α-adrenergic drugs may be helpful. Dopamine is usually the preferred agent as it may improve, or at least not worsen, the renal blood flow. β-Adrenergic stimulation may be tried in the case of depressed myocardial contractility. Blood glucose control is of paramount importance to decrease mortality and morbidity in critically ill patients (Hotchkiss and Karl, 2002). Discoveries related to the link between coagulation and inflammation have been particularly exciting, leading to the development of recombinant activated protein C (Griffin et al., 2006). This serine protease is one of the most important inhibitors of coagulation; it can improve the microcirculation, reduce the endothelial cell permeability, and enhance the endothelial cell survival. Promising results have been obtained in a few transplant recipients with severe sepsis (Kulkarni et al., 2003; Grochowiecki et al., 2006).

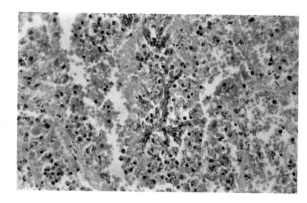

Figure 9.7 Postmortem tissue from a case of invasive pulmonary aspergillosis: hyphae of *Aspergillus fumigatus*, septate, uniform in width (3–6 μm), with dichotomous branches, infiltrating the necrotic tissue. H & E ×40. (Courtesy of Dr MA Viviani, Ospedale Maggiore, Milan.)

Fungal infections

Fungal infections occur in about 5% of renal transplant recipients. With the exception of cryptococcal infection, which usually develops later, most of these infections develop within the first 6 months after transplantation. The intensity of immunosuppression and broad-spectrum antibiotic therapy may favor the development of fungal infections. The four major fungal etiologies of pneumonia in renal transplant recipients are *Aspergillus* species, *Histoplasma capsulatum*, *Coccidioides immitis*, and *Cryptococcus neoformans*. Unfortunately, recognizing the fungal etiology is not easy. Sputum cultures are rarely diagnostic, and the yield of bronchoscopy with bronchoalveolar lavage is often discouraging (Vilchez *et al*., 2002b).

Aspergillosis

Aspergillus species (Figure 9.7) can be found as saprophytes, but may cause systemic mycoses with very high mortality. *A. fumigatus* is the most common pathogen, but *A. flavus*, *A. niger*, and other species can cause disease.

The main risk factors for post-transplant *Aspergillus* infection are CMV disease, chronic liver, disease and hyperglycemia (John *et al*., 2003). The most frequent complication is *pneumonia*, caused by the inhalation of spores. Occasionally the portal of infection may be the paranasal sinus, gastrointestinal tract, skin, or palate. Pneumonia occurs usually between 2 weeks and 6 months after transplantation. In the lung, *Aspergillus* species cause a patchy infiltration followed by consolidation and abscess formation (Figure 9.8). The first symptoms are a dry cough, with or without hemoptysis, dyspnea, and fever, although some patients may remain apyretic. The *diagnosis* may be difficult. Hyphae may be seen upon direct microscopy of sputum or a bronchial brushing specimen. However, sputum cultures are rarely diagnostic, and the yield of bronchoscopy with bronchoalveolar lavage is often discouraging (Vilchez *et al*., 2002b). In difficult cases, percutaneous needle aspiration and transbronchial biopsy may be required. Demonstration of the galactomannan antigen in the serum has high sensitivity and specifity but a predictive value of only 68% (Maertens *et al*., 1999). Real-time PCR is also highly sensitive and specific (Kami *et al*., 2001) for the diagnosis of *Aspergillus*. In a few cases, fungi may be recovered from the blood (Alexander, 2002). *Aspergillus sinusitis* may be characterized by a ball of hyphae, or granulomatous inflammation with spread to the orbit and brain (Figure 9.9). In immunosuppressed renal transplant recipients, infection may progress to hematogenous spread, leading to *invasive aspergillosis*. The *mortality* is extraordinarily high.

Successful *treatment* depends on three factors: early diagnosis, aggressive antifungal therapy, and the ability to reduce immunosuppression (Patterson, 1999). Until recently, *amphotericin B* at doses ranging between 1.0 and 1.5 mg/kg per day was the drug of choice. However, a major disadvantage of amphotericin B is its nephrotoxicity. The new lipid-based amphotericin B, even at higher doses, has a lower risk of nephrotoxicity (Singh *et al*., 2001). The greatest renal protection is from therapy initiated with lipid-associated amphotericin, as opposed to switching for toxicity (Fishman, 2002). Because of these characteristics, lipid-based amphotericin is currently preferred, although it is not clear whether, with higher doses of this

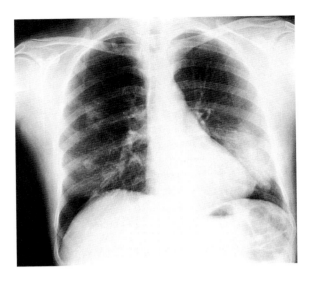

Figure 9.8 *Aspergillus* pneumonia. Patchy consolidation with faded margins

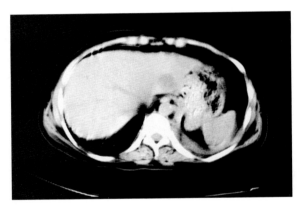

Figure 9.9 Diffuse aspergillosis. Localization in the liver. Hypodense lesion with sharp margins

agent, the efficacy is better than with conventional amphotericin B (Zak and Kusne, 1998). Itraconazole at a dose of 200 mg three times per day for 3 days, followed by a maintenance dose of 200–400 mg per day, may be used in patients who do not tolerate amphotericin B, but the results are not very promising (Rex *et al.*, 2001). The new antifungal agent *voriconazole* (6 mg/kg/12 h the first day then 3 mg/kg/12 h) proved to be superior to amphotericin B in the treatment of invasive aspergillosis (Herbrecht *et al.*, 2002). Caspofungin (70 mg/day then 50 mg/day), echinocandin, and pneumocandin are also effective. In patients with invasive aspergillosis, a combination of voriconazole and caspofungin might be considered as the preferable therapy (Singh *et al.*, 2006).

Histoplasmosis

Infection with *Histoplasma capsulatum* is relatively frequent in endemic areas (Americas, Africa). It usually presents with fever, malaise, myalgias, non-productive cough, arthralgias, and erythematosus skin lesions. *Pneumonia* is frequent. Chest radiography shows hilar adenopathy and small, irregular, and disseminated infiltrates that may eventually accumulate calcium. Chronic pneumonia usually manifests as an interstitial pneumonitis, but in 20% of the cases, can produce cavitation. Recovery of *H. capsulatum* in lung biopsy (Figure 9.10) is diagnostic. *Acute disseminated histoplasmosis* may be mistaken for military tuberculosis.

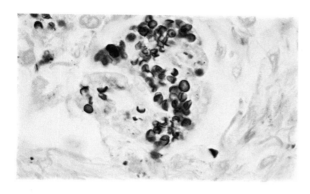

Figure 9.10 Disseminated histoplasmosis: alveolar macrophages packed with round to oval yeast-like cells of *Histoplasma capsulatum var capsulatum*, 2–4 μm in diameter. GMS × 100. (Courtesy of Dr MA Viviani, Ospedale Magglore, Milan.)

Symptoms include fever, jaundice, anemia, hepatosplenomegaly, and lympadenopathy. Some patients may show indurated ulcers of the tongue, mouth, or nose. However, histoplasmosis may affect any *system* or *organs*, leading to meningitis, gastrointestinal disease, endocarditis, hepatitis, Addison's disease, ocular disease, tibial involvement, etc. The *diagnosis* is particularly difficult in non-endemic areas. A positive *H. capsulatum* culture, an antibody titer higher than 1 : 32, or a four-fold increase over the basal level can also be regarded as diagnostic.

Treatment relies on amphotericin B or its lipid product, which is the drug of choice for cases of acute pneumonitis. Itraconazole (400 mg per day) or ketoconazole (400 mg per day) for at least 6 months can cure some 65–80% of cases (Wheat, 1994).

Cryptococcosis

Cryptococcus neoformans infection is usually acquired by the inhalation of fungus. It usually occurs more than 6 months after kidney transplantation. The majority of renal transplant recipients show a *disseminated disease* with neurological, pulmonary, and cutaneous symptoms (Vilchez et al., 2003).

*Meningoencephaliti*s is the most frequent complication of cryptococcosis (Perfect, 1989). The initial symptoms include headache, irritability, dementia, confusion, and blurred vision. With the progression of infection, coma and signs of brain-stem compression appear. Fever and nucal rigidity are often absent. Asymmetric cranial nerve palsies occur in about one quarter of patients. Lumbar puncture is needed for diagnosis. An India-ink smear of centrifuged spinal fluid sediment may reveal encapsulated yeasts in at least half of patients. Capsular antigen may be detected in cerebrospinal fluid by latex agglutination.

Cryptococcal *pneumonia* may result from the reactivation of a latent focus in the lung, or as an acute primary pulmonary infection (Alexander, 2005). Cryptococcus pneumonia presents with cough, chest pain, mucopurulent expectoration, hemoptysis, and dyspnea. Fever may be absent, and some transplant patients may be completely asymptomatic (Mueller and Fishman, 2003). Chest radiography may show a single nodule, or focal or lobar infiltrates, but none of the findings in chest radiographs and CT scans are pathognomonic (Vilchez et al., 2002b). In about 10–20% of patients there are *cutaneous nodules* that may help an early diagnosis.

The *treatment* is amphotericin B, occasionally associated with flucytosine, 25–37.5 mg every 6 hours. After 2–10 weeks, fluconazole (400 mg per day) for at leat 10 weeks is recommended. Chronic fluconazole may be continued for 6–12 months (Saag et al., 2000).

Coccidioidomycosis

Coccidioides immitis is a soil saprophyte. Infection results from the inhalation of wind-borne spores arising from soil sites. In renal transplant recipients the infection may occur in endemic areas, and can present in the form of pneumonia or disseminated disease (Braddy et al., 2006). *Pneumonia* presents with non-specific symptoms such as fever, malaise, dry cough, headache, and dyspnea. Eosinophilia and erythematosus skin lesions may be found in a few patients. X-radiologic findings show segmental

Table 9.8   X-radiologic findings in post-transplant pneumonia. Modified from Fishman and Rubin, 1988

Radiographic abnormality	Acute development	Chronic development
Nodular infiltrate	Bacteria	Fungi, *N. asteroides*, tuberculosis, *P. carinii*
Cavitation	Bacteria (*Legionella*), fungi	Tuberculosis
Peribronchovascular abnormality	Bacteria, viruses (influenza)	CMV, *P. carinii*, fungi, *N. asteroides*, tuberculosis
Consolidation	Bacteria (*Legionella*)	Fungi, *N. asteriodes*, tuberculosis, viruses, *P. carinii*
Diffuse interstitial infiltrates		CMV, *P. carinii*, fungi (rare)

pneumonitis, mild infiltrates, hilar adenopathy, and pleural effusion. Cavitation and solitary nodules (coccidioidoma) may develop in oligosymptomatic patients. The *disseminated form* is characterized by fulminant respiratory failure, disseminated intravascular coagulation and profound hypotension mimicking bacterial pneumonia and septic shock. Caspofungin, amphotericin B, and azoles are usually effective (Yamada *et al.*, 2003; Cordeiro *et al.*, 2006).

Pneumonitis

Pulmonary infection remains the most serious infectious disease in renal allograft recipients. Pneumonia prior to transplant, older age, diabetes, delayed graft function, rejection, long-term dialysis, and positive CMV serology are the main risk factors (Tveit *et al.*, 2002). Given the diverse group of potential infectious disease etiologies and the frequent lack of specificity of clinical and X-radiologic findings (Table 9.8), an aggressive diagnostic approach is often indicated. Fiberoptic bronchoscopy with transbronchial biopsy and bronchoalveolar lavage (BAL) are the most frequently used invasive techniques. Open lung biopsy and transthoracic needle aspiration may be needed in the most difficult cases.

Bacterial pneumonia

In the first month after transplantation, Gram-negative bacilli (*Escherichia coli*, *P. aeruginosa*, *Klebsiella pneumoniae*) and *S. aureus* are the most frequent causes of pneumonia. While waiting for culture results, a third-generation cephalosporin with or without an aminoglycoside can be given. Imipenem, ciprofloxacin, or vancomycin may be administered in resistant cases.

Between the second and sixth months, pneumomia may be caused by community organisms, but CMV and *P. carinii* pneumonia are also frequent. Nosocomial pneumonia has a worse prognosis than community-acquired pneumonia (Agusti *et al.*, 2003). It has been suggested that BAL be performed immediately, particularly in patients with bilateral infiltrates, to reduce drastically the immunosuppression, and that empirical erythromycin and trimethoprim–sulfamethoxazole be administered intravenously while waiting for isolation of the offending agent (Sileri *et al.*, 2002).

Legionella pneumonia

Legionella has become one of the most frequent causes of nosocomial pneumonia. In most cases, patients are contaminated from a humid environmental reservoir. In fact, *L. pneumophila* is naturally found in fresh

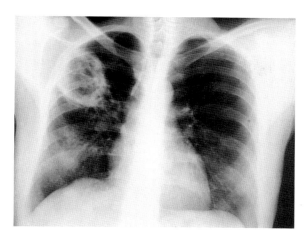

Figure 9.11 *Legionella* pneumonia. Multiple foci in the right lung with cavitation

water where the bacteria parasitize within protozoa (Steinert *et al.*, 2002). Impaired cellular immunity increases the risk of infection. Thus, organ transplant recipients are particularly vulnerable. The typical presentation is with fever >39°C, cough, and flu-like symptoms that do not respond to β-lactam antibiotics. Chest X-ray films may show irregular, nodular shadows that progress to a lobar or diffuse consolidation.

Cavitation can also occur (Figure 9.11). However, there is no specific radiographic sign. Identification of the organism may be obtained with detection of *Legionella* DNA in the serum with real-time PCR (Diederen *et al.*, 2006), or with immunochromatographic tests from sputum or biopsy samples, or by urine antigen assay. The indirect immunofluorescence antibody test or ELISA may detect 1–7 antibodies (Yzerman *et al.*, 2006). Elevated antibody titers develop only in an advanced phase of the disease. An increase of four times the titer to 1 : 128 or a single titer of 1 : 256 are diagnostic of recent exposure. Erythromycin, clarithromycin, azithromycin, and fluoroquinolones are the antibiotics of choice for legionellosis. It must be remembered that the first two agents can significantly increase blood levels of calcineurin inhibitors and mTOR inhibitors. The combination of azithromycin and fluoroquinolones is particularly promising in severe cases (Pedro-Botet and Sabria, 2005). Rifampin is also effective, and can be added to erythromycin in severe cases. As opposed to macrolides, rifampin significantly decreases the blood levels of cyclosporine or tacrolimus.

Nocardia pneumonia

The *Nocardia* species are denizens of soil and decaying plants that enter humans through inhalation or inoculation. Pulmonary nocardiosis is an important cause of opportunistic infection in immunosuppressed patients, and the incidence of this infection is increasing. Pulmonary nocardiosis typically presents as an *acute* or *subacute necrotizing pneumonia*, but may also have a *chronic* course for weeks or months. The diagnosis must be suspected in any case of chronic pneumonitis that does not respond to antibiotic therapy. The association of pneumonia with central nervous system and/or cutaneous involvement is highly suggestive for diagnosis. The X-radiologic findings are variable and not specific (Figure 9.12). Computed tomography can be useful to determine the extent of infection and the response to therapy. Usually, etiologic diagnosis requires the use of invasive procedures such as transtracheal aspiration, pulmonary needle aspiration, or biopsy. *Trimethoprim–sulfamethoxazole* is the first-line agent in the management of nocardiosis, and is usually successful when initiated early and continued for 6–12 months. However, resistance may develop with *N. farcinica* and *N. otitidiscaviarum*. Carbapenems should be used as an alternative treatment for severely ill patients (Yildiz and Doganay, 2006). Other agents are ciprofloxacin, cephalosporins, aminoglycosides, and doxycycline, but clinical data are limited (Baracco and Dickinson, 2001).

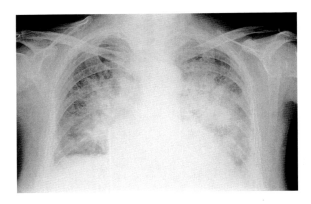

Figure 9.12 *Nocardia pneumonia*. Bilateral hilar and perihilar thickenings of different density

Acinetobacter baumannii

A. baumannii is a Gram-negative micro-organism responsible for nosocomial infections. The infection is often resistant to multiple antibiotics and is associated with increased mortality. Pneumonia is characterized by lobar consolidation and pleural effusion. About half of patients may have leukopenia. A number of patients have a fulminant course, with septic shock and respiratory failure (Leung *et al.*, 2006). A good sputum smear that contains more than 25 leukocytes per high-power field may facilitate the diagnosis (Chen *et al.*, 2001). *Imipenem* or meropenem are the antibiotics of choice. Intravenous *colistin* is effective in the case of resistance to imipenem. At high doses, however, colistin may cause nephrotoxicity. Aminoglycosides, ciprofloxacin, tetracyclines, and tigecycline may also be useful. Adequate dosing is of great importance, and the use of pharmacodynamic/pharmacokinetic principles when prescribing antibiotics increases effectiveness. The optimal duration of therapy remains unknown; several studies have supported the use of shorter courses of treatment. Alternative treatment approaches (e.g. vaccines) are under investigation.

Viral pneumonia

CMV and other herpes viruses may cause pneumonia. The diagnosis of CMV pneumonitis should be suspected in transplant patients with X-radiologic abnormalities between 1 and 4 months after transplantation. The suspicion of CMV is stronger if the patient was seronegative and received the kidney from a seropositive donor and/or if the patient was treated with antilymphocyte antibodies. The etiologic diagnosis is difficult. It may be suspected by the presence of elevated CMV antigenemia and/or by the typical histopathologic changes (cytomegaly, intracellular inclusions with peripheral chromatin clumping, intracytoplasmic inclusions) seen with bronchoscopy. However, a positive viral culture from BAL is insufficient, as it may reflect shedding from the oropharynx (Humar and Michaels, 2006). The final etiologic diagnosis may require histopathologic evidence of virus inclusions in the lung.

Community pneumonia

Pneumonia occurring after the sixth month is usually caused by community micro-organisms. The typical pathogens are *Streptococcus pneumoniae*, *Hemophylus influenzae*, and *Mycoplasma*. *Legionella* and *Chlamydia pneumoniae* are rarely found, and Gram-negative Enterobacteriaceae are restricted to high-risk patients. Cases of pneumonia due to pneumococci, *Legionella* or Enterobacteriaceae are associated with increased lethality. Viruses may be detected in nearly 15% of all pneumonia patients. Macrolides, fluoroquinolones, or doxycycline are the antibiotics of choice in the outpatient department. In hospitalized patients one of the following regimens is recommended while waiting for bacterial isolation: (1) a third-generation cephalosporin associated with a macrolide or doxycycline; (2) a fluoroquinolone agent; or (3) a β-lactamic agent plus a macrolide or doxycycline (Halm and Teirstein, 2002).

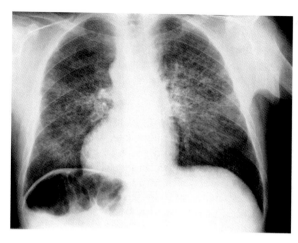

Figure 9.13 *Pneumocystis carinii* pneumonia. Interstitial pneumonitis with hilar and perihilar reticulonodular thickenings

Pneumocystis carinii pneumonia (PCP)

This is a frequent complication in transplant patients who do not receive prophylaxis with trimethoprim–sulfamethoxazole. The risk of PCP is increased in patients who have developed steroid-resistant rejection, CMV infection, or other immunomodulating infections such as tuberculosis and hepatitis C (Radisic *et al.*, 2003).

The patient with *P. carinii* pneumonia usually presents with fever and dyspnea. Physical signs are often absent on examination. Some patients may show eosinophilia. Severe hypoxemia is usually present. Interstitial pneumonia is frequent (Figure 9.13), but X-radiographic abnormalities may be variable and not specific. A correct diagnosis can be made only by BAL.

High-dose trimethoprim–sulfamethoxazole is the treatment of choice. The recommended dose is 15 mg/kg of trimethoprim, divided into 3–4 doses. A treatment of 14 days is usually sufficient. In patients allergic to sulfonamides, slow intravenous infusion of pentamidin, at doses ranging between 3 and 4 mg/kg per day according to the severity of the disease, may be indicated. Alternative treatment includes clindamycin, 900 mg every 8 hours, plus primaquine, 15 mg by mouth, every day.

Sirolimus-induced pneumonia

A few cases of interstitial pneumonitis may be caused by drugs such as beta-blockers or amiodarone. Sirolimus may also be responsible for a pneumonic illness. The presentations in these cases may range from insidious to fulminant (Haydar *et al.*, 2004). Clinical symptoms may include cough, fatigue, fever, and dyspnea. Computed tomography of the chest shows reticular and bronchiolitis obliterans-organizing pneumonia, and more rarely ground-glass opacities or lobar consolidation. Bronchoalveolar lavage may show lymphocytic or, less frequently, eosinophilic alveolitis or pulmonary hemorrhages. Discontinuation of sirolimus leads to complete recovery within 6 months (Champion *et al.*, 2006). The differential diagnosis from infectious interstitial pneumonia is important. The presence of lymphocytic alveolitis indicates sirolimus-induced pneumonia. In doubtful cases, an 'ex juvantibus' withdrawal of sirolimus may be suggested.

Tuberculosis

The *incidence* of tuberculosis is more common in transplant recipients than in the general population. Diabetes mellitus and liver disease are risk factors for post-transplant tuberculosis, and, together with co-existing infections, are also important risk factors for death (John *et al.*, 2001). The incidence of tuberculosis is more frequent in patients taking an association of tacrolimus and mycophenolate mofetil and in younger patients (Atasever *et al.*, 2005).

The *diagnosis* in transplant patients may be very difficult as the presentation can be subtle, and tuberculosis often has extrapulmonary localization at different sites. Moreover, there is an increased incidence of atypical mycobacterial infection among kidney transplant recipients.

Treatment should be the routine antitubercular therapy. In non-transplant patients a frequently used regimen consits of a 2-month initial therapy with rifampin, ethambutol, pyrazinamide, and isoniazid (INH), followed by a 4-month continuation with INH and rifampin (Small and Fujiwara, 2001). There are conflicting reports on whether *INH* may accelerate the metabolism of calcineurin inhibitors; however, no interference of INH in cyclosporine bioavailability was found in one study (Sud *et al.*, 2000). Another concern with INH is hepatotoxicity. In about 20% of patients there is a rise in serum transaminase. However, as patients remain asymptomatic, there is agreement that INH may be continued unless the levels of serum transaminases exceed 2–5-fold the normal. *Rifampin* is a potent inducer of the cytochrome P450 oxidative system, and can interfere with the bioavailability of corticosteroids, cyclosporine, tacrolimus, sirolimus, everolimus, statins, and a number of other drugs. As the use of rifampin in organ transplant recipients may result in 30% acute rejections and 20% graft failures (Singh and Paterson, 1998), it may be advisable to increase by 3–5-fold the daily dose of calcineurin inhibitors with the frequency of administration from twice to thrice daily, and to double the dose of steroids (Thomas, 2002). Alternatively, rifampin may be replaced with rifabutin, which also interferes with cytochrome P450 isoenzymes but less than rifampin (Finch *et al.*, 2002). *Pyrazinamide* may be substituted for rifampin in cyclosporine-treated patients, but liver function should be monitored in view of the hepatotoxicity of pyrazinamide. Therefore, antitubercular treatment is not easy in renal transplant recipients. Close monitoring of renal function, blood levels of calcineurin inhibitors, and particular attention to possible side-effects are needed. In patients who do not tolerate the standard regimen with INH, rifampin, and pyrazinamide, a combination of bacteriostatic drugs, ethambutol, and a fluoquinolone such as ofloxacin for 2–3 years may be effective (Rubin, 2005).

Urinary tract infections

Urinary tract infection is the most common bacterial infection following renal transplantation, although the advent of effective prophylaxis with low-dose trimethoprim–sulfamethoxazole has reduced the incidence (Brown, 2002). Vesicoureteral reflux, lymphocele, stones, and other urologic complications can favor the development of urinary tract infections as well as catheterisms and ureteral stents. Advanced age and female gender are also associated with a higher incidence of urinary tract infection (Chuang *et al.*, 2005).

Infections occurring in the *first 4–6 months* after transplantation are commonly associated with transplant pyelonephritis, bacteremia, and frequent relapse after standard antibiotic therapy for 10–14 days, even in the absence of urologic abnormalities. Asymptomatic bacteriuria requires an antibacterial treatment for at least 10 days, then a new urine culture should be carried out. Acute pyelonephritis and/or positive bacteremia require antibiotic treatment for 4–6 weeks. As most cases of urosepsis are caused by Gram-negative bacteria, the initial treatment may be based on a cephalosporin, third- or fourth-generation, imipenem, meropenem, aztreonam, or, in the most severe cases, aminoglycosides. Candidal infections usually respond to fluconazole and do not require amphotericin B administration.

In the *late period*, urinary tract infections are usually asymptomatic or oligosymptomatic and respond easily to antibacterial treatment. However, *acute pyelonephritis* may also occur, particularly in patients with stones, obstructions, or stents. Acute pyelonephritis may be associated with a rapid increase in serum creatinine, which is usually reversible if the infection is controlled. Antibiotic treatment should be prolonged, as recurrence or reinfection is frequent. Although urinary tract infection usually responds to adequate treatment, there is a mortality rate of around 3.5% for transplant patients requiring frequent hospitalizations because of recurrent infectious complications. Moreover, frequent urinary tract infections can increase the risk of chronic rejection (Schmaldienst *et al.*, 2002).

Central nervous system infections (see Chapter 16)

Apart from a few cases of early encephalitis caused by *varicella virus* or *West Nile virus* (Centers for Disease Control 2002; Iwamoto *et al.*, 2003) transmitted by blood or the transplanted organ, infections

Table 9.9   Main neurologic syndromes in renal transplant with CNS infection

Pattern	Etiological agents	Clinical features	Therapy
Acute meningitis	L. monocytogenes	Altered sensorium Headache	Ampicillin + aminoglycosides
Chronic meningitis	C. neoformans	Late occurrence, Fever, headache, altered consciousness	Amphotericin B + flucytosine
Focal brain abscess	Aspergillus Toxoplasma L. monocytogenes N. asteroides	Seizures Cranial nerve palsies	Amphotericin B or ampicillin or trimethoprim–sulfamethoxazole
Multifocal leukoencephalopathy	JC virus Herpes virus	Progressive dementia	Cidofovir?

of the central nervous system (CNS) in renal transplant recipients typically present between *1 and 12 months* following transplantation. The presentation of CNS infection in transplant patients may be different from that in normal patients. The onset may be subacute and systemic signs may be lacking. The most reliable *symptoms* that may demonstrate the presence of a CNS infection are headache, alteration in mental status, focal neurologic deficit, and unexplained fever. Patients with such an array of symptoms should receive computed tomography of the head and a lumbar puncture.

Wound infections

Wound infection was frequent in the past, but has become a rare complication today in renal transplantation. The administration of intraoperative and perioperative intravenous antibiotics, meticulous surgery, and less aggressive use of corticosteroids have contributed to the declining incidence of wound infection. However, a delay in the diagnosis or management of this complication can result in significant morbidity to the recipient. Important predisposing factors are wound hematomas, urine leaks, and lymphocele, the last being more frequent in patients treated with sirolimus (Langer and Kahan, 2002). Superficial wound infections develop a mean of 11.9 days after transplantation, while infections below the fascia develop after 39.2 days (Humar *et al.*, 2001). Some investigators found that obesity is a major risk factor for wound infection (Singh *et al.*, 2005), while others reported similar incidence and severity of wound complications in obese and in non-obese renal transplant recipients (Howard *et al.*, 2002). The treatment should consist of surgical drainage. Antibiotic therapy is advisable, but deep wound infections are often polymicrobial in origin and difficult to treat.

References

Abbott KC, Oliver JD, Hypolite I, et al. Hospitalization for bacterial septicemia after renal transplantation in the United States. Am J Nephrol 2001; 21: 120–7.

Agusti C, Rano A, Sibila O, Torres A. Nosocomial pneumonia in immunosuppressed patients. Infect Dis Clin North Am 2003; 17: 785–800.

Aitken C, Hawrami K, Miller C, et al. Simultaneous treatment of cytomegalovirus and varicella zoster infections in a renal transplant recipient with ganciclovir: use of viral load to monitor response to treatment. J Med Virol 1999; 59: 412–14.

Alexander BD. Diagnosis of fungal infections: new technologies for the mycology laboratory. Transpl Infect Dis 2002; 4 (Suppl 3): 32–7.

Alexander BD. Cryptococcosis after solid organ transplantation. Transpl Infect Dis 2005; 7: 1–3.

Annane D, Cavaillon JM. Corticosteroids in sepsis from bench to bedside? Shock 2003; 20: 197–207.

Atasever A, Bacakoglu F, Toz H, et al. Tuberculosis in renal transplant recipients on various immunosuppressive regimens. Nephrol Dial Transplant 2005; 20: 797–802.

Balfour HH Jr. Antiviral drugs. N Engl J Med 1999; 340: 1255–68.

Baracco GJ, Dickinson GM. Pulmonary nocardiosis. Curr Infect Dis 2001; 3: 286–92.

Barsoum NR, Bunnapradist S, Mougodil S, et al. Treatment of parvovirus B-19 (PV B-19) infection allows for successful kidney transplantation without disease recurrence. Am J Transplant 2002; 2: 425–8.

Barton TL, Roush MK, Dever LL. Seizures associated with ganciclovir therapy. Pharmacotherapy 1992; 12: 413–15.

Berger JR, Houff S. Progressive multifocal leukoencephalopathy: lessons from AIDS and natalizumab. Neurol Res 2006; 28: 299–305.

Berthoux F, Abramovicz D, Bradley B, et al. European Best Practice Guidelines for Renal Transplantation. Nephrol Dial Transplant 2002; 17 (Suppl 4): 1–67.

Bienvenu B, Martinez F, Devergie A, et al. Topical use of cidofovir induced acute renal failure. Transplantation 2002; 73: 661–2.

Binet I, Nickeleit V, Hirsch HH. Polyomavirus disease under immunosuppressive drugs. Transplantation 1999; 67: 918–22.

Bjorang O, Tveitan I, Midvedt K, et al. Treatment of polyomavirus infection with cidofovir in a renal-transplant recipient. Nephrol Dial Transplant 2002; 17: 2023–5.

Blum A, Peleg A, Weinberg M. Anti-cytomegalovirus (CMV) IgG antibody titer in patients with risk factors for atherosclerosis. Clin Exp Med 2003; 3: 157–60.

Boivin G, Gayette N, Gilbert C, et al. Absence of cytomegalovirus resistance mutations after valganciclovir prophylaxis in a prospective multicenter study of solid-organ transplant recipients. J Infect Dis 2004; 189: 1615–18.

Bone RC, Balk RA, Cerra FB, et al. Definition for sepsis and organ failures and guidelines for the use of innovative therapies in sepsis. Chest 1992; 101: 1644–55.

Braddy CM, Heilman RL, Blair JE. Coccidioidomycosis after renal transplantation in an endemic area. Am J Transplant 2006; 6: 340–5.

Brennan DC. Cytomegalovirus in renal transplantation. J Am Soc Nephrol 2001; 12: 849–55.

Briggs JD. Causes of death after renal transplantation. Nephrol Dial Transplant 2001; 16: 1545–9.

Brown PD. Urinary tract infections in renal transplant recipients. Curr Infect Dis Rep 2002; 4: 525–8.

Campistol JM, Gutierrez-Dalmau A, Torregrosa JV. Conversion to sirolimus: a successful treatment for posttransplantation Kaposi's sarcoma. Transplantation 2004; 77: 760–2.

Cathomas G, Tamm M, McGandy CE, et al. Transplantation-associated malignancies: restriction of human herpesvirus 8 to Kaposi's sarcoma. Transplantation 1997; 64: 175–8.

Centers for Disease Control. USPHS/IDSA guidelines for the prevention of opportunistic infections in persons infected with human immunodeficiency virus. A summary. MMWR Morb Mortal Wkly Rep 1995; 44 (RR-8): 1–34.

Centers for Disease Control. West Nile virus infection in organ donor and transplant recipients – Georgia and Florida 2002. JAMA 2002; 288: 1465–6.

Chakrabarti S, Collingham KE, Osman H, et al. Cidofovir as primary pre-emptive therapy for post-transplant cytomegalovirus infections. Bone Marrow Transplant 2001; 28: 878–81.

Champion L, Stern M, Israel-Biet D, et al. Brief communication: sirolimus-associated pneumonitis: 24 cases in renal transplant recipients. Ann Intern Med 2006; 144: 505–9.

Chaves Tdo S, Lopes MH, de Souza VA, et al. Seroprevalence of antibodies against varicella-zoster virus and response to the varicella vaccine in pediatric renal transplant patients. Pediatr Transplant 2005; 9: 192–6.

Chen MZ, Hsueh PR, Lee LN, et al. Severe community-acquired pneumonia due to *Acinetobacter baumannii*. Chest 2001; 120: 1072–7.

Chuang P, Parikh CR, Langone A. Urinary tract infections after renal transplantation: a retrospective review at two US transplant centers. Clin Transplant 2005; 19: 230–5.

Clark DA. Human herpesvirus 6 and human herpesvirus 7: emerging pathogens in transplant patients. Int J Hematol 2002; 76 (Suppl 2): 246–52.

Comoli P, Labirio M, Basso S, et al. Infusion of autologous Epstein Barr virus (EBV)-specific cytotoxic T cells for prevention of EBV-related lymphoproliferative disorder in solid organ transplant recipients with evidence of active virus replication. Blood 2002; 99: 2592–8.

Cordeiro RA, Brilhante RS, Rocha MF, et al. In vitro activities of caspofungin, amphotericin B and azoles against Coccidioides posadasii strains from Northeast Brazil. Mycopathologia 2006; 161: 21–6.

Deray G, Martinez F, Katalama C, et al. Foscarnet nephrotoxicity: mechanism, incidence and prevention. Am J Nephrol 1989; 9: 316–21.

Descoeudres B, Giannini O, Graf T, et al. No effect of sirolimus for Kaposi sarcoma in a renal transplant recipient. Transplantation 2006; 81: 1472–4.

Diederen BM, de Jong CM, Kluytmans JA, et al. Detection and quantification of Legionella pneumophila DNA in serum: case reports and review of the literature. J Med Microbiol 2006; 55: 639–42.

Drachenberg CB, Papadimitriou JC, Hirsch HH, et al. Histological patterns of polyomavirus nephropathy: correlation with graft outcome and viral load. Am J Transplant 2004; 4: 2082–92.

Dunn DL, Mayoral JL, Gillingham KJ, Loeffler CM. Treatment of invasive CMV disease in solid organ transplant patients with ganciclovir. Transplantation 1991; 51: 98–102.

Emery VC, Hassan-Walker AF. Focus on new drugs in development against human cytomegalovirus. Drugs 2002; 62: 1853–8.

Fehr T, Bossart W, Wahe C, Binswanger U. Disseminated varicella infection in adult renal allograft recipients: four cases and a review of the literature. Transplantation 2002; 73: 608–11.

Fields BS, Benson RF, Besser RE. Legionella and Legionnaires' disease: 25 years of investigation. Clin Microbiol Rev 2002; 15: 506–26.

Fietze E, Prosch S, Reinke P, et al. Cytomegalovirus infection in transplant recipients: the role of tumor necrosis factor. Transplantation 1994; 58: 675–80.

Finch CK, Chrisman CR, Baciewicz AM, Self TH. Rifampin and rifabutin drug interactions: an update. Arch Intern Med 2002; 162: 985–92.

Fishman JA. Overview: fungal infections in the transplant patient. Transpl Infect Dis 2002; 4 (Suppl 3): 3–11.

Fishman JA, Rubin RH. Infection in organ-transplant recipients. N Engl J Med 1998; 338: 1741–51.

Freifeld AG, Iwen PC, Lesiak BL, et al. Histoplasmosis in solid organ transplant recipients at a large Midwestern university transplant center. Transpl Infect Dis 2005; 7: 109–15.

Funch DP, Walker AM, Schneider G, et al. Ganciclovir and acyclovir reduce the risk of post-transplant lymphoproliferative disorder in renal transplant recipients. Am J Transplant 2005; 5: 2894–900.

Furth SL, Hogg RJ, Tarver J, et al. Varicella vaccination in children with chronic renal failure. A report of the Southwest Pediatric Nephrology Study Group. Pediatr Nephrol 2003; 18: 33–8.

Geddes CC, Church CC, Collide T, et al. Management of cytomegalovirus infection by weekly surveillance after renal transplant: analysis of cost, rejection and renal function. Nephrol Dial Transplant 2003; 18: 1891–8.

Geel A, Zuidema W, van Gelder T, et al. Successful vaccination against varicella zoster virus prior to kidney transplantation. Transplant Proc 2005; 37: 952–3.

Gerna G, Baldanti F, Grossi P, et al. Diagnosis and monitoring of human cytomegalovirus infection in renal transplant recipients. Rev Med Microbiol 2001; 12: 155–75.

Goldstein SL, Somers MJ, Lande MB, et al. Acyclovir prophylaxis of varicella in children with renal disease receiving steroids. Pediatr Nephrol 2000; 14:305–8.

Gourishankar S, McDermid JC, Jhangri GS, Preiksaitis K. Herpes zoster infection following solid organ transplantation: incidence, risk factors and outcomes in the current immunosuppressive era. Am J Transplant 2004; 4: 108–15.

Griffin JH, Fernandez JA, Mosnier LO, et al. The promise of protein C. Blood Cells Mol Dis 2006; 36: 211–16.

Grochowiecki T, Nazarewski S, Meszaros J, et al. Use of drotrecogin alpha (recombinant human activated protein C, rhAPC) in the treatment of severe sepsis induced by graft pancreatitis after simultaneous pancreas and kidney transplantation: a case report. Transplant Proc 2006; 38: 276–9.

Grossi P, Minoli L, Percivalle E, et al. Clinical and virological monitoring of human cytomegalovirus infection in 294 heart transplant recipients. Transplantation 1995; 59: 847–52.

Halm EA, Teirstein AS. Management of community-acquired pneumonia. N Engl J Med 2002; 347: 2039–45.

Hammoud Z, Parenti DM, Simon GL. Abatement of cutaneous Kaposi's sarcoma associated with cidofovir treatment. Clin Infect Dis 1998; 26: 1233.

Hariharan S. BK virus nephritis after renal transplantation. Kidney Int 2006; 69: 655–62.

Haydar AA, Denton M, West A, et al. Sirolimus-induced pneumonitis: three cases and a review of the literature. Am J Transplant 2004; 4: 137–9.

Herbrecht R, Denning DW, Patterson TF, et al. Voriconazole versus amphotericin B for primary therapy of invasive aspergillosis. N Engl J Med 2002; 347: 408–15.

Hirsch HH, Knowles W, Dickermann M. Prospective studies of polyomavirus type BK replication and nephropathy in renal transplant recipients. N Engl J Med 2002; 347: 527–30.

Hirsch HH, Brennan DC, Drackenberg CD, et al. Polyoma virus-associated nephropathy in transplantation: interdisciplinary analyses and recommendations. Transplantation 2005; 79: 1277–86.

Holmes RD, Orban-Eller K, Karrer FR, et al. Response of elevated Epstein–Barr virus DNA levels to therapeutic changes in pediatric liver transplant patients: 56-month follow-up and outcome. Transplantation 2002; 74: 367–72.

Hotchkiss RS, Karl IE. The pathophysiology and treatment of sepsis. N Engl J Med 2002; 348: 138–50.

Howard RJ, Thai VB, Patton PR, et al. Obesity does not portend a bad outcome for kidney transplant recipients. Transplantation 2002; 73: 53–5.

Humar A, Ramcharan T, Denny R, et al. Are wound complications after a kidney transplant more common with modern immunosuppression? Transplantation 2001; 72: 1920–3.

Humar A. Michaels M; AST ID Working Group on Infectious Disease Monitoring. American Society of Transplantation recommendations for screening, monitoring and reporting of infectious complications in immunosuppression trials in recipients of organ transplantation. Am J Transplant 2006; 6: 262–74.

Humar A, Hebert D, Dele DH, et al. A randomized trial of ganciclovir versus ganciclovir plus immune globulin for prophylaxis against Epstein–Barr virus related posttransplant lymphoproliferative disorder. Transplantation 2006; 81: 856–61.

Ince C. The microcirculation is the motor of sepsis. Crit Care 2005; 9 (Suppl 4): S13–19.

Iwamoto M, Jernigan BD, Guasch A, et al. Transmission of West Nile virus from an organ donor to four transplant recipients. N Engl J Med 2003; 348: 2196–203.

John GT, Shankar V, Abraham AM, et al. Risk factors for post-transplant tuberculosis. Kidney Int 2001; 60: 1148–53.

John GT, Shankar V, Talaulikar G, et al. Epidemiology of systemic mucoses among renal transplant recipients in India. Transplantation 2003; 75: 1544–51.

Kaden J, Zwerenz P, Lambrecht H, Dostat R. Lipopolysaccharyde as a new reliable marker after kidney transplantation. Transplant Int 2002; 15: 163–72.

Kalpoe JS, Schippers EF, Eling Y, et al. Similar reduction of cytomegalovirus DNA load by oral valganciclovir and intravenous ganciclovir on pre-emptive therapy after renal and renal–pancreas transplantation. Antivir Ther 2005; 10: 119–23.

Kami M, Fukui T, Ogawa S, et al. Use of real-time PCR on blood samples for diagnosis of invasive aspergillosis. Clin Infect Dis 2001; 33: 1504–12.

Keating MR. Antiviral agents. Mayo Clin Proc 1992; 67: 160–8.

Ketteler M, Kunter U, Floege J. An update of herpes virus infections in graft recipients. Nephrol Dial Transplant 2003; 18: 1703–6.

Kiberd BA. Screening to prevent polyoma virus nephropathy: a medical decision analysis. Am J Transplant 2005; 10: 2410–16.

Koralnik IJ. Overview of the cellular immunity against JC virus in progressive multifocal leukoencephalopathy. J Neurovirol 2002; 8 (Suppl 2): 59–65.

Kulkarni S, Naureckas E, Cronin DC 2nd. Solid-organ transplant recipients treated with drotrecogin alfa (activated) for severe sepsis. Transplantation 2003; 75: 899–901.

Kumar J, Shaver MJ, Abul-Ezz S. Long-term remission of recurrent parvovirus-B associated anemia in a renal transplant recipient induced by treatment with immunoglobulin and positive seroconversion. Transplant Infect Dis 2005; 7: 30–3.

Kuypers DR, Vandooren AK, Luret E, et al. Adjuvant low-dose cidofovir therapy for BK polyomavirus interstitial nephritis in renal transplant recipients. Am J Transplant 2005; 5: 1997–2004.

Langer RM, Kahan BD. Incidence, therapy and consequences of lymphocele after sirolimus–cyclosporine–prednisone immunosuppression in renal transplant recipients. Transplantation 2002; 74: 804–8.

Larson EL. APIC guidelines for handwashing and hand antisepsis in health care settings. Am J Infect Control 1995; 23: 251–69.

Leung WS, Chu CM, Tsang KY, et al. Fulminant community-acquired Acinetobacter baumannii pneumonia as a distinct clinical syndrome. Chest 2006; 129: 102–9.

Limaye AP. Ganciclovir-resistant cytomegalovirus in organ transplant recipients. Clin Infect Dis 2002; 35: 866–72.

Lin WR, Lin HH, Lee SS, et al. Comparative study of the efficacy and safety of valacyclovir versus acyclovir in the treatment of herpes zoster. J Microbiol Immunol Infect 2001; 34: 138–42.

Ljungman P. Prophylaxis against herpes virus infections in transplant recipients. Drugs 2001; 61: 187–96.

Luppi M, Barozzi P, Rasini V, et al. Severe pancytopenia and hemophagocytosis after HHV8 primary infection in a renal transplant patient successfully treated with foscarnet. Transplantation 2002; 74: 131–2.

Lynfield R, Herrin JT, Rubin RH. Varicella in pediatric renal transplant recipients. Pediatrics 1992; 98: 25–31.

Maertens J, Verhaegen J, Demuyinck H, et al. Autopsy controlled prospective evaluation of serial screening for circulating galactomannan by a sandwich enzyme-linked immunoadsorbent assay for haematological patients at risk for invasive aspergillosis. J Clin Microbiol 1999; 37: 3223–8.

Majewski M, Korecka M, Joergensen J, et al. Immunosuppressive TOR kinase inhibitor everolimus (RAD) suppresses growth of cells derived from posttransplant lymphoproliferative disorder at allograft-protecting doses. Transplantation 2003; 75: 1710–17.

Mannon RB, Hoffmann SC, Kampen RL, et al. Molecular evaluation of BK polyomavirus nephropathy. Am J Transplant 2005; 12: 2883–93.

Marty FM, Rubin RH. The prevention of infection post-transplant: the role of prophylaxis, preemptive and empiric therapy. Transpl Int 2006; 19: 2–11.

McLaughlin K, Wu C, Fick G, et al. Cytomegalovirus seromismatching increases the risk of acute renal allograft rejection. Transplantation 2002; 74: 813–16.

Mohsin N, Budruddin M, Pakkyara A, et al. Complete regression of visceral Kaposi's sarcoma after conversion to sirolimus. Exp Clin Transplant 2005; 3: 366–9.

Mueller MJ, Fishman JA. Asymptomatic pulmonary cryptococcosis in solid organ transplantation: report of four cases and review of the literature. Transpl Infect Dis 2003; 5: 140–3.

Murray BM, Amsterdam D, Gray V, et al. Monitoring and diagnosis of cytomegalovirus infection in renal transplantation. J Am Soc Nephrol 1997; 8: 1448–57.

Nepomuceno RR, Balatoni CE, Natkunam Y, et al. Rapamycin inhibits the interleukin 10 signal transduction pathway and the growth of Epstein Barr virus B-cell lymphomas. Cancer Res 2003; 63: 4472–80.

Nickeleit V, Steiger J, Mihatsch MJ. BK virus infection after kidney transplantation. Graft 2002; 5 (Suppl): S46–57.

Nickeleit V, Singh HK, Mihatsch MJ. Polyomavirus nephropathy: morphology, pathophysiology, and clinical management. Curr Opin Nephrol Hypertens 2003; 12: 599–606.

Olson AD, Shope TC, Flynn JT. Pretransplant varicella vaccination is cost-effective in pediatric renal transplantation. Pediatr Transplant 2001; 5: 44–50.

Paya CV. Indirect effects of CMV in the solid organ transplant patient. Transpl Infect Dis 1999; 1 (Suppl 1): 8–12.

Paya CV. Prevention of fungal infecton in transplantation. Transpl Infect Dis 2002; 4 (Suppl 3): 46–51.

Patterson TF. Approach to fungal diagnosis in transplantation. Transpl Infect Dis 1999; 1: 262–72.

Pedro-Botet ML, Sabria M. Legionellosis. Semin Respir. Crit Care Med 2005; 26: 625–34.

Perfect JR. Cryptococcosis. Infect Dis Clin North Am 1989; 51: 277–89.

Radisic M, Lattes R, Chapman JF, et al. Risk factors for Pneumocystis carinii pneumonia in kidney transplant recipients: a case-control study. Transpl Infect Dis 2003; 5: 84–93.

Ramos E, Drachenberg CB, Papadimitriou JC, et al. Clinical course of polyoma virus nephropathy in 67 renal transplant patients. J Am Soc Nephrol 2002; 13: 2145–51.

Randhawa PS, Vats A, Zygmunt D, et al. Quantitation of viral DNA in renal allograft tissue from patients with BK virus nephropathy. Transplantation 2002; 74: 485–8.

Randhawa P, Uhrmacher J, Pasculle W, et al. A comparative study of BK and JC virus infections in organ transplant recipients. J Med Virol 2005; 77: 238–43.

Razonable RR, Brown RA, Wilson J, et al. The clinical use of various blood compartments for cytomegalovirus (CMV) DNA quantitation in transplant recipients with CMV disease. Transplantation 2002; 73: 968–73.

Regamey N, Tamm M, Wernli M, et al. Transmission of human herpesvirus 8 from renal transplant donors to recipients. N Engl J Med 1998; 339: 1358–63.

Reusser P. Oral valganciclovir: a new option for creatinine of cytomegalovirus infection and disease in immunocompromised hosts. Expert Opin Invest Drugs 2001; 10: 1745–53.

Rex JH, Walsh TJ, Nettleman M, et al. Need for alternative trial designs and evaluation strategies for therapeutic studies of invasive mycosis. Clin Infect Dis 2001; 33: 95–106.

Risi GF, Tomascak V. Prevention of infection in the immunocompromised host. Am J Infect Control 1998; 26: 594–606.

Rubin RH. Impact of cytomegalovirus infection on organ transplant recipients. Rev Infect Dis 1990; 12 (Suppl 7): S754–66.

Rubin RH. Infectious disease complications of renal transplantation. Kidney Int 1993; 44: 221–36.

Rubin RH. Infections in the organ transplant recipient. In Rubin RH, Young LS, eds. Clinical Approach to Infection in the Compromised Host, 3rd edn. New York: Plenum Publishing, 1994; 629–705.

Rubin RH, Fishman JA. A consideration of potential donors with active infection – is this a way to expand the donor pool? Transpl Int 1998; 11: 333–5.

Rubin RH. Overview: pathogenesis of fungal infections in the organ transplant recipient. Transpl Infect Dis 2002; 4 (Suppl 3): 12–17.

Rubin RH. Principles of antimicrobial therapy in the transplant patient. Transpl Infect Dis 2004; 6: 97–100.

Rubin RH. Management of tuberculosis in the transplant recipient. Am J Transplant 2005; 5: 2599–600.

Saag MS, Graybill RJ, Larsen RA, et al. Practice guidelines for the management of cryptococcal disease. Clin Infect Dis 2000; 30: 710–18.

Sagedal S, Nordal KP, Hartmann A, et al. The impact of cytomegalovirus infection and disease on rejection episodes in renal allograft recipients. Am J Transplant 2002; 2: 850–6.

Sanchez-Fructuoso AI, Prats D, Naranjo P, et al. Influenza virus immunization effectivity in kidney transplant patients subjected to two different triple-drug therapy immunosuppression protocols: mycophenolate versus azathioprine. Transplantation 2000; 69: 436–9.

Schmaldienst S, Dittrich E, Horl WH. Urinary tract infections after renal transplantation. Curr Opin Urol 2002; 12: 125–30.

Schmidt A, Oberbaum R. Bacterial and fungal infections after renal transplantation. Curr Opin Urol 1999; 9: 45–9.

Segarra-Newnham M, Salazar MI. Valganciclovir: a new oral alternative for cytomegalovirus retinitis in human immunodeficiency virus-seropositive individuals. Pharmacotherapy 2002; 22: 1124–8.

Shroff R, Trompeter R, Cubitt D, et al. Epstein–Barr virus monitoring in paediatric renal transplant recipients. Pediatr Nephrol 2002; 17: 770–5.

Sileri P, Pursell KJ, Coady NT, et al. A standardized protocol for the treatment of severe pneumonia in kidney transplant recipients. Clin Transplant 2002; 16: 450–4.

Singh D, Lawen J, Alkhudair W. Does pretransplant obesity affect the outcome in kidney transplant recipients? Transplant Proc 2005; 37: 717–20.

Singh N, Carrigan DR. Human herpesvirus-6 in transplantation: an emerging pathogen. Ann Intern Med 1996; 124: 1065–71.

Singh N, Paterson DL. Mycobacterium tuberculosis infection in solid organ transplant recipients: impact and implications for management. Clin Infect Dis 1998; 27: 1266–77.

Singh N, Paterson DL, Gayowski T, et al. Preemptive prophylaxis with a lipid preparation of amphotericin B for invasive fungal infections in liver transplant recipients requiring renal replacement therapy. Transplantation 2001; 71: 910–13.

Singh N, Yu VL. Severing the Gordian knot of prevention of cytomegalovirus in liver transplant recipients: the principle is the sword. Liver Transpl 2005; 11: 891–4.

Singh N, Limaye AP, Forrest G, et al. Combination of voriconazole and caspofungin as primary therapy for invasive aspergillosis in solid organ transplant recipients: a prospective, multicenter, observational study. Transplantation 2006; 81: 320–6.

Slifkin M, Doron S, Snydman DR. Viral prophylaxis in organ transplant patients. Drugs 2004; 64: 2763–92.

Small PM, Fujiwara PI. Management of tuberculosis in the United States. N Engl J Med 2001; 345: 189–200.

Squifflet JP, Legendre C. The economic value of valacyclovir prophylaxis in transplantation. J Infect Dis 2002; 186 (Suppl 1): S116–22.

Stallone G, Schena A, Infante B, et al. Sirolimus for Kaposi's sarcoma in renal-transplant recipients. N Engl J Med. 2005; 352: 1317–23.

Steinert M, Hentschel U, Hacker J. Legionella pneumophila: an aquatic microbe goes astray. FEMS Microbiol Rev 2002; 26: 149–62.

Strippoli G, Hodson E, Jones C, Craig J. Pre-emptive treatment for cytomegalovirus viremia to prevent cytomegalovirus disease in solid organ transplant recipients. Transplantation 2006; 81: 139–45.

Sud K, Muthukumar T, Singh B, et al. Isoniazid does not affect bioavailability of cyclosporine in renal transplant recipients. Methods Find Exp Clin Pharmacol 2000; 22: 647.

Tan HH, Goh CL. Viral infections affecting the skin in organ transplant recipients: epidemiology and current management strategies. Am J Clin Dermatol 2006; 7: 13–29.

Tanabe K, Tokumoto T, Ishikawa N, et al. Comparative study of cytomegalovirus (CMV) antigenemia assay, polymerase chain reaction, serology, and shell vial assay in the early diagnosis and monitoring of CMV infection after renal transplantation. Transplantation 1997; 64: 1721–5.

Thomas P. Post-transplant tuberculosis. Saudi. J Kidney Dis Transplant 2002; 13: 445–50.

Tong CY, Cuevas LE, Williams H, et al. Prediction and diagnosis of cytomegalovirus disease in renal transplant recipients using qualitative polymerase chain reaction. Transplantation 2000a; 69: 985–91.

Tong CY, Bakran A, Williams H, et al. Association of human herpesvirus 7 with cytomegalovirus disease in renal transplant recipients. Transplantation 2000b; 70: 213–16.

Tong CY, Bakaran A, Peiris JS, et al. The association of viral infection and chronic allograft nephropathy with graft dysfunction after renal transplantation. Transplantation 2002; 27: 576–8.

Toschi E, Sgadari C, Monini P, et al. Treatment of Kaposi's sarcoma – an update. Anticancer Drugs 2002; 13: 977–87.

Tveit DJ, Hypolite IO, Poropatich RK, et al. Hospitalizations for bacterial pneumonia after renal transplantation in the United States. J Nephrol 2002; 15: 255–62.

Van der Berg APM, Van der Bij W, Van Son WJ, et al. Cytomegalovirus antigenemia as a useful marker of symptomatic cytomegalovirus infection after renal transplantation: a report of 130 consecutive patients. Transplantation 1989; 48: 991–5.

Varga M, Reimport A, Hidvegi M, et al. Comparing cytomegalovirus prophylaxis in renal transplantation: single center experience. Transpl Infect Dis 2005; 7: 63–7.

Vats A. BK virus-associated transplant nephropathy: need for increased awareness in children. Pediatr Transplant 2004; 8: 421–5.

Vats A, Shapiro R, Randhawa PS, et al. Quantitative viral load monitoring and cidofovir therapy for the management of BK virus-associated nephropathy in children and adults. Transplantation 2003; 75: 105–12.

Vilchez RA, McCurry K, Dauber J, et al. Influenza virus infection in adult solid organ transplant recipients. Am J Transplant 2002a; 2: 287–91.

Vilchez RA, Fung J, Kusne S. Cryptococcosis in organ transplant recipients. Am J Transplant 2002b; 2: 575–80.

Vilchez R, Shapiro R, McCurry K, et al. Longitudinal study of cryptococcosis in adult solid-organ transplant recipients. Transpl Int 2003; 16: 336–40.

Vliegen I, Duijvestijn A, Graves G, et al. Cytomegalovirus infection aggravates atherogenesis in apoE knockout mice by both local and systemic immune activation. Microbes Infect 2004; 6: 17–24.

Wadei HM, Rule AD, Lewin M, et al. Kidney transplant function and histological clearance of virus following diagnosis of polyomavirus-associated nephropathy (PVAN). Am J Transplant 2006; 6: 1025–32.

Wagner HJ, Fischer L, Jabs WJ, et al. Longitudinal analysis of Epstein–Barr viral load in plasma and peripheral blood mononuclear cells of transplanted patients by real-time polymerase chain reaction. Transplantation 2002; 74: 656–64.

Wheat J. Histoplasmosis: recognition and treatment. Clin Infect Dis 1994; 19 (Suppl1): S19–26.

Wheeler AP, Bernard GR. Treating patients with severe sepsis. N Engl J Med 1999; 340: 207–14.

Woeltje FK, Mathew A, Rothstein M, et al. Tuberculosis infection and anergy in hemodialysis patients. Am J Kidney Dis 1998; 31: 848–52.

Yamada H, Kotaki H, Takahashi T. Recommendations for the treatment of fungal pneumonias. Expert Opin Pharmacother 2003; 4: 1241–58.

Yildiz O, Doganay M. Actinomycoses and Nocardia pulmonary infections. Curr Opin Pulm Med 2006; 12: 228–34.

Young NS, Brown KE. Parvovirus B19. N Engl J Med 2004; 350: 586–97.

Yzerman EP, den Boer JW, Lettinga KD, et al. Sensitivity of three serum antibody tests in a large outbreak of Legionnaires' disease in The Netherlands. J Med Microbiol 2006; 55: 561–6.

Zak MB, Kusne S. Should liposomal amphotericin B products be first line therapy for invasive aspergillosis in solid organ transplant recipients? Curr Opin Organ Transplant 1998; 3: 127–9.

Zanetta G, Maurice-Estepa L, Mousson C, et al. Foscarnet-induced crystalline glomerulonephritis with nephrotic syndrome and acute renal failure after kidney transplantation. Transplantation 1999; 67: 1376–8.

CARDIOVASCULAR COMPLICATIONS

Cardiovascular disease is a frequent cause of morbidity after kidney transplantation. Its impact on patient and graft survival is becoming more and more important as the age of the recipient and the allograft longevity are progressively increasing. Death with a functioning allograft is now a leading cause of renal allograft failure, especially in the late post-transplant period (Kasiske, 2002; Cecka, 2003). Although infection and malignancies greatly contribute to post-transplant mortality, the most common cause of death after renal transplantation is cardiovascular disease (Rigatto, 2003; Cecka, 2003). Thus, further improvement in long-term renal allograft survival may also depend on our ability to reduce cardiovascular morbidity and mortality.

More than 20 years ago, up to 246 atherogenic risk factors were identified in the general population (Hopkins and Williams, 1981), and the number continues to grow, although most risk factors do not fully account for the occurrence of cardiovascular disease. In the renal transplant patient, not only most of the traditional risk factors that may affect the general population but also a number of atherogenic risks related to previous dialysis, abnormal renal function, and use of immunosuppressive drugs are frequently present (Figure 10.1).

In this chapter, we deal with the most important *modifiable* risk factors involved in post-transplant cardiovascular disease, keeping in mind that cardiovascular disease is the result of interaction among a number of genetic, environmental, and acquired conditions.

Pre-transplant risk factors

Traditional risk factors

Many kidney transplant recipients are already affected by cardiovascular disease before transplantation (Wheeler and Steiger, 2000; Rice et al., 2002). *Traditional risk factors* are especially prevalent among patients with chronic renal diseases. Nevertheless, these factors account for about half of cardiovascular complications in dialysis patients (Zoccali et al., 2005).

Diabetes mellitus

A growing number of renal transplant candidates are diabetic. Although progress in diagnosis, prevention, and treatment has considerably improved the life expectancy of renal transplant patients with diabetes, nevertheless, the risk of *cardiovascular death*, in particular from cardiac infarct, remains higher for diabetic than for non-diabetic transplant recipients (Aakhus et al., 1999; Tyden et al., 1999; Viberti, 2001; Hypolite et al., 2002; Pilmore, 2006).

Several mechanisms may contribute to accelerated atherosclerosis and cardiovascular disease in patients with type II diabetes. They include elevated levels of serum tryglicerides and VLDL cholesterol (Gervaise et al., 2000), hyperinsulinemia (Haffner, 1999), glycation of lipoproteins (Aso et al., 2000; Bonora et al., 2000), elevated systolic blood pressure (Adler et al., 2000), hyperglycemia (Stratton et al., 2000) , and renal dysfunction (Bo et al., 2006). On the other hand, not only overt diabetes but also glucose intolerance may contribute to the formation of atherosclerotic plaque, by causing glycation of LDL cholesterol (Raj et al., 2000) and favoring a procoagulant state (Schneider, 2005).

Silent myocardial infarct is relatively frequent in diabetic transplant patients (Carlström et al., 1999). This complication should be suspected whenever symptoms of left ventricular failure appear suddenly. *Cardiomyopathy* may also develop in diabetics with an apparently normal heart and with normal coronarography. *Peripheral obliterative arteriopathy* is frequent. Apart from cardiovascular complications, diabetes may also expose transplant patients to retinopathy, neuropathy, foot ulcers, and infections.

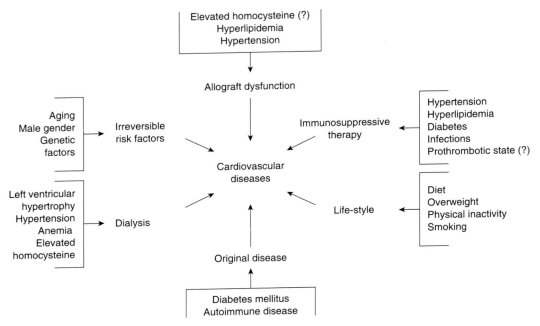

Figure 10.1   Risk factors for cardiovascular disease in transplant patients

Smoking

Cigarette-smoking increases the risk of cardiovascular disease in the general population. Smoking may also have adverse effects on renal function (Ritz *et al.*, 1998). Smoking is nephrotoxic in patients with diabetic and non-diabetic renal disease, and the potential mehanisms of smoking-induced renal damage are an increase in blood pressure and alteration of intrarenal hemodynamics, as well as activation of the sympathetic nervous, renin–angiotensin, and endothelin systems (Orth *et al.*, 2001).

In retrospective observational studies in kidney transplant recipients, cigarette-smoking has been linked to cardiovascular disease (Ponticelli *et al.*, 2002), decreased patient survival, and decreased graft survival (Kasiske and Klinger, 2000). The increase in graft failure was due to an increase in deaths. The magnitude of the negative impact of smoking on decreased patient survival after kidney transplantation is quantitatively similar to that of diabetes (Cosio *et al.*, 1999).

Non-traditional risk factors

Among non-traditional risk factors, *chronic renal insufficiency per se* may be responsible for the atherosclerotic burden (Kennedy *et al.*, 2001; Go *et al.*, 2004). In some patients, previous treatment with *steroids* or *immunosuppressive agents* may also contribute to the high cardiovascular morbidity, but the major role is played by dialysis-related factors (Table 10.1). There is a relationship between *time on dialysis* and posttransplant patient mortality (Meier-Kriesche and Kaplan, 2002; Ponticelli *et al.*, 2002). Increasing time on dialysis increases the risk of left ventricular hypertrophy and cardiomegaly. These relationships are statistically independent of other cardiovascular risk factors (Cosio *et al.*, 1998). *Left ventricular hypertrophy* is the most important cause of cardiovascular morbidity in dialysis patients. A number of factors – including arterial hypertension, chronic volume overload, arteriovenous fistula, and anemia (London, 2003; Locatelli *et al.*, 2005; Agarwall *et al.*, 2006) – may contribute to left ventricular enlargement and hypertrophy. Many dialysis patients suffer from *malnutrition-inflammation*, a condition that is now considered an important contributor to premature atherosclerosis, being interrelated to insulin resistance, oxidative stress, and endothelial

Table 10.1   Traditional and specific risk factors for cardiovascular diseases in uremic patients

Major risk factors in the general population	Specific uremia-related risk factors
Cigarette-smoking	Previous steroid therapy
Hypertension	Reduced renal function
Elevated serum cholesterol	Left ventricular hypertrophy
Elevated LDL cholesterol	Lipoprotein(a)
Low HDL cholesterol	Inflammation-malnutrition
Diabetes mellitus	Vascular calcifications
Advancing age	Hyperhomocysteinemia
Familial history of CVD	Time on dialysis

dysfunction (Stenkivel, 2005). Uremia is typically associated with abnormalities in calcium and phosphorus metabolism. There is evidence that disorders of calcium homeostasis (Goodman et al., 2000; Raggi et al., 2002) together with iatrogenic calcium overload (Derici and El Nahas, 2006) may promote *vascular calcification* and cardiac dysfunction (Rostand, 2000). *Elevated lipoprotein(a)*, which is frequently observed in uremic patients, has been associated with increased cardiovascular risk in end-stage renal disease patients, and the increased oxidative stress of lipids can contribute to atherogenesis (Kendrick, 2001). *Hyperhomocysteinemia* is constant and severe in patients with end-stage renal disease (van Guldener and Robinson, 2000; Hoffer et al., 2001; Bostom et al., 2001). The impact of hyperhomocysteinemia on accelerated atherosclerosis in dialysis patients has been ambiguous, masked by the concomitant malnutrition-inflammation state. However, recent papers clearly document a strong association between hyperhomocysteinemia and cardiovascular morbidity in dialysis patients who do not present with malnutrition-inflammation (Ducloux et al., 2006; Zoccali and Mallamaci, 2006). A *cardiovascular event before transplantation* increases by 2.6-fold the risk of developing post-transplant cardiovascular disease (Ponticelli et al., 2002). Epidemiological studies suggested an association between *antiphospholipid antibodies* (aPL) and atherosclerosis (Sherer and Schoenfeld, 2003). It has been speculated that aPL make atherosclerotic lesions more prone to rupture than in normal atherosclerosis (Frostegard, 2005). There is little information on the atherogenic role of aPL in transplant recipients. However, a study found that the presence of aPL was an independent cardiovascular risk factor in renal transplant patients (Ducloux et al., 2003).

As many uremic patients have clinically silent cardiac disease (Cice et al., 2003; Mohi-ud-din et al., 2005), transplant candidates should be screened for cardiovascular disease, and attempts should be made to modify the potential risk factors before transplantation in order to reduce post-transplant morbidity and mortality (Pascual et al., 2002). Pre-transplant screening, based on risk stratification (standard, moderate, high), may detect pre-existing disease and may identify patients likely to benefit from therapeutic strategies designed to reduce cardiovascular disease prevalence (see Chapter 3).

Risk factors after transplantation

After renal transplantation, hypertension, glucose intolerance, lipid abnormalities, and a proinflammatory state may worsen or develop *de novo* as a result of immunosuppressive therapy and/or graft dysfunction. On the other hand, volume overload, anemia, abnormalities in calcium and phosphate metabolism, and left ventricular hypertrophy may improve. As a consequence, while there is a peak of cardiovascular mortality in the early post-transplant period, the relative risk of death from cardiovascular complications tends to decline over time, when compared with dialysis patients (Meier-Kriesche et al., 2004).

Graft dysfunction

There is growing evidence that renal dysfunction is a powerful independent predictor of fatal and non-fatal cardiovascular events in the general population (Go *et al.*, 2004) and in patients who have suffered a myocardial infarction (Anavekar *et al.*, 2005). Studies in patients with chronic kidney disease suggest that a heightened risk of cardiovascular events becomes evident even with mild renal dysfunction, e.g. with creatinine levels as low as 1.4 mg/dl or creatinine clearance <60 ml/min) (Manjunath *et al.*, 2003; Vanholder *et al.*, 2005). Also in renal transplant recipients it has been demosnstrated that elevated serum creatinine is a major risk factor for cardiovascular events (Ponticelli *et al.*, 2002; Fellstrom *et al.*, 2005; Jardine *et al.*, 2005). Mechanisms by which renal dysfunction increases the cardiovascular risk are not completely elucidated. However, it is likely that the association of graft dysfunction with traditional risk factors – such as arterial hypertension, glucose intolerance, abnormal lipoprotein – and non-traditional factors – such as anemia, oxidative stress, inflammation, hyperhomocysteinemia – may contribute to the development of cardiovascular complications in patients with elevated serum creatinine levels.

Acute rejection

The number of acute rejection episodes has been found to be positively correlated with post-transplantation cardiovascular risk independent of graft function and proteinuria (Fellstrom *et al.*, 2004). It is possible that acute rejection episodes and their treatment, particularly those necessitating high doses of corticosteroids, may contribute to cardiovascular risk by causing endothelial cell damage.

Proteinuria

Patients with late persistent proteinuria have a poor prognosis not only because of reduced graft survival, but also because persistent proteinuria is an independent risk factor for increased cardiovascular morbidity and mortality in renal transplant patients (Roodnat *et al.*, 2001; Fernandez-Fresnedo *et al.*, 2002).

Post-transplant *de novo* diabetes mellitus

After transplantation, pre-existing diabetes may be aggravated or *de novo* diabetes may develop. Understanding of the incidence of post-transplant diabetes is confounded by the lack of consensus on defining diabetes (Cosio *et al.*, 2001a). Some definitions exclude patients with impaired glucose tolerance or with non-insulin-dependent diabetes. Such patients, however, share the same level of risk for long-term microvascular and macrovascular complications as those who have developed insulin-dependent diabetes. At any rate, a number of papers have pointed out that up to 20–25% of patients may develop *de novo* diabetes after transplantation, and about 45% may show abnormal glucose tolerance (Van Duijnhoven *et al.*, 2002; Kasiske *et al.*, 2003; Mathew *et al.*, 2003). Most cases of post-transplant diabetes develop within 1 year of kidney transplantation. However, cases of *de novo* diabetes have been reported even years after transplantation (Paolillo *et al.*, 2001). Post-transplant diabetes may have a deleterious impact on *patient survival*, increasing the risk of death by 1.55–2.54 times (Revanur *et al.*, 2001; Gonzalez-Posada *et al.*, 2004), and *graft survival*. The risk of graft loss was reported to be between 1.68 (Gonzalez-Posada *et al.*, 2004) and 3.7 times (Miles *et al.*, 1998) greater for diabetics, independent of age, sex, and race. Impaired graft function in diabetics was attributed to more severe hypertension, use of lower doses of immunosuppressive agents, and development of diabetic nephropathy.

Risk factors for post-transplant diabetes (Table 10.2)

A number of patients who developed post-transplant diabetes had evidence of glucose intolerance or insulin resistance before transplantation (Pesavento *et al.*, 2003). Hispanics, African-Americans, overweight patients (Kasiske *et al.*, 2003), HCV-positive patients (Fabrizi *et al.*, 2005), and those with a family history of diabetes (Martinez-Castelao *et al.*, 2005) are at higher risk of developing diabetes after transplantation. Incorrect nutrition, overweight, and physical inactivity may favor the development of diabetes after transplantation, but the main factors responsible are corticosteroids and calcineurin inhibitors. The principal mechanisms of

Table 10.2   Risk factors for post-transplant diabetes mellitus

Use of calcineurin inhibitors
Corticosteroid dose and duration
Ethnicity (Afro-American, Hispanic)
Diabetes pre-transplant
Family history of diabetes
Older age
HCV positivity
High body mass index

corticosteroid-induced diabetes are increased insulin resistance (Weir, 2001) and an increase in body weight (Jindal, 1994). There is evidence of a dose–response relationship between steroids and diabetes (Hjelmesaeth *et al*., 2001), the risk being higher in patients with familial predisposition, in Afro-American males, in patients with HLA A30 and BW42 antigens, and in elderly subjects (Sumrani *et al*., 1991). The *calcineurin inhibitors* cyclosporine and tacrolimus both have diabetogenic properties, which can be worsened by the concomitant use of high doses of corticosteroids. Insulin secretion from β-cells is Ca^{2+}-dependent. Normally, glucose enters the β-cell and is transformed into glucose-6-phosphate with consequent activation of glycolysis and generation of ATP. The intracellular increase in ATP favors membrane depolarization and the entrance of extracellular Ca^{2+} ions together with the release of Ca^{2+} from the intracellular deposits. These processes cause the release of insulin from the granules, where it is contained, and its extrusion from the cell. The interference of calcineurin inhibitors with the latter mechanism inhibits insulin production from β-cells (Gillison *et al*., 1991; Drachenberg *et al*., 1999). Tacrolimus has a diabetogenic dose-dependent activity superior to that of cyclosporine (Filler, 2000; Kasiske *et al*., 2003; Martinez-Castelao *et al*., 2005; Wong *et al*., 2005), perhaps because tacrolimus also exerts a direct toxicity on islet cells (Tamura *et al*., 1995).

Prevention of post-transplant diabetes

Transplant candidates, particularly those at increased risk for post-transplant diabetes, should undergo an *oral glucose tolerance test* before transplantation to identify undiagnosed diabetes or impaired glucose tolerance. Doses of *calcineurin inhibitors* and *corticosteroids* should be as low as possible in patients with glucose intolerance in order to minimize the risk of post-transplant diabetes. Such a policy is not easy to realize because of the risk of rejection. However, in a number of patients, corticosteroids can be avoided and calcineurin inhibitors can be minimized (Montagnino et al., 2005; Alexander et al., 2006) without hampering the long-term graft survival. *Diet* and *physical exercise* should be recommended to prevent diabetes. Overweight patients, who are at greater risk for type II diabetes, should be encouraged to lose weight (Marchetti, 2001).

Treatment

In order to prevent atherosclerotic complications, the American Diabetes Association (2003) recommended good glycemic control and aggressive treatment of associated cardiovascular risk factors with more stringent target levels for lipids and blood pressure than those recommended for the general population (Table 10.3). With a multifactorial strategy the risk of cardiovascular disease among patients with type II diabetes could be reduced (Gaede *et al*., 2003; Solomon, 2003). A hypocaloric/hypolipidic diet, light or moderate physical exercise, weight loss, and cessation of smoking should be encouraged. Blood pressure control is also of paramount importance. ACE inhibitors and angiotensin receptor blockers (ARB), either alone or in combination (Taal and Brenner, 2003), may have the advantage of renoprotection. However, these agents often have to be associated with other antihypertensive agents to obtain optimal control of blood pressure.

If there is moderate fasting hyperglycemia (140–230 mg/dl), an oral hypoglycemic agent should be prescribed. The most commonly used agent is *sulfonylurea*, an insulin secretagog. A limit of this agent is

Table 10.3   Target levels of risk factors in patients with diabetes according to recommendations of the American Diabetes Association

Blood pressure below 130/80 mmHg
Low-density lipoprotein cholesterol below 100 mg/dl (2.6 mmol/l)
Triglycerides below 150 mg/dl (1.7 mmol/l)
High-density lipoprotein cholesterol above 40 mg/dl (1.1 mmol/l)
Glycosylated hemoglobin below 7%

represented by the possibility that in the long-term the overstimulated pancreatic β-cells may show a progressive reduction in insulin production. Moreover, recent data indicate that sulfonylurea can increase the risk of cardiovascular disease (Simpson *et al.*, 2006). *Biguanides* inhibit gluconeogenesis and glucose absorption while stimulating glycolysis. The *α-glucose inhibitors* reduce gastrointestinal absorption of carbohydrates. *Metformin* can decrease the risk of cardiovascular disease. Of interest, this protective effect is independent of glycemia (Johnson *et al.*, 2002a). The *thiazolidinediones* decrease plasma insulin levels, improve endothelial function, decrease vascular inflammation, and decrease C-reactive protein levels, effects that are potentially beneficial in patients with heart failure (Fonseca, 2003). Weight gain and peripheral edema are recognized side-effects of these drugs, particularly when used in combination with insulin. The *glinides* stimulate rapid insulin secretion dependent on ambient glucose. These drugs have the advantage of prompt action; however, they have little efficacy in patients with high levels of glycosylated hemoglobin. A combination with insulin sensitizers may be useful and well tolerated in diabetic renal transplant patients (Turk *et al.*, 2006).

When selecting an appropriate oral hypoglycemic agent for transplant recipients with impaired renal function, it is important to take into account the danger of serious adverse effects such as *lactic acidosis* with metformin and severe *hypoglycemia* with sulfonylureas (Harrower, 1996). Among the sulfonylureas, glipizide is less likely to cause hypoglycemia and does not interfere with cyclosporine pharmacokinetics (Sagedal *et al.*, 1998). The majority of patients may be safely treated with the insulin-sensitizer rosiglitazone, with or without sulfonylurea. After the expected 3–6-week delay in the onset of rosiglitazone action, most patients with post-transplant diabetes will no longer require long-term insulin therapy (Villanueva and Baldwin, 2005). However, these agents may further aggravate cardiac conditions when given to diabetic patients with heart failure (Fornarow, 2004).

About 50% of diabetics require *insulin* treatment. The dose and type of insulin should be decided on an individual basis, as insulin requirements depend on the patient's diet, amount of exercise, and renal function. Tapering of corticosteroids also requires an adjustment of insulin dosage. In establishing the treatment, one should recall that the target levels for glucose controls vary greatly among diabetologists. Probably it is safer to obtain acceptable glucose levels rather than insist on 'ideal' lower glucose levels (Table 10.4). In non-expert hands, the latter policy might expose the patient to hypoglycemia, which may be dangerous, and, if frequent, portends a serious and even fatal outcome. For the same reason, attention should be paid to the Somogyi effect and the 'dawn phenomenon'. It is therefore recommended to keep early-morning values of glycemia at over 65 mg/dl.

Arterial hypertension

Arterial hypertension plays a major role in morbidity and mortality associated with cardiovascular disease. A number of papers have reported that about 67–90% of patients become hypertensive after kidney transplantation (Midtvedt and Neumayer, 2000; Schwenger *et al.*, 2001; Miller, 2002). Few studies, however, reported results of continuous ambulatory blood pressure measurements that provide a better assessment of the diurnal variation, a predictor of cardiovascular mortality (Castillo-Lugo and Vergne-Marini, 2005).

Table 10.4 Acceptable blood glucose concentration in a diabetic patient

	mg/dl	mmol/l
Fasting	70–120	3.9–6.66
Preprandial	70–120	3.9–6.66
Postprandial (1–2 h)	<200	<11.1
Early morning (3–4 a.m.)	>65	>3.6

Table 10.5 Potential mechanisms responsible for renal vasoconstriction caused by cyclosporine

Increased production of endothelin-1
Activation of renin–angiotensin system
Reduced production of nitric oxide
Increased production of TGFβ_1
Prostaglandin imbalance
Increased sympathetic activity

Causes of post-transplant hypertension

Cyclosporine may cause renal vasoconstriction through several mechanisms (Bartholomeusz *et al.*, 1998; Koomans and Ligtenberg, 2000; Morales *et al.*, 2001) (Table 10.5). As a consequence, there is a reduction of glomerular filtration rate and of renal blood flow. In turn, these functional abnormalities lead to a retention of salt and water, to an increase in extracellular fluids, and to an increased cardiac output. The apparently normal production of renin by the allograft and by the native kidney is inappropriately elevated in a setting character-ized by extracellular fluid expansion, collaborating with hypertension (Curtis, 1998). *Tacrolimus* also produces clinical post-transplant hypertension via mechanisms similar to those of cyclosporine, although hypertension is less common in patients given tacrolimus than in those receiving cyclosporine (Henry, 1999; Margreiter, 2002).

Corticosteroids can cause hemodynamic modifications, hormonal changes, and further retention of water and salt. Logistic regression analyses showed that corticosteroids are independently associated with post-transplant hypertension (Ponticelli *et al.*, 1993; Ratcliffe *et al.*, 1996). The effect largely depends on the dosage. In fact, a maintenance dose of prednisone of less than l0 mg/day appears to have little if any role in contributing to post-transplant hypertension (Ratcliffe *et al.*, 1996).

There is general agreement that *allograft dysfunction* (Ratcliffe *et al.*, 1996; Curtis, 1997; Cosio *et al.*, 2001b) is strongly associated with arterial hypertension.

The *native kidney* and pre-transplant hypertension have been identified as independent variables asso-ciated with post-transplant hypertension (Ponticelli *et al.*, 1993). It is possible to speculate that the native kidney may still produce renin, which, although normal in absolute terms, might be inappropriately elevated in the presence of an increased extracellular volume (Curtis, 1998).

Allograft artery stenosis accounts for only a minority of cases, 2–10% in the different series (Van Ypersele de Strihou and Pochet, 1992). There are three main locations for graft artery stenosis: (1) at the site of anastomosis, probably as a consequence of the surgical technique; (2) distal from the site of anas-tomosis, the cause of which is still ill-defined; and (3) at the distal arterial branches, where multiple stenoses can be seen, probably as an expression of chronic rejection (Roberts *et al.*, 1989). CMV infection and delayed graft function were risk factors significantly associated with renal transplant artery stenosis in a multivariate analysis (Audard *et al.*, 2006). The diagnosis of graft artery stenosis may be suspected in the presence of severe hypertension, if there is a bruit at the auscultation and/or in the case of a rapid deterioration of renal function after the administration of ACE inhibitors or ARB. Duplex Doppler ultrasonography of the allograft artery (de Morais *et al.*, 2003) is an excellent method for screening patients with transplant artery stenosis. Magnetic resonance imaging can also depict and characterize this complication (Akbar *et al.*, 2005), but the final diagnosis should be made using angiography.

A rare cause of *de novo* hypertension is represented by a *post-biopsy arteriovenous fistula*. The diversion of blood flow from normal renal structures, caused by the abnormal communication between artery and vein, may result in local ischemia and renin-mediated hypertension.

It has also been shown that patients who receive the kidney from a subject of a *hypertensive family* have a higher probability of developing arterial hypertension after transplantation than patients who receive a kidney from a member of a normotensive family (Guidi *et al.*, 1996).

Consequences of post-transplant hypertension

Arterial hypertension is a strong risk factor for *ischemic heart disease* (Kasiske 2002), *congestive heart failure* (Rigatto *et al.*, 2002), *coronary heart disease* (Kendrick, 2001), and *stroke* (Miller, 2002). Angiotensin II, which is often elevated in patients with hypertension, can contribute to atherogenesis by stimulating the growth of smooth muscle cells and lipoxygenase activity which, in turn, can increase inflammation and the oxidation of LDL. Hypertension also has proinflammatory effects on the endothelium, with increased formation of hydrogen peroxide and free radicals in plasma (Ross, 1999). A major consequence of hypertension is *left ventricular hypertrophy*, which is an important risk factor for a variety of cardiovascular sequelae, such as angina pectoris, myocardial infarction, stroke, congestive heart failure, arrhythmias, and sudden death. The mechanisms by which left ventricular hypertrophy is associated with the increased risk of cardiovascular complications are not fully understood (Mosterd *et al.*, 1999), but it must be pointed out that an adequate antihypertensive treatment may obtain regression of left ventricular hypertrophy and reduce the risk of cardiovascular complications (Sharp and Mayet, 2002). Hypertension can also be harmful for the long-term *kidney graft outcome*. A retrospective study showed that increased levels of systolic and diastolic blood pressure after transplantation were significantly associated with an increased risk of graft failure. Hypertension was an independent risk factor for graft failure, even when serum creatinine concentrations were normal and when patients had never been treated for rejection crisis (Opelz *et al.*, 1998).

Treatment (Table 10.6)

As transplant recipients with hypertension are at risk for cardiovascular morbidity and mortality, aggressive means should be used to lower the blood pressure. In this regard, Opelz *et al.* (2005) reviewed the outcome for 24 404 first cadaver transplant recipients and showed that lowering the systolic blood pressure, even after several years of post-transplant hypertension, was associated with improved patient and graft survival. The American Society of Transplantation recommends routine screening for hypertension and maintenance of blood pressure < 140/90 mmHg after renal transplantation (Kasiske *et al.*, 2000a), but the ideal goal should be to lower blood pressure to < 130/85 mmHg, and to 125/75 mmHg in patients with proteinuria (Mailloux and Levey, 1998). Unfortunately, however, as many as 50% of transplant patients have systolic blood pressure > 140 mmHg (Opelz et al., 1998; Kasiske et al., 2004).

Modifying *life-style* is the first measure to be taken for hypertension in renal transplant recipients. Weight control, moderate sodium restriction, low fat intake, physical exercise, and cessation of smoking are strongly recommended. As both calcineurin inhibitors and corticosteroids may cause salt- and water-dependent hypertension, *salt restriction* appears to be a rational therapeutic maneuver. However, too a severe salt restriction, if coupled with diuretic therapy, may cause a drop in glomerular filtration rate because of the impaired capacity of hemodynamic adaption of the transplanted kidney (Schweitzer *et al.*, 1991). Moreover, diuretics may synergize with calcineurin inhibitors in causing hypomagnesemia.

Most patients require the use of antihypertensive agents. The choice depends on the efficacy and tolerance in the individual patient (Table 10.7). Since increased renal vascular resistance is a prominent feature of post-transplant hypertension, drugs that lower the systemic blood pressure and increase the renal

Table 10.6   Potential causes and treatments of post-transplant hypertension

Cause	Treatment
Renal artery stenosis	Revascularization
Post-biopsy arteriovenous fistula	Embolization
Native kidney	Nephrectomy
Calcineurin inhibitors	Reduce the dose
Corticosteroids	Reduce the dose
Graft dysfunction	Antihypertensive agent

Table 10.7   Main antihypertensive agents used in renal transplant recipients

Drugs	Advantages	Side-effects
Calcium channel blockers (CCB)	Reduce arteriolar vasoconstriction Reverse ventricular hypertrophy	Peripheral edema Gastroesophageal reflux Gingival hypertrophy All CCB but nifedipine and felodipine increase cyclosporine blood levels
ACE inhibitors, ARB	Prevent heart failure Prevent intimal thickening Antiproteinuric effect	Small increase in serum creatinine Anemia Oligoanuria in transplant artery stenosis
Beta-blockers	Cardioprotective	Hyperlipidemia Interference with glucose metabolism Hypoglycemia in diabetic patients

blood flow may have a specific indication. At least in theory, *calcium channel blockers* could be the drugs of choice, as they may protect from vasoconstriction caused by calcineurin inhibitors (Rahn *et al.*, 1999). By modulating calcium flux, calcium antagonists may diminish the vascular smooth muscle reactivity to vaso-constrictive stimuli, so reversing the increase in renal vascular resistance induced by calcineurin inhibitors, particularly at the preglomerular level (English *et al.*, 1987). In a randomized, prospective trial, the use of calcium channel blockers in cyclosporine-treated renal recipients resulted in a significantly better allograft function at 2 years, and this effect was independent of blood pressure lowering (Kuypers *et al.*, 2004). Moreover, nifedipine treatment could reverse ventricular hypertrophy in renal transplant recipients (Midtvedt *et al.*, 2001). On the other hand, the management of post-transplant hypertension with these agents may be difficult. Calcium antagonists can cause severe peripheral edema, and, in combination with cyclosporine, may worsen gingival hyperplasia, constipation, or gastroesophageal reflux as a result of smooth-muscle relaxation (Demme, 2001). Non-dihydropyridinic calcium antagonists, such as verapamil and diltiazem, and some dihydropyridinic types such as amlodipine and nicardipine, can increase the blood levels of cyclosporine (Pesavento et al., 1996). Instead, nifedipine and felodipine do not interfere with the metabolism of cyclosporine. It is still a matter of controversy whether the use of dihydropyridinic calcium channel blockers may cause an increased risk of cardiovascular events in high-risk patients (Furberg et al., 1995) as well as in renal transplant recipients (Kasiske et al., 2000b).

Angiotensin-converting enzyme inhibitors (ACEI) and *angiotensin II receptor rblockers* (ARB) are effective in reducing blood pressure in renal transplant patients (Mourad et al., 1993; Burnier and Brunner, 1998; Holgado et al., 2001). ARB are well tolerated and, unlike ACEI, they do not interfere with bradykinin production and therefore cause dry cough less frequently than do ACEI. Both agents may worsen renal function in patients with transplant artery stenosis (Olyaei et al., 1999), and also, rarely, in patients without any evidence of transplant artery or articular stenosis (Curtis et al., 1993). Moreover, ACEI and ARB may cause hyperkalemia (Formica et al., 2006) and may induce anemia (Curtis, 1997). On the other hand, this class of drugs has demonstrated a number of effects that may be of benefit to transplant recipients (Stigant et al., 2000). ACEI reduce mortality following myocardial infarction, improve symptoms, and prolong the survival of patients with heart failure (Elliott, 1998; Yusuf et al., 2000). ARB and ACEI may also prevent heart failure in patients with left ventricular dysfunction, and may favor the regression of left ventricular hypertrophy (Suwelack et al., 2000; Hernandez et al., 2000; Midtvedt et al., 2001). ACE inhibitors in renal transplant recipients have also been shown to prevent an increase in the thickening of the intima–media complex of the carotid artery, as measured by ultrasound, suggesting a role in the prevention of atherosclerosis (Cieciura et al., 2000). An additional benefit of these agents is their antiproteinuric effect (Hausberg et al., 1999). Whether ACE inhibitors may also prevent chronic allograft failure (Danovitch, 2001) is still unproven.

Other antihypertensive agents can be useful in reducing the post-transplant cardiovascular risk. *Beta-blockers* may be cardioprotective, and should be considered as first-line therapy for post-transplant hypertension in patients with concomitant coronary heart disease. However, these agents may contribute to adverse effects on lipids (Elliott, 1998) and glucose metabolism (Gress et al., 2000). *Loop diuretics* can help to treat hyperkalemia and hypercalcemia, while *distal tubule diuretics* can help to combat bone disease by minimizing urinary calcium loss (Demme, 2001). However, diuretics can also contribute to adverse effects on lipids and may have other adverse metabolic effects, such as hyperuricemia.

Centrally acting drugs and *α-adrenergic receptor blockers* may be used either alone or in various combinations. In many cases, several drugs have to be used simultaneously to achieve good control of post-transplant hypertension. In the most severe cases, the powerful vasodilator *minoxidil* has to be added to control refractory hypertension.

Whenever possible, reduction of cyclosporine, tacrolimus, or corticosteroids should be taken into account if other measures are ineffective. *Bilateral nephrectomy* should be reserved primarily for patients with a history of severe hypertension before transplantation and for patients with refractory hypertension (Fricke et al., 1998). In proven *transplant artery stenosis*, percutaneous transluminal angioplasty (PTA) or surgery is indicated if stenosis narrows the artery by more than 80% (Rao, 1998; Olyaei et al., 1999). In most cases, PTA represents the first approach (Figure 10.2). Percutaneous transluminal angioplasty with or without stents has been used successfully, with reduction of blood pressure and improvement of graft function (Beecroft et al., 2004). Because of the risk of graft loss associated with surgical intervention, surgery should be considered a second option in patients in whom PTA or stenting has failed. However, successful surgery significantly reduces the risk of restenosis in comparison with PTA (Voiculescu et al., 2005). Embolization may repair an arteriovenous fistula, with improvement of hypertension (Figure 10.3).

Hyperlipidemia

The prevalence of lipid abnormalities in renal transplant recipients has been reported to range from about 40–60% in patients treated with cyclosporine or tacrolimus (Satterthwaite et al., 1998) up to 80% in those given sirolimus (Chueh and Kahan, 2003). There is a significant elevation in total cholesterol levels, due to elevations in LDL cholesterol, but significant increases in very-low-density lipoprotein (VLDL)

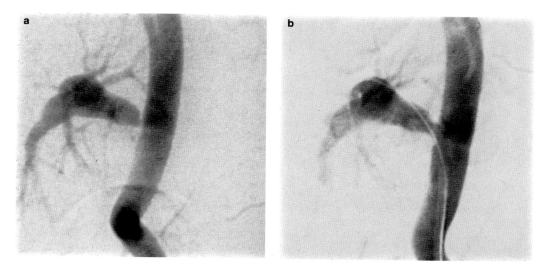

Figure 10.2 (a) Transplant artery stenosis at the beginning of the artery, (b) Correction of stenosis by PTA. (Courtesy of Dr A Nicolini, Ospedale Magglore, Milan.)

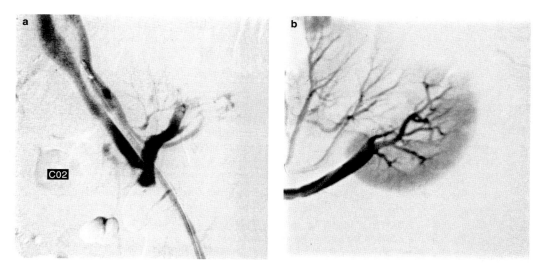

Figure 10.3 (a) Postbiopsy arteriovenous fistula in a transplanted kidney (angiography with CO_2 technique). (b) Correction of fistula by embolization. (Courtesy of Dr Nicolini, Ospedale Maggiore, Milan.)

cholesterol and VLDL triglycerides are also common, and are more severe with sirolimus or everolimus than with cyclosporine and with cyclosporine than with tacrolimus. In addition to elevations in tryglycerides and total cholesterol and its subfractions, elevated apolipoprotein B and lipoprotein(a) and increased LDL oxidation have been reported (Bosmans et al., 2001). Changes in HDL cholesterol post-transplantation are more variable. No significant changes in HDL cholesterol levels have been reported. The more atheroprotective HDL subfractions, HDL2 and HDL3, are significantly decreased in transplant recipients (Kobashigawa and Kasiske, 1997). Changes in lipids are typically observed during the first 3–6 months after transplantation, and persist even 10 or more years post-transplantation (Fellstrom et al., 2004).

Table 10.8   Possible causes of post-transplant hyperlipidemia

Unmodifiable factors	Life-style	Allograft complications	Drugs
Genetic predisposition	Obesity	Graft dysfunction	Corticosteroids
Age	Diet	Proteinuria	Calcineurin inhibitors (cyclosporine, tacrolimus)
	Physical activity	Diabetes	mTOR antagonists (sirolimus, everolimus)
			Beta-blockers
			Diuretics

Etiopathogenesis

A number of factors may contribute to lipid abnormalities (Table 10.8). Among other factors, immunosuppressive drugs such as corticosteroids, calcineurin inhibitors, and anti-mTOR (mammalian target of rapamycin) agents are heavily implicated in the development of hyperlipidemia, usually in a dose-dependent fashion. *Corticosteroids* may enhance the activity of acetyl coenzyme A carboxylase and free fatty acid synthetase, may increase the hepatic synthesis of VLDL, may downregulate LDL receptor activity of 3-hydroxy-3-methylglutaryl coenzyme A (HMG-CoA) reductase, and may inhibit lipoprotein lipase (Kobashigawa and Kasiske, 1997). The final result is increased levels of VLDL, total cholesterol, and triglycerides and decreased levels of high-density lipoproteins. *Cyclosporine* may inhibit the enzyme 26-hydroxylase, so decreasing the synthesis of bile acids from cholesterol and the transport of cholesterol to the intestines. Cyclosporine also binds to the LDL receptor, which results in increased serum levels of LDL cholesterol, and impairs the clearance of VLDL and LDL by decreasing lipoprotein lipase activity (Kobashigawa and Kasiske, 1997). Moreover, cyclosporine causes significant alterations in the susceptibility of LDL to oxidation, and may directly or indirectly cause the elevation of homocysteine levels (Fellstrom *et al.*, 2004). Of note, hypercholesterolemia is significantly less frequent in transplant patients given *tacrolimus* than in those treated with cyclosporine (Johnson *et al.*, 2000; Artz *et al.*, 2003). *Sirolimus* and *everolimus* almost regularly increase serum cholesterol and triglyceride levels. The changes in blood lipids are related to trough levels and persist over time (Chueh and Kahan, 2003). The mechanisms for hyperlipidemia caused by these anti-mTOR agents rely probably on the alteration of the insulin signaling pathway, which may cause an increase of adipose tissue lipase activity, a decrease of lipoprotein lipase activity, and increased hepatic synthesis of triglyceride (Morrissett *et al.*, 2003). Little is known about the influence of sirolimus on the oxidative modification of LDL or on blood homocysteine levels. Of interest, the anti-mTOR agents may inhibit vascular endothelial proliferation, probably through their interference with p70 S6 kinase, an essential step for endothelial cell cycle progression in response to stimuli (Vinals *et al.*, 1999). Whether these latter characteristics may result in a better atherosclerotic profile in renal transplant recipients is still unknown.

Clinical consequences

A large number of epidemiologic studies have documented the relationship between elevated total cholesterol, triglycerides, LDL, and the development of cardiovascular disease. Low levels of HDL are also associated with an increased cardiovascular risk. The oxidative metabolism of LDL appears to be the final common pathway in the relationship between hyperlipidemia and the development of atherosclerosis (Griendling and Alexander, 1997). An *atherogenic role* for lipid disturbances has also been recognized in transplant patients (Abdulmassih *et al.*, 1992; Kasiske, 2001). A number of studies reported an association between hyperlipidemia and *chronic renal allograft rejection* (Dimèny *et al.*, 1993; Isoniemi *et al.*,

Table 10.9 Main general approaches for treating post-transplant hyperlipidemia

General measures
Physical exercise
Low calorie intake

Hypertriglyceridemia
Avoid alcohol and simple sugars. Limit fat intake
Use fibrates or fish oil
Reduce corticosteroids or cyclosporine

Hypercholesterolemia
Avoid saturated fats (milk, cheese, butter, chocolate, shellfish, fatty meat)
Use polyunsaturated fats (corn oil, safflower oil)
Use statins or bile acid sequestrants
Reduce corticosteroids or cyclosporine

1994; Massy and Kasiske, 1996; Wissing *et al.*, 2000; Stephan *et al.*, 2002), suggesting that lipoprotein abnormalities may influence the progression of chronic renal allograft nephropathy. However, the association between chronic renal allograft rejection and hyperlipidemia may be the consequence rather than the cause of renal failure. In fact, renal dysfunction, proteinuria, and the additional immunosuppression often used in patients with chronic allograft nephropathy may explain the association with hyperlipidemia without necessarily implicating lipid abnormalities in the pathogenesis of chronic rejection.

Treatment

As hyperlipidemia occurs early in most renal transplant patients, the clinical assessment and treatment of hyperlipidemia should be initiated soon after transplantation (Andany and Kasiske, 2001). Potential strategies include changes in the life-style, reduced doses of immunosuppressive agents, and lipid-lowering agents (Table 10.9).

General measures include physical activity and diet. Regular physical activity should be recommended to transplant recipients. Patients with hypertriglyceridemia should be placed on a hypocaloric diet that restricts the intake of simple sugars and alcohol, in addition to limiting fat intake to less than 30% of total daily calories. This diet may obtain weight loss and resolution or improvement of hypertriglyceridemia. Dietary modification is also the safest form of treatment for elevated LDL cholesterol. Patients should be placed on a hypocaloric diet, low in cholesterol and in saturated fats but high in polyunsaturated fats. A similar diet given for 10–12 weeks obtained a 10% reduction of plasma LDL cholesterol levels (Barbagallo *et al.*, 1999). Unfortunately, many hyperlipidemic renal transplant recipients show poor compliance to the diet in the long term, and it has been suggested that dietary modification might be largely ineffective in renal transplant recipients because impaired renal function contributes strongly to hyperlipidemia in these patients (Tonstad *et al.*, 1995).

Tailoring of the immunosuppressive regimen may be considered, including a switch to agents with less propensity for causing hyperlipidemia. As corticosteroids can worsen lipid profiles, avoiding or reducing the dose of corticosteroids can help in minimizing hyperlipidemia. Randomized, controlled studies reported that renal transplant patients receiving steroid-free immunosuppression had a lower risk of hyperlipidemia (Montagnino *et al.*, 2005; Pascual *et al.*, 2005; Rostaing *et al.*, 2005) and of cardiovascular complications (Ponticelli *et al.*, 1997; Montagnino *et al.*, 2001) than patients given steroids. If steroid-free immunosuppression is considered unsafe in a particular patient, prednisone may be replaced by less

Table 10.10   Initiation of treatment and goal levels according to National Cholesterol Education Program (NCEP) guidelines. Risk factors are age (>45 years in men; >55 years in women); family history of premature coronary heart disease; smoking; hypertension; diabetes mellitus; HDL cholesterol <35 mg/dl (0.91 mmol/l)

LDL cholesterol		
Treatment initiation level (mg/dl (mmol/l))	**Goal level (mg/dl (mmol/l))**	**Concomitant risk factors**
≥190 (≥4.9)	≤160 (≤4.1)	Absent
≥160 (≥4.1)	≤130 (≤3.4)	Two or more

hyperlipidemic corticosteroids. Deflazacort, an oxazoline derivative of prednisone, induces less hyperglycemia and hyperlipidemia than the glucocorticoids commonly used (Ferraris *et al.*, 2000). Conversion from cyclosporine to tacrolimus can also lower cholesterol, LDL, and apolipoprotein B (McCune *et al.*, 1998; Artz *et al.*, 2003).

Hypolipidemic drugs may be considered when LDL cholesterol exceeds 190 mg/dl, or even at lower levels if there are other risk factors (Table 10.10). The HMG-CoA reductase inhibitors (or statins) have almost completely replaced older and less effective drugs such as bile acid sequestrants, and nicotinic acid. The *statins* (lovastatin, pravastatin, simvastatin, fluvastatin, atorvastatin, rosuvastatin) may reduce LDL cholesterol concentrations by roughly 35–40% at optimal dosage. This reduction of LDL cholesterol is accompanied by an increase in HDL cholesterol concentration of about 10% and, frequently, by a slight decrease in triglyceride concentration (Arnadottir and Berg, 1997). Since the rate of endogenous cholesterol synthesis is higher at night, statins should be given at night. Simvastatin and pravastatin should be taken on an empty stomach or at bedtime, as food decreases their absorption (Knopp, 1999), while atorvastatin may be taken at any time in a single daily administration. A retrospective study showed that renal transplant patients treated with statins had a 24% better survival than those who did not receive these drugs (Cosio *et al.*, 2002). In a randomized controlled trial, 2102 renal transplant patients were assigned to fluvastatin or placebo. A reduction of 32% in LDL cholesterol was observed in the fluvastatin arm. Although no significant reduction in coronary intervention procedures or general mortality was seen, there were significantly fewer cardiac deaths and non-fatal myocardial infarcts in patients assigned to fluvastatin (Holdaas *et al.*, 2003).

Statins are generally well tolerated, but *myopathy* and *rhabdomyolysis* may occur, particularly in elderly patients and in those with renal, hepatic, and thyroid dysfunction and hypertriglyceridemia (Table 10.11). New findings suggest that exercise, Asian race, and perioperative status may also increase the risk of statin muscle toxicity (Antons *et al.*, 2006). The risk of myopathy and rhabdomyolysis can also be potentiated by drugs metabolized by the P450 enzyme system (Clark, 2003), such as cyclosporine, tacrolimus, and sirolimus. Adjusting the statin dosage, avoiding inappropriately high concentrations of calcineurin inhibitors and anti-mTOR agents, avoiding medications known to increase the risk of myopathy (gemfibrozil, nicotinic acid), and performing regular check-ups of creatinine kinase concentrations allow safe treatment of renal transplant recipients with different statins. As statins and calcineurin inhibitors are both metabolized by the P450 cytochrome enzymatic system, bilateral *pharmacokinetic interactions* are likely to occur. However, the relevance of these interactions has been differently estimated. In combination with cyclosporine (CsA), the area under the curve (AUC) of fluvastatin increased two-fold, and CsA doses needed to be reduced, in one study (Schrama *et al.*, 1998), while no difference in the AUC of CsA was seen in another study (Goldberg and Roth,

Table 10.11   Cholesterol-lowering drugs

Drug(s)	Suggested dose	Side-effects
HMG-CoA reductase inhibitors		
Fluvastatin	20–40 mg/day	Rhabdomyolysis
Lovastatin	10–20 mg/day	Myopathy
Pravastatin	10–20 mg/day	Increase of transaminases
Simvastatin	10–20 mg/day	Interference with cyclosporine metabolism
Bile acid resin		
Cholestiramine	4–6 g/day	Flatulence, constipation, hypersensivity, interaction with fat-soluble drugs
Colestipol	5–15 g/day (space dose by 2 h with interacting drugs)	
Nicotinic acid	250–500 mg/day	Flushing, gastrointestinal disturbance, glucose intolerance, gout, liver damage; cyclosporine and steroids may exacerbate side-effects

1996). The AUC may increase by three-fold for simvastatin when administered together with CsA (Arnadottir and Hultberg, 1997), but no difference in CsA blood levels was seen in a randomized trial between transplant patients given or not given simvastatin (Lepre *et al.*, 1999). Some authors reported a ten-fold increase of the AUC also for pravastatin (Schrama *et al.*, 1998); others, however, did not find any interference of cyclosporine with the AUC of pravastatin (Knopp, 1999). Also for atorvastatin, the AUC of CsA was reported to be elevated in some studies but not in others (Asberg, 2003). At any rate, to prevent any possible side-effects, the dose of statin should not exceed 10–20 mg/day for lovastatin, simvastatin, atorvastatin, and pravastatin, and 20–40 mg/day for fluvastatin (Goldberg and Roth, 1996; Malyszko *et al.*, 2002).

Statins can also have other *protective effects* on cardiovascular disease and allograft dysfunction. These agents may inhibit smooth muscle proliferation, may improve endothelial cell function, and may reduce thrombogenicity (Fellstrom *et al.*, 2004). In two controlled trials, kidney transplant patients randomly allocated to pravastatin had a lower incidence of acute rejection and needed fewer courses of OKT3 and methylprednisolone pulses than patients not receiving pravastatin (Katznelson *et al.*, 1996; Kasiske *et al.*, 2001). The introduction of therapy with HMG-CoA reduction inhibitors early after cardiac transplantation significantly decreased the frequency of coronary artery disease compared with its introduction more than 3 years after transplantation (Kato *et al.*, 2000).

Ezetimide, a novel cholesterol absorption inhibitor usually given at a dose of 10 mg per day, could significantly reduce hypercholesterolemia and hypertriglyceridemia in renal transplant recipients already given maximal doses of statins. The drug was well tolerated by most patients, without changes in renal function (Kohnle *et al.*, 2006). Large interpatient variability of measurable immunosuppressant levels was seen, but no serious adverse events were attributed to a change in levels (Langone and Chuang, 2006). The possibility of combining statins that inhibit cholesterol synthesis with ezetimide that inhibits cholesterol absorption may help in normalizing serum cholesterol and LDL levels.

The *fibrates* (clofibrate, bezafibrate, fenofibrate, ciprofibrate, and gemfibrozil) induce a reduction in hepatic VLDL synthesis and an increase in lipoprotein lipase activity, thereby causing a reduction in triglyceride concentration and an increase in HDL cholesterol concentration. Plasma LDL cholesterol concentration falls as well, but not as markedly as with statin treatment. Thus, fibrates may be indicated in patients with hypertriglyceridemia, but not in those with hypercholesterolemia. Fibrates may cause myopathy and rhabdomyolysis. These side-effects are dose-dependent, and are more frequent in patients with renal insufficiency or in those given statins. A number of patients may also show a mild, reversible increase in plasma creatinine levels during treatment with fenofibrate, bezafibrate, and ciprofibrate but not with gemfibrozil (Broeders et al., 2000). Probably there is little interaction between fibrates and CsA (Asberg, 2003), but, to be on the safe side, in transplant patients we prefer not to exceed a daily dose of 900 mg for gemfibrozil, 400 mg for bezafibrate, or 200 mg for fenofibrate.

Fish oil may result in a decrease in serum triglyceride levels by reducing hepatic triglyceride production. Fish oil may also have beneficial effects on platelet aggregation, blood pressure, and graft function. It can be used for cases of isolated hypertriglyceridemia or as a complement to a statin in the case of combined hyperlipidemia. In patients given the old formulation of CsA (van der Heide et al., 1993), fish oil can increase blood levels of CsA, but this effect has been reported to be smaller with Neoral® (Asberg, 2003).

Other classes of lipid-lowering drugs are now used less frequently. The *bile sequestrants* cholestyramine and colestipol bind with bile acid, interrupt bile acid recirculation, and increase hepatic bile acid synthesis and LDL receptor activity (Grundy, 1994). These agents are effective in lowering cholesterol when administered at adequate doses, but adequate doses are difficult to achieve due to frequent gastrointestinal side-effects. Although these agents may interfere with the absorption of lipid-soluble drugs, with a consequent decreased CsA concentration, such an effect was not found in a study in renal transplant patients (Jensen et al., 1995). At any rate, drugs should be taken 2 hours before or 4–6 hours (minimum 2 hours) after the ingestion of cholestiramine or colestipol. *Nicotinic acid* reduces LDL, increases HDL cholesterol levels, and reduces triglyceride levels (Grundy, 1994). This drug may have many adverse effects which limit its clinical use. They include flushing, gastrointestinal disturbances, altered glucose tolerance, and increased incidence of gout in cyclosporine-treated patients.

In summary, hyperlipidemia is common after transplantation. Hyperlipidemia may be prevented by an appropriate diet and by reducing the dose of corticosteroids, cyclosporine, and sirolimus, whenever possible. Besides weight reduction and a low-fat diet, a low dose of HMG-CoA reductase inhibitor appears to be the first-line treatment for reducing LDL cholesterol levels. Ezetimide may be added in patients with more severe hypercholesterolemia. If predominant hypertriglyceridemia is present, low calorie intake, low-fat diet, and, in some cases, fish oil may help to reduce trglyceride levels. Gemfibrozil may also lower triglyceride levels, but the dose should be reduced in patients with decreased renal function.

Hyperhomocysteinemia

Homocysteine is a sulfur-containing amino acid that results from the demethylation of methionine. The degradation pathways of homocysteine are mediated by either remethylation to methionine or cystathionine formation (Figure 10.4). Homocysteine may damage vascular endothelial cells, is prothrombotic, increases collagen production, and decreases the availability of nitric oxide (Ross, 1999; Abdelfatah et al., 2002; Perna et al., 2003). In the general population, observational studies have shown a link between increased levels of plasma homocysteine and cardiovascular disease (Pasceri and Willerson, 1999; Clarke et al., 2003). Elevated levels of homocysteine, two- to four-fold above normal, are common in renal transplant recipients (Suliman et al., 2000; Ducloux et al., 2001; Friedman et al., 2002).

Etiology

The main determinant of homocysteine levels in renal transplant recipients seems to be renal function, and only to a lesser degree vitamin status (Bostom, 2000; Stein et al., 2001). Several investigators have demonstrated a relationship between cyclosporine treatment and homocysteine levels, including a relationship between cyclosporine dose or blood concentrations and homocysteine levels (Arnadottir et al., 1998; Cole

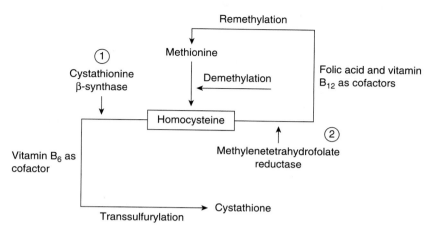

Figure 10.4 Homocysteine metabolism. Homocysteine is formed by demethylation of the essential amino acid methionine. Two enzymes are particularly important: (1) cystathionine β-synthase converts homocysteine to cystathione using vitamin B_6 as cofactor via transsulfurylation. (2) Methylenetetrahydrofolate reductase remethylates homocysteine to methionine using folic acid and vitamin B_{12} as cofactors via remethylation

et al., 1998), but there are also studies where such relationships have not been shown (Forsyte, 2001). In one study, no difference in homocysteine levels was seen between patients treated with cyclosporine or tacrolimus (Fernandez-Miranda et al., 2000).

The total homocysteine plasma level of an individual is influenced by genetic factors, and many polymorphisms have been identified (Sunder-Plassmann and Fodinger, 2003). There is a variant of the gene encoding methylenetetrahydrofolate reductase (MTHFR) involved in the enzymatic remethylation and therefore elimination of homocysteine. This variant, consisting of a cytosine (C) to thymidine (T) transition at nucleotide position 677 (C677T variant), leading to the exchange of a highly conserved alanine to valine in the mature protein, has been associated with reduced activity and increased thermolability of this enzyme in lymphocyte extracts. This mutation lowers the levels of the active form of folate and increases total plasma homocysteine both in subjects with normal kidney function and in renal transplant patients (Födinger et al., 1999).

Clinical consequences

Whether hyperhomocysteinemia in renal transplant recipients is an innocent marker of renal dysfunction or an important risk factor for atherosclerosis is still discussed. Retrospective studies concluded that plasma levels of homocysteine are correlated neither with patient nor with graft survival (Dimény et al., 1998; Hagen et al., 2001), while other investigators reported that hyperhomocysteinemia represents an independent variable associated with cardiovascular events (Ducloux et al., 2000).

Treatment

Because plasma folate and vitamin B_{12} levels are inversely related to fasting plasma total homocysteine levels, whereas plasma vitamin B_6 levels are inversely associated with a post-methionine-loading increase in plasma total homocysteine levels, supplementation with these vitamins might theoretically improve the homocysteine metabolism (Massy, 2003). In renal transplant recipients with mild hyperhomocysteinemia, high-dose folic acid (Arnadottir and Hultberg, 1997) or a combination of folic acid (5.0 mg/day), vitamin B_6 (50 mg/day), and vitamin B_{12} (0.4 mg/day), given for 6 weeks, could reduce fasting and post-methionine-loading total homocysteine levels by at least 25%, with 75% of patients achieving normalization of their total homocysteine levels (Sunder-Plassmann et al., 2000; Bostom et al., 2001). A similar supplementation with vitamins and folic acid for 6 months significantly reduced the mean carotid intimal thickness in 28 hyperhomocysteinemic renal transplant recipients, while untreated controls showed a significant increase of carotid intimal thickness (Marcucci et al., 2003). On the other hand, in three large randomized trials that investigated the effects of homocysteine-lowering therapy with vitamin B_6, vitamin B_{12}, and folic acid in non-transplanted subjects with known cardiovascular disease, no difference in cardiovascular events could be seen after a reduction in homocysteine concentration (Toole et al., 2004; Lann et al., 2006; Bona et al., 2006). Possible explanations for failure are: (1) folic acid may promote cell proliferation, thus favoring the formation of atherosclerotic plaque, (2) folic acid and vitamin B_{12} increase the methylation potential, which plays a role in atherogenesis, and (3) folic acid and vitamin B_{12} favor the methylation of L-arginine to asymmetric dimethyl-arginine, which inhibits the activity of nitric oxide synthase and is associated with an increased risk of vascular disease (Loscalzo, 2006). It now appears clear that treatment with folic acid, vitamin B_6, and vitamin B_{12} does not provide benefit, and is not the therapeutic solution for preventing cardiovascular disease.

Systemic inflammation and prothrombotic state

Atherosclerosis is now recognized as a chronic inflammatory disease (Ross, 1999; Libby et al., 2002). The potential mechanisms arise from the immune and inflammatory response to oxidative stress and/or infection. Chlamydia pneumoniae, Helicobacter pylori, and cytomegalovirus (Bruggeman et al., 1999; Humar et al., 2000) have been identified in atherosclerotic plaques. It is likely that an immune response mounted against antigens of pathogenic organisms cross-reacts with homologous host proteins, such as heat-shock proteins or stress-induced proteins (Lamb et al., 2003). Both innate and acquired immunity have been shown to be involved in the atherogenesis. Innate immunity contributes with phagocytic leukocytes, complement, and cytokines. Adaptive immunity modulates the progression with its T cells, antibodies, and immunoregulatory cytokines (Hansson et al., 2002). The consequent inflammation may alter the plaque stability. Unstable plaques have increased leukocyte infiltrates in them, and T cells and macrophages predominate at the rupture sites. As inflammatory stimuli are frequent in transplant patients, it is reasonable to think that they may strongly contribute to accelerated atherosclerosis.

A number of systemic inflammatory markers, such as C-reactive protein, fibrinogen, and CD40 ligand (CD40L) cytokine have been correlated with cardiovascular disease events. The C-reactive protein (CRP) level is an acute-phase reactant that increases markedly during an inflammatory response. A new use for this old test (high-sensitivity CRP) has gained momentum in recent years as a result of observations that even minor elevations of CRP are predictive of cardiovascular events (Ridker et al., 2002). C-reactive protein not only may be a marker of low-grade chronic systemic inflammation, but also may be a strong independent predictor of future myocardial infarction and stroke among apparently healthy subjects (Ridker, 2001). An association between elevated levels of CRP and cardiac events has been found in renal transplant recipients (Ducloux et al., 2005). Recent experimental studies showed that CRP is not only a reliable marker of inflammation and a good predictor of cardiovascular events, but might also be responsible for vascular damage. By binding to ligands exposed in damaged tissue and then activating complement, human CRP increases myocardial and cerebral infarct in rats exposed to ligation of coronary or cerebral arteries. The administration of an inhibitor of CRP may abrogate the increase in infarct size produced by CRP, opening new therapeutic possibilities (Pepys et al., 2006).

CD40 ligand (CD40L) is a trimeric, transmembrane protein of the tumor necrosis factor family, and, together with its receptor, CD40 is an important contributor to the inflammatory processes that lead to atherosclerosis, plaque destabilization, and thrombosis. Whether elevated serum levels of CD40L are associated with an increased risk of coronary events or ischemic stroke is still uncertain (Varo et al., 2003; Tanne et al., 2006). Other inflammatory markers such as pregnancy-associated plasma protein and osteoprotegerin have been found to be strong predictors of cardiovascular events in renal transplant recipients (Lauzurica et al., 2005; Hjelmesaeth et al., 2006).

Elevated plasma levels of coagulation factors such as fibrinogen, factor VII, and von Willebrand factor are associated with an increased risk of acute stroke and coronary artery disease in the general population (Frishman, 1998). These factors are elevated in renal transplant patients, and were found to be higher in those who had cardiovascular events than in those who had not (Irish and Green, 1997). Impaired fibrinolysis, with an increased risk of thrombosis and atherosclerosis, may also occur in renal transplant patients as a consequence of the elevated plasminogen activator inhibitor levels. Steroid-free immunoosuppression may restore better fibrinolytic capacity (Sartori *et al.*, 2003). Cyclosporine, tacrolimus, and sirolimus may significantly enhance platelet aggregation and secretion in response to physiological agonists (Babinska *et al.*, 1998). All these abnormalities might realize a *prothrombotic state* in renal transplant recipients that may contribute to atherogenesis, cardiovascular complications, and the development of chronic allograft nephropathy.

Treatment

Low-dose aspirin is the most widely used medication to prevent cardiovascular disease. It has had a greater effect on patients with cardiovascular disease than any other drug. Aspirin may exert multiple actions, but probably its preventive role in atherosclerotic events lies mainly on the inhibition of platelet aggregation. In the general population there is agreement that aspirin should be recommended to diabetics and in subjects at cardiovascular risk, although in people with platelet non-responsiveness aspirin is unable to prevent cardiovascular complications (Makaryus, 2006). Unless there are clinical contraindications, low-dose aspirin may be recommended in renal transplant recipients, particularly when presenting cardiovascular risk factors.

Statins can not only reduce serum cholesterol levels but also have additional effects on the process of atherosclerosis. These agents can inhibit the production of additional mevalanate products such as isoprenoids, which influence cell proliferation processes (Maron *et al.*, 2000); can activate endothelial NO synthase (Laufs *et al.*, 1998); can have beneficial effects on the vasculature independent of cholesterol lowering (O'Driscoll *et al.*, 1997); can reduce serum C-reactive protein (Jialal *et al.*, 2001); can act on the coagulation system (Rosenson *et al.*, 1998); and can reduce the expression of CD40–CD40L in endothelial cells (Schonbeck *et al.*, 2002; Alber *et al.*, 2006).

Chronic ACE inhibition has beneficial effects on fibrinolysis, coagulation, inflammatory processes (Schieffer *et al.*, 2000), coronary endothelial vasodilator dysfunction, and myocardial blood flow (Schächinger and Zeiher, 2002). Like ACE inhibitors, angiotensin II receptor blockers are also able to improve endothelial dysfunction, and decrease stroke in hypertensive patients and cardiovascular events in hypertensive diabetes (Dahlof *et al.*, 2002; Lindholm *et al.*, 2002).

Oxidative stress

Prior to the development of atherosclerotic plaques, endothelial vasodilator function is impaired early in the process of atherogenesis. The endothelium not only is a layered single-cell mechanical barrier between the blood and the vessel wall, but also regulates various important functions of the vasculature, such as vasomotion and, therefore, blood flow regulation, as well as hemostasis and wall proliferation processes (Schächinger and Zeiher, 2002). To control vasomotor tone, the endothelium releases a variety of substances, such as prostacyclin, hyperpolarizing factor, endothelin, and, most important, nitric oxide (Fleming and Busse, 1999).

A balance between the levels of superoxide and the release of nitric oxide has a critical role in the maintenance of normal endothelial function (Higashi *et al.*, 2002). An imbalance leads to vasoconstriction and vascular injury. Many factors are reported to be responsible for stimulating the production of superoxide or for reducing the production of nitric oxide: hypertension (McIntyre *et al.*, 1999), hypercholesterolemia and smoking (Schächinger and Zeiher, 2002), renovascular hypertension (Higashi *et al.*, 2002), diabetes (Sowers, 2002), and anemia (Campise *et al.*, 2003). Most renal transplant recipients with stable graft function show a pattern of *oxidative stress* which is counterbalanced by an enhancement of antioxidant mechanisms (Campise *et al.*, 2003). In the long term, however, the antioxidant capacity may tend to run low, hence exposing the patient to the damage of oxidant stress. In this regard, it should be remembered that there is an association between the oxidation of lipids and atherosclerosis, and that oxidized lipoproteins are more common in renal transplant recipients than in the general population (Varghese *et al.*, 1999; Kasiske, 2002). Unfortunately, as pointed out above, large randomized trials failed to show any protective effect of antioxidative vitamins, probably because, in the presence of oxidative stress, the radical α-tocopherol produces further radicals which might result in enhanced, rather than reduced, oxidative stress within the vessel wall (Carr *et al.*, 2000).

Anemia

Anemia, which is frequent after kidney transplantation (Vanrenterghem et al., 2003), is an independent risk factor for cardiac events in renal transplant recipients, probably by causing left ventricular hypertrophy coupled with an inadequate oxygen supply (Rigatto et al., 2002). On the other hand, as red blood cells represent a paramount antioxidant system, anemia may also lead to the depletion of glutathione-mediated antioxidant mechanisms with consequent prevalence of oxidative atherogenic factors (Campise et al., 2003). In a retrospective study, it was found that the percentage of hypochromic cells was an independent risk factor for mortality in kidney transplant recipients (Winkelmayer et al., 2004).

Obesity

There are a number of transplant patients who are already obese before transplantation, and other patients become obese after transplantation. In one study, only 9% of transplant recipients were obese before transplant, but there were 30% transplant recipients who were obese 7 years after receiving a renal transplantation (Armstrong et al., 2005). Obesity is often associated with lipoprotein abnormalities, elevated concentrations of plasminogen activator inhibitor-1, insulin resistance, increased left ventricular mass, left ventricular wall thickness, and left ventricular cavity size (Abate, 1999). These abnormalities may account for a close relationship between the excessive accumulation of body fat and premature cardiovascular morbidity and mortality (Yan et al., 2006).

In obese transplant patients (body mass index greater than 30), a number of investigators have reported lower patient and graft survival (Halme et al., 1997; Pischon and Sharma, 2001; De Mattos et al., 2003) when compared with non-obese patients. Others, however, did not find different patient and graft survival rates, although obese recipients more frequently developed diabetes (Johnson et al., 2002b; Howard et al., 2002; Armstrong et al., 2005). Nevertheless, cardiovascular events represent the leading cause of death in obese transplant recipients (Pischon and Sharma, 2001). The high incidence of post-transplant diabetes may contribute to the elevated cardiovascular risk in this population. To reduce the risk for morbidity after transplantation, a thorough evaluation of the cardiovascular state and appropriate dietetic measures are recommended in obese candidates for transplantation. Efforts should be made to avoid body weight increase after transplantation.

Uric acid

There is a complex but potentially direct causal role for uric acid in the pathogenesis of hypertension and atherosclerosis. However, the role of uric acid and its relation to cardiovascular disease and hypertension remains controversial. Recently, however, several lines of evidence have suggested that increased serum uric acid may be a significant modifiable risk factor. Increased serum uric acid is an independent predictor of cerebrovascular or cardiac events (Hayden and Tyagi, 2004; Erdogan et al., 2005). It is likely that uric acid may have a direct action on smooth muscle and vascular endothelial cells. Preliminary clinical trial results suggest that agents that lower serum uric acid may lower the blood pressure in adolescents with elevated serum uric acid levels (Feig et al., 2006). Should preliminary data be confirmed, serum uric acid will represent a possible new and intriguing target for the reduction of morbidity and mortality associated with hypertension and cardiovascular disease.

Conclusions and recommendations

The risk factors for cardiovascular disease can be grouped into two broad categories: *unmodifiable factors* such as age, male gender, menopause, and family history of premature heart disease; and *potentially modifiable factors* such as cigarette-smoking, physical inactivity, overweight, diabetes, high blood pressure, high blood cholesterol level, and immunosuppressive regimens (Table 10.12). Today there is strong evidence that the risk of cardiovascular disease falls significantly if a patient quits smoking, reduces excess alcohol, has an active life-style, and reduces their weight.

Table 10.12   Measures for prevention of cardiovascular complications after renal transplantation

Patient habit	General measure	Aggressive treatment
Smoking cessation	Avoid/minimize steroid	Glucose intolerance
Ideal body weight	Minimize CNI dose	Arterial hypertension
Healthy diet	Low-dose aspirin	Hyperlipidemia
Physical activity	Check compliance	Anemia
Compliance with therapy		Hyperuricemia (?)

CNI, calcineurin inhibitors

Transplant candidates should be screened for cardiovascular disease as part of the pre-transplant evaluation. Smoking cessation, maintenance of ideal body weight, healthy diet, and physical activity should be recommended (Rigatto, 2005). The aggressive management of cardiovascular risk factors before transplantation is likely to play a critical role in preventing cardiovascular disease after the transplant (Jardine, 2000). Glycemic control should be maximized by using all available measures. If possible, the use of corticosteroids and calcineurin inhibitors should be minimized, to prevent the development of post-transplant diabetes, especially in high-risk groups. The treatment of hypertension should be aggressive; the blood pressure should be kept lower than 130/80 mmHg, and should not exceed 120/80 in patients at high risk such as diabetics, those with more than 500 mg/day of urine protein excretion, those with more than two risk factors for cardiovascular disease, or those with target organ damage. An aggressive intervention for lipid level control is recommended; statins are preferred, but for recipients of calcineurin inhibitors the dose should be reduced by 50%. In some recipients at high risk for cardiovascular disease, a tailored immunosuppressive protocol to minimize post-transplant lipid increase should be considered. Prevention and treatment of anemia may also be useful. Studies have shown that low-dose aspirin is effective in preventing recurrent cardiovascular events. A low dose of aspirin (65–85 mg) appears to be as effective as higher doses (Johnson et al., 1999). Because platelets of renal transplant patients tend to have increased aggregability, it seems reasonable to recommend daily low-dose aspirin for renal transplant patients.

In summary, all efforts should be made to convince the transplant patient to modify diet and life-style and to adhere to drug prescriptions. The reduction of cardiovascular morbidity can improve not only life expectancy and the quality of life of the transplant recipient, but also their allograft function and survival.

References

Aakhus S, Dahl K, Widerne TE. Cardiovascular morbidity and risk factors in renal transplant patients. Nephrol Dial Transplant 1999; 54: 648–54.

Abate N. Obesity as a risk factor for cardiovascular disease. Am J Med 1999; 107 (Suppl 2A): 125–35.

Abdelfatah A, Ducloux D, Toubin G, et al. Treatment of hyperhomocysteinemia with folic acid reduces oxidative stress in renal transplant recipients. Transplantation 2002; 73: 663–5.

Abdulmassih Z, Chevalier A, Bader C, et al. Role of lipid disturbances in the atherosclerosis of renal transplant patients. Clin Transplant 1992; 6: 106–13.

Adler AI, Stratton IM, Neil HA, et al. Association of systolic blood pressure with macrovasular and microvascular complications of type 2 diabetes (UKPD 36): prospective observational study. BMJ; 2000; 321: 412–19.

Agarwal R, Brim NJ, Mahenthiran J, et al. Out-of-hemodialysis-unit blood pressure is a superior determinant of left ventricular hypertrophy. Hypertension 2006; 47: 62–8.

Akbar SA, Jafri SZ, Amendola MA, et al. Complications of renal transplantation. Radiographics 2005; 25: 1335–56.

Alber HF, Frick M, Suessenbacher A, et al. Effect of atorvastatin on circulating proinflammatory T-lymphocyte subsets and soluble CD40 ligand in patients with stable coronary artery disease – a randomized, placebo-controlled study. Am Heart J 2006; 151: 139.

Alexander JW, Goodman HR, Cardi M, et al. Simultaneous corticosteroid avoidance and calcineurin inhibitor minimization in renal transplantation. Transpl Int 2006; 19: 295–302.

American Diabetes Association. Standards of medical care for patients with diabetes mellitus. Diabetes Care 2003; 26 (Suppl 1): S33–50.

Anavekar NS, McMurray JJV, Velazquez EJ, et al. Relation between renal dysfunction and cardiovascular outcomes after myocardial infarction. N Engl J Med 2005; 351: 1285–95.

Andany MA, Kasiske BL. Dyslipidemia and its management after renal transplantation. J Nephrol 2001; 14 (Suppl 4): S81–8.

Antons KA, Williams CD, Baker SK, Phillips PS. Clinical perspectives of statin-induced rhabdomyolysis. Am J Med 2006; 119: 400–9.

Armstrong KA, Campbell SB, Hawley CM, et al. Obesity is associated with worsening cardiovascular risk factors and proteinuria progression in renal transplant recipients. Am J Transplant 2005; 5: 2710–18.

Arnadottir M, Berg AL. Treatment of hyperlipidemia in renal transplant recipients. Transplantation 1997; 63: 339–45.

Arnadottir M, Hultberg B. Treatment with high-dose folic acid effectively lowers plasma homocysteine concentration in cyclosporine-treated renal transplant recipients. Transplantation 1997; 64: 1087.

Arnadottir M, Hultberg B, Walberg J, et al. Serum total homocysteine concentration before and after renal transplantation. Kidney Int 1998; 54: 1380–4.

Artz MA, Boots JM, Ligtenberg G, et al. Improved cardiovascular risk profile and renal function in renal transplant patients after randomized conversion from cyclosporine to tacrolimus. J Am Soc Nephrol 2003; 14: 1880–8.

Asberg A. Interactions between cyclosporin and lipid-lowering drugs: implications for organ transplant recipients. Drugs 2003; 663: 367–78.

Aso Y, Inukai T, Tayama K, Takemura Y. Serum concentrations of advanced glycation endproducts are associated with the development of atherosclerosis as well as diabetic microangiopathy in patients with type 2 diabetes. Acta Diabetol 2000; 37: 87–92.

Audard V, Matignon M, Hemery F, et al. Risk factors and long-term outcome of transplant renal artery stenosis in adult recipients after treatment by percutaneous transluminal angioplasty. Am J Transplant 2006; 6: 95–9.

Babinska A, Markell MS, Salifu MO, et al. Enhancement of human platelet aggregation and secretion induced by rapamycin. Nephrol Dial Transplant 1998; 13: 3153–9.

Barbagallo CM, Gefalù AB, Gallo S, et al. Effects of Mediterranean diet on lipid levels and cardiovascular risk in renal transplant recipients. Nephron 1999; 82: 199–204.

Bartholomeusz B, Hardy KJ, Nelso AS, Philips PA. Modulation of nitric oxide improves cyclosporine A-induced hypertension in rats and primates. J Hum Hypertens 1998; 12: 839–44.

Beecroft JR, Rajan DK, Clark TW, et al. Transplant renal artery stenosis: outcome after percutaneous intervention. J Vasc Interv Radiol 2004; 15: 1407–13.

Bo S, Ciccone G, Gancia R, et al. Mortality within the first 10 years of the disease in type 2 diabetic patients. Nutr Metabol Cardiovasc Dis 2006; 16: 8–12.

Bona KH, Njolstad I, Ueland PM. Homocysteine lowering and cardiovascular events after acute myocardial infarction. N Engl J Med 2006; 354: 1578–88.

Bonora E, Kiechl S, Oberhollenzer F, et al. Impaired glucose tolerance, type II diabetes mellitus and carotid atherosclerosis: prospective results from the Bruneck Study. Diabetologia 2000; 43: 156–64.

Bosmans JL, Holvoet P, Dauwe SE, et al. Oxidative modification of low-density lipoproteins and the outcome of renal allografts at 1½ years. Kidney Int 2001; 59: 2346–56.

Bostom AG. Homocysteine 'expensive creatinine' or important modifiable risk factor for arteriosclerotic outcomes in renal transplant recipients? J Am Soc Nephrol 2000; 11: 149–51.

Bostom AG, Shemin D, Gohh RY, et al. Treatment of hyperhomocysteinemia in hemodialysis patients and renal transplant recipients. Kidney Int 2001; 78 (Suppl): S246–52.

Broeders N, Knoop C, Antoine M, et al. Fibrate-induced increase in urea and creatinine: is gemfibrozil the only innocuous agent? Nephrol Dial Transplant 2000; 15: 1993–9.

Bruggeman CA, Marjorie HJ, Nelissen-Vrancken G. Cytomegalovirus and atherogenesis. Antiviral Res 1999; 43: 135–44.

Burnier M, Brunner HR. Angiotensin II receptor antagonists in hypertension. Kidney Int 1998; 54 (Suppl 68): S107–11.

Campise M, Bamonti F, Novembrino C, et al. Oxidative stress in kidney transplant patients. Transplantation 2003; 76: 1474–8.

Carlström J, Nordén G, Mjörnstedt L, Nyberg G. Increasing prevalence of cardiovascular disease in kidney transplant patients with type 1 diabetes. Transplant Int 1999; 12: 176–81.

Carr AC, Zhu BZ, Frei B. Potential antiatherogenic mechanisms of ascorbate (vitamin C) and alfa-tocopherol (vitamin E). Circ Res 2000; 87: 349–54.

Castillo-Lugo JA, Vergne-Marini P. Hypertension in kidney transplantation. Semin Nephrol 2005; 4: 252–60.

Cecka JM. The OPTN/UNOS renal transplant registry in Cecka JM, PI Terasaki PI, eds. Cllinical Transplants 2003. Los Angeles: UCLA, 2003: 1–12.

Chueh SC, Kahan BD. Dyslipidemia in renal transplant recipients treated with a sirolimus and cyclosporine-based immunosuppressive regimen: incidence, risk factors, progression, and prognosis. Transplantation 2003; 76: 375–82.

Cice G, Di Benedetto A, D'Andrea A, et al. Sustained-release diltiazem reduces myocardial ischemic episodes in end-stage renal disease: a double-blind, randomized, cross-over, placebo-controlled trial. J Am Soc Nephrol 2003; 14: 1006–11.

Cieciura T, Senatorski G, Rell K, et al. Influence of angiotensin-converting-enzyme inhibitor treatment of the carotid artery intima-media complex in renal allograft recipients. Trasplant Proc 2000; 32: 1335–6.

Clark LT. Treating dyslipidemia with statins: the risk–benefit profile. Am Heart J 2003; 145: 387–90.

Clarke R, Lewington S, Landray M. Homocysteine, renal function, and risk of cardiovascular disease. Kidney Int 2003; 63 (Suppl 84): S131–3.

Cole DE, Ross HJ, Evroski J, et al. Correlation between total homocysteine and cyclosporine concentration in cardiac transplantation recipients. Clin Chem 1998; 44: 2307–12.

Cosio FG, Alamir A, Yim S, et al. Patient survival after renal transplantation: I. The impact of dialysis pre-transplant. Kidney Int 1998; 53: 767–72.

Cosio FG, Falkentrain MF, Pesavento TE, et al. Patient survival data after renal transplantation: II. The input of smoking. Clin Transplant 1999; 13: 336–41.

Cosio FG, Pesavento FE, Osei K, et al. Post-transplant diabetes mellitus: increasing incidence in renal allograft recipients transplanted in recent years. Kidney Int 2001a; 59: 732–7.

Cosio FG, Pelletier RP, Pesavento TE, et al. Elevated blood pressure predicts the risk of acute rejection in renal allograft recipients. Kidney Int 2001b; 59: 1158–64.

Cosio FG, Pesavento TE, Pelletier RP, et al. Patient survival data after renal transplantation: III. The effect of statins. Am J Kidney Dis 2002; 40: 638–43.

Curtis JJ. Treatment of hypertension in renal allograft patients: does drug selection make a difference? Kidney Int 1997; 63 (Suppl): S75–7.

Curtis JJ. Posttransplant hypertension. Transplant Proc 1998; 30: 2009–11.

Curtis JJ, Laskow PA, Jones PA, et al. Captopril-induced fall in glomerular filtration rate in cyclosporine-treated hypertensive patients. J Am Soc Nephrol 1993; 3: 1570–4.

Dahlof B, Devereux RB, Kyeldsen SE, et al. Cardiovascular morbidity and mortality in Losartan Intervention For Endpoint reduction in hypertension study (LIFE): a randomised trial against atenolol. Lancet 2002; 359: 995–1003.

Danovitch GM. Can ACE-inhibitors prevent chronic allograft failure? Am J Kidney Dis 2001; 37: 866–70.

Demme RA. Hypertension in the kidney transplant patient. Graft 2001; 4: 248–55.

De Mattos AM, Shibagaki Y, Russo K, et al. Study 2: relationship between pretransplant obesity and posttransplant cardiovascular events, diabetes mellitus, and graft and patient survival in renal transplant recipients. Transplant Rev 2003; 17 (Suppl 2): S38–9.

de Morais RH, Muglia VF, Mamere AE, et al. Duplex Doppler sonography of transplant renal artery stenosis. J Clin Ultrasound 2003; 31: 135–41.

Derici U, El Nahas AM. Vascular complications in uremia: old concepts and new insights. Semin Dial 2006; 19: 60–8.

Dimény E, Fellstrom B, Larsson E, et al. Hyperlipoproteinemia in renal transplant recipients: is there a linkage with chronic vascular rejection? Transplant Proc 1993; 25: 2065–6.

Dimény E, Hultberg B, Wahlberg J, et al. Serum total homocysteine does not predict outcome in renal transplant recipients. Transplantation 1998; 12: 563–8.

Drachenberg CB, Klassen DK, Weir MR, et al. Islet cell damage associated with tacrolimus and cyclosporine: morphological features in pancreas allograft biopsies and clinical correlation. Transplantation 1999; 68: 396–402.

Ducloux D, Motte G, Challier B, et al. Serum total homocysteine and cardiovacular disease occurrence in chronic, stable renal transplant recipients: a prospective study. J Am Soc Nephrol 2000; 11: 134–7.

Ducloux D, Motte G, Massy ZA. Hyperhomocysteinemia as a risk factor after renal transplantation. Ann Transplant 2001; 6: 40–2.

Ducloux D, Bourrinet E, Motte G, Chalopin JM. Antiphospholipid antibodies as a risk factor for atherosclerotic events in renal transplant recipients. Kidney Int 2003; 64: 1065–70.

Ducloux D, Kazory A, Chalopin JM. Posttransplant diabetes mellitus and atherosclerotic events in renal transplant recipients: a prospective study. Transplantation 2005; 79: 438–43.

Ducloux D, Klein A, Kazory A, et al. Impact of malnutrition on the association between hyperhomocysteinemia and mortality. Kidney Int 2006; 69: 331–5.

Elliott WJ. Traditional drug therapy of hypertension in transplant recipients. J Hum Hypertens 1998; 12: 845–9.

English J, Evan A, Houghton D, Bennett W. Cyclosporine induces acute renal dysfunction in the rat. Evidence of arteriolar vasoconstriction with preservation of tubular function. Transplantation 1987; 44: 135–41.

Erdogan D, Gullu H, Caliskan M, et al. Relationship of serum uric acid to measures of endothelial function and atherosclerosis in healthy adults. Int J Clin Pract 2005; 59: 1276–82.

Fabrizi F, Martin P, Dixit V, et al. Post-transplant diabetes mellitus and HCV seropositive status after renal transplantation: meta-analysis of clinical studies. Am J Transplant 2005; 5: 2433–40.

Feig DI, Mazzali M, Kang DH, et al. Serum uric acid: a risk factor and a target for treatment? J Am Soc Nephrol 2006; 17 (Suppl 2): S69–73.

Fellstrom B, Holdaas H, Jardine A. Cardiovascular disease in renal transplantation: management by statins. Transplant Rev 2004; 18: 122–8.

Fellstrom B, Jardine AG, Soveri I, et al. Renal dysfunction is a strong and independent risk factor for mortality and cardiovascular complications in renal transplantation. Am J Transplant 2005; 8: 1986–91.

Fernandez-Fresnedo G, Escallada R, Rodrigo E, et al. The risk of cardiovascular disease associated with proteinuria in renal transplant patients. Transplantation 2002; 73: 1345–8.

Fernandez-Miranda C, Gomez P, Diaz-Rubio P, et al. Plasma homocysteine levels in renal transplanted patients on cyclosporine or tacrolimus therapy: effect of treatment with folic acid. Clin Transplant 2000; 14: 110–14.

Ferraris JR, Pasqualini T, Legal S, et al. Effect of deflazacort versus methylprednisone on growth, body composition, lipid profile, and bone mass after renal transplantation. The Deflazacort Study Group. Pediatr Nephrol 2000; 14: 682–8.

Filler G. Tacrolimus reversibly reduces insulin secretion in paediatric renal transplant recipients. Nephrol Dial Transplant 2000; 15: 867.

Fleming I, Busse R. NO: the primary EDRF. J Mol Cell Cardiol 1999; 31: 5–14.

Födinger M, Wölfe G, Fischer G, et al. Effect of MTHFR 677C>T on plasma total homocysteine levels in renal graft recipients. Kidney Int 1999; 55: 1072–80.

Fonseca VA. Management of diabetes mellitus and insulin resistance in patients with cardiovascular disease. Am J Cardiol 2003; 92: 50J–60J.

Formica RN Jr, Friedman AL, Lorber MI, et al. A randomized trial comparing losartan with amlodipine as initial therapy for hypertension in the early post-transplant period. Nephrol Dial Transplant 2006; 21: 1389–94.

Fornarow GC. Approach to the management of diabetic patients with heart failure: role of thiazolidinediones. Am Heart J 2004; 148: 551–8.

Forsyte JL. Graft function and other risk factors as predictors of cardiovascular disease outcome. Transplantation 2001; 72 (Suppl): S16–19.

Fricke L, Diehn C, Steinhoff J, et al. Treatment of post-transplant hypertension by laparoscopic bilateral nephrectomy? Transplantation 1998; 65: 1182–7.

Friedman AN, Rosenberg IH, Selhub J, et al. Hyperhomocysteinemia in renal transplant recipients. Am J Transplant 2002; 2: 308–13.

Frishman WH. Biologic markers as predictors of cardiovascular disease. Am J Med 1998; 104: S18–27.

Frostegard J. Atherosclerosis in patients with autoimmune disorders. Arterioscler Thromb Vasc Biol 2005; 9: 1776–85.

Furberg CD, Psaty BM, Meyer JV. Nifedipine: dose-related increase in mortality in patients with coronary heart disease. Circulation 1995; 92: 1326–31.

Gaede P, Vedel P, Larsen N, et al. Multifactorial intervention and cardiovascular disease in patients with type 2 diabetes. N Engl J Med 2003; 348: 383–93.

Gervaise N, Garrigue MA, Lasfargues G, Lecomte P. Triglycerides, apo C3 and Lp B: C3 and cardiovascular risk in type II diabetes. Diabetologia 2000; 43: 703–8.

Gillison SL, Bartlett ST, Curry DL. Inhibition by cyclosporine of insulin secretion: a beta cell-specific alteration of islet tissue function. Transplantation 1991; 52: 890–5.

Go A, Chertow GM, Fan D, et al. Chronic kidney disease and the risks of death, cardiovascular events and hospitalization. N Engl J Med 2004; 351: 1296–305.

Goldberg R, Roth D. Evaluation of fluvastatin in the treatment of hypercholesterolemia in renal transplant recipients taking cyclosporine. Transplantation 1996; 62: 1559–64.

Gonzalez-Posada JM, Hernandez D, Bayes Genis B, et al. Impact of diabetes mellitus on kidney transplant recipients in Spain. Nephrol Dial Transplant 2004; 19 (Suppl 3): 57–61.

Goodman WG, Goldin J, Kuizon BD, et al. Coronary-artery calcification in young adults with end-stage renal disease who are undergoing dialysis. N Engl J Med 2000; 342: 1478–83.

Gress TW, Nieto FJ, Shahar E, et al. Hypertension and antihypertensive therapy as risk factors for type 2 diabetes mellitus. N Engl J Med 2000; 342: 905–12.

Griendling KK, Alexander RW. Oxidative stress and cardiovascular disease. Circulation 1997; 96: 3264–5.

Grundy SM. National Cholesterol Education Program. Second report of the expert panel on detection, evaluation, and treatment of high blood cholesterol in adults (Adult Treatment Renal II). Circulation 1994; 99: 1329.

Guidi E, Menghetti D, Milani S, et al. Hypertension may be transplanted with the kidney in humans: a long-term historical prospective follow-up of recipients grafted with kidney coming from donors with or without hypertension in their families. J Am Soc Nephrol 1996; 7: 1131–8.

Haffner SM. Epidemiology of insulin resistance and its relation to coronary artery disease. Am J Cardiol 1999; 84: 11J–14J.

Hagen W, Fodinger M, Heinz G, et al. Effect of MTHFR genotypes and hyperhomocysteinemia on patient and graft survival in kidney transplant recipients. Kidney Int 2001; 78 (Suppl): S253–7.

Halme L, Eklund B, Killonen L, Salmela K. Is obesity still risk factor in renal transplantation? Transpl Int 1997; 10: 284–8.

Hansson GK, Libby P, Schonbeck U, Yan ZQ. Innate and adaptive immunity in the pathogenesis of atherosclerosis. Circ Res 2002; 91: 281–91.

Harrower AD. Pharmacokinetics of oral antihyperglycemic agents in patients with renal insufficiency. Clin Pharmacokinet 1996; 2: 111–19.

Hausberg M, Barenbrock M, Hohage H, et al. ACE inhibitor versus beta-blocker for the treatment of hypertension in renal allograft recipients. Hypertension 1999; 33: 862–8.

Hayden MR, Tyagi SC. Uric acid: a new look at an old risk marker for cardiovascular disease, metabolic syndrome, and type 2 diabetes mellitus: the urate redox shuttle. Nutr Metab 2004; 1: 1–10.

Henry ML. Cyclosporine and tacrolimus (FK 506). A comparison of efficacy and safety profiles. Clin Transplant 1999; 13: 209–20.

Hernandez D, Lacalzada J, Salido E, et al. Regression of left ventricular hypertrophy by lisinopril after renal transplantation: role of ACE gene polymorphism. Kidney Int 2000; 58: 889–97.

Higashi Y, Sasaki S, Nakagawa K, et al. Endothelial function and oxidative stress in renovascular hypertension. N Engl J Med 2002; 346: 1954–62.

Hjelmesaeth J, Hartmann A. Kofstad J, et al. Tapering of prednisolone and cyclosporin the first year after renal transplantation: the effect on glucose tolerance. Nephrol Dial Transplant 2001; 16: 829–35.

Hjelmesaeth J, Ueland T, Flyvbjerg A, et al. Early posttransplant osteoprotegerin levels predict long-term (8-year) patient survival and cardiovascular death in renal transplant patients. J Am Soc Nephrol 2006; 17: 1746–54.

Hoffer LJ, Robitaille L, Elian KM, et al. Plasma reduced homocysteine concentrations are increased in end-stage renal disease. Kidney Int 2001; 59: 372–7.

Holdaas P, Fellstrom B, Jardine AG, et al. Effect of fluvastatin on cardiac outcomes in renal transplant recipients: a multicentre, randomised, placebo controlled trial. Lancet 2003; 36: 2024–31.

Holgado R, Anaja F, Del Castillo D. Angiotensin II type 1 (AT1) receptor antagonists in the treatment of hypertension after renal transplantation. Nephrol Dial Transplant 2001; 16 (Suppl 1): 117–20.

Hopkins PN, Williams RR. A survey of 246 suggested coronary risk factors. Atherosclerosis 1981; 40: 1–52.

Howard RJ, Thai VB, Patton PR, et al. Obesity does not portend a bad outcome for kidney transplant recipients. Transplantation 2002; 73: 53–5.

Humar A, Gillingham K, Payne WD, et al. Increased incidence of cardiac complications in kidney transplant recipients with cytomegalovirus disease. Transplantation 2000; 70: 310–13.

Hypolite IO, Bucci J, Hshieh P, et al. Acute coronary syndromes after renal transplantation in patients with end-stage renal disease resulting from diabetes. Am J Transplant 2002; 2: 274–81.

Irish AB, Green FR. Environmental and genetic determinants of the hypercoagulable state and cardiovascular disease in renal transplant recipients. Nephrol Dial Transplant 1997; 12: 167–73.

Isoniemi H, Nurminen M, Tikkanen MJ, et al. Risk factors predicting chronic rejection of renal allografts. Transplantation 1994; 57: 68–72.

Jardine A. Pretransplant management of ESRD patients to minimize posttransplant risk. Transplantation 2000; 70: S46–50.

Jardine A, Fellstrom B, Logan JO. Cardiovascular risk and renal transplantation: post hoc analysis of the Assessment of Lescol in Renal Transplantation (ALERT) study. Am J Kidney Dis 2005; 46: 529–36.

Jensen RA, Lal SM, Diaz-Arias A, et al. Does cholestyramine interfere with cyclosporin absorption? A prospective study in renal transplant patients. ASAIO J 1995; 41: M704–6.

Jialal I, Stein D, Balis, et al. Effect of hydroxymethyl glutaryl coenzyme A reductase inhibitor therapy on high sensitive C-reactive protein levels. Circulation 2001; 103: 1933–5.

Jindal RM. Posttransplant diabetes mellitus. A review. Transplantation 1994; 58: 1289–98.

Johnson C, Ahsan N, Gonwa T, et al. Randomized trial of tacrolimus (Prograf) in combination with azathioprine or mycophenolate mofetil versus cyclosporine (Neoral) with mycophenolate mofetil after cadaveric kidney transplantation. Transplantation 2000; 69: 834–41.

Johnson DW, Isbel NM, Brown AM, et al. The effect of obesity on renal transplant outcomes. Transplantation 2002b; 74: 675–81.

Johnson ES, Lanes SF, Wentworth CE, et al. A metaregression analysis of dose–response effect of aspirin on stroke. Arch Intern Med 1999; 159: 1248–53.

Johnson JA, Majumdar SR, Simpson SH, Toth EL. Decreased mortality associated with the use of metformin compared with sulfonylurea in the type 2 diabetes. Diabetes Care 2002a; 25: 2244–8.

Kasiske BL, Chakkera H, Roel J, et al. Explained and unexplained ischemic heart disease risk after renal transplantation. J Am Soc Nephrol 2000b; 11: 1735–43.

Kasiske BL. Epidemiology of cardiovascular disease after renal transplantation. Transplantation 2001; 72: S5–8.

Kasiske BL. Ischemic heart disease after renal transplantation. Kidney Int 2002; 61: 356–69.

Kasiske BL, Ballantyne CM. Cardiovascular risk factors associated with immunosuppression in renal transplantation. Transplant Rev 2002; 1: 1–21.

Kasiske BL, Klinger D. Cigarette smoking in renal transplant recipients. J Am Soc Nephol 2000; 11: 753–9.

Kasiske BL, Vasquez HA, Harmon WE, et al. Recommendations for the outpatient surveillance of renal transplant recipients. American Society of Transplantation. J Am Soc Nephrol 2000a; 11 (Suppl): S1–86.

Kasiske BL, Heim-Duthoy KL, Singer GG, et al. The effect of lipid-lowering agents on acute renal allograft rejection. Transplantation 2001; 72: 223–7.

Kasiske BL, Snyder JJ, Gilbert D, Matas AJ. Diabetes mellitus after kidney transplantation in the United States. Am J Transplant 2003; 3: 178–85.

Kasiske BL, Anjum S, Shah R, et al. Hypertension after kidney transplantation. Am J Kidney Dis 2004; 43: 1071–81.

Kato T, Tokoro T, Namii Y, et al. Early introduction of HMG-CoA reductase inhibitors could prevent the incidence of transplant coronary artery disease. Transplant Proc 2000; 32: 331–3.

Katznelson S, Wilkinson AH, Kobashigawa JA, et al. The effect of pravastatin on acute rejection after kidney transplantation: a pilot study. Transplantation 1996; 61: 1469–74.

Kendrick E. Cardiovascular disease and the renal transplant recipient. Am J Kidney Dis 2001; 38 (Suppl 6): S36–43.

Kennedy R, Case C, Fathi R, et al. Does renal failure cause an atherosclerotic milieu in patients with end-stage renal disease? Am J Med 2001; 110: 198–204.

Knopp RM. Treatment of lipid disorder. N Engl J Med 1999; 341: 498–511.

Kobashigawa JA, Kasiske BL. Hyperlipidemia in solid organ transplantation. Transplantation 1997; 63: 331–8.

Kohnle M, Pietruck F, Kribben A, et al. Ezetimibe for the treatment of uncontrolled hypercholesterolemia in patients with high-dose statin therapy after renal transplantation. Am J Transplant 2006; 6: 205–8.

Koomans HA, Ligtenberg G. Mechanisms and consequences of arterial hypertension after renal transplantation. Transplantation 2001; 72 (Suppl 6): S9–12.

Kuypers DR, Neumayer HH, Fritsche L, et al. Calcium channel blockade and preservation of renal graft function in cyclosporine-treated recipients: a prospective randomized placebo-controlled 2-year study. Transplantation 2004; 78: 1204–11.

Lamb DJ, El-Sankary W, Ferns GA. Molecular mimicry in atherosclerosis: a role for heat shock proteins in immunisation. Atherosclerosis 2003; 167: 177–85.

Langone AJ, Chuang P. Ezetimibe in renal transplant patients with hyperlipidemia resistant to HMG-CoA reductase inhibitors. Transplantation 2006; 81: 804–7.

Laufs U, La FataV, Plutzky J, Liao JK. Upregulation of endothelial nitric oxide synthase by HMG CoA reductase inhibitors. Circulation 1998; 97: 1129–35.

Lauzurica R, Pastor C, Bayes B, et al. Pretransplant pregnancy-associated plasma protein-a as a predictor of chronic allograft nephropathy and posttransplant cardiovascular events. Transplantation 2005; 80: 1441–6.

Lepre F, Rigby R, Hawley C, et al. A double blind controlled trial for the treatment of dyspilidaemia in renal allograft recipients. Clin Transplant 1999; 13: 520–6.

Libby P, Ridker PM, Maseri A. Inflammation and atherosclerosis. Circulation 2002; 105: 1135–43.

Lindholm LM, Ibsen H, Dahlof B, et al. Cardiovascular morbidity and mortality in patients with diabetes in the Losartan Intervention For Endpoint reduction in hypertension study (LIFE): a randomized trial against atenolol. Lancet 2002; 359: 1004–10.

Locatelli F, Pozzoni P, Del Vecchio L. Anemia and heart failure in chronic kidney disease. Semin Nephrol 2005; 25: 392–6.

London GM. Left ventricular hypertrophy: why does it happen? Nephrol Dial Transplant 2003; 18 (Suppl 8): 2–6.

Lonn E, Yusuf S, Arnold MJ, et al.; Hope 2 Investigators. Homocysteine lowering with folic acid and B vitamins in vascular disease. N Engl J Med 2006; 354: 1567–77.

Loscalzo J. Homocysteine trials: clear outcomes for complex reasons. N Engl J Med 2006; 354: 1629–31.

Mailloux LU, Levey AS. Hypertension in patients with chronic renal disease. Am J Kidney Dis 1998; 32 (Suppl): S120–41.

Makaryus AN. Aspirin resistance, an emerging, often overlooked, factor in the management of patients with coronary artery disease. Clin Cardiol 2006; 29: 144–8.

Malyszko J, Malyszko JS, Brzosko S, et al. Effect of fluvastatin on homocysteine and serum lipids in kidney allograft recipients. Ann Transplant 2002; 7: 52–4.

Manjunath G, Tighiouart H, Ibrahim H, et al. Level of kidney function as a risk factor for atherosclerotic cardiovascular outcomes in the community. J Am Coll Cardiol 2003; 41: 47–55.

Marchetti P. Strategies for risk reduction and management of post-transplant diabetes mellitus. Transplant Proc 2001; 33 (Suppl 5A): 27S–31S.

Marcucci R, Zanazzi M, Bertoni E, et al. Vitamin supplementation reduces the progression of atherosclerosis in hyper-homocysteinemic renal trasplant recipients. Transplantation 2003; 75: 1551–5.

Margreiter R; European Tacrolimus vs Ciclosporin Microemulsion Renal Transplantation Study Group. Efficacy and safety of tacrolimus compared with ciclosporin microemulsion in renal transplantation: a randomised multicentre study. Lancet 2002; 359: 741–6.

Maron DJ, Fazio S, Linton MF. Current perspective on statins. Circulation 2000; 101: 207–13.

Martinez-Castelao A, Hernandez MD, Pascual J, et al. Detection and treatment of post kidney transplant hyper-glycemia: a Spanish multicenter cross-sectional study. Transplant Proc 2005; 37: 3813–16.

Massy ZA. Potential strategies to normalize the levels of homocysteine in chronic renal failure patients. Kidney Int 2003; 63 (Suppl 84): S134–6.

Massy ZA, Kasiske BL. Post-transplant hyperlipidemia: mechanisms and management. J Am Soc Nephrol 1996; 7: 971–7.

Massy ZA, Chadefaux-Vekemans B, Chevalier A, et al. Hyperhomocysteinemia: a significant risk factor for cardiovascular disease in renal transplant recipients. Nephrol Dial Transplant 1994; 9: 1103–8.

Mathew TH, Rao M, Job V, et al. Post-transplant hyperglycemia: a study of risk factors. Nephrol Dial Transplant 2003; 18: 164–71.

McCune TR, Thacker LR, Peters TG, et al. Effects of tacrolimus on hyperlipidemia after successful renal transplantation. Transplantation 1998; 65: 87–92.

McIntyre M, Bohr DF, Dominiczak AF. Endothelial function in hypertension: the role of superoxide anion. Hypertension 1999; 34: 539–45.

Meier-Kriesche HU, Kaplan B. Waiting time on dialysis as the strongest modifiable risk factor for renal transplant outcomes: a paired donor kidney analysis. Transplantation 2002; 74: 1377–81.

Meier-Kriesche HU, Schold JD, Srinivas TR, et al. Kidney transplantation halts cardiovascular disease progression in patients with end-stage renal disease. Am J Transplant 2004; 10: 1662–8.

Midtvedt K, Hartmann A. Hypertension after kidney transplantation: are treatment guidelines emerging? Nephrol Dial Transplant 2002; 17: 1166–9.

Midtvedt K, Neumayer HH. Management strategies for post-transplant hypertension. Transplantation 2000; 70: SS64–9.

Midtvedt K, Ihlen H, Hartmann A, et al. Reduction of left ventricular mass by lisinopril and nifedipine in hypertensive renal transplant recipients: a prospective randomized double-blind study. Transplantation 2001; 72: 107–11.

Miles AMV, Sumrani N, Horowitz R, et al. Diabetes mellitus after renal transplantation. Transplantation 1998; 65: 380–4.

Miller LW. Cardiovascular toxicity of immunosupressive agents. Am J Transplant 2002; 2: 807–18.

Mohi-ud-din K, Bali HK, Benerjee S, et al. Silent myocardial ischemia and high-grade ventricular arrhythmias in patients on maintenance hemodialysis. Ren Fail 2005; 27: 171–5.

Montagnino G, Tarantino A, Segoloni G, et al. Long-term results of a randomized study comparing three immunosuppressive schedules with cyclosporine in cadaveric kidney transplantation. J Am Soc Nephrol 2001; 12: 2163–9.

Montagnino G, Sandrini S, Casciani C. A randomized trial of steroid avoidance in renal transplant patients treated with evertolimus and cyclosporine. Transplant Proc 2005; 37: 788–90.

Morales JM, Andres A, Rengel M, Rodicio JL. Influence of cyclosporin, tacrolimus and rapamycin on renal function and arterial hypertension after renal transplantation. Nephrol Dial Transplant 2001; 16 (Suppl 1): 121–4.

Morrisett JD, Abdel-Fattah G, Kahan BD. Sirolimus changes lipid concentrations and lipoprotein metabolism in kidney transplant recipients. Transplant Proc 2003; 35: 143S.

Mosterd A, D'Agostino RB, Silbershatz H, et al. Trends in the prevalence of hypertension, antihypertensive therapy and left ventricular hypertrophy from 1950 to 1989. N Engl J Med 1999; 340: 1221–7.

Mourad G, Ribstein J, Mimran A. Converting-enzyme inhibitor versus calcium antagonist in cyclosporine-treated renal transplants. Kidney Int 1993; 43: 419–25.

O'Driscoll G, Green D, Taylor RR. Simvastatin, an HMC CoA reductase inhibitor improves endothelial function within one month. Circulation 1997; 95: 1126–31.

Olyaei AJ, de Mattos AM, Benne WM. A pratical guide to the management of hypertension in renal transplant recipients. Drugs 1999; 58: 1011–27.

Opelz G, Wujciak T, Ritz E. Association of chronic kidney graft failure with recipient blood pressure. Kidney Int 1998; 53: 217–22.

Opelz G, Dohler B; Collaborative Transplant Study. Improved outcomes after renal transplantation associated with blood pressure control. Am J Transplant 2005; 11: 2725–31.

Orth SR, Viedt C, Ritz E. Adverse effects of smoking in the renal patient. J Exp Med 2001; 194: 1–15.

Paolillo JA, Boyle GJ, Law YM, et al. Posttransplant diabetes mellitus in pediatric thoracic organ recipients receiving tacrolimus-based immunosuppression. Transplantation 2001; 71: 252–6.

Pasceri V, Willerson JT. Homocysteine and coronary heart disease: a review of the current evidence. Semin Intern Cardiol 1999; 4: 121–8.

Pascual J, Quereda C, Zamora J. Updated metaanalysis of steroid withdrawal in renal transplant patients on calcineurin inhibitors and mycophenolate mofetil. Transplant Proc 2005; 37: 3746–8.

Pascual M, Theruvath T, Kawai T, et al. Strategies to improve long-term outcomes after renal transplantation. N Engl J Med 2002; 346: 580–90.

Pepys MB, Hirschfield GM, Tennent GA, et al. Targeting C-reactive protein for the treatment of cardiovascular disease. Nature 2006; 440: 1217–21.

Perez-Fontan M, Rodriguez-Carmona A, Falcon TG, Valdés E. Early proteinuria in renal transplant recipients treated with cyclosporine. Transplantation 1999; 67: 561–8.

Perna AF, Ingrosso D, Lombardi C, et al. Possible mechanisms of homocysteine toxicity. Kidney Int 2003; 63 (Suppl 84): S137–40.

Pesavento TE, Jones PA, Julian BA, Curtis JJ. Amlodipine increases cyclosporine levels in hypertensive renal transplant patients. Results of a prospective study. J Am Soc Nephrol 1996; 7: 831–5.

Pesavento TE, Henry ML, Falkenhain ME, Ferguson RM. Study 3: Post-transplant diabetes mellitus: evidence for glucose intolerance and insulin resistance existing before transplantation. Transplant Rev 2003; 17 (suppl 2): S39.

Pilmore H. Cardiac assessment for renal transplantation. Am J Transplant 2006; 6: 659–65.

Pischon T, Sharma AM. Obesity as a risk factor in renal transplant patients. Nephrol Dial Transplant 2001; 16: 14–17.

Ponticelli C, Montagnino G, Aroldi A. Hypertension after transplantation. Am J Kidney Dis 1993; 21 (Suppl 2): S73–8.

Ponticelli C, Tarantino A, Segoloni GP, et al. A randomized study comparing three cyclosporine-based regimens in cadaveric renal transplantation. J Am Soc Nephrol 1997; 8: 638–46.

Ponticelli C, Villa M, Cesana B, et al. Risk factors for late kidney allograft failure. Kidney Int 2002; 62: 1848–54.

Raggi P, Boulay A, Chasan-Taber S, et al. Cardiac calcifications in adult hemodialysis patients. A link between end-stage renal disease and cardiovascular disease? J Am Coll Cardiol 2002; 39: 695–701.

Rahn KH, Barenbrock M, Frtischka E, et al. Effect of nitrendipine on renal function in renal transplant patients treated with cyclosporine: a randomised trial. Lancet 1999; 354: 1415–20.

Raj DSC, Choudhury D, Welbourne TC, Levi M. Advanced glycation end products. A nephrologist's perspective. Am J Kidney Dis 2000; 35: 365–80.

Rao VK. Post-transplant medical complications. Surg Clin North Am 1998; 78: 113–32.

Ratcliffe PJ, Dudley CRK, Higgins RM, et al. Randomized controlled trial of steroid withdrawal in renal transplant recipients receiving triple immunosuppression. Lancet 1996; 348: 643–8.

Revanur VK, Jardine AG, Kingsmore DB, et al. Influence of diabetes mellitus on patient and graft survival in recipients of kidney transplantation. Clin Transplant 2001; 15: 89–94.

Rice M, Martin J, Hathaway D, Tolley E. Prevalence of cardiovascular risk factors before kidney transplantation. Prog Transplant 2002; 12: 299–304.

Ridker PM. High-sensivity C-reactive protein. Circulation 2001; 103: 1813–17.

Ridker PM, Hennekens CH, Rifai N, et al. Hormone replacement therapy and increased plasma concentration of C-reactive protein. Circulation 1999; 100: 713–16.

Ridker PM, Rifai N, Buring JE, Cook NR. Comparison of C-reactive protein and low-density lipoprotein cholesterol levels in the prediction of first cardiovascular events. N Engl J Med 2002; 347: 1557–65.

Rigatto C, Parfrey P, Foley R, et al. Congestive heart failure in renal transplant recipients: risk factors, outcomes and relationship with ischemic heart disease. J Am Soc Nephrol 2002; 13: 1084–90.

Rigatto C. Clinical epidemiology of cardiac disease in renal transplant recipients. Semin Dial 2003; 16: 106–10.

Rigatto C. Management of cardiovascular diseases in renal transplant recipients. Cardiol Clin 2005; 23: 331–42.

Ritz E, Benck U, Franek E, et al. Effects of smoking on renal hemodynamics in healthy volunteers and in patients with glomerular disease. J Am Soc Nephrol 1998; 9: 1798–804.

Roberts JP, Ascher NL, Feyd DS, et al. Transplant artery stenoses. Transplantation 1989; 48: 580–3.

Roodnat JI, Mulder PGH, Rischen-Vos J, et al. Proteinuria after renal transplantation affects not only graft survival but also patient survival. Transplantation 2001; 72: 438–44.

Rosenson RS, Tangney CC. Antiatherothrombotic properties of statins. Implication of cardiovascular event reduction. JAMA 1998; 279: 1643–80.

Ross R. Atherosclerosis. An inflammatory disease. N Engl J Med 1999; 340: 115–26.

Rostaing L, Cantarovich D, Mourad G, et al. Corticosteroid-free immunosuppression with tacrolimus, mycophenolate mofetil, and daclizumab induction in renal transplantation. Transplantation 2005; 79: 807–14.

Rostand SG. Coronary heart disease in chronic renal insufficiency: some management considerations. J Am Soc Nephrol 2000; 11: 1948–56.

Sagedal S, Aasberg A, Hartmann A, et al. Glipizide treatment of post-transplant diabetes does not interfere with cyclosporine pharmacokinetics in renal allograft recipients. Clin Transplant 1998; 6: 553–6.

Sartori TM, Rigotti P, Marchini F, et al. Plasma fibrinolytic capacity in renal transplant recipients: effect of steroid-free immunosuppression therapy. Transplantation 2003; 75: 994–8.

Satterthwaite R, Aswad S, Sunga V, et al. Incidence of new-onset hypercholesterolemia in renal transplant patients treated with FK506 or cyclosporine. Transplantation 1998; 65: 446–9.

Schieffer B, Schieffer E, Hilfiker-Kleiner D, et al. Expression of angiotensin II and interleukin 6 in human coronary artherosclerotic plaques: potential implication for inflammation and plaque instability. Circulation 2000; 101: 1372–8.

Schneider DC. Abnormalities of coagulation, platelet function, and fibrinolysis associated with syndromes of insulin resistance. Coron Artery Dis 2005; 16: 473–6.

Schrama YC, Hené RJ, De Jonge N, et al. Efficacy and muscle safety of fluvastatin in cyclosporine-treated cardiac and renal transplant recipients. Transplantation 1998; 66: 1175–81.

Schonbeck U, Gerdes N, Varo N, et al. Oxidized low-density lipoproteins augment and 3-hydroxy-3-methylglutaryl coenzyme A reductase inhibitor limit CD40 and CD40L expression in human vascular cells. Circulation 2002; 106: 2888–93.

Schweitzer E, Matas AJ, Gillingham KG, et al. Cause of renal allograft loss. Progress in the 1980s, challenges for the 1990s. Ann Surg 1991; 214: 679–88.

Schwenger V, Zeier M, Ritz E. Hypertension after renal transplantation. Ann Transplant 2001; 6: 25–30.

Shächinger V, Zeiher A. Atherogenesis – recent insights into basic mechanisms and their clinical impact. Nephrol Dial Transplant 2002; 17: 2055–64.

Sharp A, Mayet J. Regression of left ventricular hypertrophy: hoping for a longer life. J Renin Angiotensin Aldosterone Syst 2002; 3: 141–4.

Sherer Y, Schoenfeld Y. Antiphospholipid antibodies: are they pro-atherogenic or an epiphenomenon of atherosclerosis? Immunobiology 2003; 207: 13–16.

Simpson SH, Majumdar SR, Tsuyuki RT, et al. Dose–response relation between sulfonylurea drugs and mortality in type 2 diabetes mellitus: a population-based cohort study. CMAJ 2006; 174: 169–74.

Solomon CG. Reducing cardiovascular risk in type 2 diabetes. N Engl J Med 2003; 348: 457–9.

Sowers JR. Hypertension, angiotensin II, and oxidative stress. N Engl J Med 2002; 346: 1999–2001.

Stein G, Muller A, Busch M, et al. Homocysteine, its metabolites, and B-group vitamins in renal transplant patients. Kidney Int 2001; (Suppl 78): S262–5.

Stenkivel P. Inflammation in end stage renal disease – a fire that burns within. Clin Nephrol 2005; 149: 185–9.

Stephan A, Barbari A, Karam A, et al. Hyperlipidemia and graft loss. Transplant Proc 2002; 34: 2423–5.

Stigant CE, Cohen J, Vivera M, Zaltzman JS. ACE inhibitors and angiotensin II antagonists in renal transplantation: an analysis of safety and efficacy. Am J Kidney Dis 2000; 35: 58–63.

Stratton IM, Adler AI, Neil HA, et al. Association of glycaemia with macrovascular and microvascular complication of type 2 diabetes (UKPDS 35): prospective observational study. BMJ 2000; 321: 405–12.

Suliman ME, Qureshi AE, Barany P, et al. Hyperhomocysteinemia, nutritional status, and cardiovascular disease in hemodialysis patients. Kidney Int 2000; 57: 1727–35.

Sunder-Plassmann G, Floth A, Fodinger M. Hyperhomocysteinemia in organ transplantation. Curr Opin Urol 2000; 10: 89–94.

Sunder-Plassmann G, Fodinger M. Genetic determinants of the homocysteine level. Kidney Int 2003; 63 (Suppl 84): S141–4.

Suwelack B, Gerardt U, Hausberg M, et al. Comparison of quinapril versus atenolol: effects on blood pressure and cardiac mass after renal transplantation. Am J Cardiol 2000; 86: 583–5.

Taal MW, Brenner BM. Combination ACEI and ARB therapy: additional benefit in renoprotection. Curr Opin Nephrol Hypertens 2002; 11: 377–81.

Tamura K, Fujimura T, Tsutsumi T, et al. Transcriptional inhibition of insulin by FK506 and possible involvement of FK506 binding protein-12 in pancreatic beta-cell. Transplantation 1995; 59: 1606–13.

Tanne D, Haim M, Goldbourt U, et al. CD40 ligand and risk of ischemic stroke or coronary events in patients with chronic coronary heart disease. Int J Cardiol 2006; 107: 322–6.

Tonstad S, Holdaas H, Gorbitz C, Ose L. Is dietary intervention effective in post transplant hyperlipidemia? Nephrol Dial Transplant 1995; 10: 82–5.

Toole JF, Malinow MR, Chambless LE, et al. Lowering homocysteine in patients with ischemic stroke to prevent recurrent stroke, myocardial infarction, and death; the Vitamin Intervention for Stroke Prevention (VISP) randomized trial. JAMA 2004; 291: 565–75.

Turk T, Pietruck F, Dolff S, et al. Repaglinide in the management of new-onset diabetes mellitus after renal transplantation. Am J Transplant 2006; 6: 842–6.

Tyden G, Bolinder J, Solders G, et al. Improved survival in patients with insulin-dependent diabetes mellitus and end-stage diabetic nephropathy 10 years after combined pancreas and kidney transplantation. Transplantation 1999; 67: 645–8.

van der Heide JJ, Bilo HJ, Donker JM, et al. Effect of dietary fish oil on renal function and rejection in cyclosporine-treated recipients of renal transplants. N Engl J Med 1993; 329: 769–73.

Van Duijnhoven EM, Cristiaans MHL, Boots JMM, et al. Glucose metabolism in the first 3 years after renal transplantation in patients receiving tacrolimus versus cyclosporine-based immunosupression. J Am Soc Nephrol 2002; 13: 213.

van Guldener C, Robinson K. Homocysteine and renal disease. Semin Thromb Hemost 2000; 26: 313–24.

Vanholder R, Massy Z, Argiles A, et al. Chronic kidney disease as cause of cardiovascular morbidity and mortality. Nephrol Dial Transplant 2005; 20: 1048–56.

Vanrenterghem Y, Ponticelli C, Morales J, et al. Prevalence and management of anemia in renal transplant recipients: a European Survey. Am J Transplant 2003; 3: 835–45.

Van Ypersele de Strihou C, Pochet JM. Hypertension in the transplant patient. In Cameron JS, Davison AM, Kerr D, et al., eds. Oxford Textbook of Clinical Nephrology. Oxford: Oxford University Press, 1992; 1594–602.

Varghese Z, Fernando RL, Turakhia G, et al. Calcineurin inhibitors enhance low-density lipoprotein oxidation in transplant patients. Kidney Int 1999; 56 (Suppl 71): S137–40.

Varo N, de Lemos JA, Libby P, et al. Soluble CD40 risk prediction after acute coronary syndrome. Circulation 2003; 108: 1049–52.

Viberti G. Diabetes mellitus: a major challenge in transplantation. Transplant Proc 2001; 33 (Suppl 5A): 3S–7S.

Villanueva G, Baldwin D. Rosiglitazone therapy of posttransplant diabetes mellitus. Transplantation 2005; 80: 1402–5.

Vinals F, Chambard JC, Pouyssegur J. p70 S6 kinase-mediated protein synthesis is a critical step for vascular endothelial cell proliferation. J Biol Chem 1999; 274: 26776–82.

Voiculescu A, Schmitz M, Hollenbeck M, et al. Management of arterial stenosis affecting kidney graft perfusion: a single-centre study in 53 patients. Am J Transplant 2005; 5: 1731–8.

Weir M. Impact of immunosuppressive regimens on post-transplant diabetes mellitus. Transplant Proc 2001; 33 (Suppl 5A): 23S–6S.

Wheeler DC, Steiger J. Evolution and etiology of cardiovascular disease in renal transplant recipients. Transplantation 2000; 70 (Suppl): SS41–5.

Winkelmayer WC, Lorenz M, Kramar R, et al. Percentage of hypochromic cells is an independent risk factor for mortality in kidney transplant recipients. Am J Transplant 2004; 12: 2075–81.

Wissing KM, Abramowicz D, Broeders N, Vereerstraeten P. Hypercholesterolemia is associated with increased kidney graft loss caused by chronic rejection in male patients with previous acute rejection. Transplantation 2000; 70: 464–72.

Wong YT, Del-Rio-Martin J, Jaques B, et al. Audit of diabetes in a renal transplant population. Transplant Proc 2005; 37: 3283–5.

Yan LL, Daviglus ML, Liu K, et al. Midlife body mass index and hospitalization and mortality in older age. JAMA 2006; 295: 190–8.

Yusuf S, Sleight P, Pogue J, et al. Effects of an angiotensin–converting-enzyme inhibitor, ramipril, on cardiovascular events in high–risk patients. The Heart Outcomes Prevention Evaluation Study Investigators. N Engl J Med 2000; 342: 145–53.

Zoccali C, Tripepi C, Mallamaci F. Predictors of cardiac death in ESRD. Semin Nephrol 2005; 25: 358–62.

Zoccali C, Mallamaci F. Homocysteine and risk in end-stage renal disease: a matter of context. Kidney Int 2006; 69: 204–6.

11 MALIGNANCY

Cancer represents a major cause of morbidity and mortality for renal transplant recipients. In Europe, the overall prevalence of cancer after renal transplantation is between 20 and 30% at 10 years, and can reach 40% at 20 years (Berhoux et al., 2002). In the USA, the adjusted death rate from cancer for renal transplant patients is 1.4 per 1000 person-years (Ojo et al., 2000). In Australia and New Zealand, the cumulative risk of tumors other than those of the skin is 40% by 30 years after transplantation, whereas 75% of renal allograft recipients have skin cancer (Sheil, 2002).

After transplantation, a pre-existing tumor may recur, or cancer may be transmitted by the donor organ. However, the main category of cancer is that which develops *de novo* following a kidney transplant.

Pre-existing cancers

One of the major problems for transplant clinicians is to assess the degree of risk associated with a previous history of cancer in a kidney transplant candidate. In many cases there is no relationship between cancer and the development of renal failure, but a number of patients enter end-stage renal failure either as a consequence of nephrotoxic antineoplastic treatments or because they were affected by renal carcinomas. Moreover, the risk of cancer is higher in dialysis patients than in the general population (Maisonneuve et al., 1999), cancer of the kidney and bladder being the most frequent in dialysis patients. The excess risk might be attributed to underlying renal or urinary tract disease, or the effect of loss of renal function on the kidney and bladder, and to the increased susceptibility to viral carcinogenesis.

Some 10 years ago, the Cincinnati Transplant Tumor Registry (CTTR) reported a *recurrence rate* of 21% in 1297 renal transplant recipients with cancer treated before transplantation (Penn, 1997a). However, more recent data from the Organ Procurement and Transplantation Network/United Network for Organ Sharing (OPTN/UNOS) reported a smaller number of recurrent malignancies, 106 in 1358 (7.8%) kidney transplant recipients with a history of previous cancer (Kauffman et al., 2005a).

The risk of recurrence is related to a number of factors (Table 11.1). Generally speaking, factors contributing to low recurrence rates are a *favorable histology* (in situ carcinomas or low-grade malignancy), *small sized* tumors, and a *long time* interval between treatment of the malignancy and transplantation. The *type* of cancer is also important.

The prognosis of *renal carcinomas* depends on tumor stage, morphologic features, histologic grade, and the type and histologic pattern of tumor cells (Cohen and McGovern, 2005). Greatly different is the risk of post-transplant recurrence between symptomatic and incidental renal carcinomas. The CTTR registry reported a recurrence rate of 23% in patients who had received nephrectomy before transplantation, while of 70 patients with incidental renal carcinomas, discovered on a work-up or nephrectomy for unrelated reasons, none had a recurrence after transplantation (Penn, 1997a). There is no evidence that the waiting time may influence the risk of recurrence after transplantation (Hanaway et al., 2005).

Bladder carcinoma has a cumulative risk of recurrence of 15%, the risk being low for patients with localized mucosal bladder tumors. Although a prolonged waiting time does not decrease the risk for recurrence (Hanaway et al., 2005), a waiting time of 2 years for patients with T3–T4 carcinoma may be advisable.

Endometrial tumors of stage I, well differentiated, and with a proliferation depth of less than half that of the myometrium are at low risk of recurrence in women younger than 45 years (Pellerin and Finan, 2005). The risk of recurrence in postmenopausal women also depends on whether the cancer is

Table 11.1   Factors influencing the risk of post-transplant recurrence of pre-existing tumors

Litlle risk of recurrence	High risk of recurrence
In situ cancer	Widespread cancer
Low-grade malignancy at histology	High-grade malignancy at histology
Small size of tumor	Size >5 cm
Long interval between tumor discovery and transplantation	Short interval between tumor discovery and transplantation
Incidental tumors	Lung, breast, prostate, intestine
Non-melanoma skin cancer	Myeloma, lymphoma

estrogen-correlated or not (Marchetti *et al.*, 2005). *In situ cervical squamous* or *adenocarcinomas* are also considered to have a low risk of recurrence, although these tumors still carry some risk of mortality (Sherman *et al.*, 2005).

The risk of recurrence for seminoma or non-seminoma tumors of the *testis* is also low, being, respectively, 3.4% and 7.4% when patients are transplanted after an interval of at least 2 years, and 0.26% and 3.3% when the interval exceeds 5 years (Kauffman *et al.*, 2005a).

Papillary thyroid carcinoma usually has a favorable prognosis. Although recurrence can occur even after many years, the low recurrence rate and mortality associated with this disease do not justify a mandatory waiting time (Hanaway *et al.*, 2005).

There is a high risk of late recurrence for *lung cancer*, *breast cancer*, and *myeloma*. These patients should be carefully monitored even years after transplantation. Localized *carcinoma of the prostate* may recur in about 12% of cases after transplantation (Penn, 1997a). Regular measurement of prostate-specific antigen and ultrasonography are recommended in these patients. *Hodgkin's lymphoma* and *non-Hodgkin's lymphoma* have a rate of recurrence of 9% and 11%, respectively (Troffe *et al.*, 2004). Other reports, however, reported no case of recurrence in patients who lost their first transplant because of lymphoma and who were retransplanted after an appropriate disease-free interval (Karras *et al.*, 2004). It is to be pointed out, however, that some cases of post-transplant lymphoproliferative disorders were probably infectious complications associated with Epstein–Barr virus rather than true malignant complications (Hanaway *et al.*, 2005).

Non-melanoma skin cancer may have a high risk of recurrence after transplantation, particularly in patients living in sunny areas. However, this is not considered a contraindication to transplantation, in view of the possibility of early diagnosis and eradication of these tumors. *Melanoma* may recur in 10–19% of cases after transplantation. The mortality after recurrence is very high (Penn, 1996; Chapman *et al.*, 2001).

In summary, patients with a pre-existing cancer are at variable risk of recurrence after transplantation. For cancers with a higher recurrence rate, a waiting period of at least 5 years before transplantation is recommended, due to the possibility that immunosuppression may stimulate the growth of dormant metastases. Moreover, as it has been demonstrated in the general population (Dong and Hemminki, 2001), it is likely that also transplant recipients with pre-existing cancer are more susceptible to the development of *de novo* cancer. For these reasons, careful monitoring of these patients is highly recommended, particularly in the long term. The choice of immunosuppressive therapy should take into account the possibility of avoiding or minimizing the use of powerful biological reagents and calcineurin inhibitors that may favor the onset of tumors. There is mounting evidence that mTOR (mammalian target of rapamycin) inhibitors may have antiangiogenic activity (Guba *et al.*, 2002) and may interfere with the proliferation of cancer cells, especially in the presence of an overactivity of phosphatidylinositol

3 kinase (PI3k) or of a loss of PTEN, the physiologic suppressor of the PI3k-driven cascade of kinases (Brennan *et al.*, 2002; Ponticelli, 2004). On the basis of their properties, both sirolimus and everolimus are now used for adjuvant therapy of a number of cancers in the general population. While waiting for these results, it is of note that a significant reduction of the incidence of tumors in renal transplant recipients has been reported after the introduction of mTOR inhibitors (Kauffman *et al.*, 2005b; Campistol *et al.*, 2006).

Transmission of cancer from donors

Organ donation may involve the risk of transmitting malignancy (Penn, 1997b). A report investigated the risk of donor-related malignancies in patients transplanted between 1994 and 2001 in the USA. The cadaveric donor-related tumor rate was 0.04% (14 of 34 .993), with a mortality rate of 46% (Kauffman *et al.*, 2002).

Renal carcinomas have high rates of transmission and of distant metastases. However, survival has been reported in a few recipients in whom malignancy was confined to the renal graft or the immediate surroundings (Sheil, 2001). In these cases, prompt identification and excision of the lesion at the time of surgery allowed no recurrence of malignancy after a mean follow-up of 79 months. Allograft nephrectomy, discontinuation of immunosuppression, and local radiation therapy gave good results in most cases of local spread of tumor, while 67% of recipients with widespread metastases died of cancer and only 27% of them had complete remission following treatment.

Malignant *melanomas* and *choriocarcinomas* are the most dangerous donor neoplasms, with high rates of distant metastases and mortality in the recipient. The measurement of β-human chorionic gonadotropin is useful in order to exclude the presence of choriocarcinomas in female donors with menstrual irregularities following pregnancy or abortion.

Donors with primary *brain tumors* have been accepted in the past because of the rarity of extra-renal spread. However, more recent experience has shown the possibility of metastasis for brain tumors not only in the presence of risk factors such as cell type, grade of tumor, history of craniotomy, and presence of shunts, but even in the absence of risk factors (Detry *et al.*, 2000). For this reason, donors with intracranial bleeding, but no evidence of hypertension, intracranial aneurysm, or arteriovenous malformation, should be carefully screened in order to exclude the presence of occult primary neoplasias.

Error in the diagnosis of donor brain-death due to brain tumors has significant and often fatal consequences. A donor-related transmission rate of 74% was identified among donors with a misdiagnosed brain death. Sixty-four per cent of recipients suffered diffuse metastatic disease. The overall survival was poor, with a 5-year survival rate of 32% (Buell *et al.*, 2005).

Transmission of *HHV-8 virus* from the donor, with a potential risk of Kaposi's sarcoma for the recipient, has also been demonstrated (Regamey *et al.*, 1998).

De novo cancers

Epidemiology

Immunosuppressed transplant recipients have a 3–4-fold increased risk of developing tumors (Penn, 2000), but the risk of developing certain cancers is increased several hundred-fold. Non-Hodgkin's lymphoma, Kaposi's sarcoma, and carcinoma of the kidney, liver, skin, lip, vulva, and perineum are much more frequent among transplant recipients, with an incidence varying from 6 to 0.5% (Table 11.2).

Compared with the general population, after renal transplantation, the risk of developing Kaposi's sarcoma increases by 400–1000 times, vulvar and anal carcinoma by 100 times, non-Hodgkin's lymphoma by 28–49 times, hepatocellular carcinoma by 20–38 times, and labial carcinoma by 29 times. The risk of *in situ* cervical uterine carcinoma increases from 3.3 (Fairley *et al.*, 1994) to 16 times (Penn, 1990), while that of renal carcinoma increases by 30–40 times (Penn, 1998a). Skin and lip cancers account for 36–46% of total cancers (Penn, 1998a; Montagnino *et al.*, 1996), and are even more frequent in sunny countries (Sheil, 2001). However, some neoplasias that are common among the general population

Table 11.2 Comparison between the incidence of cancer in renal transplant recipients and in the general population

Higher incidence
    Kaposi's sarcoma (400–1000 times)
    Skin carcinomas (100 times)
    Vulvar, anal carcinomas (100 times)
    Non-Hodgkin's lymphoma (28–49 times)
    Hepatic carcinoma (20–38 times)
    Labial carcinoma (29 times)
    Renal carcinoma (8.9 times)

Lower incidence (?)
    Breast carcinoma
    Prostate carcinoma
    Lung carcinoma
    Colon carcinoma
    Bladder carcinoma
    Uterus carcinoma
    Rectum carcinoma

(carcinoma of the prostate, breast, lung, colon, rectum, bladder, and uterus) showed a lower incidence among transplant recipients in the CCTR registry (Penn, 1996). These data are at odds with those of two other major registries, the Nordic Renal Transplant Registry (NRTR) (Birkeland *et al.*, 1995) and the Australia/New Zealand Transplant Registry (ANZTR) (Sheil, 2002), showing an increased incidence of nearly all types of cancers in renal transplant recipients. This might be explained by differences in the studied population, differences in the criteria for cancer inclusion, and differences in the average age of patients at transplantation (Penn, 1999).

Etiopathogenesis

Several factors may favor the development of post-transplant cancer (Table 11.3).

Immunosuppressive therapy

Immunosuppressive therapy is one of the most important causative factors. The risk of tumor is clearly related to the intensity of immunosuppression, while there is no evidence that immunosuppressive drugs exert a specific oncogenic effect (Birkeland and Hamilton-Dutoit, 2003).

    Calcineurn inhibitors (CNI) can promote cancer progression by interfering with immunesurveillance and with antiviral activity. CNI may also exert a direct cell-autonomous effect via transforming growth factor-β (TGFβ) stimulation, independent of its effect on the host's immune system (Hojo *et al.*, 1999). Some studies found no difference in the incidence of neoplasia between transplant patients treated with *azathioprine* (Aza) and those treated with cyclosporine (CsA), at least up to 10 years (Penn, 1990; London *et al.*, 1995; Montagnino *et al.*, 1996), while other studies found an increased incidence of cancer in the CsA era (Tremblay *et al.*, 2002). In particular, Kaposi's sarcoma is 400–500 times more frequent among graft recipients treated with Aza and steroids than in the general population (Harwood *et al.*, 1979), and about 1000 times more frequent among CsA-treated renal transplant recipients (Cockburn and Krupp, 1989). Neoplasias tend to develop after a relatively short period of time in transplanted patients treated with CsA, on average 60–67 months after transplantation (Penn, 1986; Montagnino *et al.*, 1996). Kaposi's

Table 11.3 Risk factors for the development of post-transplant cancer

Immunosuppressive therapy
Transplant duration
Viral infections
Age
Duration of uremia
Chronic antigenic stimuli
Genetic predisposition
Previous malignancy
Environment
Ethnicity

sarcoma and lymphoma have the shortest mean time of appearance (21 and 33 months, respectively) while hepatobiliary and vulvar/perineal carcinoma have the longest (82 and 112 months, respectively) (Penn, 1996). The incidence of post-transplant lymphoproliferative disorders (PTLD) seems to be disturbingly higher in the series from the USA. This difference is probably accounted for by the large use of sequential immunosuppression with *antilymphocyte antibodies* in the USA (Bustami *et al.*, 2004), while sequential immunosuppression is used more rarely in Europe (London *et al.*, 1995). Once again, it seems that this effect is related to the more powerful immunosuppression caused by these agents rather than to a specific oncogenic effect (Opelz and Dohler, 2004). Indirect confirmations of the role played by the intensity of immunosuppression are given by the observation that patients who received pre-dialysis immunosuppression were at increased risk for cancer after transplantation (Hibberd *et al.*, 2002), and by the CTS (Collaborative Transplant Study) data showing a higher incidence of cancer in heart and lung transplant recipients, who usually receive stronger immunosuppression (Figure 11.1). On the other hand, a large cohort study showed that *mycophenolate mofetil* (MMF) is not associated with an increased risk of lymphoma or other malignancies post-renal transplant, and may even be associated with a lower risk in some populations (Robson *et al.*, 2005). The *mTOR inhibitors*, sirolimus and everolimus, might exert a protective effect against cancer. Indeed, mTOR acts as a sensor of mytogenic stimuli regulating cellular growth and division. Thus, mTOR is potentially an attractive target for molecular-targeted treatment (Houghton and Huang, 2004). Kauffmann *et al.* (2005a) reviewed the data for 33 249 patients who received a cadaver renal transplant from July 1996 to December 2001. Data were censored at 963 days to allow comparable follow-up time among drug treatment groups. The incidence rates of any *de novo* post-transplant malignancy were 0.60% with sirolimus/everolimus, given either alone or in combination with CNI, and 1.81% with cyclosporine/tacrolimus, the difference being significant. The rates of a *de novo* solid tumor were 0%, 0.47%, and 1.00%, respectively. The relative risk associated with sirolimus/everolimus immunosuppression for any *de novo* cancer was 0.39, and for *de novo* solid cancer was 0.44. In another review, Campistol *et al.* (2006) reported a lower risk of skin and non-skin malignancies at 5 years after renal transplantation in patients who withdrew cyclosporine after 3 months while continuing with sirolimus, compared with those who received sirolimus combined with cyclosporine.

Transplant duration

Post-transplant neoplasias increase with time, as shown by all the registries. This can be explained by the length of continuous antigenic stimulation, by the natural aging process of the grafted population, and/or by the increased time of exposure to immunosuppressive agents and viral pathogens. An important role is played by prolonged exposure to the sun, which accounts for the extremely high incidence of skin tumors in long-term transplanted patients living in sunny countries (Sheil, 2002).

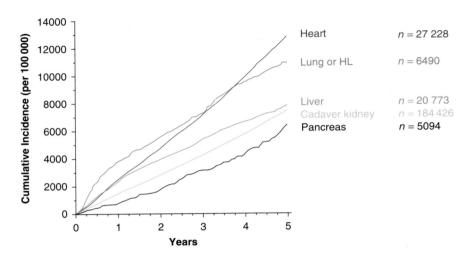

Figure 11.1 Increasing risk of cancer with time: all types of malignant tumors. Heart and lung transplant recipients who are usually given stronger immunosuppression have an increased risk of developing cancer. From CTS, Collaborative Transplant Study. E-51109-0205

Viral infections

Viral infections can favor neoplastic tissue development and can be involved in a number of different types of cancer (Table 11.4). At least 15% of all cancers are associated with viral infections (zur Hausen, 1991). Human papilloma virus (HPV) has been implicated in skin, oropharynx, esophagus, uterine, anal, and bladder cancers (Daneshpouy et al., 2001; Boukamp, 2005; Patel et al., 2005). Epstein–Barr virus (EBV) is the main etiologic agent in the genesis of post-transplant lymphoproliferative diseases (Ho et al., 1988). The role of hepatitis viruses B and C in hepatocellular carcinoma is well recognized. Finally, human herpes virus 8 (HHV-8) has been found by polymerase chain reaction (PCR) in all forms of Kaposi's sarcoma (Shalling et al., 1995; Sarid et al., 2002).

Potential mechanisms that may trigger cell proliferation may derive from apoptosis, oncogenes, and mutations in tumor suppressor genes. It has been suggested that *apoptosis* is a protective host response to eliminate virus-infected cells. Some viruses (such as cytomegalovirus and EBV) can modulate apoptosis by inhibition, thus allowing the virus to complete its replication cycle before the cell dies. Bcl-2 proto-oncogene, which regulates the effector phase of apoptosis and positively promotes cell proliferation, is strongly expressed in patients with PTLD (Chetty et al., 1996). *Oncogenes* can interact with tumorigenesis, for example TP53, which encodes p53, a protein that regulates progression of the cell cycle in the G_1–S stage. *Mutations* in suppressor genes may also play an oncogenic role. In the absence of mutations, p53 behaves as an oncosuppressor gene. However, if mutations occur, as has been documented in most Burkitt's lymphomas (Cherney et al., 1997) as well as in cutaneous lesions (Gibson et al., 1997), p53 becomes a dominant oncogene. Normal cells with DNA damage show an upregulation of p53 and stop at this stage for repair, while cells with mutant p53 let damaged DNA proceed, leaving random oncogenetic changes to occur (Fisher, 1994). Some oncogenic adenoviruses and human papilloma viruses produce proteins capable of downregulating p53 protein. Another major oncogenic factor is represented by late membrane protein, which is encoded by EBV (Lu et al., 2005).

Besides viruses, attention has also been focused on other microbial agents such as *Helicobacter pylori*, which might be implicated in the induction of lymphomas associated with the gastric mucosa (Hsi et al., 2000; Aull et al., 2003).

Table 11.4 Etiologic role of viruses in post-transplant cancers

Cancer	Virus
Lymphoma	Epstein–Barr virus, CMV (?)
Kaposi's sarcoma	Human herpes virus 8
Vulva, perineum carcinoma	Human papilloma virus
Liver carcinoma	Hepatitis B and C virus
Oropharynx, esophagus carcinoma	Human papilloma virus
Bladder carcinoma	Human papilloma virus
Leukemia	HTLV 1 and 2
Cervix carcinoma	Human papilloma virus
Skin cancer	Human papilloma virus

Age

Age is a well-known predisposing factor to cancer. Together with heart disease and stroke, cancer accounts for 75% of all deaths among the elderly general population. Aging is characterized by reduced reparative cell proliferation and DNA repair after exposure to environmental factors, such as ultraviolet radiation (Wei et al., 1993). Moreover, the longer is the exposure to oncogenic factors (iatrogenic and viral), the higher is the probability of developing a neoplasia.

Duration of uremia

Another possible predisposing role for cancer development may be played by the prolonged uremic status before transplantation. Bladder and kidney cancers are particularly frequent in dialysis patients (Stewart et al., 2003), and are more frequent in patients with a long duration of renal disease (Peces et al., 2004). Some tumors, such as hepatic, thyroid, or colon adenocarcinomas, are as frequent among dialysis patients as in the transplanted population (Brunner et al., 1995), and other malignancies also, such as anogenital cancers, seem to have a similar incidence among dialysis patients and transplant recipients (Fairley et al., 1994). There are a number of possible predisposing factors for the development of tumors in patients with end-stage renal disease: (1) uremia, which may be considered a state of immune deficiency; (2) a possible linkage between kidney disease and the risk of cancer (Birkeland, 1998); (3) previous immunosuppression used to treat many kidney diseases such as primary glomerulonephritis, lupus nephritis, vasculitis, mixed connective tissue diseases, etc.; (4) impaired DNA repair mechanisms and reduced antioxidant defense (Vamvakas et al., 1998); and (5) the prolonged use of potentially oncogenic drugs, such as analgesic drugs (Stewart et al., 2003).

Chronic antigenic stimulation

Chronic antigenic stimulation by the foreign allograft coupled with inadequate cytotoxic T cell activity caused by concomitant immunosuppressive therapy may represent an important cause of neoplastic tissue development. It has been proposed that host–donor microchimerism might favor lymphoma development (Nalesnik and Starzl, 1997), and that microchimerism might be one explanation for the preferential occurrence of malignancies in the transplanted graft itself, arising from donor cells (Goldstein et al., 1996). An alternative pathogenetic role for the local effect of cytokines or other tumor-promoting interactions at the site of the grafted organ is also possible.

Genetic predisposition

It is well known that some tumors may have a genetic predisposition. In organ transplant recipients, HLA antigens, such as B27 and DR7, have been found to be associated with a higher incidence of skin cancer (Bouwes-Bavinck et al., 1991). Interleukin-10 promoter polymorphisms can increase the susceptibility to squamous-cell skin cancer in renal transplant recipients (Alamartine *et al.*, 2003). Five of eight renal transplant patients who developed Kaposi's sarcoma harbored either genetic or antigenic markers of their matched donors (Barozzi *et al.*, 2003). In transplant patients living in Cape Town, squamous-cell cancer and basal-cell cancer of the skin were the most common cancers in white patients, while no case occurred in non-white patients. On the other hand, Kaposi's sarcoma was the most common cancer in non-white renal allograft recipients, in whom it accounted for almost 80% of all cancers (Moosa, 2005). Taken together, these data suggest that genetic factors are important determinants of cancer development after renal transplantation.

Previous malignancy

The incidence of *de novo* transplant malignancies is significantly higher for patients with a positive previous malignancy. According to the OPTN/UNOS database, *de novo* tumors developed in 7.8% of deceased donor transplant recipients with a history of previous malignancy and in 2.8% of patients reporting no previous malignancy (Kauffman *et al.*, 2005).

Environment

A clear example of the importance of the environment is given by skin tumors, which are by far more frequent in sunny countries.

Ethnicity

Some tumors, such as Kaposi's sarcoma, have a racial distribution, and are frequently reported in Arabic, Jewish, and Mediterranean populations (Qunibi *et al.*, 1988; Montagnino *et al.*, 1994), while papers from large series of renal transplant recipients from Northern countries reported either exceptional (Odajnyk and Muggia, 1985) or no cases of Kaposi's sarcoma (Vogt *et al.*, 1990). This difference may be accounted for by different ethnicity. However, environmental factors might be equally important in the induction of Kaposi's sarcoma, since its increased incidence among Mediterranean transplant recipients might be related to the increased incidence of HHV-8 infection in these populations.

Lymphoproliferative disorders

Malignant lymphomas are neoplastic transformations of cells resident in lymphoid tissues. The two major variants of lymphoma are non-Hodgkin's lymphoma (NHL) and Hodgkin's disease. NHL is the second most common malignancy in renal transplant patients after skin and lip cancers (Penn, 1998b), while Hodgkin's disease is only slightly more common in transplanted patients than in the general population (Birkeland *et al.*, 1995; Caillard *et al.*, 2006).

The *incidence* of PTLD in adult renal transplant recipients ranges between 1.3 (Leblond *et al.*, 1995) and 14% (Wasson *et al.*, 2006). About 85% of PTLD are represented by B-cell lymphoma and express CD20, while T-cell lymphoma and Hodgkin's disease are more rare. An American survey reported an almost doubled risk of PTLD in renal transplant recipients treated with antilymphocyte antibodies (Bustami *et al.*, 2004). Opelz *et al.* (2006) also reported that the standardized incidence ratio of lymphoma compared with a similar non-transplant population was more than 20 for patients who received induction with antithymocyte globulins, and 9.4 for patients with no induction. The highest rate of PTLD is in the first 12–24 months (Faull *et al.*, 2005; Smith *et al.*, 2006). In the Australia/New Zealand register there was another cluster of PTLD, 5–10 years after transplantation (Faull *et al.*, 2005).

B-cell lymphomas

Pathogenesis

Most PTLD are B-cell lymphomas caused by *Epstein–Barr virus* (EBV), which is generally of recipient origin (Gulley *et al.*, 2003). B cells acutely infected by EBV express about 90 transformation-associated viral genes, which may serve as targets for the immune system. Acute infection is kept under control by natural killer (NK) cells and by EBV-specific CD4+ or CD8+ cytotoxic T lymphocytes (CTL). In healthy subjects, very few B lymphocytes harbor EBV DNA. This pool is maintained in part by a lytic infection cycle, which

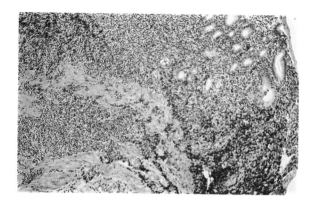

Figure 11.2 Marginal zone extranodal lymphoma (MALT-associated) localized to the antral gastric region. Observe the infiltration through the muscolaris mucosae (Courtsey of Professor R. Buffa, University of Milan.)

provides virus for the infection of new cells (Campe *et al.*, 2003). Latently infected B cells express only a limited number of genes: EBV nuclear antigen-1 (EBNA-1) and latent membrane protein 2 (LMP-2). This restricted gene expression is a mechanism through which the virus evades host responses. Moreover, EBNA-1 is required for the viral DNA to maintain itself in actively dividing lymphocytes and can reduce the surface expression of MHC class I and adhesion molecules, while LMP-2 allows the virus to limit its gene expression in the latency phase (Cohen, 1997). These latently infected B lymphocytes are immortalized through the production of an EBV-encoded gene, BCRF1, which has more than 80% amino acid identity with IL-10 (Moore *et al.*, 1990), which inhibits the synthesis of interferon-γ (IFNγ) by lymphocytes and NK cells. The inhibition of IFNγ can favor the outgrowth of EBV-transformed B cells. Moreover, EBV generates a polypeptide analogous in structure and bioactivity to interleukin-10. This cytokine has been suggested to have an important role in EBV-induced PTLD and graft tolerance by inducing anergy to donor-specific alloantigens through its suppressive effects on macrophage and T lymphocyte functions (Birkeland *et al.*, 1999). All these factors impair the ability of the immune system to eliminate the virus, and lead to the development of polyclonal polymorphic hyperplasia that may evolve into a more malignant monoclonal tumor. Moreover, LMP-1 acts as an oncogene. It binds to several tumor-necrosis-factor receptors, and this results in the activation of nuclear factor-κB transcription, upregulation of cellular adhesion molecules, cytokine production, and B-cell proliferation. Finally, LMP-1 encodes at least two proteins that inhibit apoptosis, bcl-2 and delta20 (Kulwichit *et al.*, 1998).

Of interest, the incidence of PTLD is increased 7–10-fold in patients who have had symptomatic *cytomegalovirus* (CMV) disease. In addition, EBV replication is regularly observed in patients with CMV infection (Tolkoff-Rubin and Rubin, 1998).

Bacterial infections caused by *Helicobacter pylori* or *Campylobacter jejuni* may be associated with a particular type of PTLD named mucosa-associated lymphoid tissue lymphoma, or *MALToma* (Figure 11.2). In the gastric form, CD4+ T cells that encounter *H. pylori* antigens stimulate the proliferation of neoplastic B cells which differentiate into mature plasma cells (Parsonnet and Isaacson, 2004). In immunoproliferatve small intestinal disease, in response to *C. jejuni*, lymphoma cells synthesize α heavy chains (Lecuit *et al.*, 2004; Parsonnet and Isaacson, 2004). MALToma may occur in kidney transplant recipients, and is usually less aggressive than other PTLD (Hsi *et al.*, 2000).

In *CsA-treated* patients, the incidence of PTLD is related to the dose of CsA (Gaya *et al.*, 1995). While the risk of PTLD development with *tacrolimus* seems to be comparable to that observed with CsA in some series (Armitage *et al.*, 1993), Opelz and Dohler, 2004) reported that treatment with tacrolimus increased the risk by approximately two-fold. Theoretically, the use of *sirolimus* or *everolimus*, which inhibit IL-10 signal transduction and the growth of EBV-cell lymphoma (Majewski *et al.*, 2000; Nepomuceno *et al.*, 2003), should reduce the risk of PTLD.

A peculiar feature of PTLD is the high incidence in the *pediatric population*, where PTLD represent 53% of malignancies, while in adults, PTLD represent 15% of neoplasias (Penn, 1998b). The increased

Table 11.5 Main clinical characteristics of post-transplant lymphoproliferative disorders

Cellular derivation	85% B cell
	12–14% T cell
Classification	Polymorphic diffuse B-cell hyperplasia
	Polyclonal polymorphic B-cell lymphoma
	Monoclonal polymorphic B-cell lymphoma
General symptoms	Fever, nightly sweating, weight loss, anemia
Localized signs	Uncommon, but lymphadenopathy frequent
Extranodal disease	Common
Gastrointestinal	47–53%
Renal	12–23%
Pulmonary	15–38%
Central nervous system	12%
Skin	Uncommon
Bone	Uncommon
Hepatosplenic	Uncommon

incidence of PTLD in the pediatric population has been attributed to the higher rate of primary EBV infection after transplantation (Dror *et al.*, 1999), and to the higher amount of lymphoid tissue than in adults.

Clinical presentation

The clinical presentation is variable (Table 11.5). In some cases, lymphoma presents as a benign infectious *mononucleosis-like* syndrome. Sometimes the patient complains of *fever, night sweats,* and *weight loss* greater than 10% of body weight. In other cases, the presentation is *dramatic*, because of intestinal perforation. The development of PTLD may be preceded by the appearance of a monoclonal immunoglobulin peak. On the other hand, most kidney transplant recipients showing monoclonal peaks did not develop any PTLD after years of follow-up (Radl *et al.*, 1985).

Post-transplant lymphoproliferative diseases may involve *multiple organs* in about half of cases, or cause *extranodal masses* with a higher extranodal involvement than in the general population (Penn and First, 1986). About 70% of PTLD occur in *extranodal* localizations (Bates *et al.*, 2003), particularly in the gastrointestinal system, in the kidney, in the central nervous system, or in the lungs (Figure 11.3). Some 10% of PTLD present with gastrointestinal symptoms (Nash *et al.*, 2000). A frequent localization is in the small intestine. A particular type of mucosa-associated lymphoid tissue (MALT) gastric lymphoma can develop in carriers of *H. pylori*. In 12–23% of cases the kidney is affected by lymphomatous cells, which may cause acute renal failure. Kidney biopsy can allow early diagnosis in these cases (Tornroth *et al.*, 2003). Central nervous system involvement is associated with lymphoid infiltration in other organs in 10–15% of cases, while in 12–14% of cases the brain is the only involved site, versus a 1–2% prevalence of unique central nervous system localization in the general population. The differential diagnosis from cerebral abscesses may be difficult in the case of an isolated cerebral lymphoma (Snanoudj *et al.*, 2003).

Classification

Most PTLD cells observed in patients with solid organ allografts are of host origin. Morphologic classification has defined three main features for PTLD (Table 11.6).

Polymorphic diffuse B-cell hyperplasia, which prevalently invades the oropharynx and lymph nodes. It is characterized by the presence of differentiated plasmacytes and by the absence of atypia or necrosis;

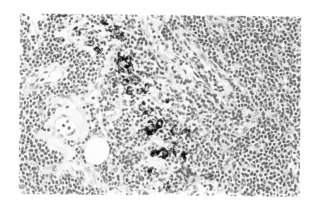

Figure 11.3 Low-grade, non-Hodgkin's B lymphoma in lung parenchyma. The general architecture is completely substituted by proliferation of lymphoid infiltrate. (Courtesy of Professor R. Buffa, University of Milan.)

Table 11.6 Categories of post-transplant lymphoproliferative disorders

Polymorphic diffuse B-cell hyperplasia (retention of the underlying architecture)
Affects mostly children and adolescents
Develops shortly after transplantation
Is polyclonal
Multiple EBV infections
Good prognosis
Often regresses after stopping immunosuppression

Polyclonal polymorphic B-cell lymphomas (obliteration of the underlying architecture)
Extranodal diffusion
Mean age 40 years
Develops shortly after transplantation
Polyclonal or monoclonal
Single EBV infection

Monoclonal polymorphic B-cell lymphomas (architecture similar to usual lymphoma)
Frequent in lymph nodes, but also extranodal
Mean age 55 years
Develops late after transplantation
Always monoclonal
Single EBV infection

polyclonal polymorphic B-cell lymphomas, which may arise in lymph nodes or various extranodal sites, are characterized by nuclear atypia of the large cells and extensive necrosis; *monoclonal polymorphic B cell lymphomas* or *immunoblastic lymphomas* are characterized by a disseminated disease, are monoclonal, and present one or more alterations of oncogene or tumor suppressor genes. While polymorphic lesions may be polyclonal, monomorphic lesions are always monoclonal (Knowles *et al.*, 1995; Whiting and Hanto, 1998), although this view has been challenged (Dror *et al.*, 1999).

The Society of Hematopathology (Harris *et al.*, 1997) suggested that patients with PTLD should be investigated for the *clonality* of lymphoproliferation through cell typing of surface and cytoplasmic

Table 11.7   Categories of post-transplant lymphoproliferative disorders according to the Society for Hematopathology Workshop (Harris et al., 1997)

Early lesions
  Reactive plasmacytic hyperplasia
  Infectious mononuclesis-like

Polymorphic PTLD
  Polyclonal
  Monoclonal

Monomorphic PTLD
  B cell lymphoma
    diffuse large-cell lymphoma (immunoblastic, centroblastic, anaplastic)
    Burkitt's/Burkitt's-like lymphoma
  T cell lymphoma
    peripheral T cell lymphoma, unspecified type (usually large-cell)
    anaplastic large-cell lymphoma (T/null)
    other types (e.g. T/NK)

Other
  T cell-rich/Hodgkin's disease-like large B cell lymphoma
  Plasmacytoma-like
  Myeloma

immunoglobulins, cytogenetic analysis of metaphase preparations, and immunoglobulin gene rearrangement analysis by blot hybridization and analysis of tandem repeats of EBV genomes (Table 11.7). Clonality is an important prognostic factor, since polyclonal lesions respond better to treatment. Also, clonal cytogenetic abnormalities (gene rearrangements) revealed by metaphase examination of biopsy specimens (Hanto *et al.*, 1989) may disclose the malignant transformation of benign polyclonal B-cell proliferation into malignant monoclonal lymphoma. Recently, Timms *et al.* (2003) provided evidence that PTLD can arise from a broad range of target B cells and not only from the pool of antigen-selected memory cells that EBV colonizes in immunocompetent subjects. Thus, there seems not to be any barrier to the EBV-induced transformation of naive B cells *in vivo*. EBV may also infect cells with many replacement mutations in framework regions. These PTLD are less responsive to treatment, since B cells that survive non-productive rearrangements may evade T-cell control.

EBV PCR monitoring of PTLD patients has been reported to have a high specificity (100%) but a low sensitivity (39%). Therefore, its usefulness for screening is reduced. However, PCR may be helpful to monitor the clinical course and response to therapy in patients with PTLD (Tsai *et al.*, 2002).

T-cell lymphomas

T-cell lymphomas represent only 12–14% of lymphoproliferative disorders in renal transplant recipients. Most PTLD are αβ T-cell lymphomas. The percentage of T-cell PTLD induced by EBV ranges between 20% (Van Gorp *et al.*, 1994) and 38% (Dockrell *et al.*, 1998). Most tumors are peripheral T-cell lymphomas with extranodal presentation, and are monoclonal.

Etiopathogenesis

The role of EBV infection is less relevant for T-cell than for B-cell lymphomas. Prolonged *immunosuppression* may favor an impaired clearance of pathogens, which, in turn, provides excessive antigenic stimulation of T cells with the development of malignant clones. In this regard, it is to be noted that half of the T-cell PTLD in Japan had a proven human T-lymphotropic virus type 1 (HTLV-1) genome in the tumor tissue and seropositivity for HTLV-1 (Hoshida et al., 2002). *Mutations of the p53 gene* may also concur with the overgrowth of malignant clones, as they have been detected in most cases of T-cell PTLD together with mutations of other oncogenes, in contrast to what happens in T-cell lymphomas occurring in immunocompetent subjects (Hoshida et al., 2002). These mutations of the p53 gene may also account for the transition from polymorphic to monomorphic PTLD.

Clinical presentation

T-cell lymphomas usually occur late after transplantation (Hanson et al., 1997; Albalate et al., 1998). They are frequently extranodal and are clinically characterized by fever, anemia, thrombocytopenia, and neutropenia. Some patients present with non-specific symptoms, pancytopenia, and/or liver dysfunction, with no obvious lymphadenopathy. The course is aggressive with a poor prognosis (Rajakariar et al., 2004). In rare cases, T-cell PTLD may be associated with a hemophagocytic syndrome (Peeters et al., 1997). A few cases of $\gamma\delta$ T-cell lymphomas have also been reported in transplant patients, with either hepatosplenic or mucocutaneous involvement (Ross et al., 1994; Roncella et al., 2000).

Treatment

According to the European Best Practice Guidelines (Berthoux et al., 2002), the management of PTLD should start with *prophylaxis*. Heavy immosuppression should be avoided whenever possible. The use of powerful antilymphocyte antibodies should be discouraged in EBV-negative recipients and should not be prolonged in other cases. Blood EBD load should be monitored, and immunosuppressive therapy should be modulated accordingly. Polymorphic diffuse B-cell hyperplasia still seems to be dependent upon active viral replication. In this case, the use of acyclovir or valacyclovir, which inhibit EBV DNA replication, may be sufficient to treat the disease. However, acyclovir has no effect on the latent EBV genome in non-producer cell lines. EBV replication in these cells occurs only during host cell proliferation and depends on host DNA polymerase, and is presumably unaffected by acyclovir (Birkeland et al., 1999). Antiviral therapy directed against CMV may also be useful in view of the pathogenetic role of CMV infection (Table 11.8).

A *sequential treatment* approach has been suggested, according to the stage of the disease (Davis et al., 1998; Whiting and Hanto, 1998). In these cases, as well as in cases with cytogenetic abnormalities, massive *reduction* or *withdrawal of immunosuppression* is the first therapeutic step (Starzl et al., 1984; Swinnen et al., 1995). It has been recommended either to maintain only steroids or to decrease CNI by 50%, with cessation of azathioprine and mycophenolic acid (Berthoux et al., 2002). Treatment with acyclovir/valacyclovir or ganciclovir/valganciclovir may also be useful. The response is particularly good in low-risk patients (Tsai et al., 2001) and in patients with MALToma when minimization of immunosuppression is associated with the eradication of *H. pylori* (Aull et al., 2003) or *C. jejuni* (Lecuit et al., 2004) by antibiotic therapy.

A second step consists of the introduction of *interferon-α 2b*, which may increase the activity of cytotoxic T lymphocytes against EBV and may render B lymphoma cells susceptible to anti-IgM-induced apoptosis (Hayashida et al., 2006). Interferon-α 2b does not increase infections, but may expose patients to an increased risk of rejection. Interferon-α gives a rapid response – within 3 weeks in approximately 50% of patients (Davis et al., 1998) – thus enabling decisions about alternative treatments to be made quickly.

Chemotherapy with various schemes is indicated when interferon-α 2b fails or when the disease has a rapid progression, as in cases of Burkitt's lymphoma-like disease. Encouraging results have been obtained with the ProMACE-CytaBOM regimen (Swinnen et al., 1995). On day 1, cyclophosphamide, 650 mg/m^2, adriamycin, 25 mg/m^2, and VP16 (etoposide), 120 mg/m^2, are given intravenously, while oral prednisone is started at a dose of 60 mg/m^2 and continued for 14 days. At day 8, cytarabine, 300 mg/m^2, bleomycin, 5 mg/m^2, vincristine, 1.4 mg/m^2, methotrexate, 120 mg/m^2, and leucovorin, 25 mg/mq every 6 h, are administered intravenously. At day 22, a new cycle is started again. The mortality with this regimen is about 25%,

Table 11.8 Prophylaxis of post-transplant lymphoproliferative disorders

General measures for prophylaxis of EBV and CMV infection
  avoid heavy immunosuppression
  do not use ATG/OKT3 in EBV-negative patients
  Monitor EBV and CMV viral load
  modulate immunosuppression according to the viral load
  acyclovir/valacyclovir for EBV
  ganciclovir/valganciclovir for CMV

but survivors achieve complete remission without relapse after a median follow-up of 64 months. During treatment, the other immunosuppressive agents are stopped without risk of rejection, in contrast to the CHOP (cyclophosphamide, adriamycin, vincristine, and prednisone) regimen (Swinnen, 1997).

The association of interferon-α may further improve the results of chemotherapy in difficult cases (Liu *et al.*, 2006). Chemotherapy associated with *radiation therapy* or with resection of localized disease plus withdrawal of immunosuppression is mandatory in patients with monoclonal lesions containing clonal cytogenetic abnormalities in most cells. With this sequential approach, up to 76% of patients were successfully treated in one series (Davis *et al.*, 1998), while in a pediatric series (Dror *et al.*, 1999), up to 80% of patients, including those with monomorphic or monoclonal lesions, achieved complete or partial remission without receiving systemic chemotherapy. Bexarotene, a novel synthetic retinoid analog, has been used successfully in a pancreas and kidney transplant patient who proved to be refractory to chemotherapy and reduced immunosuppression (Tsai *et al.*, 2005).

Alternative treatments with *monoclonal antibodies* (MAB) may also give promising results. The combination of anti-CD21 (the EBV receptor) and anti-CD24 (a pan-B-cell antibody) MAB resulted in complete remission in 61% of 58 patients with PTLD. A poor response was observed in patients with multivisceral disease, late onset, and CNS involvement. Only 8% of patients had a relapse (Beukerron *et al.*, 1998). *Rituximab*, a MAB directed against the CD20 antigen of B cells, has been used increasingly in the treatment of CD20-positive lymphoma. Most patients were treated with the standard dose of 375 mg/m^2 once a week for four consecutive weeks. Complete response was seen in 50–63% of cases of PTLD (both polymorphic and monomorphic) occurring in carriers of solid organ transplantation (Milpied *et al.*, 2000; Oertel *et al.*, 2005). When compared with cytotoxic chemotherapy, rituximab had comparable rates of remission but reduced toxicity and mortality (Svoboda *et al.*, 2006). However, resistance may occur in patients with fulminant disease, in EBV-negative cases, and in those with variable expression of CD20 by neoplastic cells or with an elevated apoptotic threshold (Smith, 2003). In these cases the addition of chemotherapy may improve the results (Gulley *et al.*, 2003).

A more recent approach may consist of the infusion of autologous *EBV-specific cytotoxic T lymphocytes* (CTL). Five patients with disseminated monoclonal or localized polyclonal PTLD unresponsive to the reduction of immunosuppression received 4–5 courses of reduced-dosage polychemotherapy, accompanied by rituximab on the first day of each course, while localized disease was removed surgically. At treatment completion, autologous EBV-specific CTL were infused. All patients showed a complete response to treatment, without therapy-related toxicity or rejection, and remission persisted with good renal function at a median follow-up of 31 months (Comoli *et al.*, 2005).

In summary, the treatment of PTLD may follow different steps (Table 11.9). A high percentage of PTLD may be prevented through the use of antiviral agents, such as acyclovir, valacyclovir, or ganciclovir. In the case of development of PTLD, the first therapeutic measure should consist of reducing immunosuppression and adding interferon-α, which may obtain resolution in some cases. In patients who do not respond, encouraging results may be obtained with rituximab. Chemotherapy, radiation therapy, or hemotherapy should be reserved for patients who fail rituximab (Svoboda *et al.*, 2006).

Table 11.9   Possible steps for treatment of post-transplant
lymphoproliferative disorders

Massive reduction or withdrawal of immunosuppressive therapy. Antiviral therapy
Interferon-α
Chemotherapy
Chemotherapy associated with local resection, radiation therapy, interferon-α
Monoclonal antibodies directed against CD20, or CD21, or CD24
Infusion of specific cytotoxic T lymphocytes

Kaposi's sarcoma

Kaposi's sarcoma (KS) is a multicentric vascular tumor of viral etiology, which mainly affects immunosuppressed individuals. KS presents with red-purple or blue-brown macules, plaques, and nodules of the skin and mucous membranes, but can also extend to abdominal viscera and lungs.

Epidemiology

Kaposi's sarcoma is a rare tumor, representing 0.01–0.06% of tumors in the general population, but its prevalence increases with immunosuppression. Regamey et al. (1998) found a seroprevalence of HHV-8 in 6.4% of patients at the time of transplantation, which rose to 17.7% at 1 year after transplantation. The incidence is higher among transplant recipients treated with CsA than in those given Aza and steroids. Kaposi's sarcoma shows a geographic distribution, with a prevalence of 4–7.8% among Arab and Mediterranean renal transplant patients (Qunibi et al., 1988) and of 0.4% among transplanted patients from northern and western countries (Odajnyk and Muggia, 1985). The risk ratio for KS among 6596 Australian recipients of cadaver donor renal allografts has been calculated to be more than 1000 (Sheil et al., 1993), while in Italian experiences the risk ratio for KS ranged between 113 (Serraino et al., 2005) and 225 (Montagnino et al., 1994). The male/female ratio, which is usually 9–15 : 1 in the general population, decreases after transplantation to 2.2–3 : 1. The age of onset is much younger among transplant recipients than in the general population.

Etiopathogenesis

Identification of the novel human herpes virus HHV-8 (Chang et al., 1994; Moore and Chang, 1995) has allowed better understanding of the pathogenesis of KS. In fact, HHV-8 can be found in all forms of KS (Hengge et al., 2002). However, the presence of HHV-8 is not sufficient per se to cause the development of KS. The development of KS requires the reactivation of HHV-8, which can be triggered by a compromised host immune response and/or the evasion of infected cells by the host NK cell-driven response (Sirianni et al., 2002). Hypotheses for how HHV-8 can be oncogenic are wide-ranging. The virus might either exert a direct oncogenic effect or mediate the development of neoplasia by interfering with IL-6, chemokine, and Ox-2 homologs. It has been shown that in HIV-related KS, multiple lesions in the same patient arise from a single clone of cells (Rabkin et al., 1997). Thus, the current hypothesis is that each lesion arises from a monoclonal population of circulating progenitor cells, transformed by HHV-8, that home to multiple local sites, develop into spindle cells, and proliferate.

Clinical features

Kaposi's sarcoma generally occurs a short period after transplantation, usually earlier in CsA-treated than in azathioprine-treated patients. Histologically, KS is characterized by angioproliferation of the upper dermis, constituted by a mixed cellular population comprising infiltrating lymphocytes, proliferating fibroblasts,

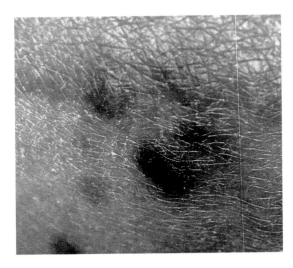

Figure 11.4 Nodular Kaposi's sarcoma: the elementary lesions consist of violaceous nodules, elevated upon the skin surface

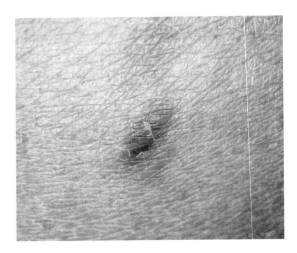

Figure 11.5 Epidemic-like type of Kaposi's sarcoma: this kind of lesion is frequently observed in CsA-treated patients. Lesions consist of oval and fusiform maculae, distributed along the lines of skin cleavage. A single lesion may be present

endothelial cells, and characteristic eosinophilic 'spindle cells' that have immunochemical and ultrastructural features of endothelial cells.

Clinically, KS can manifest with papular or nodular red-bluish *cutaneous* lesions (Figure 11.4). The cutaneous lesions may be firm or compressible, and may even appear initially as a dusky stain, especially about the toes. Lesions may be single (Figure 11.5) or multiple, and may occur not only in the skin and but also in the *oropharyngeal mucosa.* At times, lesions may become nodular, and, with advanced disease, the lesions may become confluent, with large plaques developing, particularly in the legs. Lymphatic involvement is not unusual, and KS may present as lymphadenopathy in its more severe manifestations, also in the *visceral mucosae.* The trachea, lungs, and gastrointestinal tract are frequently involved. Extensive parenchymal or pleural involvement of the lung may result in life-theratening compromise. In about a quarter of cases, visceral KS is not associated with cutaneous lesions.

Table 11.10   Possible steps for treatment of post-transplant Kaposi's sarcoma

Reduction of immunosuppression
   if no result pass to the second step
Conversion to sirolimus or everolimus
   if no result pass to the third step
Complete withdrawal of immunosuppression
   if no result pass to the fourth step
Cidofovir or foscarnet
   if no result pass to the fifth step
Interferon-α
   if no result pass to chemotherapy
Chemotherapy

Prognosis

The forms of KS confined to the skin and/or lymph nodes and/or which have minimal oral involvement usually have a good prognosis, as they may respond to a reduction of immunosuppression. The forms associated with edema or ulceration, extensive oral or gastrointestinal involvement, or other non-nodal viscera are more aggressive, and carry a poorer prognosis, with a high risk of death. Early diagnosis is therefore important. Transplanted patients with suspect cutaneous lesions should be seen by a dermatologist in order to have an early diagnosis and prompt therapeutic measures (Montagnino and Bencini, 1994). Diagnosis may be difficult in those patients with visceral localization of KS who do not display any cutaneous lesions. However, about half of them have lesions in the oral mucosa, which may favor the diagnosis. In order to exclude visceral involvement, a complete staging should be performed via chest X-radiographic examination, abdominal ultrasound scan, or computed tomography, gastroscopy, and colonoscopy.

Therapy

There are several options for the treatment of post-transplant KS (Table 11.10). Many patients with non-visceral lesions have complete or partial remission of KS following *withdrawal* or *reduction of immuno-suppressive therapy*. In single-center series (Duman *et al.*, 2002, Firoozan *et al.*, 2005), 90% of patients had a regression or complete healing of their lesions after the reduction of immunosuppression, and about two-thirds maintained their graft function after mean follow-ups of 41–46 months since Kaposi's sarcoma diagnosis and immunosuppressive therapy withdrawal. Therefore, this maneuver should be attempted as a first-line treatment in all cases. Circumscribed lesions usually stop or heal simply by reducing the CsA dosage. More widespread and severe cutaneous lesions, in the presence of oral mucosa localizations, require complete CsA withdrawal. Of interest, the withdrawal of cyclosporine and its replacement with *sirolimus* led to a complete resolution of KS in a number of renal transplant recipients (Campistol *et al.*, 2004; Stallone *et al.*, 2005). However, some cases failed to respond (Descoeudres *et al.*, 2006). In cases of visceral lesions that do not respond to conversion to sirolimus, immunosuppressive agents should be gradually withdrawn, while maintaining only small doses of prednisone. The reintroduction of immunosuppression at low doses should be done with caution and only after healing has been documented. In fact, the reintroduction or increase of immunosuppressive therapy can result in a fatal reactivation with visceral involvement after a partial regression of KS.

Table 11.11	Main risk factors for skin cancer
Exposure to ultraviolet B rays (sunlight)	
Older age	
Caucasian race (pale skin)	
Immunosuppression	
Genetic predisposition	
Virus infection (papilloma virus)	
Smoking	

The introduction of novel *antiviral agents* has prompted new therapeutic options in these patients. Adefovir, an acyclic nucleoside phosphonate (ANP) with both antiretrovirus and antiherpes virus activity, was shown effectively to block HHV-8 DNA replication *in vitro* (Neyts and De Clercq, 1997). The ANP analogs *cidofovir* and *foscarnet* are two other agents that have shown potent anti-HHV-8 activity *in vitro* (Medveczky *et al.*, 1997; Willers *et al.*, 1999), while ganciclovir showed an intermediate strength against HHV-8. Preliminary clinical trials (Little *et al.*, 2003) and single-case reports seem to confirm the efficacy of cidofovir and foscarnet.

Interferon should be started in cases which do not respond to the cessation of immunosuppression (Krown *et al.*, 2006). *Chemotherapy* has also been used. Vincristine, vinblastine, bleomycin, doxorubicin, and etoposide alone or in combination have showed comparable efficacy (Arican *et al.*, 2000). Good results have been reported with paclitaxel alone in two patients with generalized cutaneous and visceral KS not responding to withdrawal of immunosuppression (Patel *et al.*, 2002).

Skin cancer

Skin cancers are also described in Chapter 17. Here, only their etiology and incidence in the transplant population are commented upon. Cutaneous cancers represent the most common type of neoplasia after organ transplantation, being extremely common in countries with high *sunlight exposure* and in patients with a *light complexion*. In the transplant population, such cancers appear at an earlier age, behave more aggressively, and may appear at multiple sites (Rubel *et al.*, 2002; Euvrard *et al.*, 2003).

Etiopathogenesis

Several factors may contribute to the development of post-transplant skin cancer (Table 11.11).

The *ultraviolet* (UV) component of sunlight plays a crucial role. Exposure to UVB results in the production of pyrimidine dimers and photogroups which can lead to the mutation of different genes (Freeman *et al.*, 1989). In skin cancer, the most frequent UV-induced mutation is that of the p53 gene (Sarasin and Gigliola-Mari, 2002). This gene orchestrates the response of epidermal cells to UV-induced DNA damage. The dysfunction of p53 is an important early step in the formation of skin cancer. UVB also favors induction of the matrix metalloproteinase family, which degrades the macromolecules of the extracellular matrix (Brenneisen *et al.*, 2002). This results in premature aging and carcinogenesis.

It is well known that *older age* is an independent risk factor for skin cancer, and this has also been demonstrated in transplant patients (Ramsay *et al.*, 2000).

Race is a well-known factor influencing the risk for skin cancer. Caucasian people are more susceptible to skin neoplasia than are black subjects.

The role of *immunosuppression* is clearly demonstrated by the observation that even in areas with reduced sunlight exposure, such as Finland, transplantation increases the occurrence of cutaneous tumors by 20 times in comparison with the general population (Kyllonen *et al.*, 1994). The longer is the immunosuppression the higher is the risk. In an Australian single-center series, the incidence of non-melanoma skin cancer was around 19% in the first 5 years after transplantation and 47% after 20 years or more (Carroll *et al.*, 2003).

Genetic predisposition may also play a role. In some populations, an increased frequency of cutaneous neoplasias has been found among patients homozygous for HLA-B27 and HLA-DR7 (Bouwes-Bavinck *et al.*, 1991). Recent data reported that an interleukin-10 gene polymorphism may contribute to the development of skin squamous-cell carcinomas in transplant recipients (Alamartine *et al.*, 2003).

Viruses are a major etiologic factor; cutaneous tumors may develop from papilloma virus-induced warts, through a neoplastic transformation induced by sunlight exposure and prolonged immunosuppression (Stockflet *et al.*, 2002).

Finally, as for other tumors, *smoking* is an independent risk factor also for skin cancer (De Hertog *et al.*, 2001).

Types of skin cancer

Squamous-cell carcinomas (SCC)

SCC are the most frequent cancers in the transplanted population, with an increase of 40–250 times the reported incidence in the general population. Cancer is often preceded by precancerous lesions such as keratoacanthosis, epidermodysplasia verruciformis, or actinic porokeratosis, or by extensive atrophic cutaneous areas. These lesions may appear in multiple parts of the body, either exposed to sunlight or not. While in the general population cancerous lesions develop around the seventh to eighth decade of life, in transplant recipients they tend to appear around the fourth to fifth decade, with a more aggressive evolution than in the general population. According to the CTTR (Penn, 1995b, 1998a), lymph nodal metastases are observed in 5.8% of cutaneous neoplasias, 75% of them being due to squamous-cell carcinomas. Moreover, 5.1% of patients with cutaneous tumors die, 60% of deaths being caused by squamous-cell carcinoma, only 33% by malignant melanomas. These lesions should therefore be accurately evaluated by a dermatologist in order to prevent their evolution into malignant lesions. Especially in patients under long-term immunosuppression, sun exposure of areas affected by these precancerous conditions should be strongly contraindicated.

Basal-cell carcinomas

Basal-cell cancers are the second most frequent cutaneous neoplastic lesions in transplanted patients, occurring ten times more frequently than in the normal population. In normal subjects, basal-cell carcinomas usually outnumber squamous-cell carcinomas by 5:1, while in the transplant population the opposite has been observed, with a squamous/basal-cell carcinoma ratio of 1.8:1 (Penn, 1990).

Melanomas

Melanomas represent 5.3% of all skin cancers in transplant recipients (Penn, 1995b). A predisposing condition is represented by cutaneous nevi (Grob *et al.*, 1996; Gulec *et al.*, 2002). Unlike squamous-cell and basal-cell carcinomas, which are correlated with total cumulative exposure to ultraviolet radiation, melanomas are associated with intense intermittent sun exposure (Bentham and Aase, 1996; Gilchrest *et al.*, 1999), being most common in patients with indoor occupations who occasionally expose themselves to high sun radiation during vacations. While in the general population melanomas are rarely observed in youth, in the CTTR experience, 54% of melanomas occurred in pediatric recipients, at a mean age of 12 years. Melanomas appear on average 63 months after transplantation. It is difficult to assess the prognosis of post-transplant melanoma from the available studies, as the number of patients is small and the follow-ups are short. In a large French study, of 17 patients with melanoma, four died, while 12 were still alive 3 years after removal of the tumor without reduction of immunosuppression (Leveque *et al.*, 2000).

Therapy

Preventive measures are important. Transplant patients should be made aware of the skin cancer risk and should be advised to *avoid excessive sun exposure* and to apply sun-protective lotions to the most exposed areas (forehead, neck, forearms, hands, and shoulders). Most squamous and basal cell carcinomas usually heal after surgical removal. However, most patients with cutaneous neoplasias also display multiple precancerous lesions, which should be treated in order to prevent recurrence of carcinomas. Whenever possible, a gradual *reduction of immunosuppression* may be considered. Systemic *retinoids* may slow down the progression of dysplastic lesions to cancer (McNamara *et al.*, 2002). Retinoids do not interfere with immunosuppression, but may be burdened by undesired untoward effects such as liver toxicity and hyperlipidemia, and should therefore be prescribed only in cases of actinic keratoses or multiple skin cancers.

Renal carcinoma

According to the CTTR, renal carcinomas represent 14% of all tumors (Penn, 1995b). Most renal carcinomas in renal transplant recipients occur in the native kidney, although about 10% of them may involve the transplanted kidney (Moudouni *et al.*, 2005).

This elevated prevalence may be explained by the high number of renal tumors in patients with end-stage renal failure. Denton *et al.* (2002), by reviewing the pathology of 260 ipsilateral native nephrectomies before transplantation, found 0.6% cases of oncocytoma, 4.2% of renal cell carcinoma, 14% of adenoma, and 33% of acquired cystic kidney disease, a well-known predisposing factor for the development of renal carcinomas (Kliem *et al.*, 1997), which is strongly associated with the duration of renal disease (Peces *et al.*, 2004).

The *prognosis* for patients with renal cancer is closely related to tumor size and extension outside Gerota's fascia. Tumors less than 7 cm, without local extension, carry a 95% 5-year survival; tumors larger than 7 cm without local invasion have a 88% survival at 5 years, while the 5-year survival drops to 20% for cancer involving adjacent structures (Javidan *et al.*, 1999).

Experimental studies showed that rapamune is very effective in halting the progression of renal carcinoma and in inhibiting metastasis (Luan *et al.*, 2003). Clinical studies also showed that CCI-779, a novel mTOR antagonist, demonstrated antitumor activity and encouraging survival in patients with advanced renal cell carcinoma (Atkins *et al.*, 2004). Moreover, rapamune in combination with Iressa® may be useful in renal cell carcinoma associated with von Hippel–Lindau mutations (Gemmill *et al.*, 2005). On the basis of these results, it may be suggested that an *anti-mTOR agent* be given for primary immunosuppression in renal transplant recipients with a history of renal malignancy.

Prostate carcinoma

With the aging of renal transplant recipients, the risk of prostate cancer increases. A questionnaire reported an incidence of 0.65% per year in French transplant centers, much higher than the incidence observed in the general population (Cormier *et al.*, 2003) The median age was 58 years (range 41–70), and the median time after transplantation was 60 months (range 1–156 months). It is even possible that this high prevalence was underestimated, as it was somewhat higher in a center that performed routine PSA testing (Malavaud *et al.*, 2000). The rate of poorly differentiated tumors was higher than in the general population. A Gleason score higher than 7 is predictive of a bad prognosis and a poor response to radiation therapy. For transplant patients younger than 70 years, surgery is mandatory. Radiotherapy or radioactive seed is indicated in cases of poor cardiac reserve or poor general condition.

Carcinoma of the liver

Hepatocellular carcinomas account for almost 90% of post-transplant liver carcinomas. Most other carcinomas are bile-duct cell carcinomas (cholangiocarcinomas). Some cases of primary leiomyosarcoma have also been reported (Fuijta *et al.*, 2002). Chronic liver disease of any type predisposes to the development of carcinoma. However, apart from a few cases secondary to hemochromatosis, most cases of post-transplant hepatocellular cancer develop in carriers of HBV (Tang *et al.*, 1999) and HCV infection (Nakayama *et al.*, 2000), the risk being roughly proportional to the duration of infection. Some cases of primary leiomyosarcoma have also been reported (Fuijta *et al.*, 2002).

The clinical *diagnosis* may be difficult, as signs and symptoms may be attributed to the underlying primary disease. Anemia and increased liver enzymes are not specific signs. The appreciation of a tender mass in the liver at palpation and a hemoperitoneum at paracentesis are the most valuable clinical features, which occur, however, at an inoperable stage. The most reliable indicators are serum α-fetoprotein, which shows very high levels in about 70% of cases, and imaging procedures. Transplant patients who are HBV- or HCV-positive should have α-fetoprotein levels measured at least every 6 months, and should receive a liver ultrasonography at least once a year in order to detect early an underlying hepatocellular carcinoma. Percutaneous liver biopsy in the area of previously localized nodules or masses can be diagnostic.

Gynecological carcinomas

In transplant recipients, these carcinomas occur at an earlier age than in the general population (Penn, 1995b). About one-third of patients have *in situ* lesions. The cancer is often preceded by condilomas or papilloma virus infections, which may induce cervical cancer through inactivation of the retinoblastoma suppressor gene (Cohen *et al.*, 2003). Vulva and perineum carcinomas may be multifocal, with involvement also of the vagina and uterine cervix (Penn, 1986). Transplanted women frequently show endometrial hyperplasia (Bobrowska *et al.*, 2006) and diffuse uterine adenomatous tumors (Cheng and Wee, 2003). Carcinomas of the uterine cervix represent 11% of neoplasias among transplant recipients (Penn, 1995b). This underlines the importance of accurate gynecological screening in order to diagnose any precancerous lesion early.

A gynecological examination performed every 3 years is fundamental for early diagnosis of papilloma virus infections and genital dysplasias. The visit should include a Pap test, colposcopy, and histologic evaluation of anogenital dysplastic lesions. Since a Pap test may give a high proportion of false-positive reactions, annual colposcopy with epithelial dyeing using acetic acid and toluidine blue should be performed. All abnormal areas should be biopsied, and the dysplastic or papilloma virus-infected areas should be treated with laser vaporization or electroresection or with 5-fluorouracil topical ointments.

Miscellaneous tumors

A number of neoplasias (hepatomas, histiocytomas, fibrosarcomas, mesotheliomas, etc.) have too low an incidence to be correctly evaluated from a statistical point of view. The Australia/New Zealand Registry reported an increased risk for thyroid carcinoma (risk ratio of 5.2, with an attributable risk of 17.2 cases per 10 000) in renal transplant recipients, many of whom presented with lymphatic metastasis (Pond *et al.*, 2005). The same registry reported an increased incidence of endocrine carcinomas (289 times), leukemia (5.6 times), and carcinomas of the digestive system (2.5 times) and respiratory system (twice), as compared with the general population (Sheil *et al.*, 1993). Nevertheless, a recent review concluded that there is no increased risk of colorectal cancer among transplant recipients (Saidi *et al.*, 2003). A review of the United States Renal Data System reported a low rate of lymphoid leukemias (0.2%) and myelomas (0.24%), with a possible association between myeloma and hepatitis C virus (Caillard *et al.*, 2006).

In order to reduce the increased risk of cancer in transplant recipients, some guidelines should be followed. They include regular surveillance, dietetic and other life-style measures, and appropriate treatment of viral infections (Table 11.12).

Table 11.12 Main recommendations to a transplant recipient for prevention or early detection of cancers

Regular surveillance (once a year)
Dermatological evaluation
Gynecological evaluation (colposcopy)
Prostatic evaluation (PSA, ultrasonography)
Native kidney ultrasonography
Occult blood in the stools

Life habits
Stop smoking
Minimize sun exposure
Reduce the intake of fats
Minimize salt-cured and smoked food
Use alcohol in moderation
Self-examination of breasts and testes
Do not underevaluate febrile episodes (viral infections?)

References

Alamartine E, Berthoux P, Mariat C, et al. Interleukin-10 promoter polymorphism and susceptibility to skin squamous cell carcinoma after renal transplantation. J Invest Dermatol 2003; 120: 99–103.

Albalate M, Octavio JG, Echezarreta G, et al. Diffuse T-cell lymphoma in a kidney graft recipient 17 years after transplantation. Nephrol Dial Transplant 1998; 13: 3242–4.

Arican A, Karakayali H, Bilgin N, Haberal M. Results of treatment in renal transplant patients with Kaposi sarcoma: one center experience. Transplant Proc 2000; 626–8.

Armitage JM, Fricker FJ, DelNido P, et al. A decade (1982 to 1992) of pediatric cardiac transplantation and the impact of FK 506 immunosuppression. J Thorac Cardiovasc Surg 1993; 105: 464–72.

Atkins MB, Hidalgo M, Stadler WM, et al. Randomized phase II study of multiple dose levels of CCI-779, a novel mammalian target of rapamycin kinase inhibitor, in patients with advanced refractory renal cell carcinoma. J Clin Oncol 2004; 22: 909–18.

Aull MJ, Buell JF, Peddi VR, et al. MALToma: a Helicobacter pylori-associated malignancy in transplant patients. Transplantation 2003; 75: 225–8.

Barozzi P, Luppi M, Facchetti F, et al. Post-transplant Kaposi sarcoma originates from the seeding of donor-derived progenitors. Nat Med 2003; 9: 554–61.

Bates WD, Gray DNR, Dada MA, et al. Lymphoproliferative disorders in Oxford renal transpant recipients. J Clin Pathol 2003; 56: 439–46.

Bentham G, Aase A. Incidence of malignant melanoma of the skin in Norway, 1955–1989: associations with solar ultraviolet radiation, income and holidays abroad. Int J Epidemiol 1996; 25: 1132–8.

Berthoux F, Abramowicz D, Bradley B, et al. European Best Practice Guidelines for Renal Transplantation (Part 2). Nephrol Dial Transplant 2002; 17 (Suppl 4): 1–67.

Beukerron M, Jais JP, Leblond V, et al. Anti-B-cell monoclonal antibody treatment of severe posttranplant B-lymphoproliferative disorder: prognostic factors and long-term outcome. Blood 1998; 92: 3137–47.

Birkeland SA, Storm HH, Lamm LU, et al. Cancer risk after renal transplantation in the Nordic countries, 1964–1986. Int J Cancer 1995; 60: 183–9.

Birkeland SA, Bendtzen K. Interleukin 10 and Epstein Barr virus induced posttransplant lymphoproliferative disorder. Transplantation 1996; 61: 1425–6.

Birkeland SA. Malignancies occurring de novo after transplantation. Curr Opin Organ Transplant 1998; 3: 82–9.

Birkeland SA, Bendtzen K, Møller B, et al. Interleukin-10 and posttransplant lymphoproliferative disorder after kidney transplantation. Transplantation 1999; 67: 876–81.

Birkeland SA, Hamilton-Dutoit S. Is posttransplant lymphoproliferative disorder (PTLD) caused by any specific immunosuppressive drug or by the transplantation per se? Transplantation 2003; 76: 984–8.

Bobrowska K, Kaminski P, Cyganek A, et al. High rate of endometrial hyperplasia in renal transplanted women. Transplant Proc 2006; 38: 177–9.

Boukamp P. Non-melanoma skin cancer: what drives tumor development and progression? Carcinogenesis 2005; 26: 1657–67.

Bouwes-Bavinck JN, Vermeer BJ, Van der Woude FJ, et al. Relation between skin cancer and HLA antigens in renal transplant recipients. N Engl J Med 1991; 325: 843–8.

Brennan P, Mehl AM, Jones M, Rowe M. Phospatydilinositol 3-kinase is essential for the proliferation of lymphoblastoid cells. Oncogene 2002; 21: 1263–71.

Brenneisen P, Sies H, Scharfetter-Kochanek K. Ultraviolet B-irradiation and matrix metalloproteinases: from inducton via signaling to initial events. Ann NY Acad Sci 2002; 973: 31–43.

Brunner FP, Landais P, Selwood NH on behalf of the EDTA-ERA Registry Committee. Malignancies after renal transplantation: the EDTA-ERA Registry experience. Nephrol Dial Transplant 1995; 10 (Suppl 1): 74–80.

Buell JF, Gross T, Alloway RR, et al. Central nervous system tumors in donors: misdiagnosis carries a high morbidity and mortality. Transplant Proc 2005; 37: 583–4.

Bustami RT, Ojo AO, Wolfe RA, et al. Immunosuppression and the risk of post-transplant malignancy among cadaveric first kidney transplant recipients. Am J Transplant 2004; 4: 87–93.

Caillard S, Agodoa LY, Bohen E, Abbott K. Myeloma, Hodgkin disease and lymphoid leukemia after renal transplantation: characteristics, risk factors and prognosis. Transplantation 2006; 81: 888–95.

Campe H, Jaeger G, Abu-Ajram C, et al. Serial detection of Epstein–Barr virus DNA in sera and peripheral blood lymphocyte samples of pediatric renal allograft recipients with persistent mononucleosis-like symptoms defines patients at risk to develop lymphoproliferative disease. Pediatr Transplant 2003; 7: 46–52.

Campistol JM, Gutierrez-Dalmau A, Torregrosa JV. Conversion to sirolimus: a successful treatment for posttransplantation Kaposi's sarcoma. Transplantation 2004; 77: 760–2.

Campistol J, Eris J, Oberbauer R, et al. Sirolimus therapy after early cyclosporine withdrawal reduces the risk of cancer in adult renal transplantation. J Am Soc Nephrol 2006; 17: 581–9.

Carroll RP, Ramsay HM, Fryer AA, et al. Incidence and prediction of nonmelanoma skin cancer post-renal transplantation. A prospective study in Queensland Australia. Am J Kidney Dis 2003; 41: 676–83.

Chang Y, Cesarman E, Pessin MS, et al. Identification of herpes-virus-like DNA sequences in AIDS-associated Kaposi's sarcoma. Science 1994; 266: 1865–9.

Chapman JR, Sheil AGR, Disney APS. Recurrence of cancer after renal transplantation. Transplant Proc 2001; 33: 1830–1.

Cheng CL, Wee A. Diffuse uterine adenomatoid tumor in an immunosuppressed renal transplant recipient. Int J Gynecol Pathol 2003; 22: 198–201.

Cherney BW, Bhatia KG, Sgadari C, et al. Role of the p53 tumor suppressor gene in the tumorgenicity of Burkitt's lymphoma cells. Cancer Res 1997; 57: 2508–15.

Chetty R, Biddolph S, Kaklamanis L, et al. Bcl-2 proteins strongly expressed in post-transplant lymphoproliferative disorders. J Pathol 1996; 180: 254–8.

Cockburn IT, Krupp P. The risk of neoplasms in patients treated with cyclosporine. J Autoimmun 1989; 2: 723–31.

Cohen HT, McGovern FJ. Medical progress: renal-cell carcinoma. N Engl J Med 2005; 353: 2477–90.

Cohen JI. Epstein–Barr virus and the immune system. Hide and seek. JAMA 1997; 278: 510–13.

Cohen Y, Singer G, Lavie O, et al. The RASSF1A tumor suppressor gene is commonly inactivated in adenocacinoma of the uterine cervix. Clin Cancer Res 2003; 9: 2981–4.

Comoli P, Maccario R, Locatelli F. Treatment of EBV-related post-renal transplant lymphoproliferative disease with a tailored regimen including EBV-specific T cells. Am J Transplant 2005; 5: 1415–22.

Cormier L, Lechevallier E, Barrou B, et al. Diagnosis and treatment of prostate cancers in renal-transplant recipients. Transplantation 2003; 75: 237–9.

CTS, Colloborative Transplant Study. E-51109-0205.

Daneshpouy M, Socie G, Clavel C, et al. Human papillomavirus infection and anogenital condyloma in bone marrow transplant recipients. Transplantation 2001; 71: 167–9.

Davis CL, Wood BL, Sabath DE, et al. Interferon-α treatment of posttransplant lymphoproliferative disorder in recipients of solid organ transplants. Transplantation 1998; 66: 1770–9.

De Hertog S, Wensveen CA, Bastiaens MT, et al. Relation between smoking and skin cancer. J Clin Oncol 2001; 19: 231–8.

Denton MD, Magee CC, Ovuworie C, et al. Prevalence of renal cell carcinoma in patients with ESRD pre-transplantation: a pathologic analysis. Kidney Int 2002; 61: 2201–9.

Descoeudres B, Giannini O, Graf T, et al. No effect of sirolimus for Kaposi sarcoma in a renal transplant recipient. Transplantation 2006; 81: 1472–4.

Detry O, Honore P, Hans MF, et al. Organ donors with primary central nervous system tumor. Transplantation 2000; 70: 244–8.

Dockrell DH, Stricklar JG, Paya CV. Epstein–Barr virus-induced T-cell lymphoma in solid organ transplant recipients. Clin Infect Dis 1998; 26: 180–2.

Dong C, Hemminki K. Second primary neoplasms in 633,964 cancer patients in Sweden, 1958–1996. Int J Cancer 2001; 93: 155–61.

Dror Y, Greenberg M, Taylor G, et al. Lymphoproliferative disorders after organ transplantation in children. Transplantation 1999; 67: 990–8.

Duman S, Toz H, Asci G, et al. Successful treatment of Kaposi's sarcoma by reduction of immunosuppression. Nephrol Dial Transplant 2002; 17: 892–6.

Euvrard S, Kanitakis J, Claudy A. Skin cancer after renal transplantation. N Engl J Med 2003; 348: 1681–91.

Fairley CK, Sheil AGR, McNeil JJ, et al. The risk of anogenital malignancies in dialysis and transplant patients. Clin Nephrol 1994; 41: 101–5.

Faull R, Hollett P, McDonald S. Lymphoproliferative disease after renal transplantation in Australia and New Zealand. Transplantation 2005; 80: 193–7.

Firoozan A, Hosseini Moghaddam SM, Einollahi B, et al. Outcome of Kaposi's sarcoma and graft following discontinuation of immunosuppressive drugs in renal transplant recipients. Transplant Proc 2005; 37: 3061–4.

Fisher DE. Apoptosis and cancer. Cell 1994; 8: 539–42.

Freeman SE, Hacham H, Gange RW, et al. Wavelength dependence of pyrimidine dimer formation in DNA of human skin irradiated in situ with ultraviolet light. Proc Natl Acad Sci USA 1989; 86: 5605–9.

Fujita H, Kiriyama M, Kawamura T, et al. Primary hepatic leiomyosarcoma in a woman after renal transplantation: report of a case. Surg Today 2002; 32: 446–9.

Gaya SB, Rees AJ, Lechler RJ, William G, Mason PD. Maligant disease in patients with long-terrm renal transplants. Transplantation 1995; 59: 1705–9.

Gemmill RM, Zhou M, Costa L, et al. Synergistic growth inhibition by Iressa and rapamycin is modulated by VHL mutations in renal cell carcinoma. Br J Cancer 2005; 92: 2266–77.

Gibson GE, O'Grady A, Kay EW, et al. p53 tumor suppressor gene protein expression in premalignant and malignant skin lesions of kidney transplant recipients. J Am Acad Dermatol 1997; 36: 924–31.

Gilchrest BA, Eller MS, Geller AC, Yaar M. The pathogenesis of melanoma induced by ultraviolet radiation. N Engl J Med 1999; 340: 1341–8.

Goldstein DJ, Austin JHM, Zuech N, et al. Carcinoma of the lung after heart transplantation. Transplantation 1996; 62: 772–5.

Grob JJ, Bastuji-Garin S, Vaillant R, et al. Excess of nevi related to immunodeficiency: a study in HIV-infected patients and renal transplant recipients. J Invest Dermatol 1996; 107: 694–7.

Guba M, von Breitenbuch P, Steinbauer M, et al. Rapamycin inhibits primary and metastatic tumor growth by antiangiogenesis: involvement of vascular endothelial growth factor. Nat Med 2002; 8: 128–35.

Gulec AT, Seckin D, Saray Y, et al. Number of acquired melanocytic nevi in renal transplant recipients as a risk factor for melanoma. Transplant Proc 2002; 34: 2136–8.

Gulley ML, Swinnen LJ, Plaisance KT, et al. Tumor origin and CD20 expression in posttransplant lymphoproliferative disorder occurring in solid organ transplant recipients: implication for immune based therapy. Transplantation 2003; 79: 959–64.

Hanaway M, Weber S, Buell JF, et al. Risk for recurrence and death from preexisting cancers after transplantation. Transplant Rev 2005; 19: 151–63.

Hanson MN, Morrison VA, Peterson BA, et al. Post-transplant T-cell lymphoproliferative disorders are aggressive late complications of solid organ transplantation. Blood 1997; 89: 3626–33.

Hanto DW, Birkenbach H, Frizzera G, et al. Confirmation of the heterogeneity of posttransplant Epstein–Barr virus associated B-cell proliferations by immunoglobulin gene rearrangement analyses. Transplantation 1989; 47: 458–64.

Harris NL, Ferry JA, Swerdlow SH. Post transplant lymphoproliferative disorders: summary of Society for Hematopathology Workshop. Semin Diagn Pathol 1997; 14: 8–14.

Harwood AR, Osaba D, Hofstades SL, et al. Kaposi's sarcoma in recipients of renal transplants. Am J Med 1979; 67: 759–65.

Hayashida M, Hoshika A, Kanetaka Y, et al. IFN-alpha sensitizes daudi B lymphoma cells to anti-IgM induced loss of mitochondrial membrane potential through activation of c-Jun NH(2)-terminal kinase. J Interferon Cytokine Res 2006; 26: 421–9.

Hennge UR, Ruzicka T, Tyring SK, et al. Update on Kaposi's sarcoma and other HHV8 associated diseases. Part 2: Pathogenesis, Castleman's disease and pleural effusion lymphoma. Lancet Infect Dis 2002; 2: 344–52.

Hibberd AD, Trevillian PR, Wlodarzcy KJH, et al. Predialysis immunosuppression is an independent risk factor for some cancers in renal transplantation. Transplant Proc 2002; 33: 1846–7.

Ho M, Jaffe R, Miller G, et al. The frequency of Epstein–Barr virus infection and associated lymphoproliferative syndrome after transplantation and its manifestation in children. Transplantation 1988; 45: 719–27.

Hojo M, Morimoto T, Maluccio M, et al. Cyclosporine induces cancer progression by a cell-autonomous mechanism. Nature 1999; 397: 530–4.

Hoshida Y, Hongyo T, Nakatsuka SI, et al. Gene mutations in lymphoproliferative disorders of T and NK/T cell phenotypes developing in renal transplant patients. Lab Invest 2002; 82: 257–64.

Houghton PJ, Huang S. mTOR as a target for cancer therapy. Curr Top Microbiol Immunol 2004; 279: 339–59.

Hsi ED, Singleton TP, Swinnen L, et al. Mucosa-associated lymphoid tissue-type lymphomas occurring in post-transplantation patients. Am J Surg Pathol 2000; 24: 100–6.

Javidan J, Stricker HJ, Timboli P, et al. Prognostic significance of 1997 TNM classification of renal cell carcinoma. J Urol 1999; 162: 1277–81.

Karras A, Thervet E, Le Meur Y, et al. Successful renal retransplantation after post-transplant lymphoproliferative disease. Am J Transplant 2004; 4: 1904–9.

Kauffman HM, McBride MA, Cherikh WS, et al. Transplant tumor registry: donor related malignancy. Transplantation 2002; 74: 358–62.

Kauffman HM, Cherikh WS, McBride MA, et al. Transplant recipients with a history of malignancy: risk of recurrent and de novo cancers. Transplant Rev 2005a; 19: 55–64.

Kauffman HM, Cherick WS, Cheng BD, et al. Maintenance immunosuppression with target-of-rapamycin inhibitors is associated with a reduced incidence of de novo malignancies. Transplantation 2005b; 80: 883–9.

Klein G, Klein E. Immune surveillance against virus-induced tumors and non-rejectability of spontaneous tumors: contrasting consequences of host versus tumor evolution. Proc Natl Acad Sci USA 1977; 74: 2121–5.

Kliem V, Kolditz M, Behrend M, et al. Risk of renal cell carcinoma after kidney transplantation. Clin Transplant 1997; 11: 255–8.

Knowles DM, Cesarman E, Chadburn A, et al. Correlative morphologic and molecular genetic analysis demonstrates three distinct categories of posttransplantation lymphoproliferative disorders. Blood 1995; 85: 552–65.

Krown SE, Lee JY, Lin L, et al. Interferon-alpha2b with protease inhibitor-based antiretroviral therapy in patients with AIDS-associated Kaposi sarcoma: an AIDS malignancy consortium phase I trial. J Acquir Immune Defic Syndr 2006; 41: 149–53.

Kulwichit W, Edwards RH, Davenport EM, et al. Expression of the Epstein–Barr virus latent membrane protein 1 induces B-cell lymphoma in transgenic mice. Proc Natl Acad Sci USA 1998; 95: 11963–8.

Kyllonen L, Pukkala E, Ekund B. Cancer incidence in a kidney-transplanted population. Transpl Int 1994; 7 (Suppl 1): S350–2.

Leblond V, Sutton L, Dorent R, et al. Lymphoproliferative disorders after organ transplantation: a report of 24 cases observed in a single institution. J Clin Oncol 1995; 13: 961–8.

Lecuit M, Abachin E, Martin A, et al. Immunoproliferative small intestinal disease associated with Campylobacter jejuni. N Engl J Med 2004; 350: 239–48.

Leveque L, Dalac S, Dompmartin A, et al. Melanoma in orgin transplant patients. Ann Dermatol Venered 2000; 127: 160–5.

Little RF, Merced-Galindez F, Staskus K, et al. A pilot study of cidofovir in patients with Kaposi sarcoma. J Infect Dis 2003; 187: 149–53.

Liu Q, Fayad L, Cabanillas F, et al. Improvement of overall and failure-free survival in stage IV follicular lymphoma: 25 years of treatment experience at The University of Texas M.D. Anderson Cancer Center. J Clin Oncol 2006; 24: 1582–9.

London NJ, Farmey SM, Will EJ, et al. Risk of neoplasia in renal transplant patients. Lancet 1995; 346: 403–6.

Lu ZX, Ye M, Yan GR, et al. Effect of EBV LMP1 targeted DNAzymes on cell proliferation and apoptosis. Cancer Gene Ther 2005; 12: 647–54.

Luan FL, Ding R, Sharma VK, et al. Rapamycin is an effective inhibitor of human renal cancer metastasis. Kidney Int 2003; 63: 917–26.

Maisonneuve P, Agodoa L, Gellert R, et al. Cancer in patients on hemodialysis for end stage renal disease: an international collaborative study. Lancet 1999; 354: 93–9.

Majewski M, Korecka M, Kossev P, et al. The immunosuppressive macrolide RAD inhibits growth of human Epstein–Barr virus-transformed B lymphocytes in vitro and in vivo: a potential approach to prevention and treatment of posttransplant lymphoproliferative disorders. Proc Natl Acad Sci USA 2000; 97: 4285–90.

Malavaud B, Hoff M, Miedouge M, et al. PSA-based screening for prostate cancer in renal transplantation. Transplantation 2000; 69: 2461–2.

Marchetti M, Vasile C, Chiarelli S. Endometrial cancer: asymptomatic endometrial findings. Characteristics of postmenopausal endometrial cancer. Eur Gynaecol Oncol 2005; 26: 479–84.

McNamara IN, Muir J, Galbraith AJ. Acitretin for prophylaxis of cutaneous malignancies after cardiac transplantation. J Heart Lung Transplant 2002; 21: 1201–5.

Medveczky MM, Horvath E, Lund T, Medveczky PG. In vitro antiviral drug sensitivity of the Kaposi's sarcoma-associated herpesvirus. AIDS 1997; 11: 1327–32.

Milpied N, Vasseur B, Parquet N, et al. Humanized anti-CD20 monoclonal antibody (rituximab) in posttransplant B-lymphoproliferative disorder: a retrospective analysis on 32 patients. Ann Oncol 2000; 11 (Suppl 1): 113–16.

Montagnino G, Bencini PL. Cutaneous and mucosal nodules in a transplant patient. Nephrol Dial Transplant 1994; 9: 1503–4.

Montagnino G, Bencini PL, Tarantino A, et al. Clinical features and course of Kaposi's sarcoma in kidney transplant patients: report of 13 cases. Am J Nephrol 1994; 14: 121–6.

Montagnino G, Lorca E, Tarantino A, et al. Cancer incidence in 854 kidney transplant recipients from a single institution: comparison with normal population and with patients under dialytic treatment. Clin Transplant 1996; 10: 461–9.

Moore KW, Vieira P, Fiorentino DF, et al. Homology of cytokine synthesis inhibitory factor (IL-10) to the Epstein–Barr virus gene BCRF1. Science 1990; 248: 1230–4.

Moore PS, Chang Y. Detection of herpesvirus-like DNA sequences in Kaposi's sarcoma in patients with and without HIV infection. N Engl J Med 1995; 332: 1181–5.

Moosa MR. Racial and ethnic variations in incidence and pattern of malignancies after kidney transplantation. Medicine (Baltimore) 2005; 84: 12–22.

Moudouni SM, Tligui M, Doublet JD, et al. Nephron-sparing surgery for de novo renal cell carcinoma in allograft kidneys. Transplantation 2005; 80: 865–7.

Nakayama E, Akiba T, Marumo F, Sato C. Prognosis of anti-hepatitis C virus antibody-positive patients on regular hemodialysis therapy. J Am Soc Nephrol 2000; 11: 1896–902.

Nalesnik MA, Starzl TE. On the crossroad between tolerance and posttransplant lymphoma. Curr Opin Organ Transplant 1997; 2: 30–5.

Nash CL, Price LM, Stewart DA, et al. Early gastric post-transplantation lymphoproliferative disorder and H. pylori after kidney transplantation: a case report and review of the literature. Can J Gastroenterol 2000; 14: 721–4.

Nepomuceno RR, Balaton CE, Natkunam Y, et al. Rapamycin inhibits the interleukin 10 signal transduction pathway and the growth of Epstein Barr virus B-cell lymphomas. Cancer Res 2003; 63: 4472–80.

Neyts J, De Clercq E. Antiviral drug susceptibility of human herpesvirus 8. Antimicrob Agents Chemother 1997; 41: 2754–6.

Odajnyk C, Muggia FM. Treatment of Kaposi's sarcoma: overview and analysis by clinical setting. J Clin Oncol 1985; 3: 1277–85.

Oertel SH, Verschuuren E, Reinke P, et al. Effect of anti-CD20 antibody rituximab in patients with posttransplant lymphoproliferative disorder (PTLD). Am J Transplant 2005; 5: 2901–6.

Ojo AO, Hanson JA, Wolfe RA, et al. Long-term survival in renal transplant recipients with graft function. Kidney Int 2000; 57: 307–13.

Opelz G, Dohler B. Lymphomas after solid organ transplantation: a collaborative transplant study report. Am J Transplant 2004; 4: 222–30.

Opelz G, Naujokat C, Daniel V, et al. Disassociation between risk of graft loss and risk of non-Hodgkin lymphoma with induction agents in renal transplant recipients. Transplantation 2006; 81: 1227–33.

Parsonnet J, Isaacson PG. Bacterial infection and MALT lymphoma. N Engl J Med 2004; 350: 213–15.

Patel N, Salifu M, Sumrani N, et al. Successful treatment of post-renal transplant Kaposi's sarcoma with paclitaxel. Am J Transplant 2002; 2: 877–9.

Patel HS, Silver AR, Northover JM. Anal cancer in renal transplant patients. Int J Colorectal Dis 2005; 16: 1–5.

Peces R, Martinez-Ara J, Miguel JL, et al. Renal cell carcinoma co-existent with other renal disease: clinicopathological features in pre-dialysis patients and those receiving dialysis or renal transplantation. Nephrol Dial Transplant 2004; 19: 2789–96.

Peeters P, Sennesael J, De Raeve H, et al. Hemophagocytic syndrome and T-cell lymphoma after kidney transplantation: a case-report Transpl Int 1997; 10: 471–4.

Pellerin GP, Finan MA. Endometrial cancer in women 45 years of age or younger: a clinicopathological analysis. Am J Obstet Gynecol 2005; 193: 1640–4.

Penn I. Cancers of anogenital region in renal transplant recipients. Analysis of 65 cases. Cancer 1986; 58: 611–16.

Penn I. Cancers complicating organ transplantation. N Engl J Med 1990; 323: 1767–9.

Penn I. Malignancy after immunosuppressive therapy: how can the risk be reduced? Clin Immunother 1995a; 9: 207–18.

Penn I. Primary kidney tumors before and after renal transplantation. Transplantation 1995b; 59: 480–5.

Penn I. Malignant melanoma in organ allograft recipients. Transplantation 1996; 61: 274–8.

Penn I. Evaluation of transplant candidates with pre-existing malignancies. Ann Transplant 1997a; 2: 14–17.

Penn I. Transmission of cancer from organ donors. Ann Transplant 1997b; 2: 7–12.

Penn I. De novo cancers in organ allograft recipients. Curr Opin Organ Transplant 1998a; 3: 188–96.

Penn I. The role of immunosuppression in lymphoma formation. Semin Immunopathol 1998b; 20: 343–55.

Penn I. Posttransplant malignancies. Transplant Proc 1999; 31: 1260–2.

Penn I. Post-transplant malignancy: the role of immunosuppression. Drug Saf 2000; 23: 101–13.

Penn I, First, MR. Development and incidence of cancer following cyclosporine therapy. Transplant Proc 1986; 18 (Suppl 1): 210–15.

Pond F, Serpell JW, Webster A. Thyroid cancer in the renal transplant population: epidemiological study. ANZ J Surg 2005; 75: 106–9.

Ponticelli C. The pleiotropic effects of mTOR inhibitors. J Nephrol 2004; 17: 762–8.

Qunibi W, Akhtar M, Sheth K, et al. Kaposi's sarcoma: the most common tumor after renal transplantation in Saudi Arabia. Am J Med 1988; 84: 225–32.

Rabkin CS, Janz S, Lash A, et al. Monoclonal origin of multicentric Kaposi's sarcoma lesions. N Engl J Med 1997; 336: 988–93.

Radl J, Valentijn RM, Haaijman JJ, Paul LC. Monoclonal gammopathies in patients undergoing immunosuppressive treatment after renal transplantation. Clin Immunol Immunopathol 1985; 37: 98–102.

Rajakariar R, Bhattacharyya M, Norton A, et al. Post transplant T-cell lymphoma: a case series of four patients from a single unit and review of the literature. Am J Transplant 2004; 4: 1534–8.

Ramsay HM, Fryer AA, Reece S, et al. Clinical risk factors associated with nonmelanoma skin cancer in renal transplant recipients. Am J Kidney Dis 2000; 36: 167–76.

Regamey N, Tamm M, Wernli M, et al. Transmission of human herpesvirus 8 infection from renal transplant donors to recipients. N Engl J Med 1998; 138: 301–3.

Robson R, Cecka JM, Opelz G, et al. Prospective registry-based observational cohort study of the long-term risk of malignancies in renal transplant patients treated with mycophenolate mofetil. Am J Transplant 2005; 5: 2954–60.

Roncella S, Cutrona G, Traini M, et al. Late Epstein–Barr virus infection of a hepatosplenic γδ T-cell lymphoma arising in a kidney transplant recipient. Hematologica 2000; 85: 256–62.

Ross CW, Schnitzer B, Shaldon S, et al. Gamma/delta T-cell post-transplantation lymphoproliferative disorder primarily in the spleen. Am J Clin Pathol 1994; 102: 310–15.

Rubel JR, Milford EL, Abdi R. Cutaneous neoplasms in renal transplant recipients. Eur J Dermatol 2002; 12: 532–5.

Saidi RF, Dudrick PS, Goldman MH. Colorectal cancer after renal transplantation. Transplant Proc 2003; 35: 1410–12.

Sarasin A, Gigliola-Mari G. P53 gene mutations in human skin cancers. Exp Dermatol 2002; 11 (Suppl 1): 44–7.

Sarid R, Kelpfish A, Schattner A. Virology, pathogenetic mechanisms and associated diseases of Kaposi's sarcoma-associated herpesvirus (human herpesvirus 8) Mayo Clin Proc 2002; 77: 941–9.

Serraino D, Piselli P, Angeletti C, et al. Risk of Kaposi's sarcoma and of other cancers in Italian renal transplant patients. Br J Cancer 2005; 92: 572–5.

Shalling M, Ekman M, Kaaya E. A role for a new herpes virus (KSHV) in different forms of Kaposi's sarcoma. Nat Med 1995; 1: 707–8.

Sheil AG. Donor-derived malignancy in organ transplant recipients. Transplant Proc 2001; 33: 1827–9.

Sheil AG. Organ transplantation and malignancy: inevitable linkage. Transplant Proc 2002; 34: 2436–7.

Sheil AG, Disney APS, Mathew TH, Amiss N. De novo malignancy emerges as a major cause of morbidity and late failure in renal transplantation. Transplant Proc 1993; 25: 1383–4.

Sherman ME, Wang SS, Carreon J, Devesa SS. Mortality trend for cervical squamous and adenocarcinoma in the United States. Relation to incidence and survival. Cancer 2005; 103: 1258–64.

Sirianni MC, Vicenzi L, Topino S, et al. NK cell activity controls human herpesvirus 8 latent infection and is restored upon highly active antiretroviral therapy in AIDS patients with regressing Kaposi's sarcoma. Eur J Immunol 2002; 32: 2711–20.

Smith J, Rudser K, Gillen D, et al. Risk of lymphoma after transplantation varies with time: an analysis of the United States Renal Data System. Transplantation 2006; 81: 175–80.

Smith MR. Rituximab (monoclonal anti-CD20 antibody): mechanisms of action and resistance. Oncogene 2003; 22: 7359–68.

Snanoudj R, Durrbach A, Leblond V, et al. Primary brain lymphomas after kidney transplantation: presentation and outcome. Transplantation 2003; 76: 930–7.

Stallone G, Schena A, Infante B, Di Paolo S, Sirolimus for Kaposi's sarcoma in renal-transplant recipients. N Engl J Med 2005; 352: 1317–23.

Starzl TE, Nalesnik MA, Porter KA, et al. Reversibility of lymphomas and lymphoproliferative lesions developing under cyclosporin–steroid therapy. Lancet 1984; 323: 583–7.

Stewart GH, Buccianti G, Agodoa L, et al. Cancer of the kidney and urinary tract in patients on dialysis for end-stage renal disease: analysis of data from the United States, Europe, and Australia and New Zealand. J Am Soc Nephrol 2003; 14: 197–207.

Stockflet E, Ulrich C, Mayer T, Christofers E. Epithelial malignancies in organ transplant patients: clinical presentation and new methods of treatment. Recent Results Cancer Res 2002; 160: 251–8.

Svoboda J, Kotloff R, Tsai DE. Management of patients with post-transplant lymphoproliferative disorder: the role of rituximab. Transpl Int 2006; 19: 259–69.

Swinnen LJ. Treatment of organ transplant-related lymphoma. Hematol Oncol Clin North Am 1997; 11: 963–73.

Swinnen LJ, Mullen GM, Carr TT. Aggressive treatment for postcardiac transplant lymphoproliferation. Blood 1995; 86: 3333–40.

Tang S, Lo CM, Chan TM, Lai KN. Early detection of hepatocellular carcinoma in hepatitis-B-positive renal transplant recipients. J Surg Oncol 1999; 72: 99–101.

Timms JM, Bell A Flowell JR, et al. Target cell of Epstein–Barr virus (EBV) positive post-transplant lymphoproliferative disease: similarities to EBV positive Hodgkin's lymphoma. Lancet 2003; 361: 217–23.

Tolkoff-Rubin NE, Rubin RH. Viral infections in organ transplantation. Transplant Proc 1998; 30: 2060–3.

Tornroth T, Heiro M, Marcussen N, Fransilla K. Lymphomas diagnosed by percutaneous kidney biopsy. Am J Kidney Dis 2003; 42: 960–71.

Tremblay F, Fernandes M, Habbab F, et al. Malignancy after renal transplantation: incedence and role of type of immunosuppression. Ann Surg Oncol 2002; 9: 785–8.

Troffe J, Buell JJF, Woodle ES, et al. Recurrence risk after organ transplantation in patients with a history of Hodgkin disease and non-Hodgkin lymphoma. Transplantation 2004; 78: 972–7.

Tsai DE, Hardy CL, Tomaszwesky JE, et al. Reduction in immunosuppression as initial therapy for posttransplant lymphoproliferative disorders: analysis of prognostic variables and long-term follow-up of 42 adult patients. Transplantation 2001; 71: 1076–88.

Tsai DE, Nearey M, Hardy CL, et al. Use of EBV-PCR for the diagnosis and monitoring of post-transplant lymphoproliferative disorder in adult solid organ transplant patients. Am J Transplant 2002; 2: 946–54.

Tsai DE, Aqui NA, Vogl DT, et al. Successful treatment of T-cell post-transplant lymphoproliferative disorder with the retinoid analog bexarotene. Am J Transplant 2005; 5: 2070–3.

Vamvakas S, Bahner U, Heidland A. Cancer in end stage renal disease: potential factors involved. Am J Nephrol 1998; 18: 89–95.

Van Gorp J, Doornewaard H, Verdonck LF, et al. Posttransplant T-cell lymphoma. Report of three cases and a review of the literature. Cancer 1994; 73: 3064–72.

Vogt P, Frei U, Repp H, et al. Malignant tumors in renal transplant recipients receiving cyclosporin: survey of 598 first kidney transplantations. Nephrol Dial Transplant 1990; 5: 282–8.

Wasson S, Zafar MN, Best J, Reddy HK. Post-transplantation lymphoproliferative disorder in heart and kidney transplant patients: a single-center experience. J Cardiovasc Pharmacol Ther 2006; 11: 77–83.

Wei Q, Matanoski GM, Farmer ER. DNA repair and aging in basal cell carcinoma: a molecular epidemiology study. Proc Natl Acad Sci USA 1993; 90: 1614–18.

Whiting JF, Hanto DW. Cancer in recipients of organ allografts. In: Racusen LC, Solez K, Burdick JF, eds. Kidney Transplant Rejection. New York: Marcel Dekker, 1998: 577–604.

Willers CP, Reimann G, Mertins L, Brockmeyer NH. Influence of foscarnet on HIV-associated Kaposi's sarcoma derived cell lines. Eur J Med Res 1999; 14: 514–16.

zur Hausen H. Virus in human cancers. Science 1991; 254: 1167–73.

Gastrointestinal complications are frequent in renal transplant recipients and may involve any tract of the gastrointestinal tube (Helderman and Goral, 2002; Ponticelli and Passerini, 2005). Most complications are trivial and are often not referred by the patient to the transplant clinician. Nevertheless, even minor gastrointestinal symptoms may impair the psychological general well-being (Strid *et al.*, 2002). In about 10% of renal transplant patients, severe gastrointestinal disorders may develop, eventually leading to graft loss and even patient death (Sarkio *et al.*, 2004). The most frequent gastrointestinal complications in renal transplant recipients include oral lesions, esophagitis, peptic ulcer, diarrhea, colon hemorrhage, or perforation. These disorders may be related to medications, infections, and/or exacerbation of pre-existing gastrointestinal pathology.

Oral lesions

There are a number of oral lesions that may develop in renal transplant recipients (Table 12.1).

Dental problems

Most kidney transplant recipients have serious dental problems that were usually already present during dialysis. Enamel defects are common, particularly in children and young adults. They have an unusual pattern, with a much higher prevalence of diffuse opacities and enamel hypoplasia than in the normal population (Nunn *et al.*, 2000). This increased prevalence is probably due to disordered calcium and phosphate metabolism leading to demineralization. Dental and medical care should be closely integrated for renal transplant recipients to avoid the undesirable dental sequelae of, in particular, gingival overgrowth, carcinoma, and enamel hypoplasia. The last may be reparable to a high esthetic standard using dental composite filling material.

Mouth lesions

Ginigival hyperplasia is a well-known complication of cyclosporine. Risk factors for gum hyperplasia are duration of transplant, cyclosporine, serum creatinine concentration, azathioprine, and prednisone dosage (Thomason *et al.*, 2005). Moreover, gingival hyperplasia can be caused or worsened by the concomitant use of calcium channel blockers (Spoildorio *et al.*, 2002). Prevention with appropriate oral hygiene is important in controlling the inflammatory component and decreasing the severity of overgrowth. A 3–5-day treatment with azithromycin can improve subjective symptoms and the clinical picture in some patients (Nash and Zalzman, 1998; Tokgoz *et al.*, 2004). Switching from cyclosporine to tacrolimus or orthodontic therapy may be necessary in azithromycin-resistant cases. Dental disease may be responsible for malnutrition, abscess, or septicemia, and can compromise the patient's general health.

Aphtous *ulcers* are frequent and often recur in the same patient. They are usually caused by CMV. Aphtous ulcers present as well-defined circles and may be single or multiple. Ulcers can be found on all areas of the oral mucosa, except the hard palate, gingiva, and vermilion border. Biopsy specimens obtained from ulcer beds usually show intranuclear inclusions resembling an owl eye (Matsumoto *et al.*, 2004). Mouth ulcers can also be caused by drugs, being relatively frequent in patients treated with the antiproliferative mTOR (mammalian target of rapamycin) inhibitors. In a study by Van Gelder *et al.* (2003) mouth ulcers occurred in about a quarter of transplant recipients treated with sirolimus and mycophenolate mofetil (MMF) without steroids.

Herpes simplex may cause cold sores, or gingivostomatitis often accompanied by fever, malaise, and lymphadenopathy. Mucosal vesicles may also be caused by varicella zoster virus. Oral *warts* are more frequent in renal transplant recipients than in the normal population.

Table 12.1   Main oral lesions in renal transplant recipients

Demineralization	Virus-induced	Drug-induced	Malignancy	Fungal
Enamel hypoplasia	Aphtae (CMV)	Mouth ulcers (mTOR inhibitors)	Squamous-cell carcinoma	Candida albicans
	Herpes simplex (HSV-1)	Gum hypertrophy (cyclosporine, calcium channel antagonists)	Non-Hodgkin's lymphoma	
	Warts Kaposi (HHV-8) Leukoplakia (EBV)			

Oral *candidiasis* is frequent in renal transplant recipients. It can be the result of the immunosuppression or may develop after vigorous antibiotic treatment. It may cause irregular or widespread erythema, erosive changes, or a typical creamy surface. Nystatin swish and swallow every 6 hours, or cotrimazole, may be effective in preventing oral and esophageal fungal infections. *Candida*-associated denture stomatitis is particularly frequent in denture wearers taking immunosuppressive therapy (Golecka *et al.*, 2006). *Plaque-like lesions* of the oral mucosa may also be associated with bacterial overgrowth and should be treated with antibiotics and antiseptics.

Oral malignancy

Leukoplakia is a pre-cancerous lesion that may be caused by the activation of endogenous Epstein–Barr virus (EBV) or by exogenous EBV infection. Of note, EBV DNA may be detected by cytobrushing in almost 90% of renal transplant recipients (Braz-Silva *et al.*, 2006). Leukoplakia may occur in any area of the mouth. It is characterized by white plaques, and histologically by benign hyperkeratosis. In some transplant patients this lesion may rapidly progress to squamous-cell carcinoma (Hernandez *et al.*, 2003).

Kaposi's sarcoma may present as a red, purple, brown, or bluish macule or nodule, usually located on the palate or the oropharynx. (Figure 12.1).

The mouth is a rare location of *non-Hodgkin's lymphoma*, but it is more frequent in transplant patients than in the general population. Many patients with this lymphoproliferative disorder acquired an EBV infection after transplantation. *Plasmablastic lymphoma* is a recently recognized entity most often reported in the oral cavity, mainly in the setting of underlying human immunodeficiency viral infection, whereby a role for EBV and, more recently, human herpes virus 8 (HHV-8) has been described in renal transplant recipients (Yoon *et al.*, 2003).

A number of other *pre-malignant* and *malignant lesions* of the oral mucosa and of the tongue have also been reported in transplant recipients.

Esophageal disorders

The commonest esophageal disorder in renal transplant recipients is represented by *candidal esophagitis*. This usually occurs within 6 months after transplantation, and is particularly frequent in leukopenic or over-immunosuppressed patients as well as in diabetic patients and in patients debilitated from infection or other complications. The symptoms are characterized by difficult swallowing, painful swallowing, retrosternal pain, pyrosis, and odinophagia. Esophagitis may also be complicated by intractable singultus. Usually, esophagitis is associated with candidal stomatitis and epiglottitis. Occasionally, esophagitis may be complicated by fungemia. Milder cases may be treated with local nystatin. Most patients respond to treatment with

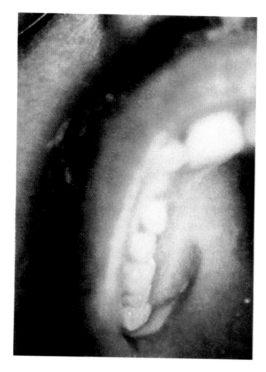

Figure 12.1 Oral Kaposi's sarcoma localized at palate

intravenous amphotericin B for 2–6 days (Frick *et al.*, 1988). Voriconazole also has a broad anti-candidal activity, but is less nephrotoxic than amphotericin B. However, a substantial reduction of mTOR antagonists and calcineurin inhibitors is required as there is a strong interaction of this triazole with drugs metabolized by the cytochrome P450 system (Mathis *et al.*, 2004). Caspofungin, an echinocandin, has been reported to be effective and well tolerated in patients given cyclosporine (Anttila *et al.*, 2003).

Other causes of esophagitis include *CMV* (Bobak, 2003) or *herpes simplex* infection (Mosiman *et al.*, 1994). The typical appearance of viral esophagitis, which occurs more frequently during periods of intensive immunosuppression, is represented by multiple erosive lesions with or without ulcers along the entire esophagus. Vesicular lesions are usually seen in case of herpetic esophagitis. However, since the endoscopic manifestation of herpetic esophagitis may be variable, the diagnosis should be confirmed by cytology, tissue studies, and viral cultures. The infection responds to specific antiviral agents, which should be started as soon as the diagnosis is confirmed, since untreated viral ulcers can progress to esophageal perforation and/or hemorrhage, which may even be fatal (Helderman and Goral, 2002).

The esophagus may be involved by *Kaposi's sarcoma*. On endoscopy, the lesions appear as multiple grayish-purple plaques. Although most lesions are asymptomatic, a digestive hemorrhage may be the first sign of the disease. Rarely, the esophagus may be the first localization of an extranodal *lymphoproliferative disorder* in renal transplant patients (Kranz *et al.*, 2006).

Stomach and duodenum disorders

Gastric discomfort

A number of transplant patients may suffer from nausea, vomiting, abdominal pain, or gastric discomfort. These symptoms may be caused by the numerous pills that some patients have to take every day, by trivial infections favored by immunosuppressive therapy, or by the specific gastric toxicity of calcineurin

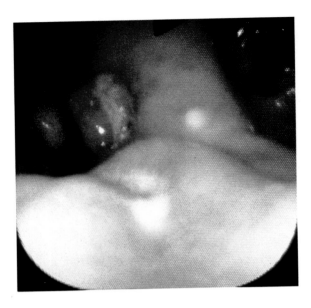

Figure 12.2 Two peptic uicers of the angulus at gastroscopy in a transplant recipient with a previous history of peptic ulcer during dialysis treatment. (Courtesy of Dr A Carrara, Ospedale Maggiore, Milan.)

inhibitors, corticosteroids, or MMF. Nausea, vomiting, dyspepsia, and anorexia are particularly frequent in patients given MMF, occurring in 49.7% of cases within the first 6 months after transplantation (Tierce et al., 2005). These complications are related to the dose of the drug and to the peak concentration of mycophenolic acid in the blood (Behrend and Braun, 2005). The gastric adverse effects are irritative in nature and are often reversible. However, in a number of patients they may require a dose change, which may increase the risk of acute rejection (Knoll et al., 2003; Tierce et al., 2005) and decrease the graft survival (Hardinger et al., 2004; Pelletier et al., 2003). As gastric symptoms are related to the peak blood concentration, it is advisable to subdivide the daily dose of MMF into two or even three administrations. Recently, an enteric-coated sodium mycophenolate has been produced that has proved to be therapeutically equivalent to MMF in de novo renal transplant patients (Salvadori et al., 2004; Massari et al., 2005). No significant differences in safety profile and the incidence of gastrointestinal adverse events were seen in randomized studies comparing MMF and sodium mycophenolate (Budde et al., 2004; Kamar et al., 2005). However, an exploratory study indicated that converting patients with moderate or severe gastrointestinal symptoms from MMF to enteric-coated mycophenolate sodium significantly reduced the symptom burden and improved patient functioning and well-being (Chan et al., 2006).

Peptic ulcer

Gastroduodenal ulcer was a frequent cause of mortality until a few years ago, accounting for about 4% of deaths after transplantation (Kestens and Alexandre, 1988). More recently, however, the prognosis has improved, and mortality or graft loss due to peptic ulcer have become exceptional. Several factors may contribute to the development of post-transplant peptic ulcer disease (Figure 12.2).

Risk factors (Table 12.2)

An important risk factor for peptic ulcer is a *history of peptic ulcer disease* (Chen et al., 2004). About 30% of renal transplant recipients have *Helicobacter pylori colonization* of the stomach (Sarkio et al., 2001). The *emotional stress* caused by the operation and by postoperative complications may also play an important role. Although the ulcerogenic role of *corticosteroids* is still controversial, the high doses of corticosteroids may contribute to the stress in favoring the development of peptic ulcer (Messman and Scholmerich, 2000). As a matter of fact, a strong association between intravenous high-dose methylprednisolone pulses and the development of peptic ulcer has been found in a series (Chen et al., 2004). *MMF*

Table 12.2 Factors predisposing to the development of peptic ulcer in renal transplant patients. Well-established factors are given in italic

General	Immunosuppressive drugs	Other drugs
History of previous ulcer	*High-dose IV corticosteroids*	*Aspirin*
H. pylori colonization	Oral corticosteroids	*NSAIDs*
Emotional stress	Mycophenolate mofetil	
Cigarette-smoking	Sirolimus	

displays a similar side-effect profile to that of *non-steroidal anti-inflammatory drugs* with 3–8% of cases of ulcer perforation or bleeding within 6 months (Bjarnason, 2001). Cases of gastrointestinal hemorrhage due to complicated gastroduodenal ulcer have also been reported in patients taking *sirolimus*, probably as a consequence of the retarded healing caused by the drug (Smith *et al.*, 2005). Finally, *cigarette-smoking* may also lead to ulceration by worsening the detrimental effects of aggressive factors and impairing the repair of gastric ulceration (Wu and Cho, 2004).

Prevention and treatment

At present the incidence of peptic ulcer has declined substantially. This is mainly due to the fact that transplant candidates are actively screened for evidence of peptic ulcer before transplantation. Patients with pre-existing ulcer are usually treated with H_2-receptor antagonists or proton-pump inhibitors. Antibiotic therapy directed to eradicate *H. pylori* further contributes to complete healing of the ulcer. Moreover, doses of corticosteroids have been considerably reduced in comparison with the past. The incidence of rejection and other complications is also reduced. Today, many transplant groups use prophylactic H_2-receptor antagonists, proton-pump inhibitors, or sucralfate after operation. The utility of this routine *prophylaxis* may be challenged, but it is a common experience that the mortality due to gastroduodenal perforation or hemorrhage falls to almost zero after the constant use of preventive anti-ulcer therapy. At any rate, there are no doubts that patients with a history of a previous ulcer should be given gastric protection for the first few months after transplantation. Considering the excellent results of non-operative ulcer therapy in transplant patients, surgery should be limited to exceptional, complicated cases.

Viral infections

Other causes of gastroduodenal disorders include *CMV* and *herpes simplex infection*. CMV infection is a frequent cause of nausea, vomiting, gastroparesis, or bleeding. In kidney transplant patients with upper gastrointestinal symptoms, 40% showed a polymerase chain reaction positive for CMV (Peter *et al.*, 2004) and 74% who received gastroscopy showed a biopsy positive for CMV (Sarkio *et al.*, 2005).

Small bowel disorders

Ulcers of the small intestine represent a rare but dreadful complication of renal transplantation. Their development may be favored by corticosteroids, sirolimus (Molinari *et al.*, 2005), or intestinal ischemia (Dee *et al.*, 2002), and even more often by CMV infection (Bobak, 2003). An increased incidence of ischemia and obstruction of the small bowel has been reported in patients with polycystic kidney disease, possibly as a consequence of circulating active secretagogs produced by extrarenal cysts (Andreoni *et al.*, 1999).

The small bowel tract more often involved is *terminal ileum*. The clinical picture consists of periumbilical colicky pain, nausea, and vomiting. Frequently the patient presents with small bowel obstruction, bleeding, or perforation. The diagnosis is difficult. Plain films of the abdomen may show signs of obstruction or perforation. Endoscopy may reveal ulcers in the high jejunum. A new non-invasive technique, wireless capsule endoscopy, allows visualization of the entire small intestine, and represents a major improvement in diagnosis. If the involved segment is perforated, stenotic, or bleeding, it should be resected.

Colon disorders

About half of renal transplant recipients presenting with lower abdominal symptoms may show abnormalities at colonoscopy (Korkmaz *et al.*, 2004). The risk of colonic complications is increased in elderly transplant patients and in those with polycystic kidney disease (Dominguez-Fernandez *et al.*, 1998).

Cecum or *ascending colon hemorrhage* can occur in association with severe CMV infection or, rarely, with zygomycosis (Echo *et al.*, 2005).

Colon perforation may complicate a diverticular disease or be a consequence of intestinal ischemia or disseminated CMV infection. In this regard, it should be noted that an increasing number of life-threatening ischemic colitis cases caused by CMV are being reported in organ transplant recipients (Maurer, 2000; Bobak, 2003; De Bartolomeis *et al.*, 2005). In patients with fever and abdominal pain, early viral detection by CMV polymerase chain reaction can be life-saving (Lee *et al.*, 2004). Rare cases of colonic perforation caused by malakoplakia have been reported (Berney *et al.*, 1999). Malakoplakia is a rare pseudotumoral inflammatory disease known to affect immunocompromised subjects, mainly with a history of recurrent *Escherichia coli* infection. The urinary tract is the most frequent site of the disease, but all organs can be involved. Colonic perforation is often fatal in transplant recipients because of the inability to contain the perforation, and only rapid diagnosis and aggressive surgical treatment can improve the prognosis.

Pseudo-obstruction is a potentially dangerous condition with symptoms, signs, and X-radiologic appearance of an acute, large bowel obstruction, but without any identifiable cause. The treatment is conservative, with nasogastric decompression and neostigmine (Remzi, 2002).

Inflammatory bowel disease in spite of immunosuppression has been reported in 14 transplant patients. Of them, nine developed ulcerative colitis and five Crohn's disease. Seven patients with ulcerative colitis remained in remission, but two patients required colectomy. Patients with Crohn's disease continued to have flares despite treatment (Riley *et al.*, 1997).

Diarrhea

Diarrhea may be defined as more than three bowel movements per day with a daily stool bulk exceeding 150 ml. Diarrhea is frequent in renal transplant recipients. The main causes of diarrhea after transplantation are: infections, immunosuppressive drugs, antibiotics, and other drugs.

Etiology

Infectious agents

Severe diarrhea is often caused by infectious agents (Maes *et al.*, 2006). A number of micro-organisms may be responsible for diarrhea: bacteria, viruses, and parasites (Table 12.3). *Enteric bacteria* responsible for diarrhea are *Shigella*, *Salmonella typhi* and *typhimurium* and *Campylobacter*.

Approximately 50% of transplant patients receiving antibiotics for any reason develop *Clostridium difficile*-associated diarrhea (Sellin, 2001). Symptoms may begin at any time during the course of antimicrobial treatment, or even after antimicrobial agents have been stopped. *Pseudomembranous colitis* is the result of a toxin-mediated enteric disease, while there is no microbial invasion of the intestinal mucosa. The most common symptom is diarrhea, often associated with fever. Dehydration, hypoalbuminemia, electrolyte disturbances, and colonic perforation, due to necrotizing colitis with gangrene, are the most frequent complications. Colonoscopy, showing a typical pseudomembranous colitis, and the identification of *C. difficile* or its toxin in the stool may confirm the diagnosis. Recurrent disease may develop in about 20% of cases. Life-threatening fulminant cases requiring colectomy have been reported in kidney and in kidney and pancreas transplant recipients (Keven *et al.*, 2004).

Table 12.3   Main micro-organisms responsible for diarrhea in renal transplant patients

Bacteria

Clostridium difficile (oral vancomycin), *Salmonella* species (fluoroquinolones), *Campylobacter jejuni*, *Listeria monocytogenes* (ampicillin–sulbactam), other enteric pathogens (*Shigella, Yersinia, E. coli*)

Viruses

CMV, herpes simplex, adenovirus, Coxsackie, rotavirus

Parasites

Cryptosporidium, Microsporidium, Isospora belli, Strongyloides stercoralis, Giardia lamblia (quinacrine, metronidazole)

The most frequent cases of acute diarrhea are of viral etiology, and typically last for a period of 1–3 days. *CMV infection* with gastrointestinal involvement is a frequent cause of diarrhea. In CMV enterocolitis, with or without fever, gastrointestinal bleeding, perforation, and toxic megacolon are possible complications. *Adenovirus, rotavirus,* and *enterovirus* may also be responsible for diarrhea.

Diarrhea due to gastrointestinal *protozoal* infection is not reported frequently in transplant patients, although T cell-associated immunity plays an important role against protection from these agents. *Cryptosporidium* is one of the most frequent protozoa causing a usually self-limiting diarrhea. In immunocompromised hosts, however, the infection may be protracted and life-threatening. In transplant patients, a course of antimicrobial therapy along with concurrent reduction in immunosuppression optimizes the immunologic status and may potentially lead to resolution of the infection (Tran *et al.*, 2005).

Drugs

Drug-induced diarrhea is also frequent. All the major immunosuppressive agents may cause diarrhea (Pescovitz and Navarro, 2001). In a meta-analysis of randomized trials that compared tacrolimus and cyclosporine, diarrhea was more frequently associated with *tacrolimus* than with *cyclosporine* (Webster *et al.*, 2005). In another study, diarrhea incidence was significantly higher with *mycophenolate mofetil* than with *azathioprine* (Wang *et al.*, 2004). It has been hypothesized that potent inhibition of the purine salvage pathway cannot keep up with the growing need for guanine nucleotides by the rapidly dividing nature of the gastrointestinal tract (Neerman and Boothe, 2003). *Sirolimus* (Vasquez, 2000) and *everolimus* (Vitko *et al.*, 2005) may also cause diarrhea, possibly as a consequence of their potent antiproliferative effects on enterocytes. *Antibiotics* are a well-recognized cause of diarrhea, by altering the gut flora. Other agents that may cause diarrhea are *colchicine* and *misoprostol*.

Differential diagnosis

The differential diagnosis between infectious disease and drug-caused diarrhea in transplant recipients is as important as it is difficult (Table 12.4). *Drug history* should be the initial step of the diagnostic approach. The *time of onset* is also important. If diarrhea occurs in the first month after transplantation, a role of immunosuppression is likely, and reduction of the drug dosage may be the first therapeutic step. Instead, if diarrhea develops after the first post-transplant month, infectious disease is probable, unless there was a recent increase in immunosuppression (Rubin, 2001). Diarrhea developing within 12 hours of a meal is likely caused by the ingestion of staphylococcal toxins. A lag period of 3 or more days after consumption of a contaminated meal is usually seen in salmonellosis. Diarrhea which develops later than 48 hours after

Table 12.4   Differential diagnosis and main characteristics of drug-induced and post-bacterial diarrhea

Drug-induced	Bacteria-induced
Characteristics	*Characteristics*
Usually within the first month	After the first month
No fever	Fever
No leukocytosis	Inflammatory cells in the stool
Precautions	*Clues to etiological diagnosis*
Check blood levels of tacrolimus (increasing)	Staphylococcal < 12 hours after meal
	Salmonella ≥ 3 days after meal
	Nosocomial > 2 days after hospitalization

hospitalization must be considered nosocomial. *Fever* is present in more than 50% of infections, while it is usually absent in drug-induced diarrhea. *Inflammatory cells* in the stool may be seen in 25–40%, and abnormality on endoscopy or computed tomography in about 50% of cases caused by infection, while they are absent in cases caused by immunosuppressive agents. As a rule, in any case of diarrhea, the *stools* should be examined for bacteria and parasites, including coccidians and *Microsporidia*. In cases of negative work-up, endoscopic assessment should be done in search of a diagnosis. Of note, while blood levels of cyclosporine under diarrhea remain stable, the blood levels of tacrolimus show a significant increase. Thus, the *blood levels of tacrolimus* should be carefully monitored, especially when MMF is withdrawn (Maes *et al.*, 2002).

Treatment

Treatment of diarrhea includes rest and large fluid intake, preferably with sugar and electrolytes. In the most severe cases, intravenous infusion of fluid and electrolytes is needed. Opioids should be avoided at the beginning, as diarrhea can eliminate toxins and micro-organisms. However, they may be of relief in cases of persisting diarrhea. The specific treatment depends on the etiology. In the case of diarrhea caused by an immunosuppressive agent, removal of the offending drug is usually sufficient to reverse the symptoms. Antibacterial (fluoroquinolones, ampicillin) or antiparasitic agents (metronidazole) may be given while waiting for the results of stool cultures. Treatment of *Clostridium difficile* consists of vancomycin given orally, 125–500 mg four times daily for 7–14 days. The addition of the probiotic agent *Saccharomyces boulardii* can reduce the risk of recurrence (Schaier *et al.*, 2004). Cholestyramine, 1 g three times daily for 5 days, may bind the toxin and may be used in milder cases.

Intestinal ischemia

Intestinal ischemia is an important cause of morbidity and mortality after kidney transplantation. It is more frequent in patients older than 40 years and in patients receiving long-term hemodialysis. The most frequent *symptoms* and *signs* are abdominal pain, fever, tenderness, and leukocytosis. However, in immunosuppressed transplant patients, the clinical presentation may be atypical with vague abdominal symptoms, fever of unknown origin (Lee *et al.*, 2004), or persistent afebrile diarrhea (Maes *et al.*, 2003). A diagnosis of intestinal ischemia should be considered in patients who develop abdominal symptoms during the early post-transplant period. *Pneumoperitoneum* may occur in about one-third of cases. Plain abdominal X-ray films, CT scan, and/or colonoscopy are helpful for a correct diagnosis. The *prognosis* is particularly severe, with a mortality rate ranging around 55% (Dee *et al.*, 2002). Aggressive diagnostic evaluation and treatment may improve the prognosis (Lederman *et al.*, 1998). *Treatment* should consist of early surgery under a broad spectrum of antibiotics and the reduction of immunosuppressive therapy.

Intestinal tuberculosis

Intestinal tuberculosis is rare. The *diagnosis* can be difficult because its symptoms and laboratory results are non-specific. In a transplant patient the disease may present with abdominal pain, digestive bleeding, weight loss, and unexplained fever. More rarely, intestinal tuberculosis is associated with massive hemorrhage, diarrhea, or severe anemia (Kandutsch *et al.*, 2004). The vague character of symptoms and the radiographic presentation of this disease, which frequently mimics many other conditions, may lead to great difficulties in its diagnosis. In most cases the diagnosis of intestinal tuberculosis in transplant patients was made post-mortem.

All levels of the gastrointestinal tract may be involved. Colonoscopy is important to confirm a suspected diagnosis. The most characteristic endoscopic findings are circular ulcers, small diverticula (3–5 mm), and sessile firm polyps. The suspected diagnosis must be confirmed by the presence of caseating granulomas and/or acid-fast bacilli. Polymerase chain reaction is currently recommended for assessing the presence of tubercle bacilli in tissue specimens obtained by endoscopic biopsy.

Gastrointestinal malignancy

Carcinoma

The risk of gastric *carcinoma* in transplant patients is similar to that observed in the general population, while that of rectal cancer is significantly reduced. However, the relative risk of anal cancer is modestly increased, particularly in renal transplant patients with papilloma virus infection (Patel *et al.*, 2005). However, the risk of colon cancer is higher than in the general population (Stewart *et al.*, 1997). Particularly elevated is the risk of anal carcinoma, which is around 100 times more frequent than in the general population (Penn, 1998).

The development of hyperplastic and multiple *gastric polyps* in organ transplant recipients has been reported in a few cases (Amaro *et al.*, 2002). The cause is unknown.

Kaposi's sarcoma

Kaposi's sarcoma may involve the gastrointestinal tract, and may rarely cause massive gastrointestinal hemorrhage (Calzone *et al.*, 2002). Gastrointestinal lesions are more responsive to liposomal doxorubicin than are cutaneous lesions (Hernandez-Morales, and Hernandez-Zaccaro, 2005).

Lymphoma

Lymphoproliferative disorders can involve the gastrointestinal tract in up to 10% of transplant recipients (Nash *et al.*, 2000). Most post-transplant lymphoproliferative disorders (PTLD) are *B cell lymphomas* associated with the Epstein–Barr virus. The risk of PTLD is particularly elevated for transplant recipients without anti-EBV antibodies, and for those treated with antilymphocyte antibodies (Opelz and Dohler, 2004). The *diagnosis* of gastrointestinal PTLD is usually difficult. The disease is often heralded by hemorrhage or by acute abdomen from perforation or obstruction. The *prevention* of PTLD relies on the prevention and treatment of EBV infection. The role of antiviral agents is still under discussion. However, a combination of reducing immunosuppression, antiviral agents, and anti-CMV immunoglobulins could obtain a significant reduction of EBV DNA levels in a consistent number of pediatric liver transplant recipients (Holmes *et al.*, 2002). Experimental studies have shown that the mTOR inhibitors sirolimus (Nepomuceno *et al.*, 2003) and everolimus (Majiewski *et al.*, 2003) can inhibit the replication of EBV, suggesting a possible role of these drugs for preventing and treating EBV infection and related disorders. The *treatment* of EBV-associated lymphoproliferative disorders may consist of different steps (see Chapter 11). The reduction or withdrawal of immunosuppression may give good results in low-risk patients (Tsai *et al.*, 2001). Antiviral treatment may have an additional protective effect. Interferon-α and chemotherapy can be effective in resistant cases. Rituximab, a monoclonal antibody directed against the CD20 antigen of B cells, can obtain a response in two-thirds of post-transplant lymphoproliferative disorders (Milpied *et al.*, 2000). However, resistance may occur (Smith, 2003). In these cases, treatment may be more effective when combined with chemotherapy (Gulley *et al.*, 2003).

Very rare cases of *T-cell intestinal lymphoma* have also been reported. The prognosis is severe, despite aggressive chemotherapy (Michael *et al.*, 2003).

A particular form of lymphoma is *MALT lymphoma*, which is associated with *Helicobacter pylori* infection in the gastric location and with *Campylobacter jejuni* in the small intestine. MALT lymphoma may respond in milder cases to a reduction of immunosuppression (Hsi *et al.*, 2000) and/or to specific antibiotics against *H. pylori* (Shehab *et al.*, 2001; Aull, 2003).

References

Amaro R, Neff GW, Karnam US, et al. Acquired hyperplastic gastric polyps in solid organ transplant patients. Am J Gastroenterol 2002; 97: 2220–4.

Andreoni KA, Pelletier RP, Elkhammas EA, et al. Increased incidence of gastrointestinal surgical complications in renal transplant recipients with polycystic disease. Transplantation 1999; 67: 262–6.

Anttila VJ, Piilonen A, Valtonen M. Co-administration of caspofungin and cyclosporine to a kidney transplant patient with pulmonary Aspergillus infection. Scand J Infect Dis 2003; 35: 893–4.

Aull MJ, Buell JF, Peddi VR, et al. MALToma: a Helicobacter pylori-associated malignancy in transplant patients: a report from the Israel Penn International Transplant Tumor Registry with a review of published literature. Transplantation 2003; 75: 225–8.

Behrend M, Braun F. Enteric-coated mycophenolate sodium: tolerability profile compared with mycophenolate mofetil. Drugs 2005; 65: 1037–50.

Berney T, Chautems R, Ciccarelli O, et al. Malakoplakia of the caecum in a kidney-transplant recipient: presentation as acute tumoral perforation and fatal outcome. Transpl Int 1999; 12: 293–6.

Bjarnason I. Enteric coating of mycophenolate sodium: a rational approach to limit topical gastrointestinal lesions and extend the therapeutic index of mycophenolate. Transplant Proc 2001; 33: 3238–40.

Bobak DA. Gastrointestinal infections caused by cytomegalovirus. Curr Infect Dis Rep 2003; 5: 101–7.

Braz-Silva PH, Ortega KL, Rezende NP, et al. Detection of Epstein–Barr virus (EBV) in the oral mucosa of renal transplant patients. Diagn Cytopathol 2006; 34: 24–8.

Budde K, Curtis J, Knoll G, et al. Enteric-coated mycophenolate sodium can be safely administered in maintenance renal transplant patients: results of a 1-year study. Am J Transplant 2004; 4: 237–43.

Calzone A, Naso P, Puliatti C. Massive gastrointestinal hemorrhage in a renal transplant recipient due to visceral Kaposi's sarcoma. Endoscopy 2002; 34: 179.

Chan L, Mulgaonkar S, Walker R, et al. Patient-reported gastrointestinal burden and health-related quality of life following conversion from mycophenolate mofetil to enteric-coated mycophenolate sodium. Transplantation 2006; 81: 1290–7.

Chen KJ, Chen CH, Cheng CH, et al. Risk factors for peptic ulcer disease in renal transplant recipients – 11 years of experience from a single center. Clin Nephrol 2004; 62: 14–20.

De Bartolomeis C, Collini A, Barni R, et al. Cytomegalovirus infection with multiple colonic perforations in a renal transplant recipient. Transplant Proc 2005; 37: 2504–6.

Dee SL, Butt K, Ramaswamy G. Intestinal ischemia. Arch Pathol Lab Med 2002; 126: 1201–4.

Dominguez- Fernandez E, Albrecht KH, Heemann U, et al. Prevalence of diverticulosis and incidence of bowel perforation after kidney transplantation in patients with polycystic kidney disease. Transpl Int 1998; 11: 28–31.

Echo A, Hovsepian RV, Shen GK. Localized cecal zygomycosis following renal transplantation. Transpl Infect Dis 2005; 7: 68–70.

Frick T, Fryd DS, Goodale RL, et al. Incidence and treatment of candida esophagitis in patients undergoing renal transplantation. Data from the Minnesota prospective randomized trial of cyclosporine versus antilymphocyte globulin-azathioprine. Am J Surg 1988; 155: 311–13.

Golecka M, Oldakowska-Jedynak E, Mierzwinska-Nastalska E, Adamczyk-Sosinska E. Candida-associated denture stomatitis in patients after immunosuppression therapy. Transplant Proc 2006; 38: 155–6.

Gulley ML, Swinnen LH, Plaisance KT, et al. Tumor origin and CD20 expression in posttransplant lymphoproliferative disorder occurring in solid organ transplant recipients: implication for immune based therapy. Transplantation 2003; 79: 959–64.

Hardinger K, Brennan DC, Lowell J, Schnitzler MA. Long-term outcome of gastrointestinal complications in renal transplant patients treated with mycophenolate mofetil. Transpl Int 2004; 17: 609–16.

Helderman JH, Goral S. Gastrointestinal complications in renal transplantation. J Am Soc Nephrol 2002; 13: 277–87.

Hernandez G, Arriba L, Jimenez C, et al. Rapid progression from oral leukoplakia to carcinoma in an immunosuppressed liver transplant recipient. Oral Oncol 2003; 39: 87–90.

Hernandez-Morales DE, Hernandez-Zaccaro AE. Gastrointestinal and cutaneous AIDS-related Kaposi's sarcoma: different activity of liposomal doxorubicin according to location of lesions. Eur J Cancer Care 2005; 14: 264–6.

Holmes DR, Orban-Eller K, Karrer FR, et al. Response of elevated Epstein–Barr virus DNA levels to therapeutic changes in pediatric liver transplant patients: 56 months follow-up and outcome. Transplantation 2002; 74: 367–72.

Hsi ED, Singleton TP, Swinnen L, et al. Mucosa-associated lymphoid tissue-type lymphomas occurring in post-transplantation patients. Am J Surg Pathol 2000; 24: 100–6.

Kamar N, Oufroukhi L, Faure P, et al. Questionnaire-based evaluation of gastrointestinal disorders in de novo renal-transplant patients receiving either mycophenolate mofetil or enteric-coated mycophenolate sodium. Nephrol Dial Transplant 2005; 10: 2231–6.

Kandutsch S, Feix A, Haas M, et al. A rare case of anemia due to intestinal tuberculosis in a renal transplant recipient. Clin Nephrol 2004; 62: 168–71.

Kestens PJ, Alexandre GPJ. Gastroduodenal complications after transplantation. Clin Transplant 1988; 2: 221–5.

Keven K, Basu A, Re L, et al. Clostridium difficile colitis in patients after kidney and pancreas–kidney transplantation. Transpl Infect Dis 2004; 6: 10–14.

Knoll GA, MacDonald I, Khan A, Van Walraven C. Mycophenolate mofetil dose reduction and the risk of acute rejection after renal transplantation. J Am Soc Nephrol 2003; 14: 2381–6.

Korkmaz M, Gur G, Yilmaz U. Colonoscopy is a useful diagnostic tool for transplant recipients with lower abdominal symptoms. Transplant Proc 2004; 36: 190–2.

Kranz B, Vester U, Becker J, et al. Unusual manifestation of posttransplant lymphoproliferative disorder in the esophagus. Transplant Proc 2006; 38: 693–6.

Lederman ED, Conti DJ, Lempert N, et al. Complicated diverticulitis following renal transplantation. Dis Colon Rectum 1998; 41: 613–18.

Lee CJ, Lian JD, Chang SW, et al. Lethal cytomegalovirus ischemic colitis presenting with fever of unknown origin. Transpl Infect Dis 2004; 6: 124–8.

Maes BD, Lemahieu W, Kuypers D. Differential effect of diarrhea on FK 506 versus cyclosporine A trough levels and resultant prevention of allograft rejection in renal transplant recipients. Am J Transplant 2002; 2: 989–92.

Maes BD, Dalle L, Geboes K, et al. Erosive enterocolitis in mycophenolate mofetil-treated renal transplant recipients with persistent afebrile diarrhea. Transplantation 2003; 75: 665–72.

Maes BD, Hadaya K, de Moor B, et al. Severe diarrhea in renal transplant patients: results of DIDACT study. Am J Transplant 2006; 6: 1466–72.

Majiewski M, Korecka M, Joergensen J, et al. Immunosuppressive TOR kinase inhibitor everolimus (RAD) suppresses growth of cells derived from posttransplant lymphoproliferative disorder at allograft-protecting doses. Transplantation 2003; 63: 4472–80.

Massari P, Duro-Garcia V, Giron F, et al. Safety assessment of the conversion from mycophenolate mofetil to enteric-coated mycophenolate sodium in stable renal transplant recipients. Transplant Proc 2005; 37: 916–19.

Mathis AS, Shah NK, Friedman GS. Combined use of sirolimus and voriconazole in renal transplantation: a report of two cases. Transplant Proc 2004; 36: 2708–9.

Matsumoto CS, Fishbein TM, Kaufman SS. Gastrointestinal infections in solid organ transplant recipients. Curr Opin Organ Transplant 2004; 9: 406–12.

Maurer JR. The spectrum of colonic complications in a lung transplant population. Ann Transplant 2000; 5: 54–7.

Messman H, Scholmerich J. Do adrenal cortical hormones influence the pathogenesis of stress ulcer? Dtsch Med Wochenschr 2000; 125: 99–100.

Michael J, Greenstein S, Schechner R. Primary intestinal posttransplant T-cell lymphoma. Transplantation 2003; 75: 2131–2.

Milpied N, Vasseur B, Parquet N, et al. Humanized anti-CD20 monoclonal antibody (rituximab) in posttransplant B-lymphoproliferative disorder: a retrospective analysis on 32 patients. Ann Oncol 2000; 11 (Suppl 1): 113–16.

Molinari M, Al-Saif F, Ryan EA, et al. Sirolimus-induced ulceration of the small bowel in islet transplant recipients: report of two cases. Am J Transplant 2005; 5: 2799–804.

Mosiman F, Cuenoud PF, Steinhauslin F, Wauters JP. Herpes simplex esophagitis after renal transplantation. Transpl Int 1994; 7: 79–82.

Nash CL, Price LM, Stewart DA, et al. Early gastric post-transplantation lymphoproliferative disorder and H. pylori after kidney transplantation: a case report and review of the literature. Can J Gastroenterol 2000; 14: 721–4.

Nash MM, Zaltzman JS. Efficacy of azithromycin in the treatment of cyclosporine-induced gingival hyperplasia in renal transplant recipients. Transplantation 1998; 65: 1611–15.

Neerman MF, Boothe DM. A possible mechanism of gastrointestinal toxicity posed by mycophenolic acid. Pharmacol Res 2003; 47: 523–6.

Nepomuceno RR, Balatoni CE, Natkuman Y, et al. Rapamycin inhibits the interleukin 10 signal transduction pathway and the growth of Epstein Barr virus B cell lymphomas. Cancer Res 2003; 63: 4472–80.

Nunn JH, Sharp J, Lambert HJ, et al. Oral health in children with renal disease. Pediatr Nephrol 2000; 14: 997–1001.

Opelz G, Dohler B. Lymphomas after solid organ transplantation: a collaborative transplant study report. Am J Transplant 2004; 4: 222–30.

Patel HS, Silver AR, Northover JM. Anal cancer in renal transplant patients. Int J Colorectal Dis 2005; 16: 1–5.

Pelletier RP, Akin B, Henry ML, et al. The impact of mycophenolate mofetil dosing patterns on clinical outcome after renal transplantation. Clin Transplant 2003; 17: 200–20.

Penn I. De novo cancers in organ allograft recipients. Curr Opin Organ Transplant 1998; 3: 188–96.

Pescovitz MD, Navarro MT. Immunosuppressive therapy and post-transplantation diarrhea. Clin Transplant 2001; 15 (Suppl 4): 23–8.

Peter A, Telkes G, Varga M, et al. Endoscopic diagnosis of cytomegalovirus infection of upper gastrointestinal tract in solid organ transplant recipients: Hungarian single experience. Clin Transplant 2004; 18: 580–4.

Ponticelli C, Passerini P. Gastrointestinal complications in renal transplantation. Transpl Int 2005; 18: 643–50.

Remzi FH. Colonic complications of organ transplantation. Transplant Proc 2002; 34: 2119–21.

Riley TR, Schoen RE, Lee RG, Rakela J. A case series of transplant recipients who despite immunosuppression developed inflammatory bowel disease. Am J Gastroenterol 1997; 92: 279–82.

Rubin RH. Gastrointestinal infectious disease complications following transplantation and their differentiation from immunosuppressant-induced gastrointestinal toxicity. Clin Transplant 2001; 15 (Suppl 4): 11–22.

Salvadori M, Holzer H, de Mattos A, et al. Enteric-coated mycophenolate sodium is therapeutically equivalent to mycophenolate mofetil in de novo renal transplant patients. Am J Transplant 2004; 4: 231–6.

Sarkio S, Rautelin H, Kyllonen L, et al. Should Helicobacter pylori infection be treated before kidney transplantation? Nephrol Dial Transplant 2001; 16: 2053–7.

Sarkio S, Halme L, Kyllonen L, Salmela K. Severe gastrointestinal complications after 1515 adult kidney transplantations. Transpl Int 2004; 17: 505–10.

Sarkio S, Halme L, Arola J, et al. Gastrointestinal cytomegalovirus infection is common in kidney transplant patients. Scand J Gastroenterol 2005; 40: 508–14.

Schaier M, Wendt C, Zeier M, Ritz E. Clostridium difficile diarrhoea in the immunosuppressed patient – update on prevention and management. Nephrol Dial Transplant 2004; 19: 2432–6.

Sellin JD. The pathophysiology of diarrhea. Clin Transplant 2001; 15 (Suppl 4): 2–10.

Shehab TM, Hsi ED, Poterucha JJ, et al. Helicobacter pylori-associated gastric MALT lymphoma in liver transplant recipients. Transplantation 2001; 71: 1172–5.

Smith AD, Bai D, Marroquin CE, et al. Gastrointestinal hemorrhage due to complicated gastroduodenal ulcer disease in liver transplant patients taking sirolimus. Clin Transplant 2005; 19: 250–4.

Smith MR. Rituximab (monoclonal anti-CD20 antibody): mechanisms of action and resistance. Oncogene 2003; 22: 7359–68.

Spoildorio LC, Spoildorio DM, Neves KA, et al. Morphological evaluation of combined effects of cyclosporine and nifedipine on gingival overgrowth in rats. J Periodontal Res 2002; 37: 192–5.

Stewart T, Henderson R, Grayson H, Opelz G. Reduced incidence of rectal cancer, compared to gastric and colonic cancer, in a population of 73 076 men and women chronically immunosuppressed. Clin Cancer Res 1997; 3: 51–5.

Strid H, Simren M, Johansson AC, et al. The prevalence of gastrointestinal disorders with impaired psychological general well–being. Nephrol Dial Transplant 2002; 8: 1434–9.

Thomason JM, Seymour RA, Ellis J. Risk factors for gingival overgrowth for patients medicated with ciclosporin in the absence of calcium channel blockers. J Clin Periodontol 2005; 32: 273–9.

Tierce JC, Porterfield-Baxa J, Petrilla AA, et al. Impact of mycophenolate mofetil (MMF)-related gastrointestinal complications and MMF dose alterations on transplant outcomes and healthcare costs in renal transplant recipients. Clin Transplant 2005; 19: 779–84.

Tokgoz B, Sari HI, Yildiz O. Effects of azithromycin on cyclosporine-induced gingival hyperplasia in renal transplant patients. Transplant Proc 2004; 36: 2699–702.

Tran MQ, Gohh RY, Morrissey PE, et al. Cryptosporidium infection in renal transplant patients. Clin Nephrol 2005; 63: 305–9.

Tsai DE, Hardy CL, Tomaszweski JE, et al. Reduction in immunosuppression as initial therapy for posttransplant lymphoproliferative disorder in adult solid organ transplant patients. Transplantation 2001; 71: 1076–88.

Van Gelder T, ter Meulen CG, Hené R, et al. Oral ulcers in kidney transplant recipients treated with sirolimus and mycophenolate mofetil. Transplantation 2003; 75: 788.

Vasquez EM. Sirolimus: a new agent for prevention of allograft rejection. Am J Health Syst Pharm 2000; 57: 437–48.

Vitko S, Margreiter R, Weimar W, et al. Three-year efficacy and safety results from a study of everolimus versus mycophenolate mofetil in de novo renal transplant recipients. Am J Transplant 2005; 10: 2521–30.

Wang K, Zhang H, Li Y, et al. Safety of mycophenolate mofetil versus azathioprine in renal transplantation: a systematic review. Transplant Proc 2004; 36: 2071–2.

Webster AC, Woodroffe RC, Taylor RS, et al. Tacrolimus versus ciclosporin as primary immunosuppression for kidney transplant recipients: meta-analysis and meta-regression of randomised trial data. BMJ 2005; 331: 810.

Wu WK, Cho H. The pharmacological actions of nicotine on the gastrointestinal tract. J Pharmacol Sci 2004; 94: 348–58.

Yoon JH, Yook JI, Kim HJ, et al. Solitary plasmacytoma of the mandible in a renal transplant recipient. Int J Oral Maxillofac Surg 2003; 32: 664–6.

13 PANCREATIC AND HEPATOBILIARY COMPLICATIONS

Pancreas

Acute pancreatitis

Post-transplantation pancreatitis is an infrequent complication with a high risk of mortality. The incidence of acute pancreatitis in renal transplant recipients ranges around 1%, with mortality in about a third of cases (Chapman *et al.*, 1991; Adani *et al.*, 2005).

Risk factors

Several factors may contribute to the pathogenesis of pancreatitis after transplantation (Table 13.1). There is a well-known association between *end-stage renal disease* and acute pancreatitis. *Hyperparathyroidism* is frequent in dialysis patients and may require time before reversing after transplantation. Hyperparathyroidism is associated with pancreatitis in 1.5–17% of cases. Although the relationship between these two entities is still under discussion, there are data suggesting that hypercalcemia, caused by hyperparathyroidism, is a major risk factor for the development of pancreatitis (Carnaille *et al.*, 1998). A number of patients developed pancreatitis after *parathyroidectomy* (Mjaland and Normann, 2000). Many dialysis patients have silent *gall-stone disease* (Badalamenti *et al.*, 1994), which may increase the risk of acute pancreatitis either by obstruction or by reflux of biliary or duodenal contents, which stimulate pancreatic secretion. A possible role has been advocated for *immunosuppressive* drugs, including corticosteroids (Buchman, 2001), azathioprine (Siwach *et al.*, 1999), cyclosporine (Ko *et al.*, 1997), tacrolimus (Nieto *et al.*, 2000; Ogunseinde *et al.*, 2003), and mycophenolate mofetil (Furst, 1999). Rare cases of acute pancreatitis have developed after the administration of OKT3 (Scheinin *et al.*, 1993) or antithymoglobulins (Lee *et al.*, 2006). Changes consistent with the presence of *cytomegalovirus* in the gland and good response to ganciclovir have been reported in patients with post-transplant pancreatitis, suggesting an involvement of viral infection (Klassen *et al.*, 2000; Sinha *et al.*, 2003). *Hypertriglyceridemia*, which may be frequent in transplant patients, is also often associated with pancreatitis (Murphy *et al.*, 2002; Grochowiecki *et al.*, 2003).

Clinical syndromes

Some patients with acute pancreatitis have mild discomfort, and recovery is uneventful. In other cases, this disorder has a rapid onset, with upper abdominal pain, vomiting, fever, tachycardia, leukocytosis, and elevation of serum levels of pancreatic enzymes. Clinical and laboratory parameters are useful for the diagnosis and prognosis (Table 13.2). Computed tomography may show edema (Figure 13.1), inflammation of the pancreas, extension of edema or fluid in peripancreatic tissue, or multiple fluid collection in the peripancreatic region. At endoscopic retrograde cholangiopancreatography (ERCP), intraparenchymal extravasation due to necrosis can be seen (Figure 13.2).

Prognosis

The severity of pancreatitis is usually assessed by contrast-enhanced computed tomography (CT) imaging (Table 13.3). The most severe cases are those associated with partial or total necrosis of the pancreas, which can be diagnosed by the lack of enhancement (Balthazar, 2002). If pancreatitis remains sterile, the overall mortality is about 10%, while it ranges between 30 and 40% if there is an infected necrosis. The differential diagnosis may be made by CT-guided fine-needle aspiration of pancreatic and peripancreatic tissue.

Table 13.1   Risk factors for post-transplant pancreatitis

Renal insufficiency
Hyperparathyroidism
Parathyroidectomy
Biliary stones
Immunosuppressive drugs
CMV infection
Hypertriglyceridemia

Table 13.2   Clinical and laboratory signs of adverse prognosis in acute pancreatitis

Clinical	Laboratory
Age >55 years	Urinary trypsinogen activating peptide ↑
Intra-abdominal pressure >25 cmH$_2$O	C-reactive protein ↑
Infection	Hematocrit >10% in 24–48 hours ↓
Hypotension	Glycemia >200 mg/dl ↑
Renal failure	Calcemia ↓
Multiorgan failure	Bicarbonate ↓

In renal transplant recipients acute pancreatitis may follow a fulminating course. These patients develop a systemic *inflammatory response* syndrome, the inflammatory cascade being triggered by cytokines, immunocytes, and the complement system. Early death is due to a multisystem organ failure, with the development of adult respiratory distress syndrome, renal failure, upper gastrointestinal bleeding, disseminated intravascular coagulation, and shock (Table 13.4). In other patients death occurs later, usually from infection. In surviving patients a number of complications may occur. Pancreatic ascites and pleural effusion may occur as a consequence of fistulas or disruption of the main pancreatic duct. Necrosis, edema, and hemorrhage in the pancreatic bed and surrounding tissues may lead to the formation of phlegmon or pseudocyst, which can be differentiated by ERCP (Figure 13.3) ultrasonography, or computed tomography. A serious complication of either phlegmon or pseudocyst is pancreatic abscess, characterized by increased pain, hectic fever, and leukocytosis.

Therapy

Specific interventions for acute pancreatitis have generally not been helpful. Resting the pancreas has not changed the course of the disease, but nasogastric suction is indicated in the case of associated ileus. Early nutritional support may aid recovery. Enteral feeding, through laparoscopic or combined endoscopic–radiologic jejeunostomy tube placement, is safe, well tolerated, and less expensive than parenteral nutrition (Mitchell *et al.*, 2003).

The *timing* and *type* of intervention in patients with acute necrotizing pancreatitis are controversial. Supportive medical therapy is generally recommended in patients with sterile acute pancreatitis, which carries a relatively low mortality. Conversely, as infected necrotizing pancreatitis is almost universally fatal without intervention, the debridement and resection of infected necrosis should be undertaken soon after its confirmation. Alternative methods of debridement are aggressive irrigation and drainage through large percutaneous catheters, and transgastric or transduodenal drainage and irrigation (Baron and Morgan, 1999).

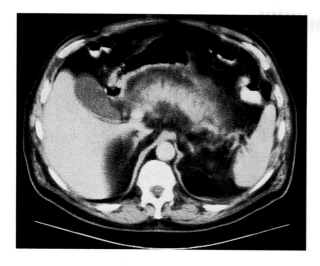

Figure 13.1 Acute pancreatitis. A diffusely enlarged pancreas with loss of cleavage plan. Exudative peripancreatic collection

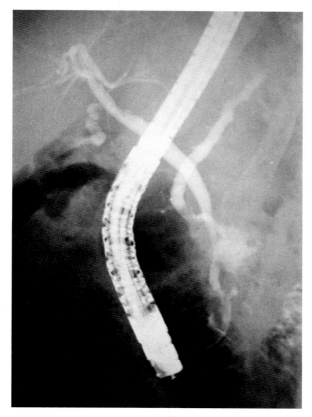

Figure 13.2 ERCP. Acute pancreatitis of the head of the pancreas with intraparenchymal extravasation due to necrosis and compression of the choledocus. (Courtesy of Dr A Carrara, Ospedale Maggiore, Milan.)

Severe acute pancreatitis requires intensive monitoring of cardiovascular, pulmonary, renal, and septic complications. The measurement of intra-abdominal pressure is also helpful. Conservative treatment includes early enteral nutrition, colloids, early continuous venovenous hemofiltration when indicated, and antibiotic prophylaxis. The early administration of imipenem, probably the antibiotic of choice, can reduce

Table 13.3 Score of lesions seen at computed tomography in patients with acute pancreatitis. From Balthazar et al., 1985

A   Normal
B   Focal or diffuse edema
C   Changes in the peripancreatic fat
D   Phlegmon or fluid collection in or around the pancreas
E   Two or more fluid collections or presence of gas in or adjacent to pancreas

Table 13.4 Main systemic and local complications of acute pancreatitis

Systemic acute complications	Local complications
Acute respiratory distress syndrome	Pancreatic abscess
Shock	Pancreatic phlegmon
Acute renal failure	Pancreatic pseudocysts
Coagulopathy	Pancreatic ascites
Gastrointestinal bleeding	Pancreatic pleural effusion
Hyperglycemia	Chronic pancreatitis
Hypocalcemia	
Sepsis	

the need for surgery and the overall number of major complications (Nordback et al., 2001). Endoscopic retrograde cholangiopancreatography and sphincterotomy in gallstone pancreatitis (Figure 13.4) result in reduced biliary sepsis.

Pharmacological treatment is still under investigation. Proteinase inhibitors such as gabexate mesylate do not seem to offer great advantage, as their use in the prevention of post-endoscopic retrograde cholangiopancreatography (ERCP) pancreatitis has been disappointing. Initial studies using ulinastatin are promising, but additional dose–response studies are needed (Hoogerwerf, 2005). Somatostatin, which may inhibit pancreatic secretion, has been proved to reduce the risk of recurrent pancreatitis (Di Francesco et al., 2006), and has been found to be effective in single case reports. Controlled trials with octreotide did not provide convincing data about its efficacy (Lamberts et al., 1996). The benefit of anti-TNF monoclonal antibodies and interleukin-10 has been documented in experimental models, but no clinical study is available (Pezzilli et al., 2006).

Late complications

Pancreatic pseudocyst

Pseudocysts of the pancreas are collections of tissue, fluid, debris, and blood, which may develop 1–4 weeks after acute pancreatitis.

Pseudocysts may be responsible for pain, caused by compression of the adjacent viscera, and may be responsible of life-threatening complications, including rupture, hemorrhage, and abscess. Echography and CT (Figure 13.5) may detect a pseudocyst, and can be useful for monitoring whether the pseudocyst may resolve or expand. Moreover, under ultrasound or CT guidance, pseudocysts may be drained either by fine needles or by tubes.

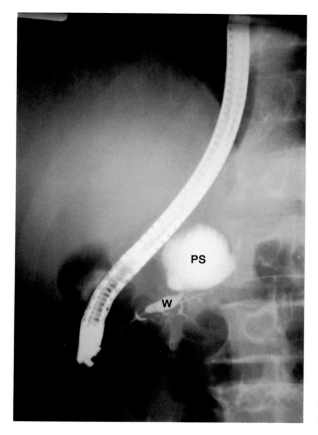

Figure 13.3 ERCP. Pancreatic pseudocyst (PS) communicating with the Wirsung duct. (Courtesy of Dr A Carrara, Ospedale Maggiore, Milan.)

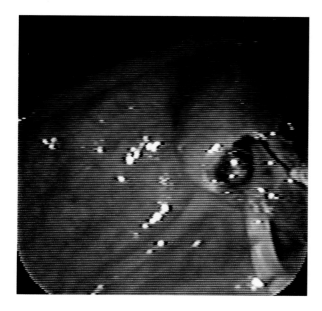

Figure 13.4 Endoscopic view of a papillosphincterotomy with removal of an ampullary impacted stone causing pancreatitis (Courtesy of Dr A Carrara, Ospedale Maggiore, Milan.)

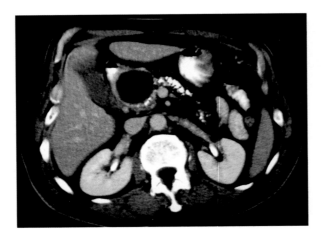

Figure 13.5 Pseudocyst of the head of pancreas at computed tomography

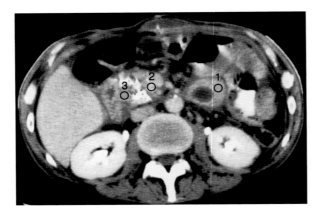

Figure 13.6 Chronic pancreatitis. Calcification of the head

Chronic pancreatitis

Chronic pancreatitis may develop as a consequence of acute pancreatitis or as chronic damage. Clinically, patients with chronic pancreatitis may present with symptoms identical to those found in acute pancreatitis, but *pain* may be absent, intermittent, or persistent. It may be diffuse to the abdomen or localized to the back or to the upper right or left quadrant. *Steatorrhea* and *diarrhea* are frequent complications. Amylases and lipases may be normal or slightly elevated. Many patients show glucose intolerance or an overt *diabetes*. About 40% of patients with chronic pancreatitis may have vitamin B$_{12}$ malabsorption. The diagnosis is usually based on the classic triad of steatorrhea, diabetes, and pancreas calcifications (Figure 13.6).

With the exception of a few cases requiring surgery for stricture of the pancreatic duct or the endoscopic removal of stones, treatment usually consists of the administration of pancreatic enzymes.

Liver complications

Viral hepatitis

Hepatitis virus infection is one of the major causes of morbidity and mortality in renal transplantation. It has been reported that up to 25% of patients have some degree of liver failure in the early post-transplant period, and liver failure is implicated as the cause of death in about 30% of these patients in the long term

Table 13.5   Main adverse prognostic factors in transplant patient carriers of viral hepatitis

Hepatitis B	Hepatitis C
Duration of viral infection	Duration of viral infection
Older age	Genotype 1a, 1b
Female sex	Alcohol consumption
HBV DNA+ at transplantation	Co-infection with HBV
HbeAg+ at transplantation	Diabetes
Chronic active hepatitis	Chronic active hepatitis
Corticosteroids (?)	Corticosteroids (?)

Table 13.6   Possible extrahepatic complications of viral hepatitis

Systemic complications	Allograft complications
Diabetes mellitus	Acute rejection
Cardiovascular disease	Membranoproliferative glomerulonephritis
Anemia	Membranous glomerulonephritis
Cryoglobulinemia	Cryoglobulinemic nephritis
Cutaneous disorders	Thrombotic microangiopathy

(Ahsan and Rao, 2002). Some factors may indicate a poor prognosis (Table 13.5). Apart from liver disease, the viruses may cause extrahepatic complications including hematologic, cutaneous, musculoskeletal, and renal disorders (Table 13.6). Most patients acquire hepatitis viruses before transplantation, mainly through blood transfusions. In a few cases, however, the infection can be transmitted via the allograft from donors with actively replicating viruses.

Hepatitis B (HBV) infection

Hepatitis B virus is a DNA virus. Some 20 years ago the incidence of HBV infection was high in dialysis patients. More recently, however, only exceptionally does a dialysis patient become infected with HBV. There are several reasons for this *reduced incidence* of HBV infection: (1) in most dialysis units HBV carriers are isolated, and prophylactic measures are taken; (2) hepatitis B virus-negative patients receive systemic vaccination against HBV; (3) The use of blood transfusion in dialysis patients is considerably reduced since recombinant human erythropoietin has been made available; and (4) there is rigorous control for hepatitis virus in the blood to be transfused.

The long-term *prognosis* for HBV-positive transplant patients is poorer than for HBV-negative transplants (Kletzmayr and Watschinger, 2002; Fabrizi *et al.*, 2005). Many HBV-positive transplant patients may remain asymptomatic for years, with a moderate elevation of alanine aminotransferase (Aroldi *et al.*, 1998; Morales, 1998), and about 3% of them may even show spontaneous disappearance of HB antigens and HBV DNA (Fornairon *et al.*, 1996). However, immunosuppressive therapy generally favors viral replication and the development of diabetes, which represents a further risk factor. In spite of good clinical conditions and mild biologic abnormalities, most patients show progressive worsening of histologic lesions from mild chronic hepatitis (Figure 13.7) to cirrhosis (Figure 13.8), which represents the first

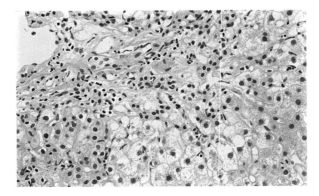

Figure 13.7 Liver biopsy in a 34-year-old HBV-positive kidney transplant recipient. Portal area shows scarce mixed inflammatory infiltrates and ductal proliferation. Periportal hepatocytes show clear cytoplasms due to cholate stasis and some tubular arrangement with perisinusoidal fibrosis. (H & E ×75)

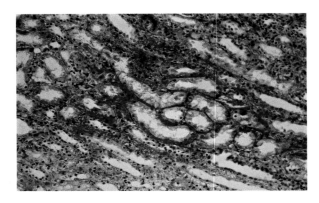

Figure 13.8 Chronic hepatitis and cirrhosis. Broad bands of fibrous tissue due to centroportal bridging necrosis, separate two parenchymal nodules. Chronotrope-anilin ×25. (Courtesy of Dr MF Donato, Ospedale Maggiore, Milan.)

cause of death for HBV-positive renal transplant recipients together with extrahepatic sepsis (Younossi *et al.*, 1999; Aroldi *et al.*, 2005). Older age, female sex, and the presence of chronic active hepatitis were found to be significantly associated with the risk of developing cirrhosis (Rao *et al.*, 1993). Other investigators found that patients with positive HBV DNA or HBeAg at transplantation had the highest risk of developing severe liver disease (Fairley *et al.*, 1991). In a few cases, the accumulation of HBV stimulates an immune response in spite of immunosuppression, leading to *fibrosing cholestatic hepatitis* and rapid progression to liver failure (Figure 13.9).

A minimal level of monitoring should include visits and repeat transaminase level measurements at 4-monthly intervals. Serial HBV DNA testing and repeat liver biopsy are not necessary. Ultrasound examination and serum α-fetoprotein testing should be evaluated at 6-monthly intervals in patients at risk of hepatocellular carcinoma, as are patients with cirrhosis.

The *treatment* of hepatitis B was disappointing until recently. The use of interferon has been limited by the frequent occurrence of rejection (Magnone *et al.*, 1995). However, the therapeutic scenario has changed more recently after the availability of three antiviral drugs. The first of these antiviral agents, *lamivudine*, has proved able to improve the manifestations of HBV involvement and to maintain most transplant patients free of viral recurrence (Goffin *et al.*, 1998; Lee *et al.*, 2001; Viganò *et al.*, 2005). The daily dose in patients with normal renal function ranges between 100 and 150 mg. In patients with renal insufficiency the dose should be modified according to the values of creatinine clearance. A daily dose of 50 mg is suggested if creatinine clearance ranges between 30 and 50 ml/min; the dose should be reduced to 25 mg if creatinine clearance is between 15 and 30 ml/min; and a daily dose of 10 mg is suggested for levels of creatinine clearance lower than 15 ml/min. Most renal transplant patients treated with lamivudine

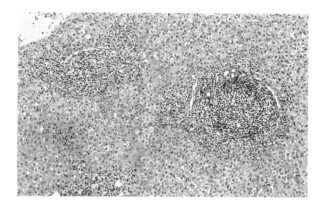

Figure 13.9 Liver biopsy taken in a 42-year-old HCV-positive woman 8 months after renal transplantation. Mild chronic active hepatitis. Enlarged portal tracts with lymphoid follicles with germinal centers and bile ducts lesions. Mild periportal piecemeal necrosis is present. In the lobule there are small foci of liver cell necrosis with modest lymphocytic reaction. H & E ×25. (Courtesy of Dr MF Donato, Ospedale Maggiore, Milan.)

achieve a rapid and durable suppression of HBV, which substantially lowers the risk of liver decompensation and death. In liver transplant recipients the combination lamivudine–immunoglobulins, although quite expensive, offers good protection from HBV-related liver failure (Dan *et al.*, 2006). Unfortunately, some 15–25% of patients develop resistance to the drug every year, due to viral mutation, reaching 80% at 4 years (Locarnini, 2005). Moreover, withdrawal of the drug may result in biochemical and virological relapse. Patients who develop resistance to lamivudine may be switched to the reverse transcriptase inhibitor *adefovir*, or to its more lipophilic prodrug adefovir dipivoxil. At an initial dose of 10 mg per day, then adjusted according to renal function, this drug proved to be safe and effective in renal transplant recipients resistant to lamivudine (Fontaine *et al.*, 2005). Adefovir has a lower frequency of resistance, reaching 40% by 4 years in non-transplant patients (Locarnini, 2005). *Entecavir*, the newest antiviral agent, is a guanosine analog with excellent activity against HBV DNA polymerase. The drug has few side-effects and has proved to be superior to lamivudine by achieving undetectable HBV DNA levels in patients with chronic hepatitis B (Chang *et al.*, 2006; Lai *et al.*, 2006). The main problem with the current therapies is that HBV can be suppressed but not eradicated, and relapse occurs when the drug is stopped. In some cases the relapse may be so severe as to cause liver decompensation and death. Thus, once treatment with antiviral agents has been begun, it should be continued indefinitely (Hoofnagle, 2006).

Hepatitis C (HCV) infection

HCV is a small RNA virus. The prevalence of HCV infection in renal transplant patients ranges between 6 and 46% (Fabrizi *et al.*, 2001), being influenced by race, geographic origin of the patient, type and duration of dialysis, number of blood transfusions, positivity for HBV infection, and the sensitivity and specifity of diagnostic tests. Several *genotypes* of HCV have been recognized. Carriers of genotypes 1a and 1b have significantly higher probability of developing chronic liver disease than do patients with other genotypes (Aroldi *et al.*, 1998; Prieto *et al.*, 1999).

Most, but not all, HCV-positive transplant patients progress to *cirrhosis*. About 50–80% of renal allograft recipients with HCV infection may remain asymptomatic and with normal serum transaminase levels for years. Some investigators interpreted these data with caution by pointing out that more than half of patients with normal liver function may show chronic liver disease at histologic examination (Berthoux, 1995; Orloff *et al.*, 1995). However, the Barcelona group showed that 15-year patient survival was significantly better in patients with normal serum levels of alanine aminotransferase (ALT) than in those with elevated ALT (Bestard *et al.*, 2005). Moreover, Perez *et al.* (2005) found a significant association between ALT levels and septal fibrosis, interface hepatitis, and confluent necrosis at liver biopsy. A correlation was also observed between ALT and staging, periportal necroinflammatory activity, and lobular necroinflammatory activity, suggesting that ALT may be a good marker for histologic lesions. On the other hand, even liver biopsy may show wide variations in severity of the lesions, depending on the indication for biopsy (mild or

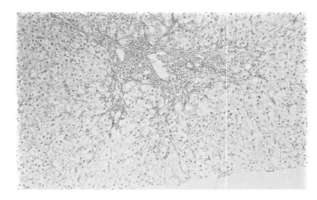

Figure 13.10 Liver biopsy showing cholestatic features in a 35-year-old man with renal transplant. Enlarged portal tract with some ductal proliferation. Periportal interface shows perihepatocyctic fibrosis spreading into the lobule. PAS ×25. (Courtesy of Dr MF Donato, Ospedale Maggiore, Milan.)

severe biochemical abnormalities) and on the timing of biopsy, an early biopsy usually showing milder lesions (Figure 13.10) than a late biopsy. Some clinical studies showed that, when patients were followed for at least 10 years, more than 50% of HCV-positive transplant patients had chronic liver disease (Vosnides, 1997). However, Kamar et al. (2005a) found that, more than 10 years after transplantation, among 52 HCV-positive transplant patients, liver fibrosis remained stable in 21 patients, progressed in another 21, and showed a regression in ten patients. In the last two groups, the progression and regression of liver fibrosis were gradual during follow-up. Ferritin levels and hepatosiderosis were significantly higher in fibrosers. Initial fibrosis stage and high diversification of the hypervariable region-1 of the HCV genome between transplantation and the first liver biopsy were independent factors associated with liver fibrosis regression.

Patient survival is lower in HCV-positive renal transplant recipients. A review of the United States Renal Data System reported that patient survival was slightly superior in HCV-positive than in HCV-negative transplant recipients (Meier-Kriesche et al., 2001). However, the results are strongly influenced by the length of follow-up. A number of reports on patients followed for 10–20 years showed a significantly higher mortality in HCV-positive than in HCV-negative renal transplant recipients (Aroldi et al., 1998; Hanafusa et al., 1998; Legendre et al., 1998; Mathurin et al., 1999). A recent meta-analysis confirmed a significantly higher risk of death in HCV-positive than in HCV-negative transplant patients (Fabrizi et al., 2005). It is unclear whether co-infection with HBV worsens the course of HCV-positive patients (Pouteil-Noble et al., 1995), may reduce the reactivation of HBV (Yen et al., 2006), or does not affect patient survival (Aroldi et al., 2005). Extrahepatic sepsis, liver failure, and cardiovascular disease accounted for most deaths in HCV-positive renal transplant recipients (Aroldi et al., 2005). The high rate of cardiovascular death reported in HCV-positive patients may probably be accounted for by the frequent association of HCV with diabetes mellitus (Noto and Raskin, 2006). While life-threatening complications usually develop in the long-term, a few patients may have a rapid evolution to liver failure (Munoz de Bustillo et al., 1998; Toth et al., 1998). Such an aggressive course seems to be more frequent in patients who acquired the virus shortly before or after transplantation (Delladetsima et al., 2006). A cholestatic syndrome with fibrosing cholestatic hepatitis at biopsy (Figure 13.11) is usually seen in these patients. Whether renal transplantation and dialysis have a different impact on patient survival of HCV-positive patients has also been investigated. Pereira et al. (1998) and Bucci et al. (2004) reported that the risk of death of renal transplant patients was considerably lower than that of dialysis patients. However, Perez et al. (2006) found that HCV-positive renal transplant patients showed a larger proportion of cases with septal fibrosis and confluent necrosis at liver biopsy than did HCV-positive patients on dialysis, suggesting that renal transplantation might lead to a more severe liver disease. This might be caused by the deleterious effect of immosuppressive therapy in transplant patients. However, it is also possible that hemodialysis may inhibit virus replication through the release of interferon-like substances during the dialysis session (Badalamenti et al., 2003).

Also, data about the influence of HCV infection on *graft survival* are conflicting. Some investigators found similar graft survival both in the short term (Corell et al., 1995) and in the long term (Aroldi

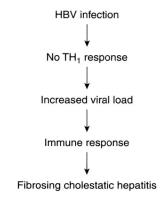

HBV infection

↓

No TH$_1$ response

↓

Increased viral load

↓

Immune response

↓

Fibrosing cholestatic hepatitis

Figure 13.11   A possible mechanism for rapid progression liver failure in HBV-positive transplant patients.

et al., 1998) between HCV+ and HCV– transplant recipients, but a meta-analysis reported reduced graft survival in HCV+ transplant patients (Fabrizi *et al.*, 2005). Of interest, in one study, pure graft survival (censored by death) was better in HCV-positive patients with elevated ALT than in those with normal ALT (Bestard *et al.*, 2005). Numerous factors may account for these conflicting results: HLA matching, severity of liver disease before transplantation, duration of HCV infection, type of immunosuppression, diabetes, etc.

The *treatment* of HCV infection in renal transplant patients is still disappointing. The reduction of immunosuppression and withdrawal of corticosteroids might theoretically reduce the virus replication, but there are no controlled trials supporting this hypothesis. On the other hand, such an approach may increase the risk of acute rejection. Interferon-α and pegylated interferons are now widely used in non-transplant HCV-positive patients. However, renal transplantation is considered a contraindication to interferon treatment (Natov and Pereira, 2002). Interferon-α is not particularly effective in eradicating the virus, may be poorly tolerated, and can also increase the expression of HLA antigens and induce acute rejection (Rostaing *et al.*, 1995; Magnone *et al.*, 1995). The association of interferon-α with ribavirin, an antiviral agent, proved to be superior to interferon alone in obtaining a sustained virologic response and histologic improvement in non-transplant patients with chronic HCV (McHutchison *et al.*, 1998; Moriyama and Arakawa, 2006). Ribavirin is usually well tolerated. However, the drug accumulates in the membrane of erythrocytes, leading to membrane fragility and, in some cases, to hemolysis and anemia. Ribavirin-induced anemia is dose-dependent, and is more frequent in patients with renal failure. When given as monotherapy in renal transplant patients, ribavirin increased liver fibrosis, as a result of hemolysis and increased levels of ferritin (Kamar *et al.*, 2005b). In spite of the increased risk of rejection caused by interferon, combined treatment with ribavirin may be suggested for patients with progressive liver disease. Newer inosine monophosphate dehydrogenase (IMPDH) inhibitors are in various stages of development. Viramidine, a liver-targeting prodrug of ribavirin, has demonstrated significant antiviral activity and erythrocyte-sparing properties. Clinical trials of merimepodib, another investigational IMPDH inhibitor, are under way (Gish, 2006).

There is some experimental (Watashi *et al.*, 2003) and clinical (Inoue *et al.*, 2003) evidence that cyclosporine may inhibit HCV RNA replication. It has also been shown that the progression of liver fibrosis may be delayed in HCV-positive liver transplant recipients (Levy *et al.*, 2004). However, there is no convincing evidence that cyclosporine has a favorable influence on the outcome of HCV-related liver disease in renal transplant recipients. Future drugs for HCV infection will belong to four main categories, including new interferons, alternatives to ribavirin, specific HCV inhibitors, and immune modulators. New treatments and vaccines might make it possible to eradicate HCV in the future (Pawlotsky, 2006).

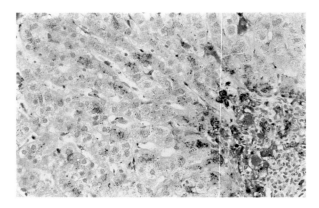

Figure 13.12 Iron overload in a 50-year-old male transplant recipient submitted to multiple transfusions before transplantation. Portal tracts and periportal areas show aggregates of iron-laden macrophages together with a moderate amount of hemosiderin in the parenchymal cells. Perl's ×75. (Courtesy of Dr MF Donato, Ospedale Maggiore, Milan.)

Hepatitis GB virus (HGBV) infection

Patients on maintenance hemodialysis are at increased risk for HGBV infection, which may be transmitted by transfusions or other means. However, there is evidence that HGBV *per se* is not associated with acute or chronic hepatitis. Even in renal transplant recipients the positivity of HGBV does not seem to affect the outcome (Murthy *et al.*, 1998; Rostaing *et al.*, 1999), although one case of acute hepatitis has been reported in a renal transplant patient (Couzi *et al.*, 2004). In a study with long-term follow-up, mean 11 years after transplantation, patient carriers of HCV and HGBV infection had lower levels of HCV RNA than patients with HCV infection alone. These data suggest an interaction between these two viruses in renal transplant recipients (De Filippi *et al.*, 2001).

Liver hemosiderosis

Normal ferritin levels range between 15 and 200 ng/ml in males and between 12 and 150 ng/ml in females. Iron overload, caused by repeated blood transfusions or by inadequate parenteral iron supplementation, may lead to massive iron deposits in parenchymal cells that are stored as insoluble granular, gold-brown aggregates known as hemosiderin (Figure 13.12). In this case, the serum ferritin level usually exceeds 800 ng/ml. In the liver, with advancing hemosiderosis, fibrosis increases and cirrhosis may develop.

Since the introduction of human recombinant erythropoietin, the incidence of hemosiderosis in dialysis and transplant patients has reduced. After transplantation, the rise in hemoglobin levels is accompanied by a decrease in serum ferritin levels, which are lowest at the sixth month. After this time, ferritin levels increase, their evolution depending on the iron status at transplantation (Teruel *et al.*, 1989). In most patients, iron overload is difficult to remove, particularly if serum ferritin levels exceed 800 ng/ml. Hemosiderosis can cause tissue fibrosis and progressive liver failure (Ogihara *et al.*, 2002).

Treatment consists of periodic phlebotomies. The removal of 300 ml of blood depletes the body of 200–250 mg of iron. Early treatment may obtain a normalization of serum ferritin (which is usually higher than 800 ng/ml) and serum transaminases. However, if hepatic fibrosis has developed, treatment is usually ineffective. Thus, particularly in polytransfused patients, regular monitoring of serum ferritin after transplantation is recommended. Magnetic resonance imaging of the liver may be a useful guide to deciding the intensity of treatment (Park *et al.*, 1994).

Hepatic veno-occlusive disease

This is a non-thrombotic obliterative process of the central or sublobular hepatic veins. The disease may be caused by pyrrolizidine alkaloids, chemotherapy, or irradiation. A score of cases have been reported in renal transplant recipients, most, but not all, treated with azathioprine and prednisone (Jeffries *et al.*, 1998; Vallet-Pichard *et al.*, 2003). A possible role for a hepatotropic viral infection has been hypothesized, as the association with cytomegalovirus infection or viral hepatitis is frequent. The clinical picture is characterized by ascites, hepatomegaly, cholestasis, and portal hypertension. At computed tomography, periportal edema, ascites, and a narrow right hepatic vein can be seen (Erturk et al., 2006). The prognosis is poor. A successful case treated with a transjugular intrahepatic portosystemic shunt has been described (Azoulay et al., 1998). As most patients die a few months after discovery of the disease, liver transplantation should be considered after the diagnosis is established.

Nodular regenerative hyperplasia

This is an unusual liver disease, histologically characterized by diffuse nodular involvement of the liver and by the absence of fibrosis. The disease may lead to intrahepatic portal hypertension and/or chronic anicteric cholestasis.

A few cases of nodular regenerative hyperplasia of the liver have been reported in renal transplant patients, some referred to azathioprine (Jones et al., 1988; Ichikawa et al., 1998), others associated with peliosis hepatitis or veno-occlusive disease (Cavalcanti et al., 1994). Previous treatment with potentially hepatotoxic drugs or coincident viral hepatitis have been implicated in the pathogenesis, but it is also possible that the disease may be triggered by autoimmune mechanisms (Youssef and Tavill, 2002). Stenosis and thromboses of small portal vessels might be responsible for the disease, leading to abnormal liver perfusion with atrophy of hypoperfused areas and regenerative hyperplasia of hyperperfused areas.

Cholelithiasis and choledocholithiasis

Some studies have found an increased risk of cholelithiasis in transplant patients. This may be due to the use of cyclosporine (Alberu et al., 2001), which augments the lithogenicity of the bile and may also induce cholestasis by inhibiting ATP-dependent bile salt transport (Kadmon et al., 1993). Other reports, however, have found that the incidence and morbidity of gallstones after transplantation are low, and hence prophylactic cholecystectomy is not justified (Greenstein et al., 1997; Melvin et al., 1998).

The administration of ursodeoxycholic acid (5–10 mg/kg per day) may dissolve cholesterol and associated gallstones and reduce cholestasis in transplant patients (Ganschow, 2002). Under treatment, the blood levels of cyclosporine should be checked, as an improvement of cholestasis and enhanced absorption of cyclosporine may increase the blood levels of the drug (Sharobeem et al., 1993). There has been some controversy about the indication for prophylactic cholecystectomy in patients with silent cholelithiasis. A decision analysis based on published studies showed that expectant management for asymptomatic cholelithiasis is favored in pancreas/renal transplant patients, resulting in 2 : 1000 deaths compared with 5 : 1000 for prophylactic cholecystectomy (Kao et al., 2005). Surgery is certainly indicated in patients with frequent symptoms, in patients with prior complications of gallstone disease, and in patients at high risk of complications (large gallstones, calcified gallbladder, etc.). Endoscopic sphincterotomy followed by stone extraction is a possible alternative in patients with common duct stones.

References

Adani GL, Baccarani U, Viale P, et al. Acute pancreatitis after kidney transplantation. Am J Gastroenterol 2005; 100: 1620–1.

Ahsan N, Rao KV. Hepatobiliary diseases after kidney transplantation unrelated to classic hepatitis virus. Semin Dial 2002; 15: 358–65.

Alberu J, Gatica M, Cachafeiro-Vilar M, et al. Asymptomatic gallstones and duration of cyclosporine use in kidney transplant recipients. Rev Invest Clin 2001; 53: 396–400.

Aroldi A, Lampertico P, Elli A, et al. Long-term evolution of anti-HCV positive renal transplant recipients. Transplant Proc 1998; 30: 2076–8.

Aroldi A, Lampertico P, Montagnino G, et al. Natural history of hepatitis B and C in renal allograft recipients. Transplantation 2005; 79: 1132–6.

Azoulay D, Castaing D, Lemoine A, et al. Successful treatment of severe azathioprine-induced hepatic veno-occlusive disease in a kidney-transplanted patient with transjugular intrahepatic portosystemic shunt. Clin Nephrol 1998; 50: 118–22.

Badalamenti S, De Fazio C, Castelnovo C, et al. High prevalence of silent gallstone disease in dialysis patients. Nephron 1994; 66: 225–7.

Badalamenti S, Catania A, Lunghi G, et al. Changes in viremia and circulating interferon-alpha during hemodialysis in hepatitis C virus-positive patients: only coincidental phenomena? Am J Kidney Dis 2003; 42: 143–50.

Balthazar EJ. Staging of acute pancreatitis. Radiol Clin North Am 2002; 40: 1199–209.

Balthazar EJ, Ranson JH, Naidich DP, et al. Acute pancreatitis: prognostic value of CT. Radiology 1985; 156: 767–72.

Baron TH, Morgan DE. Acute necrotizing pancreatitis. N Engl J Med 1999; 340: 1412–17.

Berthoux F. Hepatitis C virus infection and disease in renal transplantation. Nephron 1995; 71: 386–94.

Bestard O, Cruzado JM, Torras J, et al. Long-term effect of hepatitis C virus chronic infection on patient and renal graft survival. Transplant Proc 2005; 37: 3774–7.

Bucci JR, Lentine KL, Agodoa LY, et al. Outcomes associated with recipient and donor hepatitis C serology status after kidney transplantation in the United States: analysis of the USRDS/UNOS database. Clin Transplant 2004; 1: 51–61.

Buchman AL. Side effects of corticosteroid therapy. J Clin Gastroenterol 2001; 33: 289–94.

Carnaille B, Oudar C, Pattou F, et al. Pancreatitis and primary hyperparathyroidism: forty cases. Aust NZ J Surg 1998; 68: 117–19.

Cavalcanti R, Pol S, Carnot F, et al. Impact and evolution of peliosis hepatitis in renal transplant recipients. Transplantation 1994; 58: 315–16.

Chang TT, Gish RG, de Man R, et al. A comparison of entecavir and lamivudine for HBeAg-positive chronic hepatitis B. N Engl J Med 2006; 354: 1001–10.

Chapman WC, Nylander WA, Williams LF Sr, Richie RE. Pancreatic pseudocyst formation following renal transplantation. Clin Transplant 1991; 5: 86–9.

Corell A, Morales JM, Mandrono A, et al. Immunosuppression induced by hepatitis C virus infection reduces acute rejection. Lancet 1995; 346: 1497–8.

Couzi L, Morel D, Merville P, et al. Acute hepatitis associated with hepatitis G virus primo-infection in a renal transplant recipient. Transplantation 2004; 78: 951–3.

Dan YY, Wai CT, Yeoh KG, Lim SG. Prophylactic strategies for hepatitis B patients undergoing liver transplant: a cost-effectiveness analysis. Liver Transpl 2006; 12: 736–46.

De Filippi F, Lampertico P, Soffredini R, et al. High prevalence, low pathogenicity of hepatitis G virus in kidney transplant recipients. Dig Liver Dis 2001; 33: 477–9.

Delladetsima I, Psichogiou M, Sypsa V, et al. The course of hepatitis C virus infection in pretransplantation anti-hepatitis C virus-negative renal transplant recipients: a retrospective follow-up study. Am J Kidney Dis 2006; 47: 309–16.

Di Francesco V, Angelini G, Zoico E, et al. Effect of native somatostatin on sphincter of Oddi motility in patients with acute recurrent pancreatitis. A pilot study with ultrasound-secretin test. Dig Liver Dis 2006; 38: 268–71.

Erturk SM, Mortele KJ, Binkert CA, et al. CT features of hepatic venoocclusive disease and hepatic graft-versus-host disease in patients after hematopoietic stem cell transplantation. AJR Am J Roentgenol 2006; 186: 1497–501.

Fabrizi F, Martin P, Ponticelli C. Hepatitis C virus infection and renal transplantation. Am J Kidney Dis 2001; 38: 919–34.

Fabrizi F, Lunghi G, Poordad FF, Martin P. Management of hepatitis B after renal transplantation: an update. J Nephrol 2002; 15: 113–22.

Fabrizi F, Martin P, Dixit V, et al. HBsAg seropositive status and survival after renal transplantation: meta-analysis of observational studies. Am J Transplant 2005; 5: 2913–21.

Fairley CK, Mijch A, Gust ID, et al. The increased risk of fatal liver disease in renal transplant patients who are hepatitis B e antigen and/or HBV DNA positive. Transplantation 1991; 52: 497–500.

Fontaine H, Vallet-Pichard A, Chaix ML, et al. Efficacy and safety of adefovir dipivoxil in kidney recipients, hemodialysis patients, and patients with renal insufficiency. Transplantation 2005; 80: 1086–92.

Fornairon S, Pol S, Legendre Ch, et al. The long-term virologic and pathologic impact of renal transplantation on chronic hepatitis B infection. Transplantation 1996; 62: 297.

Furst DE. Leflunomide, mycophenolic acid and matrix metalloproteinase inhibitors. Rheumatology 1999; 38 (Suppl 2): 14–18.

Ganschow R. Cholelithiasis in pediatric organ transplantation: detection and management. Pediatr Transplant 2002; 6: 91–6.

Gish RG. Treating HCV with ribavirin analogues and ribavirin-like molecules. J Antimicrob Chemother 2006; 57: 8–13.

Goffin E, Horsmans Y, Cornu C, et al. Lamivudine inhibits hepatitis B virus replication in kidney graft recipients. Transplantation 1998; 66: 407–9.

Greenstein SM, Katz S, Sun S, et al. Prevalence of asymptomatic cholelithiasis and risk of acute cholecystitis after kidney transplantation. Transplantation 1997; 63: 1030–2.

Grochowiecki T, Szmidt J, Galazka Z, et al. Do high levels of serum triglycerides in pancreas graft recipients before transplantation promote graft pancreatitis? Transplant Proc 2003; 35: 2339–40.

Hanafusa T, Ichikawa H, Kyo M, et al. Retrospective study on the impact of hepatitis C virus infection on kidney transplant patients over 20 years. Transplantation 1998; 66: 471–6.

Hoofnagle JH. Hepatitis B – preventable and now treatable. N Engl J Med 2006; 354: 1074–8.

Hoogerwerf WA. Pharmacological management of pancreatitis. Curr Opin Pharmacol 2005; 5: 578–82.

Ichikawa Y, Kyo M, Hanafusa T, et al. A 20-year case study of a kidney transplant recipient with chronic active hepatitis C: clinical course and successful treatment for late acute rejection induced by interferon therapy. Transplantation 1998; 65: 134–8.

Inoue K, Sekiyama K, Yamada M, et al. Combined interferon alpha2b and cyclosporin A in the treatment of chronic hepatitis C: controlled trial. J Gastroenterol 2003; 38: 567–72.

Jeffries MA, McDonnell WM, Tworek JA, et al. Venoocclusive disease of the liver following renal transplantation. Dig Dis Sci 1998; 43: 229–34.

Jones MC, Best PV, Catto GRD. Is nodular regeneration of the liver associated with azathioprine therapy after renal transplantation? Nephrol Dial Transplant 1988; 3: 331–3.

Kadmon M, Klünemann C, Böhme M, et al. Inhibition by cyclosporin A of adenosine triphosphate-dependent transport from the hepatocyte to bile. Gastroenterology 1993; 104: 1507–14.

Kamar N, Rostaing L, Selves J, et al. Natural history of hepatitis C virus-related liver fibrosis after renal transplantation. Am J Transplant 2005a; 5: 1704–12.

Kamar N, Boulestin A, Selves J, et al. Factors accelerating liver fibrosis progression in renal transplant patients receiving ribavirin monotherapy for chronic hepatitis C. J Med Virol 2005b; 76: 61–8.

Kao LS, Flowers C, Flum DR. Prophylactic cholecystectomy in transplant patients: a decision analysis. J Gastrointest Surg 2005; 9: 965–72.

Klassen DK, Drachenberg CB, Papadimitriou JC, et al. CMV allograft pancreatitis: diagnosis, treatment and histologic features. Transplantation 2000; 69: 1968–71.

Kletzmayr J, Watschinger B. Chronic hepatitis B virus infection in renal transplant recipients. Semin Nephrol 2002; 22: 375–89.

Ko CW, Gooley T, Schoch HG, et al. Acute pancreatitis in marrow transplant patients: prevalence at autopsy and risk factor analysis. Bone Marrow Transplant 1997; 20: 1081–6.

Lai C-L, Shouval D, Lok AS, et al. Entecavir versus lamivudine for patients with HBeAg-negative chronic hepatitis B. N Engl J Med 2006; 354: 1010–20.

Lamberts SWJ, van der Lely AJ, de Herder WW, Hofland LJ Octreotide. N Engl J Med 1996; 334: 246–54.

Lee WC, Wu MJ, Cheng CH, et al. Lamivudine is effective for the treatment of reactivation of hepatitis B and fulminant hepatic failure in renal transplant recipients. Am J Kidney Dis 2001; 38: 1074–81.

Lee WC, Wu MJ, Cheng CH, et al. Acute pancreatitis following antilymphocyte globulin therapy in a renal transplant recipient. Clin Nephrol 2006; 65: 144–6.

Legendre C, Garriche V, Bihan L, et al. Harmful long-term impact of hepatitis C virus infection in kidney transplant recipients. Transplantation 1998; 65: 667–70.

Levy G, Villamil F, Samuel D, et al. Results of lis2t, a multicenter, randomized study comparing cyclosporine microemulsion with C2 monitoring and tacrolimus with C0 monitoring in de novo liver transplantation. Transplantation 2004; 77: 1632–8.

Locarnini S. Molecular virology and the development of resistant mutants: implications for therapy. Semin Liver Dis 2005; 25 (Suppl 1): 9–19.

Magnone M, Holley JL, Shapiro R, et al. Interferon-alpha-induced acute renal allograft rejection. Transplantation 1995; 59: 1068–70.

Mathurin P, Mouquet C, Poynard T, et al. Impact of hepatitis B and C virus on kidney transplantation outcome. Hepatology 1999; 29: 257–63.

McHutchison JG, Gordon SC, Schiff ER, et al. Interferon alfa-2b or in combination with ribavirin as initial treatment for chronic hepatitis C. N Engl J Med 1998; 339: 1485–92.

Meier-Kriesche HU, Ojo AO, Hanson JA, Kaplan B. Hepatitis C antibody status and outcomes in renal transplant recipients. Transplantation 2001; 72: 241–4.

Melvin WS, Meier DJ, Elkhammas FA, et al. Prophylactic colecystectomy is not indicated following renal transplantation. Am J Surg 1998; 175: 317–19.

Mitchell RMS, Byrne MF, Baillie J Pancreatitis. Lancet 2003; 1: 1447–55.

Mjaland O, Normann E. Severe pancreatitis after parathyroidectomy. Scand J Gastroenterol 2000; 35: 446–8.

Morales JM. Renal transplantation in patients positive for hepatitis B or C (pro). Transplant Proc 1998; 30: 2064–9.

Moriyama M, Arakawa Y. Treatment of interferon-alpha for chronic hepatitis C. Expert Opin Pharmacother 2006; 7: 1163–79.

Munoz de Bustillo E, Ibarrola C, Colina F, et al. Fibrosing cholestatic hepatitis in hepatitis C virus-infected renal transplant recipients. J Am Soc Nephrol 1998; 9: 1109–13.

Murphy JO, Mehigan BJ, Keane FB. Acute pancreatitis. Hosp Med 2002; 63: 487–92.

Murthy BVR, Muerhoff AS, Desai SM, et al. Predictors of GBV-C infection among patients referred for renal transplantation. Kidney Int 1998; 53: 1769–74.

Natov SN, Pereira BJG. Management of hepatitis C infection in renal transplant recipients. Am J Transplant 2002; 2: 483–90.

Nieto Y, Russ P, Everson G, et al. Acute pancreatitis during immunosuppression with tacrolimus following an allogeneic umbilical cord blood transplantation. Bone Marrow Transplant 2000; 26: 109–11.

Nordback I, Sand J, Saaristo R, Paajanen H. Early treatment with antibiotics reduces the need for surgery in acute necrotizing pancreatitis: a single center randomized study. J Gastrointest Surg 2001; 5: 113–18.

Noto H, Raskin P. Hepatitis C infection and diabetes. J Diabetes Complications 2006; 20: 113–20.

Ogihara M, Yanagida T, Kamata T, et al. Prolonged liver dysfunction caused by hemosiderosis in renal transplant recipients. Int J Urol 2002; 9: 187–9.

Ogunseinde BA, Wimmers F, Washington B, et al. A case of tacrolimus (FK506)-induced pancreatitis and fatality 2 years postcadaveric renal transplant [Letter]. Transplantation 2003; 76: 448.

Orloff SL, Stempel CA, Wright TL, et al. Long-term outcome in kidney transplant patients with hepatitis C (HCV) infection. Clin Transplant 1995; 9: 119–24.

Park SB, Kim HC, Lee SH, et al. Evolution of serum ferritin levels in renal transplant recipients with severe iron overload. Transplant Proc 1994; 26: 2054–5.

Pawlotsky JM. Therapy of hepatitis C: from empiricism to eradication. Hepatology 2006; 43 (Suppl 1): S207–20.

Pereira BJG, Levey AS. Hepatitis C virus infection in dialysis and renal transplantation. Kidney Int 1997; 51: 981–99.

Pereira BJG, Natov SN, Bouthot BA, et al. Effect of hepatitis C infection and renal transplantation on survival in end-stage renal disease. Kidney Int 1998; 53: 1374–81.

Perez RM, Ferreira AS, Medina-Pestana JO, et al. Is alanine aminotransferase a good marker of histologic hepatic damage in renal transplant patients with hepatitis C virus infection? Clin Transplant 2005; 19: 622–5.

Perez RM, Ferreira AS, Medina-Pestana JO, et al. Is hepatitis C more aggressive in renal transplant patients than in patients with end-stage renal disease? J Clin Gastroenterol 2006; 40: 444–8.

Pezzilli R, Fantini L, Morselli-Labate AM. New approaches for the treatment of acute pancreatitis. JOP 2006; 7: 79–91.

Pouteil-Noble C, Tardy JC, Chossegros P, et al. Coinfection by hepatitis B virus and hepatitis C virus in renal transplantation: morbidity and mortality in 1098 patients. Nephrol Dial Transplant 1995; 10 (Suppl 6): 122–4.

Prieto M, Berenguer M, Rayon M, et al. High incidence of allograft cirrhosis in hepatitis C virus genotype 1b infection following transplantation: relationship with rejection episodes. Hepatology 1999; 29: 250–6.

Rao KV, Anderson WR, Kasiske BL, Dahl DC. Value of liver biopsy in the evaluation and management of chronic liver disease in renal transplant recipients. Am J Med 1993; 94: 241–50.

Rostaing L, Izopet J, Baron E, et al. Preliminary results of treatment of chronic hepatitis C with recombinant interferon alpha in renal transplant patients. Nephrol Dial Transplant 1995; 10: 93–6.

Rostaing L, Henry S, Cisterne JM, et al. Efficacy and safety of lamivudine on replication of recurrent hepatitis B after cadaveric renal transplantation. Transplantation 1997; 64: 1624–7.

Rostaing L, Izopet J, Arnaud C, et al. Long-term impact of superinfections by hepatitis G virus in hepatitis C virus-positive renal transplant patients. Transplantation 1999; 67: 556–60.

Scheinin S, Radovancevic B, Frazier OH. Acute pancreatitis complicating OKT3 administration for resistant cardiac rejection. Transplant Proc 1993; 25: 2368–9.

Sharobeem R, Baca Y, Furet Y, et al. Cyclosporine A and ursodeoxycholic acid interaction. Clin Transplant 1993; 7: 223–6.

Sinha S, Jha R, Lakhtakia S, Narayan G. Acute pancreatitis following kidney transplantation – role of viral infections. Clin Transplant 2003; 17: 32–6.

Siwach V, Bansal V, Kumar A, et al. Post-renal transplant-induced pancreatitis. Nephrol Dial Transplant 1999; 14: 2495–8.

Teruel JL, Lamas S, Vila T, et al. Serum ferritin levels after renal transplantation: a prospective study. Nephron 1989; 51: 462–5.

Toth MC, Pascual M, Chung RT, et al. Hepatitis C virus-associated fibrosing cholestatic hepatitis after renal transplantation. Response to interferon-alpha therapy. Transplantation 1998; 66: 1254–8.

Vallet-Pichard A, Rerolle JP, Fontaine H, et al. Veno-occlusive disease of the liver in renal transplant patients. Nephrol Dial Transplant 2003; 18: 1663–6.

Vigano M, Colombo M, Aroldi A, et al. Long-term lamivudine monotherapy in renal-transplant recipients with hepatitis-B-related cirrhosis. Antivir Ther 2005; 10: 709–13.

Vosnides GC. Hepatitis C in renal transplantation. Kidney Int 1997; 52: 843–61.

Watashi K, Hijikata M, Hosaka M, et al. Cyclosporin A suppresses replication of hepatitis C virus genome in cultured hepatocytes. Hepatology 2003; 38: 1282–8.

Yen TH, Huang CC, Lin HH, et al. Does hepatitis C virus affect the reactivation of hepatitis B virus following renal transplantation? Nephrol Dial Transplant 2006; 21: 1046–52.

Younossi ZM, Braun WE, Protiva DE. Chronic viral hepatitis in renal transplant recipients with allografts functioning for more than 20 years. Transplantation 1999; 67: 272–5.

Youssef WI, Tavill AS. Connective tissue diseases and the liver. J Clin Gastroenterol 2002; 35: 345–9.

14

SKIN COMPLICATIONS

Cutaneous or mucosal complications are frequent in renal transplant recipients. The lesions are mainly related to the prolonged use of immunosuppressive drugs, but an important contributing role may also be played by exposure to sunlight and viral infections. Cutaneous complications may be subdivided into cancerous lesions, lesions caused by drugs, infections, and miscellaneous lesions.

Cancerous lesions

Incidence

Renal transplant recipients have a high risk of skin cancer, up to 65 times more than the general population (Jensen *et al.*, 1999). The spectrum of premalignant and malignant lesions includes Kaposi's sarcoma, actinic keratosis, Bowen's disease, keratoacanthoma, porokeratosis, basal-cell carcinomas, squamous-cell carcinomas, anogenital carcinomas, and melanoma. The incidence of cancer progressively increases with the duration of follow-up after intervention. In populations with heavy exposure to sunlight, such as in Australia, there is a linear increase in the incidence of cutaneous cancer, reaching 75% at 30 years post-transplantation (Sheil, 2002). The incidence of skin neoplasms in less sunny areas, such as The Netherlands, is around 40% at 20 years, which is, however, 250 times that in the general Dutch population (Hartevelt *et al.*, 1990). In an Irish study, there was a steady increase in risk for renal transplant recipients older than 50 years in the first two post-transplant years, whereas the increased risk in younger transplant patients occurred later, but much more significantly, reaching 200 times the risk for an age-matched non-transplanted population by year 6 post-transplant (Moloney *et al.*, 2006).

Risk factors

Several factors may predispose to skin cancer (Table 14.1). The oncogenic effect of *ultraviolet B* (UVB) light is well known. Ultraviolet B radiation may favor the initiation of cancer by inducing a mutation in the p53 tumor suppressor gene, by modifying the DNA of keratinocytes and by interfering with the local immune response. Ultraviolet light has a very short penetration through garments, and is thus of concern only for exposed body surfaces. A number of factors may interfere with the oncogenic risk of prolonged exposure to sunlight. It is well known that skin tumors are rare in the black population, while they are frequent in patients with pale, thin skin. Renal transplant patients with light blond or red hair color have a triple risk of skin cancer compared with those with dark hair (Lindelof *et al.*, 2003). Also, *ultraviolet A* (UVA) radiation might exert an oncogenic effect in patients treated with *azathioprine*. Upon exposure to low levels of UVA, 6-thioguanine, an active metabolite of azathioprine, is converted into reactive oxygen species and guanine-6-sulfonate, a mutagenic compound. Under therapeutic doses of azathioprine the skin becomes more sensitive to UVA but not UVB radiation (O'Donovan *et al.*, 2005). *Genetic factors* may also play a role. A major carcinogenic factor is represented by UVB-induced free-radical damage. In normal subjects the glutathione *S*-transferase enzymes can limit the toxic effect of reactive oxygen species. The genetic variations in these enzymes are associated with the development of skin cancer (Marshall *et al.*, 2000). A genetic role is also suggested by the observation that several members of a family may develop the same type of tumor in the same area. *Ethnicity* is also important. Skin cancer occurs rarely in Asiatic transplant recipients (Hoshida *et al.*, 1997), and is exceptional in black transplant patients (Moosa and Gralla, 2005). There is increasing evidence that *human papilloma virus* (HPV) infection is involved in the development of skin cancer (Bouwes Bavinck *et al.*, 2001), while Epstein–Barr virus-positive carcinoma cells are found only

Table 14.1   Factors influencing the risk for skin tumors in renal transplant recipients

Ultraviolet B rays
  Induce mutation in tumor suppressor p53
  Modify DNA of keratinocytes
  Interfere with local immune response

Ultraviolet A rays
  Convert 6-thioguanine into ROS and mutagenic compounds

Genetic factors
  Variations in glutathione *S*-transferase
  Familial susceptibility

Ethnicity
  Skin tumors rare in Asiatic transplant patients, exceptional in black transplant patients

Viral infections
  HPV

Immunosuppressive drugs
  Reduce immune surveillance
  Favor HPV infections
  Inactivate p53 gene

rarely in renal transplant recipients (Ternesten-Bratel *et al.*, 2003). *Immunosuppression* amplifies the deleterious effect of UVB by causing dermal depletion of cells related to immune surveillance against tumor (Galvao *et al.*, 1998), favoring the papilloma virus infection (Harwood *et al.*, 2000), and inactivating the tumor suppressor gene p53 protein (Gibson *et al.*, 1997). Male sex, previous history of actinic keratosis, and Bowen's disease increase the risk of non-melanoma cancer (Carroll *et al.*, 2003).

Diagnosis

Skin cancers in renal transplant recipients have some peculiar characteristics. While in the general population basal-cell carcinomas outnumber squamous-cell carcinomas, the mean ratio being 5:1, the reverse is true in renal transplant recipients, with a ratio of 1:1.7 (Penn, 1998). Non-melanoma skin cancers occur in the normal population mostly in the seventh and eighth decades of life, whereas in transplant patients the average age is 30–40 years. Even if most skin cancers have a low grade of malignancy the mortality rate for skin neoplasms is about 5% in the renal transplant population, compared with 1–2% of all cancer deaths in the general population, mostly caused by melanoma (Penn, 1998).

Of paramount importance is the time and the accuracy of diagnosis. A report found a diagnostic accuracy only in 54% of 102 lesions that were biopsied (Cooper and Wojnarowska, 2002). This low accuracy rate implies a need for biopsy of suspicious lesions in transplant patients.

Preventive measures

To minimize the morbidity and mortality of skin cancer, some preventive measures are recommended (Table 14.2). They include diligent UV protection, with so-called broad-spectrum sunscreens that protect

Table 14.2 Main measures to prevent the risk of cancer in transplant recipients

Avoidance of sun and UV light exposure
Use of appropriate clothes, sunglasses, wide-brimmed hat, sun-protective creams
Avoidance of smoking (risk of lip cancer)
Frequent self-examination
Regular dermatological evaluation

against UVA as well as UVB radiation (Parrish, 2005). Frequent self-examination of the skin and regular dermatologic evaluation are also recommended. Unfortunately, the use of sun-protective measures such as sun avoidance and protective clothing is poor, and the use of sun barrier creams is often inappropriate (Seukeran et al., 1998).

Retinoids are molecules with effects similar to those of vitamin A. They have been proposed for chemo-prevention of non-melanoma skin cancer. The mechanisms of action of retinoids are still unknown, but it likely that these agents interfere with multiple functions. Topical retinoids – such as tretinoin, tazarotene, or adapalene – may be useful to treat actinic keratoses and also basal-cell and squamous-cell carcinomas (Stockfleth et al., 2002). Data on the use of systemic retinoids come mainly from case reports. Kovach et al. (2005) reviewed nine studies describing 111 transplant recipients. Most studies reported a decrease in the number of malignant and premalignant lesions under treatment with systemic retinoids. The most frequent side-effect was mucocutaneous dryness that often led to a dose reduction, but rarely to discontinuation. However, an increased number of cancers occurred in patients who discontinued retinoids. The authors concluded that retinoids actually have a chemopreventive effect in renal transplant recipients. Although the optimal dosage is still far from being established, the authors suggested starting with low doses, with a progressive increase to an effective dose.

Premalignant diseases

Solar keratosis

Solar keratosis, formerly known as actinic keratosis, is a premalignant condition. It is preferentially localized on sun-exposed areas, and consists of round–oval well-defined erythematous patches, with dry and keratotic adherent scale that causes bleeding if detached (Figure 14.1). Long-term evolution may be toward squamous-cell carcinoma. The histologic pattern is that of an in situ carcinoma. Particularly in sun-exposed patients, one can find hundreds of lesions. The best treatments are liquid nitrogen or electro-curettage. Widespread lesions may be treated with acitretin, which may improve the aspect of actinic keratosis by alterating the keratinization, with peeling of the stratum corneum (Smit et al., 2004). Doses of 0.4 mg/kg are poorly tolerated because of cheilitis, escessive peeling of the skin, and hair disorders. Doses of 0.2 mg/kg are better tolerated, and may significantly decrease the thickeness of the lesions, but do not influence the incidence of new skin malignancies (De Sevaux et al., 2003).

Bowen's disease

This is an intraepithelial carcinoma, which may be located on the trunk or limbs (Figure 14.2). Its clinical and histologic features are similar to those of solar keratosis. When located on the genitalia the condition is called erythroplasia of Queyrat, which presents as one or a few large plaques, and shows histologically advanced dysplasia and carries significant risk of malignancy. Good results in renal transplant recipients have been obtained with topical imiquimod, a local immune modulator which does not interfere with systemic immunity (Smith et al., 2001).

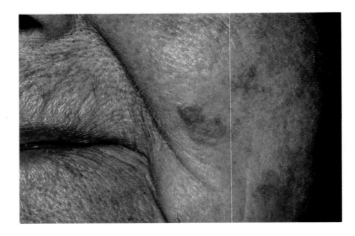

Figure 14.1 Solar keratoses: an erythmatosquamous lesion on sun-exposed areas. If inflamed, the lesion can be more infiltrated and mimic a frank squamous cell carcinoma. Palpation can reveal a keratotic, rough surface

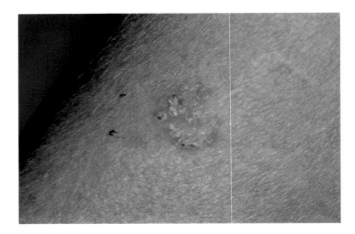

Figure 14.2 Bowen's disease. Slowly enlarging erthematosquamous patch. Hyperkeratosis and infiltration are usually not prominent

Bowenoid papulosis

Full-thickness epidermal dysplasia of the vulva or penis is usually called Bowenoid papulosis by many dermatologists, even if it should be known as grade III *vulval* or *penile intraepithelial neoplasia*. This condition is strongly associated with HPV-16 infection. In iatrogenically immunosuppressed patients, Bowenoid papulosis is refractory to treatment. The evolution to carcinoma of the vulva, perineum, scrotum, penis, perianal skin, or anus is not uncommon.

Keratoacanthoma

This is a rapidly evolving tumor of the skin, composed of keratinizing squamous cells. However, in some transplant recipients, keratoacanthoma is almost indistinguishable from squamous-cell carcinoma (Euvrard *et al.*, 2003). The tumor is benign in most cases, with spontaneous resolution. The etiology is unknown. The pathogenetic role of human papillomavirus infection is still controversial (Viviano *et al.*, 2001). The tumor usually presents most commonly on extremities as a firm, rounded, flesh-colored or red papule that in a few weeks may become 10–20 mm across. At this nodular stage, the center contains a horny plug (Figure 14.3). As the lesion matures, the accumulating keratin protrudes from the top of the lesion, resembling a crater.

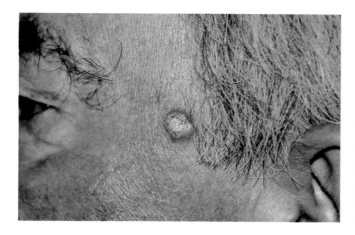

Figure 14.3 Keratoacanthoma. Keratotic nodule on the temporal area. In most cases the tumor presents as a solitary lesion. At the periphery the lesion is skin-colored to red with little teleangiectases beneath the surface. The center contains a yellowish, horny plug

The most useful clues to clinical diagnosis are well-preserved symmetry of the lesion and no infiltration at the base. Spontaneous resolution is achieved in about 3 months, with the epidermal covering receding toward the base and the horny core being shed. Multiple lesions can also occur.

Carcinomas of the vulva and perineum

The incidence of these tumors is 100-fold increased in renal transplant patients if compared with controls (Penn, 1989). One-third of patients have *in situ* lesions. Patients with invasive lesions are much younger than their counterparts in the normal population. One-third of affected patients have a history of *condylomata acuminata*.

Carcinoma of the vulva may develop either *de novo*, or from pre-existing areas of leukoplakia or pigmented papular lesions, with histologic features of Bowen's disease. The anterior vulva, and especially the labia minora, are the main areas involved. The lesion most commonly presents as an ulcerated nodule. Pre-existing Bowen's disease or leukoplakia should heighten clinical suspicion. In carcinoma of the penis, the initial lesion is almost always within the preputial sac. It may be preceded by erythroplasia, or a warty excrescence that can be misdiagnosed as a wart. *In situ* cancer may be treated with laser therapy, electrocautery, and topical fluorouracil.

Squamous-cell carcinoma (SCC) of the skin

This malignant tumor arises from the keratinocytes of the epidermis. Squamous-cell carcinoma is the *commonest malignancy* in transplant patients. It usually develops on sun-exposed sites and often coexists with a background of viral warts. In such patients, papilloma virus and sun exposure appear to act as co-carcinogens. In immunosuppressed patients, the malignancy of SCC is greater. Thus, it is extremely important that transplant recipients are strongly advised to avoid sun exposure.

Usually, SCC does not arise on healthy skin but on *sunlight-damaged skin* (Figure 14.4). These photo-induced lesions consist of solar elastoidosis of the dermis, hyperkeratosis, irregular pigmentation, and telangiectasia of the skin, or leukokeratosis of the lips. The clinical appearance can be misleading, however. The first evidence of malignancy is *induration*. Thus, any indurated lesion should be submitted to histologic analysis. The area may be plaque-like, verrucous, tumid, or ulcerated, without sharp limits, usually extending beyond the visible margins of the lesion. The edges are an opaque yellow color, and tissue around the tumor is inflamed. The most common sites are those more exposed to the sun: backs of the hands and forearms, the upper part of the face, and, in men, the pinna. In transplant patients the tumor frequently appears at multiple sites (Rubel *et al.*, 2002). Also frequent is localization on the lower lip, particularly in patients with smoking habits (De Visscher *et al.*, 1997).

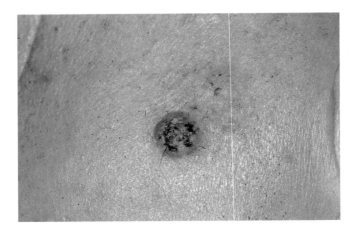

Figure 14.4 Squamous cell carcinoma. There is a photo-damaged area surrounding the tumor. The central nodule is firm, indolent, and can ulcerate

The evolution is faster than in basal-cell carcinoma but much slower than in keratoacanthoma. The prognosis is poor in transplant recipients with advanced head and neck SCC (Preciado *et al.*, 2002). Regional lymph nodes may become enlarged as the result of either infection or metastases. The effective *treatments* for the cure of SCC are: local destruction, surgery, chemotherapy, or radiotherapy. Superficial tumors can be managed with cryotherapy or electrocautery and curettage. Mohs' microsurgery is recommended for high-risk tumors. Combination chemotherapy with isotretinoin and interferon-α proved to be helpful in transplant patients with aggressive squamous-cell carcinomas (Euvrard *et al.*, 2003). However, *preventive measures* remain the most important goal.

Basal-cell carcinoma

This is a malignant tumor which rarely metastasizes. Basal-cell carcinoma is composed of pluripotential cells that form continuously during life, and, like embryonic primary epithelial germ cells, have the potential to form hair, sebaceous glands, and apocrine glands.

The presence of a large number of nevi, freckles, and solar elastosis all add to the basal-cell carcinoma risk, suggesting an etiologic role both for UV radiation and for regional factors. Basal-cell carcinoma may arise in *skin damaged* by sunlight, ionizing radiation, and scars. In renal transplant recipients, basal-cell carcinoma develops on average 6–7 years after transplantation. Patients are younger, there is a male prevalence, and in 35–40% of cases the tumor is extracephalic, not affecting the head or neck (Kanitakis *et al.*, 2003).

The early tumors are small, translucent, and pearly, with a thin epidermis and visible telangiectasia (Figure 14.5). As the mass of the tumor grows, ulceration can occur, and may re-epithelialize and break down several times before becoming permanent. Pigment, when present, is usually unevenly distributed in the tumor. In the pagetoid variant, the basal-cell carcinoma spreads only superficially, is bounded by a slightly raised thread-like margin, and has a central atrophic and scaly zone (Figure 14.6). The morpheic or sclerodermiform variant shows dense fibrosis of the stroma, producing a thick plaque rather than a tumor. Unfortunately, the diagnostic accuracy is low in renal transplant recipients, about 40% with a sensitivity of 66.6% and a specificity of 85.6% (Cooper and Wojnarowska, 2002). Thus, biopsy is recommended for any suspicious lesion.

Typically, basal-cell carcinoma runs a slow progressive course of peripheral extension, which procures the thread-like margins, the nodule with a central depression, or an expanding rodent ulcer. A patient who has one basal-cell carcinoma should always be followed, both because new tumors may develop elsewhere and because there is some risk of local recurrence. Surgery, cryosurgery, Mohs' surgical technique with pathological control of excision margins, and radiotherapy are all good therapeutic options.

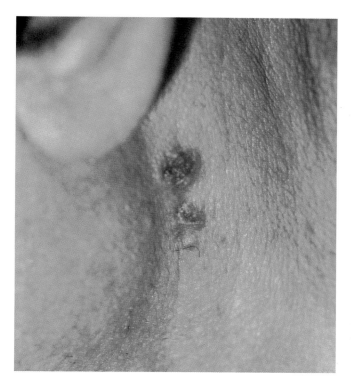

Figure 14.5 Nodular basal cell carcinoma. The lesion is firm, not tender, with a characteristic translucent aspect with waxy reflexes. When present, the pearly margin is a very useful tool for diagnosis

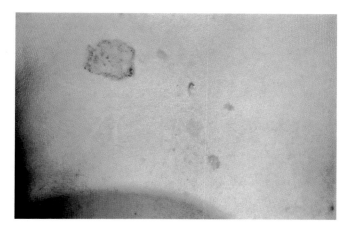

Figure 14.6 Pagetoid basal cell carcinoma on the trunk: the micronodular edge is evident. The epidermis covering the central zone is atrophic and scaly. Combined with increased vascularity, this feature gives resemblance to Paget's disease of the nipple. In poorly cared-for patients, pagetoid basal cell carcinomas may achieve a very large size

Melanoma

This highly malignant tumor arises from epidermal melanocytes. The precise cause of melanoma is unknown, but sunlight, race, and genetic predisposition are recognized risk factors. Melanomas usually develop in areas exposed to the sun intermittently, and are more common in persons with *intense intermittent exposure* to ultraviolet radiation (Gilchrest *et al.*, 1999). The incidence of melanoma in the black population is one-tenth than in the white population. Patients with melanoma can be genetically predisposed to an

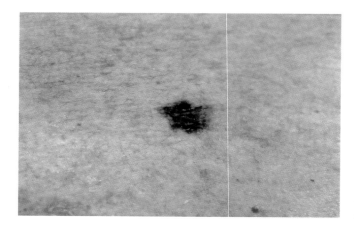

Figure 14.7 Superficial spreading melanoma. Pigmented and almost nonpalpable lesion. Asymmetry, irregular borders, irregularity in color distribution, and a diameter of 0.5 cm or more are all suspect features for a malignant lesion

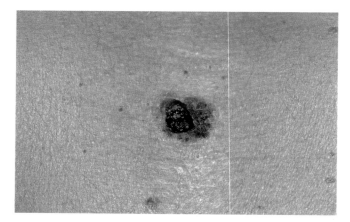

Figure 14.8 Nodular melanoma. The lesions often ulcerate. The nodular component is not in the center of the lesion, giving a more asymmetric aspect to the lesion. Color is variable from dark brown to light brown, red, blue, and black. A whitish color is sometimes visible. Amelanotic melanomas are especially difficult to diagnose clinically

aberration of cell-cycle control and transcriptional control (Halachmi and Gilchrest, 2001). The incidence of melanoma in renal transplant patients is 3–6 fold higher than in other immunosuppressed patients (Penn, 1996). In renal transplant recipients, as well as in the general population, the presence of a large number of melanocytic nevi is the best known risk factor for melanoma (Gulec *et al.*, 2002). Cases of transmission from the donor, even years after melanoma surgery, have been reported (MacKie *et al.*, 2003).

Clinicopathologically there are several forms of melanoma. Epiluminescence, which allows examination of the surface of the pigmented lesion at moderate magnifications with a small and simple hand-held device, may be a useful tool for diagnosis. *Superficial spreading melanoma* is an irregularly shaped brown lesion usually still macular and only later palpable, with variations in brown and black pigmentation (Figure 14.7). Regression may cause pigment loss. The essential pathologic features are foci of malignant melanoma cells in the dermis with areas of *in situ*, that is intraepithelial, malignant changes in the adjacent epidermis. *Nodular melanoma* (Figure 14.8) is most commonly located on the trunk, and is an elevated, dome-shaped polypoid or even pedunculated structure, often totally or partially devoid of pigment (amelanotic melanoma). Histologically, there is a focus of invasive melanoma cells in the dermis in direct contact with the epidermis, but without abnormalities of the adjacent epidermis on either side of the nodule. *Lentigo maligna melanoma* is a flat, variously pigmented, irregularly shaped lesion most commonly located on the face. With time, a raised central nodule develops. Histologically, after a long phase of *in situ* involvement, invasion into the underlying dermis will take place. *Acral lentiginous melanoma* (and subungual melanoma), found mainly on the sole of the foot, is a large macular, lentiginous pigmented area around an invasive raised tumor. The histologic pattern consists of an extensive area of lentiginous changes in the epidermis around the focus of invasive melanoma.

Whenever possible, adequate surgical excision is the basic principle of treatment. *Sentinel lymph node* biopsy, that is, biopsy of the lymph node into which drains the dye or the radiolabeled material injected at the site of the tumor, allows, if negative, avoidance of unnecessary full lymph node dissection, while it may help in diagnosing controversial melanocytic lesions (Su *et al.*, 2003). As the microenvironment of the skin may contribute to Akt-mediated melanocyte transformation (Bedogni *et al.*, 2005), there is a rationale for the use of mTOR (mammalian target of rapamycin) inhibitors for preventing recurrence in renal transplant recipients treated for a previous melanoma.

Kaposi's sarcoma

Kaposi's sarcoma (KS) is a multifocal, vascular, malignant tumor that accounts for more than 5% of malignancies in transplant patients. KS occurs endemically in tropical Africa, in some Mediterranean areas, and among Jews and Arabs, while it occurs sopradically in Europe and North America. The incidence of KS is 400–500 times greater in renal transplant patients compared with controls of the same ethnic origin (Penn, 1997). The male to female ratio is 2.8 : 1 in transplant patients, far less than the 10–15 : 1 ratio seen in the general population.

Etiopathogenesis

Kaposi's sarcoma is associated with the presence of human herpes virus 8 (HHV-8). HHV-8 has been regularly found by polymerase chain reaction in all forms of KS (classic KS, AIDS–KS, endemic KS, and organ transplant KS), in certain types of Castleman's disease, in primary effusion lymphoma (Sarid *et al.*, 2002), and in EBV-negative post-transplant lymphoproliferative disorders (Kapelushnik *et al.*, 2001). HHV-8 contains potential oncogens able to transform all lines *in vitro*. HHV-8 viremia and the detection of HHV-8 in all forms of KS makes it the candidate causative agent (Simonart *et al.*, 1998).

After transplantation, HHV-8 can reactivate quickly, the risk being higher in patients with strong immunosuppression (Eberhard *et al.*, 1999) and in the endemic areas. Increased HHV-8 DNA levels in peripheral blood lymphocytes are associated with the progression of KS (Pellet *et al.*, 2002). HHV-8 can also be transmitted through renal allografts, representing a potential risk factor for transplantation-associated KS (Regamey *et al.*, 1998), but reactivation of the virus remains the main factor responsible for the development of post-transplant KS (Andreoni *et al.*, 2001).

Clinical features

In the skin, KS lesions have a dark blue or purplish color, being initially almost macular and becoming progressively more tumid (Figure 14.9). Lesions usually begin on the extremities, most commonly on the feet, with multifocal and asymptomatic development (Figure 14.10). The rate of spread is remarkably variable. Lymph nodes, mucosal surfaces, and internal organs, particularly the small intestine, may all be involved as the disease progresses. About 60% of patients have a non-visceral KS confined to the skin, conjunctiva, or oropharyngolaryngeal mucosa. Only 10% of patients do not have skin disease.

Treatment

In transplant patients, the withdrawal or even reduction of immunosuppression may obtain improvement and even complete recovery of KS, particularly if the lesions are limited to the skin (Montagnino *et al.*, 1994; Duman *et al.*, 2002). The reduction or withdrawal of immunosuppression allows the immune system to recover sufficiently to reduce viral replication, with subsequent viral persistence and low-grade viral replication that coincides with clinical remission of the KS lesions. While some patients show progressive, irreversible allograft dysfunction, other patients may maintain stable graft function with mild immunosuppression or with small doses of prednisone alone (Montagnino *et al.*, 1994; Moosa *et al.*, 1998; Duman *et al.*, 2002).

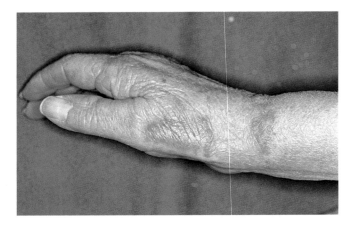

Figure 14.9 Kaposi's sarcoma. Erythematous patches of irregular, elongated with little infiltration. The surface is smooth, the consistency firm. These lesion\s are indolent and not ulcerated

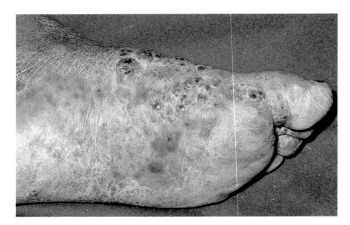

Figure 14.10 Kaposi's sarcoma. Violaceous, infiltrated, firm plaques of ecchymotic aspect on the foot with superimposed nodules. The nodules are more friable and may ulcerate. Long-standing lesions may be tender

Recently, a number of papers have documented the possibility of complete reversal of KS in renal transplant patients switched from cyclosporine to sirolimus (Campistol *et al.*, 2004; Stallone *et al.*, 2005). The improvement of lesions can probably be attributed to the antiangiogenetic effect of sirolimus, which impedes endothelial cell proliferation mediated by vascular endothelial growth factor (VEGF). In fact, VEGF activates a cascade of kinases mediated by mTOR, a serine–threonine kinase which is inhibited by sirolimus and its derivate everolimus.

Further approaches in patients who do not respond to a reduction of immunosuppression or to the introduction of mTOR antagonists may consist of antiviral therapies and/or chemotherapy. Because of the viral origin of KS, antiviral treatment is theoretically indicated. However, poor results have been obtained with ganciclovir or foscarnet. Trials with cidofovir in HIV patients showed that this agent could neither suppress the progression of KS nor decrease the viral load (Little *et al.*, 2003). Another therapeutic approach consists of the intravenous administration of liposomal tretinoin, which proved to be of benefit in AIDS patients with associated KS (Bernstein *et al.*, 2002). Among the numerous cytotoxic drugs used in KS, such as vincristine, cyclophosphamide, vinblastine, bleomycin, thalidomide, or actinomycin, comparative data have established that polyethylene glycol (PEG)-liposomal doxorubicin is the first-line treatment option in patients with advanced KS (Sharpe *et al.*, 2002). When required, treatment options include excision or radiotherapy of single lesions.

Retrasplantation in patients who have lost a previous allograft because of KS is generally not recommended. However, one retransplanted patient did not show any sign of recurrence of KS 3 years after retransplantation (Euvrard *et al.*, 2002a). The possibility of offering primary immunosuppression based on sirolimus or everolimus brings new hope for successful retransplantation in patients who have lost their first allograft because of KS.

Lymphomas

Cutaneous lymphomas are rare. Most are *B-cell lymphomas*, which present as single or multiple papules or nodules on the face, trunk, or limbs. A significant proportion of patients who present with cutaneous infiltration by B-cell lymphoma have systemic disease. Staging is therefore mandatory in these patients (Sah *et al.*, 2004). A particular form is large B-cell lymphoma of the leg, which accounts for 2% of primary cutaneous lymphomas. It usually presents in elderly patients, and manifests clinically as erythematous nodules or tumors, often unilateral, on the lower third of the legs. On rare occasions, it presents with extracutaneous dissemination. Remission of B-cell lymphoma may occur after a reduction of immunosuppressive therapy (Euvrard *et al.*, 2003). Intralesional injections of 3 million units of recombinant interferon-α (IFNα) three times per week may obtain complete tumor regression after a mean of 8.5 weeks (Cozzio *et al.*, 2006). Approximately one-third of patients with primary cutaneous lymphoma ultimately relapse, and relapse rates appear higher in those patients receiving local therapy only. Rituximab or high-dose systemic therapy and autologous stem transplantation therapy have been suggested in the more severe cases (Ingen-Housz-Oro *et al.*, 2004; Goto *et al.*, 2005)

Post-transplant *cutaneous T-cell lymphoma* is extremely rare. Ravat *et al.* (2006) reviewed the 23 cases reported in the literature. Of them, five patients had erythrodermic disease, and eight had primary cutaneous anaplastic large-cell lymphoma. In addition, there were two cases of mycosis fungoides, one case of subcutaneous panniculitis-like T-cell lymphoma, one case of CD30+ lymphomatoid papulosis, and six cases of peripheral T-cell lymphoma, of which three were CD30+ large-cell lymphomas. Seventeen cases had renal transplants and the majority received both cyclosporine and azathioprine. The sex ratio was 18:5 (male/female), and the mean age at diagnosis was 53 years. Mean time from transplantation to diagnosis was 6.4 years, and mean survival time from diagnosis was 14.5 months. However, the introduction of monoclonal antibodies for the treatment of cancer has changed the outlook for patients with T-cell malignancies. Recent studies with the single agent alemtuzumab, an anti-CD52 monoclonal antibody, have shown improved response rates and survival in patients with cutaneous T-cell lymphoma. Preliminary data also suggest that alemtuzumab may have activity in patients with heavily pretreated peripheral T-cell lymphoma who are refractory to conventional chemotherapy (Dearden, 2006).

Merkel-cell carcinoma (MCC)

Merkel-cell carcinoma is an uncommon tumor, most commonly affecting elderly Caucasians. Usually the tumor manifests as a solitary painless erythematous nodule, sometimes ulcerated, located on the head or neck. More than half of patients develop local lymph node metastases, and almost half develop distant metastases. The mortality rate is 56% within 2 years in transplant patients.

Fifty-five cases of MCC have been reported in renal transplant recipients (Euvrard *et al.*, 2002b), suggesting an increased incidence in immunosuppressed patients. Temporary regression of Merkel cell carcinoma metastases after cessation of cyclosporine has been reported (Friedlander *et al.*, 2002).

Treatment consists of surgical excision with 2 cm margins or Mohs' surgery. Lymphadenectomy with radiotherapy and chemotherapy is recommended.

Lesions caused by drugs

Immunosuppresive drugs

The immunosuppressive agents used to prevent rejection may be responsible for several lesions of the skin or mucosae.

Table 14.3 Corticosteroid-related skin abnormalities

Cushingoid appearance
  facial fullness
  buffalo hump
  increased supraclavicular and suprasternal fat
  trunkal obesity
Acne
  may evolve to acne conglobata
Bateman's purpura
  purpuric lesions either spontaneous or after minimal trauma
Striae rubrae
Facial erythrosis
Atrophic, friable skin
Telangiectasias
Hypertrichosis
  face and back

Corticosteroids

Renal transplant recipients given corticosteroid treatment may show a number of dermatologic lesions (Table 14.3). The most typical side-effect is represented by a *Cushingoid appearance*, with facial and neck fullness, buffalo hump, increased supraclavicular and suprasternal fat, and trunkal obesity. These features are usually dose-dependent, and are caused by abnormalities in the fat distribution. Cushingoid features are particularly frequent in the initial post-transplant period, when higher doses of corticosteroids are used. In the long term, some lesions may spontaneously disappear. However, some 40% of patients still maintain a Cushingoid appearance in spite of the low dosage of prednisone.

The most frequent complication of corticosteroids is *acne*, which is usually dose-related. Acne occurs early on the cheeks, forehead, chin, and chest. Rarely, the lesions may progress to nodulocystic transformation (acne conglobata). Doxicycline, 100 mg daily, may be effective in reducing acne. Severe cases can be successfully treated with isotretinoin or acitretin, a second-generation retinoid used also for progressive solar keratoses, widespread warts, or recurrent skin malignancies. The severity of acne tends to decrease when the dose of corticosteroids is reduced.

A complication seen almost constantly in patients given prolonged corticosteroid administration is so-called *Bateman's purpura* (Figure 14.11). It consists of irregular purpuric areas that develop spontaneously or after minor trauma, mainly on the extensor surfaces of the hands, forearms, and legs, often with spontaneous star-shaped pseudo-scars. *Striae rubrae* are wide and violaceous stripes, located mainly over the abdomen, thighs, and buttocks. *Facial erythrosis* and rosacea can occur. Some patients have increased *hair growth*, mainly on the face and back. Finally, the skin of corticosteroid-treated patients can become thin, *atrophic*, and *friable*. Topical retinoic acid at concentrations ranging from 0.01 to 0.05% may improve this complication. Some patients, however, complain of irritation. Ammonium lactate 6–12% creams are usually better tolerated.

Azathioprine

Azathioprine may cause *thinning of the hair* and scalp hair loss. Azathioprine may also be responsible for changes of color or texture of the hair. Actinic keratoses may occur in azathioprine-treated patients, particularly after extensive sunlight exposure.

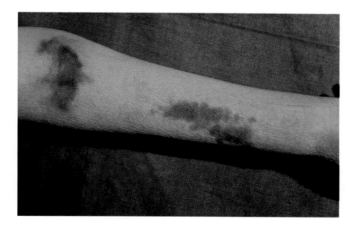

Figure 14.11 Bateman's purpura in a transplant patient receiving long-term steroid therapy

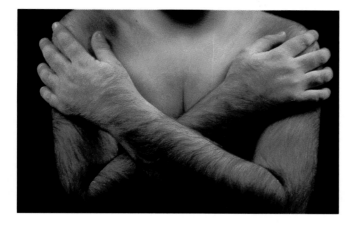

Figure 14.12 Hirsutism in a 10-year-old girl given cyclosporine

Cyclosporine

The skin is one of the principal sites of accumulation of cyclosporine. The drug, which is highly lipophilic, may be partly eliminated through the sebaceous glands. This could explain the frequent pilosebaceous lesions observed in cyclosporine-treated patients.

A frequent complication of cyclosporine is represented by *hypertrichosis*, which is usually dose-dependent (Figure 14.12). In children, however, this side-effect is more related to age than to dosage (Euvrard *et al.*, 2001). Hypertrichosis is characterized by thick and pigmented hair appearing over the trunk, back, shoulders, arms, neck, forehead, helices, and malar areas. This complication is particularly disturbing in dark-haired women and in children. A possible mechanism for cyclosporine-induced hypertrichosis is the increased activity of α-reductase, an enzyme that transforms androgens into dihydrotestosterone in peripheral tissues (Vexiau *et al.*, 1990). If so, treatment with finasteride, an inhibitor of α-reductase used successfully in patients with idiopathic hirsutism (Rittmaster, 1995), may be helpful.

Alopecia areata and universalis have also been observed. Accelerated male-pattern balding may occur. *Skin hyperpigmentation* and bullous or vegetative lesions have also been reported in cyclosporine-treated patients (Ponticelli and Zorzi, 2001).

Sebaceous hyperplasia, epidermal cysts, and *pilar keratosis* have been reported in 10–20% of patients treated with cyclosporine, but it can be difficult to discern whether these lesions should be attributed

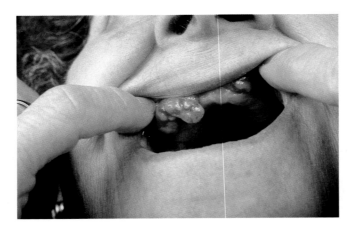

Figure 14.13 Gingival hyperplasia in cyclosporine-treated patient. Good oral hygiene can minimize this side-effect

to cyclosporine, to corticosteroids, or to both drugs. Cyclosporine may also be responsible for *acne*. However, apart from hypertrichosis, there are no major differences in skin lesions between patients treated with cyclosporine and those treated with azathioprine, at least in the early stages after transplantation (Bunney *et al.*, 1990).

Gum hyperplasia occurs in about one-third of transplant patients treated with cyclosporine. It is caused by hyperplasia of the epithelial and connective-tissue components, as well as by altered extracellular metabolism. This complication generally occurs after 3 or more months of treatment, and can be worsened by the concomitant administration of calcium channel blockers or phenytoin. The incidence of gingival hyperplasia seems to be more frequent in patients with chronic graft nephropathy (Boratynska *et al.*, 2003). Gingival overgrowth is at least partially preventable with careful oral hygiene. Initially, hyperplasia of the anterior interdental papillae occurs, which subsequently spreads to the whole gum, also involving the inner side (Figure 14.13). A 5-day treatment with Azithrocin®, a macrolide antimicrobial agent, may improve subjective symptoms and the clinical picture (Nash and Zaltzman, 1998). The most severe cases require gingivectomy. The possibility that a gingival Kaposi's sarcoma may mimic a cyclosporine-related gingival hyperplasia should be taken into account.

Tacrolimus

In spite of the similar mechanism of inhibition of calcineurin, tacrolimus gives fewer skin abnormalities and does not cause gingival hyperplasia. Cases of *alopecia* have been reported in patients treated with tacrolimus (Talbot *et al.*, 1997; Tricot *et al.*, 2005).

Sirolimus

Clinical trials have reported that the use of sirolimus is frequently associated with skin disorders, but details of the type and severity of these disorders are not provided. Follicular acneiform eruptions (Kunzle *et al.*, 2005) and ulcerating debilitating maculopapular rash (Tracey *et al.*, 2005), severe enough to necessitate the cessation of sirolimus in renal recipients, have been described.

Other drugs

Photo-damage of the head and neck, telangiectasia, and solar elastosis were found to be significantly more frequent in renal transplant recipients treated with *calcium channel blockers* than in patients who did not receive these drugs (Cooper and Wojnarowska, 2003). Gingival hyperplasia caused by cyclosporine can also be aggravated by the administration of calcium channel blockers (see above).

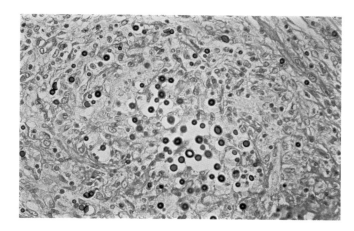

Figure 14.14 Lymphonodal cryptococcosis: pleiomorphic, single and budding yeast cells surrounded by a wife carminophilic capsule. Mayer's mucicamine. Ob x40. (Courtesy of Dr MA Viviani, Ospedale Maggiore, Milan.)

Infections

Mycotic infections

Mycotic infections account for about half of the mucocutaneous infections observed in transplant patients. *Candidiasis* of the mouth and intertriginous areas of the skin is particularly frequent in the early post-transplant period when the dosage of immunosuppressive drugs is highest. Oral rinsing with sodium bicarbonate, nystatin, or other antifungal agents may be helpful in preventing this complication.

While *disseminated fungal infections* tend to occur early, infections due to dermatophytes, that is ringworm–causing fungi, typically occur several months after transplantation. Their clinical appearance is often atypical due to the lack of erythematous changes. Lesions may present as papules, plaques, ulcers, or subcutaneous nodules (Miele *et al.*, 2002).

Pityriasis versicolor, caused by the lipophilic yeast *Pityrosporon ovale/orbiculare*, is the prevalent infection, affecting more than 30% of transplant patients (Gulec *et al.*, 2003). This complication, which can involve large areas of the trunk and flexural zones, is characterized by multiple and widespread small scaly macules, either hypopigmented or hyperpigmented. The same fungus can also cause an acneiform eruption, consisting of bland or mildly erythematosus follicular papules and pustules over the shoulders, chest, upper back, and arms (pityrosporum folliculitis). Patients may be treated with imidazole cream or selenium sulfate shampoo. Primary *cutaneous aspergillosis* is rare. It is characterized by painful erythematous plaques, and sometimes cellulitis. Disseminated aspergillosis may produce cutaneous lesions such as papulae and pustules or subcutaneous nodules. *Nocardiosis* may also present with cutaneous pustules or with particularly painful subcutaneous nodules, and is easy to biopsy (Maccario *et al.*, 1998). Cutaneous *cryptococcosis* may cause erythema nodosum-like deep nodules, whereas primary cutaneous cryptococcosis may appear as nodular, pustular, ulcerative lesions or abscesses with enlargement of the lymph nodes (Figure 14.14). Subcutaneous *pheohyphomicosis* caused by dermatiaceous fungi is a rare complication. Phycomycosis of the sinuses may manifest as facial cellulitis. Dissemination of previously localized pathogenic agents, such as *Histoplasma capsulatum*, may lead to erysipela-like lesions. Early cutaneous histoplasmosis consists of painless diffuse swelling of the affected areas, whereas older lesions are represented by multiple draining ulcers (Shuttleworth *et al.*, 1987).

Cutaneous *chromomycosis* is characterized by scaly papules that may progress to verrucous nodules or ulcerating plaques. It is caused by pigmented fungi that are common saprophytes growing in soil, vegetation, and wood. Dermal *alternariasis* can manifest as fleshy papules and nodules, smooth and firm, spreading centrifugally, with an elevated crusted border and a central area slightly depressed and atrophic.

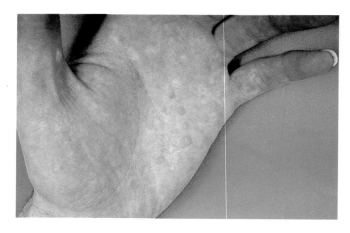

Figure 14.15 Plane warts on a hand

Whereas mucormycosis is one of the most common causes of opportunistic mycotic infection in immunosuppressed patients, cutaneous *mucormycosis* is rare. It can develop in burns and superficial wounds where spores are introduced into breaks in the skin. The clinical appearance is an erythematous macula that develops central vesiculation and necrosis. The demonstration of non-septate hyphae in smears or by culture is the most useful tool for diagnosis. *Onychomycosis* is frequent in renal transplant recipients. It is mainly caused by yeast-like fungi. Onychomycosis is more common in patients with a long duration of transplantation. It manifests mainly in distal and lateral subungual sites.

Viral infections

Herpes simplex may have a limited extension without serious consequences, but may also cause multifocal, extensive, and hemorrhagic lesions. Ulcers of the mouth and the perioral, perigenital, and perianal skin can occur in the most severe cases.

Herpes zoster can be responsible for gangrenous and hemorrhagic lesions, which usually do not extend to other areas. However, atypical herpetic infection may also cause disseminated ulcerative or necrotic skin. The administration of systemic acyclovir (5 mg/kg intravenously every 8 hours for 5 days) or valacyclovir (1 g orally three times daily for 7 days) is mandatory for patients with severe lesions (Balfour, 1999).

Varicella can occur in transplant patients, and can have a life-threatening course. Children awaiting a renal transplant should receive a specific vaccine to prevent this complication (Furth and Fivush, 2002). If varicella develops, immunosuppression should be reduced and even stopped in the most severe cases. Specific immunoglobulin infusion and acyclovir (10 mg/kg intravenously every 8 hours for 7–10 days) may improve the prognosis. Exceptional cases have been described of chronic, localized, verrucous varicella-presenting with cutaneous dissemination in varicella zoster-seronegative renal transplant patients (Jeyaratnam *et al.*, 2005).

Cutaneous manifestations caused by *cytomegaloviruses* are very rare. These consist of exanthema with vasculitis, hyperpigmented nodules and plaques, vesicobullae, and buccal and perineal ulcerations. Oral *leukoplakia*, a typical Epstein–Barr virus lesion observed mostly in patients affected by AIDS, has been also reported in HIV-negative transplant recipients (Ponticelli and Passerini, 2005).

Warts and *condylomata* caused by human papilloma virus are frequent in long-term functioning transplant patients, approaching 85% at 5 years (Leigh and Glover, 1995). They develop on sun-exposed areas, mainly in light-skinned patients (Figures 14.15 and 14.16). They are usually multiple, and their extension may be so widespread as to constitute general *verrucosis*. This is seen more frequently in long-term transplant patients (Barba *et al.*, 1997). Topical keratolytic agents or retinoic acid are the treatments of choice. Imiquimod cream 5% may be used in resistant warts (Gayed, 2002). Topical cidofovir may also be useful for the treatment of verruca vulgaris (Cha *et al.*, 2005).

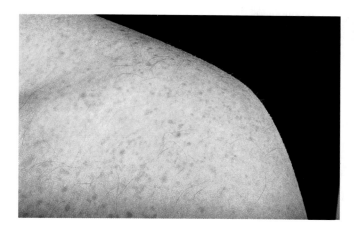

Figure 14.16 Plane warts widespread, yellow-pink, smooth-surfaces papules on limbs and trunk. Plane warts are polygonal or round in shape and may be flat or slightly elevated. Sometimes lichen planus causes difficulty in differential diagnosis

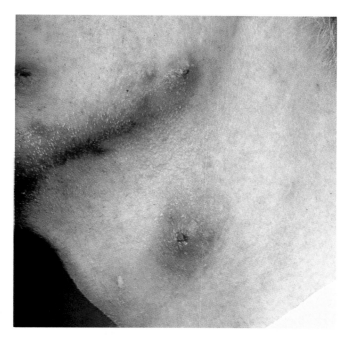

Figure 14.17 Abcessual folliculitis in a renal transplant patient. In these patients, folliculitis may be trivial, with tiny pustules on an erythmatous base. However, one can see follicular abcesses, with erythmatous, inflamed and exquisitely tender lesions that ulcerate and discharge pus

In immunosuppressed patients, there is widespread occurrence of lesions with a clinical pattern similar to *epidermodysplasia verruciformis*. This pre-cancerous condition is characterized by several widespread viral warts and pityriasis versicolor-like lesions. The infection is caused by oncogenic human papilloma virus. About 20% of renal transplant patients have antibodies against virus-like particles of epidermodysplasia verruciformis (Stark *et al.*, 1998). Extensive diffusion of *condylomata acuminata* or of molluscum contagiosum can also occur in renal transplant recipients.

Bacterial infections

Bacterial infections are usually trivial in the early period after transplantation, being represented almost exclusively by folliculitis (Figures 14.17 and 14.18). However, subcutaneous abscesses, erysipelas, and

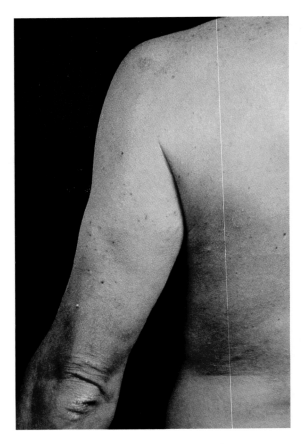

Figure 14.18 Folliculitis of limbs and trunk: the most common causative agents are Gram-positive microorganisms and yeasts. Pruritus is very variable, sometimes annoying and requiring therapy. A microbiological assessment can be rarely achieved and treatment is often empiric

impetigo, caused by Gram-positive cocci, may develop in the long term (Figure 14.19). Cutaneous infections caused by atypical mycobacteria are often manifested as spreading cellulitis around joints.

Necrotizing fasciculitis is a rare but life-threatening disorder caused by a rapidly spreading subcutaneous infection, usually sustained by polymicrobial pathogens (Seal, 2001). Clinically, necrotizing fasciculitis is characterized by progressive inflammation and extensive necrosis of the skin and soft tissue. Renal transplant patients receiving high-dose steroids are particularly susceptible to this complication. The presence of a nephrotic syndrome further increases the risk of necrotizing fasciculitis. This infection carries a high rate of mortality, ranging between 33 and 73% (Audard *et al.*, 2005). Prompt recognition and aggressive treatment, including surgical intervention with debridement of necrotic tissue and extensive fasciotomy, may improve the prognosis.

Miscellaneous lesions

Disseminated actinic *porokeratosis* may occur in up to 10% of transplant patients (Figure 14.20). It is caused by the proliferation of an abnormal clone of epidermal cells, and is characterized clinically by annular lesions surrounded by a raised keratotic ring, constituted histologically by a column of parakeratotic cells. *Norwegian scabies* is characterized by thick crusted plaques. In rare cases, transplant porokeratosis may evolve to fatal squamous-cell carcinoma (Silver and Crawford, 2003). *Urticaria* may be a cutaneous manifestation of an intestinal infestation, such as giardiasis.

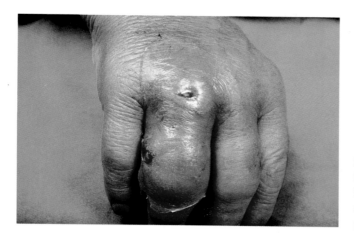

Figure 14.19 Cutaneous abcess following minor trauma in an immunosupresssed patient. Such events may have a rapid evolution and require prompt and vigorous antibiotic therapy

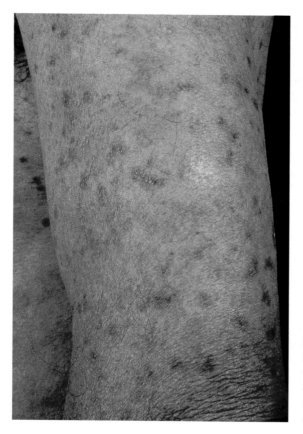

Figure 14.20 Dissemniated porokeratosis. Widely disseminated, asymptomatic, flat lesions, particularly visible on sun-exposed areas, such as extensor aspects of the limbs. A careful observation may disclose a raised, fine keratotic wall. The histological counterpart of this finding is cornoid lamella

Malakoplakia, an inflammatory disease characterized by accumulations of phagocytic macrophages, occurs primarily in immunocompromised individuals. Cutaneous involvement is rare (Lowitt *et al.*, 1996). It has been observed in the skin and subcutaneous tissues adjacent to the transplant scar. Histologically, one can find in the skin large foamy histiocytes with basophilic inclusion bodies, so-called Michaeli–Gutmann bodies, which are considered to represent the abnormal degradation of bacteria and are pathognomonic for this disease. The origin of this disorder remains unknown, although there is some evidence suggesting a possible role of Gram-negative enteric bacilli. In transplant patients the disease is related to drug-induced immunosuppression.

References

Andreoni M, Goletti D, Pezzotti P, et al. Prevalence, incidence and correlates of HHV-8/KSHV infection and Kaposi's sarcoma in renal and liver transplant recipients. J Infect 2001; 43: 195–9.

Audard V, Pardon A, Claude O, et al. Necrotizing fasciitis during de novo minimal change nephritic syndrome in a kidney transplant recipient. Transpl Infect Dis 2005; 7: 89–92.

Balfour HH Jr. Antiviral drugs. N Engl J Med 1999; 340: 1255–68.

Barba A, Tessari G, Talamini G, Chieregato GC. Analysis of risk factors for cutaneous warts in renal transplant recipients. Nephron 1997; 77: 422–6.

Bedogni B, Welford SM, Cassarino DS, et al. The hypoxic microenvironment of the skin contributes to Akt-mediated melanocyte transformation. Cancer Cell 2005; 8: 443–54.

Bernstein ZP, Chaman-Khan A, Miller KC, et al. A multicenter phase II study of the intravenous administration of liposomal tretinoin in patients with acquired immunodeficiency syndrome-associated Kaposi's sarcoma. Cancer 2002; 95: 2555–61.

Boratynska M, Radwan-Oczko M, Falkiewicz K, et al. Gingival overgrowth in kidney transplant recipients treated with cyclosporine and its relationship with chronic graft nephropathy. Transplant Proc 2003; 35: 2238–40.

Bouwes Bavinck JNB, Feltkarmp M, Struijk L, ter Scheggett J. Human papillomavirus and skin cancer risk in organ transplant recipients. J Investig Dermatol Symp Proc 2001; 6: 207–11.

Bunney MH, Benton EC, Barr BB, et al. The prevalence of skin disorders in renal allograft recipients receiving cyclosporin A compared with those receiving azathioprine. Nephrol Dial Transplant 1990; 5: 379–82.

Campistol JM, Guitierrez-Dalmau A, Torregrosa JV. Conversion to sirolimus: a successful treatment for posttransplanttaion Kaposi's sarcoma. Transplantation 2004; 7: 760–2.

Carroll R, Ramsay HM, Fryer AA. Incidence and prediction of nonmelanoma skin cancer post-renal transplantation: a prospective study in Queensland, Australia. Am J Kidney Dis 2003; 41: 676–83.

Cha S, Johnston L, Natkunam Y, Brown J. Treatment of verruca vulgaris with topical cidofovir in an immunocompromised patient: a case report and review of the literature. Transpl Infect Dis 2005; 7: 158–61.

Cooper SM, Wojnarowska F. The accuracy of clinical diagnosis of suspected premalignant and malignant skin lesions in renal transplant recipients. Clin Exp Dermatol 2002; 27: 436–8.

Cooper SM, Wojnarowska F. Photo-damage in North-European renal transplant recipients is associated with use of calcium channel blockers. Clin Exp Dermatol 2003; 28: 588–91.

Cozzio A, Kempf W, Schmid-Meyer R, et al. Intra-lesional low-dose interferon alpha2a therapy for primary cutaneous marginal zone B-cell lymphoma. Leuk Lymphoma 2006; 47: 865–9.

Dearden C. The role of alemtuzumab in the management of T-cell malignancies Semin Oncol 2006; 33 (Suppl 5): S44–52.

De Sevaux RG, Smit GV, de Jong EM, et al. Acitretin treatment of premalignant and malignant skin disorders in renal transplant recipients: clinical effects of a randomized trial comparing two doses of acitretin. J Am Acad Dermatol 2003; 49: 407–12.

De Visscher JG, Bouwes Bavinck JN, Van der Waal I. Squamous cell carcinoma of the lower lip in renal-transplant recipients. Report of six cases. Int J Oral Maxillofac Surg 1997; 26: 120–3.

Duman S, Toz H, Asci G, et al. Successful treatment of post-transplant Kaposi's sarcoma by reduction of immunosuppression. Nephrol Dial Transplant 2002; 17: 892–6.

Eberhard OK, Kliem V, Brunkhorst R. Five cases of Kaposi's sarcoma in kidney graft receipients: possible influence of the immunosuppressive therapy. Transplantation 1999; 67: 180–4.

Euvrard S, Kanitakis J, Cochat P, et al. Skin disease in children with organ transplant. J Am Acad Dermatol 2001; 44: 932–9.

Euvrard S, Kanitakis J, Bosshard S, et al. No recurrence of posttransplant Kaposi's sarcoma three years after renal transplantation. Transplantation 2002a; 73: 297–9.

Euvrard S, Kanitakis J, Claudy A. Neoplastic skin diseases in organ transplant recipients. Am J Cancer 2002b; 1: 109–20.

Euvrard S, Kanitakis J, Claudy A. Skin cancer after cancer transplantation. N Engl J Med 2003; 348: 1681–91.

Friedlander MM, Rubinger D, Rosenbaum E, et al. Temporary regression of Merkel cell carcinoma metastases after cessation of cyclosporine. Transplantation 2002; 73: 1849–50.

Furth SL, Fivush BA. Varicella vaccination in pediatric kidney transplant candidates. Pediatr. Transplant 2002; 6: 97–100.

Galvao MM, Sotto MN, Kihara SM, et al. Lymphocyte subsets and Langerhans cells in sun-protected and sun-exposed skin of immunosuppressed renal allograft recipients. J Am Acad Dermatol 1998; 38: 38–44.

Gayed SL. Topical imiquimod cream 5% for resistant perianal warts in a renal transplant patient. Int J STD AIDS 2002; 13: 501–3.

Gibson GE, O'Grady A, Kay EW p53 tumor suppressor gene protein expression in premalignant and malignant skin lesions of kidney transplant recipients. J Am Acad Dermatol 1997; 36: 924–31.

Gilchrest BA, Eller MS, Geller AC, Yaar M. The pathogenesis of melanoma induced by ultraviolet radiation. N Engl J Med 1999; 340: 1341–8.

Goto H, Nishio M, Endo T, et al. Effective in vivo purging with rituximab and autologous peripheral blood stem cell transplantation in a woman with CD5 positive primary cutaneous diffuse large B-cell lymphoma. Eur J Haematol 2005; 74: 526–8.

Gulec AT, Seckin D, Saray Y, et al. Number of acquired melanocytic nevi in renal transplant recipients as a risk factor for melanoma. Transplant Proc 2002; 34: 2136–8.

Gulec AT, Demirbilek M, Seckin D, et al. Superficial fungal infections in 102 renal transplant recipients: a case-control study. J Am Acad Dermatol 2003; 49: 187–92.

Halachmi S, Gilchrest BA. Update on genetic events in the pathogenesis of melanoma. Curr Opin Oncol 2001; 13: 129–36.

Hartevelt MM, Bouwes-Bavinck JN, Koote AM, et al. Incidence of skin cancer after renal transplantation in The Netherlands. Transplantation 1990; 49: 506–9.

Harwood CA, Surentheran T, McGregor JM, et al. Human papillomavirus infection and nonmelanoma skin cancer in immunosuppressed and immunocompetent individuals. J Med Virol 2000; 61: 289–97.

Hoshida Y, Tsukuma H, Yasunaga Y, et al. Cancer risk after renal transplantation in Japan. Int J Cancer 1997; 71: 517–20.

Ingen-Housz-Oro S, Bachelez H, Verola O, et al. High-dose therapy and autologous stem cell transplantation in relapsing cutaneous lymphoma. Bone Marrow Transplant 2004; 33: 629–34.

Jensen P, Hansen S, Moller B, et al. Skin cancer in kidney and heart transplant recipients and different long-term immunosuppression. J Am Acad Dermatol 1999; 40: 177–86.

Jeyaratnam D, Robson AM, Hextall JM, et al. Concurrent verrucous and varicelliform rashes following renal transplantation. Am J Transplant 2005; 5: 1777–80.

Kanitakis J, Alhaj-Ibrahim L, Euvrard S, Claudy A. Basal cell carcinomas developing in solid organ transplant recipients: clinicopathologic study of 176 cases. Arch Dermatol 2003; 139: 1133–7.

Kapelushnik J, Ariad S, Benharroch D, et al. Post renal transplantation human herpesvirus 8-associated lymphoproliferative disorder and Kaposi's sarcoma. Brit J Haematol 2001; 113: 425–8.

Kovach BT, Sams HH, Stasko T. Systemic strategies for chemoprevention of skin cancers in transplant recipients. Clin Transplant 2005; 19: 726–34.

Kunzle N, Venetz JP, Pascual M, et al. Sirolimus-induced acneiform eruption. Dermatology 2005; 211: 366–9.

Leigh IM, Glover MT. Skin cancer and warts in immunosuppressed renal transplant recipients. Cancer Res 1995; 139: 69–86.

Lindelof B, Granath F, Dal H, et al. Sun habits in kidney transplant recipients with skin cancer: a case-control study of possible causative factors. Acta Derm Venereol 2003; 83: 189–93.

Little RF, Merced-Galindez F, Straskus K, et al. A pilot study of cidofovir in patients with Kaposi sarcoma. J Infect Dis 2003; 187: 149–53.

Lowitt MH, Kariniemi AL, Niemi KM, Kao GF. Cutaneous malacoplakia: a report of two cases and review of the literature. J Am Acad Dermatol 1996; 34: 325–32.

Maccario M, Tortorano AM, Ponticelli C. Subcutaneous nodules and pneumonia in a kidney transplant recipient. Nephrol Dial Transplant 1998; 31: 681–6.

MacKie RM, Reid R, Junor B. Fatal melanoma transferred in a donated kidney 16 years after melanoma surgery. N Engl J Med 2003; 348: 567–8.

Marshall SE, Bordea C, Haldar NA, et al. Glutathione S-transferase polymorphism skin cancer after renal transplantation. Kidney Int 2000; 58: 2186–93.

Miele PS, Levy CS, Smith MA, et al. Primary cutaneous fungal infections in solid organ transplantation: a case series. Am J Transplant 2002; 2: 678–83.

Moloney FJ, Comber H, O'Lorcain P, et al. A population-based study of skin cancer incidence and prevalence in renal transplant recipients. Br J Dermatol 2006; 154: 498–504.

Montagnino G, Bencini PL, Tarantino A, et al. Clinical features and course of Kaposi's sarcoma in kidney transplant patients: report of thirteen cases. Am J Nephrol 1994; 14: 121–6.

Moosa MR, Treurnicht FK, Van Rensburg EJ, et al. Detection and subtyping of human herpesvirus-8 in renal transplant patients before and after remission of Kaposi's sarcoma. Transplantation 1998; 66: 214–18.

Moosa MR, Gralla J. Skin cancer in renal allograft recipients – experience in different ethnic groups residing in the same geographical region. Clin Transplant 2005; 19: 735–41.

Nash MM, Zaltzman JS. Efficacy of azithromycin in the treatment of cyclosporine-induced gingival hyperplasia in renal transplant recipients. Transplantation 1998; 65: 1611–15.

O'Donovan P, Perrett CM, Zhang X, et al. Azathioprine and UVA light generate mutagenic oxidative DNA damage. Science 2005; 309: 1871–4.

Parrish JA. Immunosuppression, skin cancer, and ultraviolet A radiation. N Engl J Med 2005; 353: 2712–13.

Pellet C, Chevret S, Frances C, et al. Prognostic value of quantitative Kaposi sarcoma-associated herpesvirus load in posttransplantation Kaposi sarcoma. J Infect Dis 2002; 186: 110–13.

Penn I. Why do immunosuppressed patients develop cancer? CRC Crit Rev Oncogen 1989; 1: 27–52.

Penn I. Malignant melanoma in organ allograft recipients. Transplantation 1996; 61: 274–8.

Penn I. Kaposi's sarcoma in transplant recipients. Transplantation 1997; 64: 669–73.

Penn I. De novo cancers in organ allograft recipients. Curr Opin Organ Transplant 1998; 4: 188–96.

Ponticelli C, Zorzi F. The skin in renal transplant recipients. In Massry SG, Glassock RJ, eds. Textbook of Nephrology. Philadelphia: Lippincott Williams and Wilkins, 2001: 1685–8.

Ponticelli C, Passerini P. Gastrointestinal complications in renal transplant recipients. Transpl Int 2005; 18: 643–50.

Preciado DA, Matas A, Adams GL. Squamous cell carcinoma of the head and neck in solid organ transplant recipients. Head Neck 2002; 24: 319–25.

Ramrakha-Jones V. Transplant patients need to be made aware of skin cancer risk. BMJ 2002; 324: 296.

Ravat FE, Spittle MF, Russell-Jones R. Primary cutaneous T-cell lymphoma occurring after organ transplantation. J Am Acad Dermatol 2006; 54: 668–75.

Regamey N, Tamm M, Wernli M, et al. Transmission of human herpesvirus 8 infection from renal-transplant donors to recipients. N Engl J Med 1998; 339: 1358–63.

Rittmaster RS. Medical treatment of androgen-dependent hirsutism. J Clin Endocrinol Metab 1995; 80: 2559–63.

Rubel JR, Milford EL, Abdi R. Cutaneous neoplasms in renal transplant recipients. Eur J Dermatol 2002; 12: 532–5.

Sah A, Barrans SL, Parapia LA, et al. Cutaneous B-cell lymphoma: pathological spectrum and clinical outcome in 51 consecutive patients. Am J Hematol 2004; 75: 195–9.

Sarid R, Kelpfish A, Schattner A. Virology, pathogenetic mechanisms and associated diseases of Kaposi's sarcoma-associated herpesvirus (human herpesvirus 8). Mayo Clin Proc 2002; 77: 941–9.

Seal DV. Necrotizing fasciitis. Curr Opin Infect Dis 2001; 14: 127–31.

Seukeran DC, Newstead CG, Cunliffe WJ. The compliance of renal transplant recipients with advice about sun protection measures. Br J Dermatol 1998; 138: 301–3.

Sharpe M, Easthope SE, Keating GM, Lamb HM. Polyethylene glycol-liposomal doxorubicin: a review of its use in the management of solid and haematological malignancies and AIDS-related Kaposi's sarcoma. Drugs 2002; 62: 2089–126.

Sheil AGR. Organ transplantation and malignancy: inevitable linkage. Transplant Proc 2002; 34: 2436–7.

Shuttleworth D, Philpot CM, Salaman JR. Cutaneous fungal infection following renal transplantation: a case control study. Br J Dermatol 1987; 117: 585–90.

Silver SG, Crawford RI. Fatal squamous cell carcinoma arising from transplant-associated porokeratosis. J Am Acad Dermatol 2003; 49: 931–3.

Simonart T, Noel JC, Van Vooren JP, Parent D. Role of viral agents in the pathogenesis of Kaposi's sarcoma. Dermatology 1998; 196: 447–9.

Smit JV, De Sevaux RG, Blokx WA, et al. Acitretin treatment in (pre)malignant skin disorders of renal transplant recipients: histology and immunohistochemical effects. J Am Acad Dermatol 2004; 50: 189–96.

Smith KJ, Germain M, Skelton H. Squamous cell carcinoma in situ (Bowen disease) in renal transplant patients treated with 5% imiquimod and 5% 5-fluorouracil therapy. Dermatol Surg 2001; 27: 561–4.

Stallone G, Schena A, Infante B, et al. Sirolimus for Kaposi's sarcoma in renal transplant recipients. N Engl J Med 2005; 352: 1317–23.

Stark S, Petridis AK, Ghim SJ, et al. Prevalence of antibodies against virus-like particles of epidermodysplasia verruciformis-associated HPV8 in patients at risk of skin cancer. J Invest Dermatol 1998; 111: 696–701.

Stockfleth E, Ulrich C, Meyer T, Christophers E. Epithelial malignancies in organ transplant patients: clinical presentation and new methods of treatment. Recent Results Cancer Res 2002; 160: 251–8.

Su LD, Fullen DR, Sondak VK, et al. Sentinel lymph node biopsy for patients with problematic spitzoid melanocytic lesions. Cancer 2003; 97: 499–507.

Talbot D, Rix D, Abusin K, et al. Alopecia as a consequence of tacrolimus therapy in renal transplantation. Transplantation 1997; 64: 1631–2.

Ternesten-Bratel A, Kjellström C, Wenberg AM, Ricksten A. Cutaneous squamoproliferative lesions in kidney transplant recipients: an investigation of specific Epstein–Barr virus expression. Acta Derm Veneorol 2003; 83: 14–17.

Tracey C, Hawley C, Griffin AD, et al. Generalized, pruritic, ulcerating maculopapular rash necessitating cessation of sirolimus in a liver transplantation patient. Liver Transpl 2005; 11: 987–9.

Tricot L, Lebbe C, Pillebout E, et al. Tacrolimus-induced alopecia in female kidney–pancreas transplant recipients. Transplantation 2005; 80: 1546–9.

Vexiau P, Fiet J, Boudou Ph, et al. Increase in plasma 5α-androstase-3α, 17β-diol glucuronide as a marker of peripheral androgen action in hirsutism: a side-effect induced by cyclosporine A. J Steroid Biochem 1990; 35: 133–7.

Viviano E, Sorce M, Mantegna M. Solitary keratoacanthomas in immunocompetent patients: no detection of papillomavirus DNA by polymerase chain reaction. New Microbiol 2001; 24: 295–7.

15 MUSCULOSKELETAL COMPLICATIONS

Skeletal complications

Most patients undergoing kidney transplantation already have some degree of renal osteodystrophy, a general term encompassing all histologic derangements of bone that may occur in uremic patients, such as hyperparathyroidism (with or without osteitis fibrosa), osteomalacia, osteosclerosis, and adynamic bone disease. In some patients more than one of these conditions may be present at the same time. After successful renal transplantation some improvement of hyperparathyroidism, aluminum-related bone disease, and amyloidosis may occur, but the introduction of immunosuppressive agents, particularly corticosteroids, may expose the patient to the risk of new bone complications, such as osteoporosis and osteonecrosis, as well as muscle and joint complications.

Osteoporosis

Osteoporosis is a systemic bone disease with qualitative and quantitative deterioration in trabecular and cortical skeleton, reduced bone mass, and a consequent increase in bone fragility and susceptibility to fractures. Bone quality cannot be measured clinically, but bone mineral density is easy to measure by dual-energy X-ray absorptiometry at the lumbar spine and proximal femur. Today, the definitions are mainly based on bone mineral density measurement. A subject is defined to have *osteopenia* if his/her T-score is between 1.0 and −2.5, while *osteoporosis* is defined by a T-score less than or equal to −2.5.

Bone loss predominantly affects *cancellous bone*. Fractures involving the long bones are more common than those involving the vertebral bodies, and usually occur more than 3 years after transplantation. Bone loss is greater during the first 6 months after transplantation, varying from 6 to 9% (Julian *et al.*, 1991; Brandenburg *et al.*, 2002; Ulivieri *et al.*, 2002), then continues at a lower rate, approximately 2% per year, in patients followed for up to 10 years after transplantation (Pichette *et al.*, 1996). In a Spanish experience, more than 50% of renal transplant recipients were osteopenic 4 years after transplantation (Marcen *et al.*, 2006). In a French study, 5 years after transplantation, 53% of patients had osteoporosis and 44% had fractures (Durieux *et al.*, 2002). The risk of osteoporotic fractures after transplantation is particularly high in diabetics and in females (Nisbeth *et al.*, 1999).

Pathogenesis

Similar to what happens in the general population, several factors may contribute to the pathogenesis of post-transplant osteoporosis (Table 15.1). *Age*, *sex*, and *postmeopausal status* are some of the most important risk factors. Low body weight, inadequate calcium intake, insufficient mobilization, smoking, and excessive alcohol consumption may also contribute to osteoporosis (Raisz, 2005). More specific factors include *end-stage renal failure* and *genetic* factors. As a matter of fact, almost half of hemodialyzed patients may show osteoporosis (Taal *et al.*, 1999; Barreto *et al.*, 2006), a finding often neglected by nephrologists. Abnormalities in vitamin D may persist for some months after transplantation, and may be responsible for reduced bone mass (De Sevaux *et al.*, 2003). Uremic children have numerous risk factors for reduced bone mass, including the underlying renal disease, nutritional deficits, and inflammation (Leonard and Bachrach, 2001). *Genetic factors* may also play a role in the degree of bone loss. Patients with the 'favorable' bb genotype for the vitamin D receptor gene have been shown to recover more bone after renal transplantation than those with Bb and BB genotypes (Torres *et al.*, 1996). *Hypophosphatemia*, which is relatively frequent in the first weeks after transplantation, may also cause a decrease in bone

Table 15.1   Factors predisposing to post-transplant osteopenia/osteoporosis

General	Transplant-related
Older age	Corticosteroids
Female sex	Genotype for vitamin D receptors
Postmenopausal status	Persistent vitamin D abnormalities
Insufficient mobilization	Persistent hyperparathyroidism
Low body weight	Cyclosporine? tacrolimus?
Inadequate calcium intake	Chronic inflammatory state
Smoking/alcohol	Hypophosphatemia

Table 15.2   Mechanisms of corticosteroid-induced osteopenia/osteoporosis

Direct effects	Indirect effects
Inhibition of osteoblast differentiation	Reduced intestinal calcium absorption
Increased proliferation of osteoclasts	Hypercalciuria
	Hypogonadism (reduced adrenal androgen and estrogen production)
	Inhibition of growth factors (growth hormone, insulin-like growth factor, transforming growth factor-β_1)

mineral density (Levi 2001; Rojas et al., 2003). A chronic inflammatory state may be a further contributor to post-transplant osteoporosis (Raisz, 2005).

However, in renal allograft recipients, the most frequent cause of osteoporosis is represented by corticosteroid treatment. In renal transplant patients, bone loss has been found to be more rapid during the first months of therapy when the doses of corticosteroids are higher (Kokado et al., 2000; Monier-Faugere et al., 2000; Mikuls et al., 2003). Other studies have pointed out that even small doses of prednisone (5 or 7.5 mg/day). when given for 1 year or more may cause substantial bone loss regardless of age, gender, or menopausal status (Staa et al., 2002; Blake and Fogelman, 2002). The pathogenesis of steroid-induced bone loss is multifactorial (Table 15.2). Pharmacological doses of corticosteroids may cause generalized defects in calcium transport across biological membranes, which may concur with other, still unknown, mechanisms in reducing the net intestinal calcium absorption. Corticosteroids also cause hypercalciuria, both by increasing bone resorption and by urinary calcium excretion. Moreover, the interference of corticosteroids with gonadotropin release and the corticosteroid-induced suppression of adrenocorticotropic hormone cause a reduced secretion of adrenal androgens and estrogens (Lane and Lukert, 1998). The resulting hypogonadal state may contribute to further bone loss. Finally, corticosteroids inhibit the secretion of growth hormone and decrease the production and/or the bioactivity of some skeletal growth factors, such as insulin-like growth factor-I and transforming growth factor-β_1. The final result is reduced bone formation. However, the main deleterious effect of corticosteroids is the direct inhibition of bone formation, as they inhibit osteoblast differentiation, induce apoptosis in mature osteoblasts as well as osteocytes (Weinstein et al., 1998; Rojas et al., 2003), and stimulate the proliferation and differentiation of human osteoclast precursors (Hirayama and Athanasou, 2002). Biochemically there is a low production of osteocalcin, a major non-collagenous bone matrix protein. Another direct effect on bone is represented by the enhancing effect on osteoclast activity and by the altered sensitivity of osteoclasts to parathyroid hormone. The sum of these direct effects of corticosteroids leads to bone loss. Corticosteroids may also indirectly favor the development of osteoporosis because they may cause proximal and systemic myopathy. Myopathy reduces physical activity and mobility, thus altering the gravitational forces on the skeleton and reducing weight-bearing activity and mobility. Myopathy may also expose the patient to fracture by increasing the propensity to fall.

The effects of other immunosuppressive agents on bone are less well known. The introduction of the calcineurin inhibitors *cyclosporine* (CsA) and *tacrolimus* has permitted a reduction in the dosage of corticosteroids during the first period of transplantation. However, an improvement in graft survival leads to a more prolonged administration of corticosteroids, with the increased risk of osteoporosis. Studies in rats showed that the administration of CsA at doses comparable to those used in transplantation can cause bone loss, mostly trabecular, accelerated bone turnover, increased bone resorption, and bone remodeling (Movsowitz *et al.*, 1988, 1989; Schlosberg *et al.*, 1989). The administration of tacrolimus caused bone loss of even greater magnitude than that described with CsA in one study (Cvetkovic *et al.*, 1994). On the other hand, another experimental study reported that the reduction of bone mass was much less severe with tacrolimus than with CsA (Inoue *et al.*, 2000). It is likely that these agents may favor the development of osteopenia by inhibiting the synthesis of calcineurin, which is an important regulator of bone formation by osteoblasts (Sun *et al.*, 2005). There is little information in humans. A cross-over study in renal transplant recipients found no difference in bone mineral density between patients given CsA alone and those given CsA or azathioprine in combination with corticosteroids (Cueto-Manzano *et al.*, 1999). On the other hand, in a prospective randomized trial, renal transplant patients assigned to receive CsA alone, without steroid, had a significant improvement of bone mineral density during the first 18 months, suggesting that CsA does not interfere with bone mineralization (Aroldi *et al.*, 1997). In the same study, patients assigned to receive CsA plus steroids after transplantation showed a significant decrease of bone mineral density. Experimental studies in rats showed that *sirolimus* does not cause bone loss, but may increase remodeling and decrease the growth rate (Bryer *et al.*, 1995). Sirolimus may also induce testicular atrophy in rats, thereby reducing sex hormones (Morris, 1992). This may theoretically expose the patient to osteopenia in the long term, but there is still no information available for humans. On the other hand, the sirolimus derivate *everolimus* directly inhibits bone resorption by osteoclasts, and thus could at least be neutral or protective for bone *in vivo*, which would favor its use in disease indications associated with bone loss (Kneissel *et al.*, 2004). *Mycophenolate mofetil* has no effect upon bone volume in rats (Dissanayake *et al.*, 1998), and no data are available in humans. *Azathioprine* has been used for many years in transplantation. Short-term studies in rats showed no effect on bone volume, but documented an increase in the number of osteoclasts (Joffe *et al.*, 1993).

In summary, many renal transplant recipients demonstrate osteoporosis. A number of factors may contribute to the development of osteoporosis and fractures. However, in renal transplant recipients these factors are probably overridden by the prominent effects of corticosteroids (Monier-Faugere *et al.*, 2000).

Prevention and treatment of bone loss

Most renal transplant patients are at increased risk of developing osteoporosis. Preventive measures and early treatment in the case of osteopenia are strongly recommended (Table 15.3). As a general rule, all patients at risk of osteoporosis should be physically active. Regular *physical activity*, including aerobic, weight-bearing, and resistance exercise is effective in increasing bone mineral density (BMD) (Rosen, 2006). Patients should also be encouraged to discontinue those *life-style habits* (tobacco and alcohol). that are risk factors for osteoporosis, and should have a diet adequate in calcium, proteins, and vitamins. *Calcium* administration at a dose of 1000 mg/day is an effective and inexpensive way of offsetting impaired calcium absorption and decreasing parathyroid secretion. Higher calcium administration (1500–2000 mg daily). may be indicated in postmenopausal women. However, the physician should keep in mind the risk of inducing hypercalciuria or hypercalcemia in transplanted patients with persistent mild hyperparathyroidism. It is therefore necessary to monitor carefully both urinary and plasma calcium.

Table 15.3		Main measures to prevent and treat post-transplant osteoporosis

Preventive measures	Osteopenia	Osteoporosis
Physical activity	The same measures as used for prevention plus	The same measures as used for osteopenia plus
Stop/minimize alcohol and tobacco use	Oral alendronate or risendronate once a week or ibandronate once a month	Intravenous pamidronate or zoledronate in the case of severe osteoporosis
Diet rich in calcium (dairy)		In the case of poor response, parathyroid hormone for 2 years
Oral calcium (1 g per day, 1.5 g in postmenopausal women)		
Calcitriol 0.5 µg/48 hours, at night		

As corticosteroids play a key role in the etiology of post-transplant bone loss, *steroid-free immunosuppression* should be considered in patients at higher risk of osteoporosis (Ponticelli and Aroldi, 2001; van den Ham et al., 2003).

All the measures that may prevent osteopenia are also useful for the *treatment* of osteoporosis. A number of drugs have been employed for the prevention of bone loss. *Vitamin D therapy* may be theoretically indicated, as calcitriol may increase calcium absorption and may also stimulate the function of osteoblasts. Moreover, vitamin D supplementation is necessary to avoid any increase of the parathyroid hormone (PTH) level (Lamy et al., 2002). In renal transplant recipients, intermittent calcitriol treatment (0.5 µg/48 h at night) and calcium supplementation for 3 months reduced bone loss and decreased PTH levels in comparison with placebo (Garcia et al., 2000). In another study, calcitriol at a dose of 0.25 µg per day plus calcium 0.5 g per day tended to maintain trabecular bone volume and to produce a wall thickness (Cueto-Manzano et al., 2000). On the other hand, late administration of calcium supplements and calcitriol did not improve post-transplant osteopenia in another study (Marcen et al., 2006).

Bisphosphonates are the treatment of choice in clinical practice. These agents bind preferentially to bones with high turnover rates, such as trabecular bone. Bisphoshonates oppose the increased bone resorption caused by corticosteroids by inhibiting osteoclast activity and by reducing the number of osteoclasts. Osteoclast survival may be decreased by destruction when contact is made with bone containing bisphosphonate or by apoptosis (Rodan and Fleisch, 1996). As a consequence, fewer osteoclasts are recruited to bone remodeling sites and the differentiation of osteoclast precursors is impaired. The number of trabecular perforations, which are the cause of reduced bone strength, is decreased. Bisphosphonates can be administered orally, but may expose the patient to upper gastrointestinal adverse effects. However, a controlled trial in non-transplant patients with osteoporosis showed that once-weekly oral alendronate, 70 mg, had an incidence of upper gastrointestinal tract side-effects comparable to that with placebo (Greenspan et al., 2002). Good results with alendronate have been reported in renal transplant recipients with high bone turnover (Cruz et al., 2002). In a controlled study, transplant recipients with osteoporosis (BMD T-score <−2.5). were randomized to be given alendronate (10 mg/day). and vitamin D (800 IU). plus calcium (2.5 g). or only vitamin D and calcium. After 1 year, patients receiving alendronate had a significantly higher increase in lumbar spine and femoral neck BMD than controls (Torregrosa et al., 2003). Another randomized trial showed that in renal transplant patients receiving CsA, azathioprine, and steroids, the mean bone density at the femoral neck decreased by 12.3% at 4 years in the group given placebo, while it did not show a significant reduction in patients who received pamidronate (0.5 mg/kg intravenously), at the time of transplantation and 1 month later

(Fan *et al.*, 2003). Potential side-effects of intravenous pamidronate are hypocalcemia in patients with vitamin D deficiency, and glomerular focal sclerosis in exceptional cases (Markowitz *et al.*, 2001). A disturbing although rare side-effect of bisphosphonates in renal transplant recipients is represented by an increase in serum creatinine. Patients receiving etidronate or clodronate more frequently showed creatinine elevations, 8% and 5% respectively, than with pamidronate, 2%, ibandronate, < 1%, or alendronate, 0% (Zojer *et al.*, 1999). Zoledronic acid is associated with the highest therapeutic ratio and a superior renal tolerability (Widler *et al.*, 2002).

Calcitonin is a specific inhibitor of bone resorption. Eel and salmon calcitonin have the highest activity/weight ratio. Pig and human calcitonins have a weaker effect. The secretion of endogenous calcitonin is modulated by blood calcium levels. Calcitonin inhibits bone resorption and thereby lowers plasma calcium. A double-blind placebo-controlled study by Adachi *et al.* (1997) concluded that calcitonin spray 200 IU/day prevented early bone loss in the lumbar spine in half of corticosteroid-treated patients. As the amino acid sequence of salmon calcitonin differs from that of the human hormone, specific antibodies may develop in most patients after the administration of salmon calcitonin. Whether these antibodies interfere with the activity of calcitonin is unclear, but it is well known that the long-term administration of salmon calcitonin can lead to resistance to the hormone and a subsequent reduction of efficacy (Plosker and McTavish, 1996). A downregulation of the skeleton receptor for calcitonin has also been hypothesized, which may provide an explanation for this 'calcitonin-escape' phenomenon (Takahashi *et al.*, 1995).

Estrogen therapy effectively prevents bone loss in postmenopausal women. Estrogen slows bone resorption, increases bone mineral density, and reduces the incidence of vertebral fractures in women with postmenopausal osteoporosis (Wells *et al.*, 2002). Although no studies regarding the effects of hormone replacement therapy in organ transplant recipients have been published, it may be rational to give estrogen replacement therapy both to premenopausal women with amenorrhea and to postmenopausal women, before and after transplantation, if no contraindication exists. Progesterone must be given concomitantly to prevent endometrial hyperplasia. However, there is concern about the possibility that estrogens may increase the risk of breast cancer and cardiovascular disease. The new selective estrogen receptor modulators, such as *raloxifene*, have proved able to maintain bone mass in postmenopausal women. They may exert fewer uterine effects with a lower risk of bleeding and, potentially, a decreased risk for breast cancer (Rosen, 2006).

Statins may increase bone mineral density and reduce the risk of fractures (Pasco *et al.*, 2002), probably through an antiresorptive effect (Rejnmark *et al.*, 2002). and/or a stimulation of bone formation (Mundy *et al.*, 1999). *Teriparatide*, a recombinant human PTH, administered subcutaneously at a dose of 40 µg per day, may produce a dramatic increase of trabecular and cortical bone density (Body *et al.*, 2002). *Strontium ranelate*, when compared with placebo, reduced the risk of new vertebral fractures and increased bone mineral density in women with postmenopausal osteoporosis given calcium and vitamin D in a *post hoc* analysis. The most frequent side-effect was diarrhea, which occurred in 6% of patients (Meunier *et al.*, 2004).

Osteonecrosis

Osteonecrosis is the death of marrow cells and the associated trabeculae and osteocytes, not due to infection. This skeletal complication has also been labeled aseptic necrosis, avascular necrosis, and osteochondritis dissecans.

Pathogenesis

The pathogenesis of osteonecrosis has been matter of discussion for years. However, there is a bulk of evidence that *corticosteroids* represent the most important risk factor for avascular necrosis. An association between osteonecrosis and the cumulative dosage of oral steroids in the first year has been reported (Inoue *et al.*, 2003; Celik *et al.*, 2006). *Overweight* may further increase the deleterious effects of corticosteroids (Tang *et al.*, 2000). Serum *parathyroid hormone* concentrations at the time of transplantation are

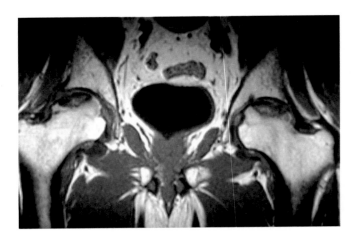

Figure 15.1 Bilateral necrosis of femoral heads in a transplant recipient (computed tomography)

also correlated with the subsequent development of osteonecrosis (Nehme *et al.*, 1989; Ferrari *et al.*, 2002), and could probably be synergistic with corticosteroids in causing avascular necrosis. A role for hypofibrinolysis conferred by a plasminogen activator inhibitor-1 gene variant has been found in Caucasian (Ferrari *et al.*, 2002). but not in Japanese renal transplant recipients (Asano *et al.*, 2004).

Prevalence and clinical features

The *prevalence* of osteonecrosis has considerably reduced in the last few years. A review of the literature including early studies showed that osteonecrosis afflicted 3–41% of kidney transplant recipients (First, 1993). However, after the introduction of cyclosporine the incidence of aseptic necrosis has decreased to 4% (Lopez-Ben *et al.*, 2004), because of lower doses of steroid, better control of pre-transplant hyper-parathyroidism, and better clinical and nutritional condition of the patient at the time of transplantation.

The *clinical symptoms* usually appear within the first year after transplantation (Marston *et al.*, 2002), but may also appear after 10 or more years. The onset of osteonecrosis is insidious, with stiffness and reduced mobility of the joint. Pain exacerbated by weight-bearing may precede X-radiographic changes. Pain may be referred from the hip to the ipsilateral knee. Effusions may develop, especially if the knee or elbow is involved. Weight-bearing bones and the femoral head are the most common sites. Other sites affected are the femoral condyle, tibial plateau, body of the talus, and humeral head. The distal tibia and humerus, proximal radius, and ulna are affected less frequently (Julian *et al.*, 1992). The disease can be multifocal.

The *diagnosis* of osteonecrosis was based on X-radiography until recently. However, computed tomography (Figure 15.1), scintigraphy combined with single-photon-emission computed tomography (SPECT), computed tomography with multiplanar reconstructions, and magnetic resonance imaging have proved to be more sensitive. Bone scintigraphy with SPECT is even more sensitive than magnetic resonance imaging in detecting osteonecrosis (Ryu *et al.*, 2002). An early diagnosis may permit less invasive treatment in the early clinical course. Several stages of osteonecrosis have been recognized (Table 15.4).

Treatment

The treatment of osteonecrosis depends on the progression of the infarct. In stages I and II, the benefit from purely *conservative management* such as limited weight-bearing and anti-inflammatory medications is short-lived. Attempts to preserve the femoral head by *core decompression* is a safe and effective procedure in the early stages (Bozic *et al.*, 1999). Surgical intervention for patients with stage III or IV is inevitably contemplated. *Total hip replacement* in renal transplant recipients allows significantly increased activity and relief from pain. However, in some patients a second operation may be needed because of septic or aseptic loosening and/or because of instability.

Table 15.4   Main clinical and radiological characteristics of the different stages of avascular necrosis of the femoral head

Staging	Symptoms	Imaging
I	Asymptomatic	Subtle mottled densities seen upon MNR imaging
II	Intermittent aching	The infarct produces a rim of increased bone density
III	Activity-related pain in the affected area	Demarcation between the infarcted segment and the subchondral bone
IV	Severe pain. Limitation of motion. Internal rotation is seriously affected	Necrotic segmental collapses, producing a flattening of the femoral head
V	Symptoms are indistinguishable from degenerative arthritis in the joint	Collapse of the femoral head. Advanced degenerative arthritis. Osteophyte formation around the femoral head
VI	Exacerbation	The acetabulum is flattened with loss of curvature. The femoral head may migrate laterally, eroding the acetabular edge

MNR, magnetic nuclear resonance

Hyperparathyroidism

In dialysis patients, parathyroid hormone (PTH). levels are usually kept at a moderately elevated level in order to promote normal bone turnover and to prevent adynamic bone disease. Therefore, a certain degree of parathyroid hyperplasia has to be accepted. In most cases, even considerable parathyroid hyperplasia can be controlled after transplantation when the functional demand for increased PTH levels is removed by the normalization of kidney function. When a renal graft starts to function properly, it does so in a setting characterized by negative calcium and positive phosphate balances, low production of cal-citriol, continuous stimulation of PTH synthesis and secretion due to the hypertrophy and hyperplasia of the parathyroid gland, and resistance to the calcemic action of PTH (Slatopolsky and Delmez, 1992). The recovery of glomerular filtration and tubular function after successful renal transplantation can correct the main causal factors of secondary hyperparathyroidism (HPTH), namely phosphate retention, decreased synthesis of calcitriol, and hypocalcemia. However, while the reversal of these abnormalities takes only a few days, months may be needed before the parathyroid functional mass improves (Bonarek et al., 1999). The higher are the serum PTH levels at transplantation the longer is the time for recovery. Concentrations above 230 pg/ml at the time of transplantation predict long-term hyperparathyroidism (Torres et al., 2002).

Pathogenesis of persistent hyperparathyroidism

In some patients, secondary HPTH is non-suppressible (Messa et al., 1998). A number of factors may be responsible for persistent hyperparathyroidism after transplantation (Table 15.5). Although some increase

Table 15.5	Factors involved in persistent post-transplant hyperparathyroidism

Poor graft function
Drugs impairing calcitriol absorption (corticosteroids). or inhibiting calcitriol synthesis (ketoconazole)
Underexpression of calcium-sensing receptors
Underexpression of vitamin D receptors

in PTH levels may be seen in long-term renal transplant patients with glomerular filtration rates higher than 70 ml/min (Montalban et al., 2003), the most important factor for the persistence of HPTH is represented by *poor graft function*. As serum calcitriol levels correlate with renal function (Martin-Malo et al., 1996), the normal production of calcitriol by the graft can favor the involution of HPTH, but, in patients with poor renal allograft function, calcitriol production may be insufficient to inhibit parathyroid secretion. The use of drugs that impair intestinal calcium absorption (*corticosteroids*) or block calcitriol synthesis (*ketoconazole*). can also interfere with the involution of HPTH after transplantation. In patients with persistent HPTH, the set-point for calcium-controlled PTH secretion may be shifted around higher calcium values, with further slowing in HPTH involution. This increase in the set-point may be the result of an underexpression of some autocrine/paracrine factors, such as *calcium-sensing receptors* (Kifor et al., 1996), and/or of *vitamin D receptors* (Korkor 1987; Drueke 1995). Therefore, not only the increased parathyroid mass, but also the altered quality of the parathyroid mass, might be responsible for uncontrollable hyperparathyroidism after kidney transplantation (Lewin et al., 2006).

Clinical course of persistent HPTH

Generally, the time-course and degree of persistent post-transplant hyperparathyroidism are correlated with the duration and intensity of pre-transplant HPTH and with the volume of parathyroid glands (McCarron et al., 1982; Parfitt, 1997). *X-radiographic alterations* in persistent post-transplant hyperparathyroidism are similar to those seen in dialysis patients with signs of accelerated bone resorption (Figure 15.2). and osteosclerosis. Persistent mild *hypercalcemia* (10.5–12 mg/dl). generally resolves within a year, but in about 4–10% of recipients it continues over the next 2 years and finally resolves without specific intervention. *Hypophosphatemia* may be another manifestation of persistent hyperparathyroidism during the first year after transplantation. It may be enhanced by the coexistence of severe hyperphosphaturia, due to tubular dysfunction, inappropriately low levels of vitamin D_3, and/or cyclosporine (Levi, 2001). Whether or not hypophosphatemia may be responsible for osteomalacia is still under discussion.

The most severe form of persistent HPTH is represented by an autonomous pattern of PTH secretion called *tertiary HPTH*, which occurs in fewer than 2% of patients after transplantation. It may be caused by the enlargement of all parathyroid glands in about one-third of cases or by two- or single-gland enlargement (Nichol et al., 2002). (Figure 15.3). Tertiary HPTH is usually associated with overt hypercalcemia because of the enhanced sensitivity of peripheral target organs (particularly the bone) to PTH action. Rarely, *hypercalcemia* exceeds 13 mg/dl, becoming symptomatic. Severely hypercalcemic patients may develop polyuria, polydipsia, hypertension, pruritus, and 'red eyes', and may suffer from nausea, vomiting, or neurologic disorders, including somnolence and mental confusion. Hypercalcemia may also cause an acute and reversible decline in renal function or chronic nephropathy (Zeiden et al., 1991). A few cases of recurrent bouts of bradycardia, often leading to asystole requiring cardiopulmonary resuscitation, have been described. In the reported cases, hypercalcemic-induced bradycardia was refractory to hydration, loop diuresis, atropine, and external pacing. Bisphosphonate (Jeffries et al., 2005) and the calcimimetic cinacalcet (Apostolou et al., 2006). have been successfully administered in some cases, but other patients

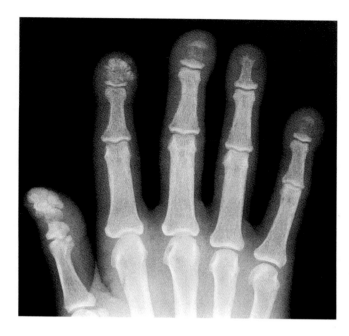

Figure 15.2 Severe hyperparathyroidism in a dialysis patient. Acroosteolysis of the terminal phalanges. Subperiostial resorption, cortical thinning and fluffy trabecular structure

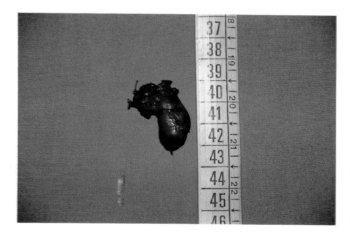

Figure 15.3 A large parathyroid adenoma removed from a transplant recipient with persistent hyperparathyroidism

failed to respond (Drueke, 2006). Exceptionally, hypercalcemia may cause *calciphylaxis* with peripheral ischemic necrosis due to vascular calcification.

Parathyroidectomy or medical treatment?

The serum parathyroid concentration above which hyperparathyroidism may cause severe complications has not been defined. This is an important practical problem, since post-transplant parathyroid surgery may expose the patient to the risk of prolonged although reversible renal allograft dysfunction (Garcia *et al.*, 2005) and, more important, to refractory hypocalcemia and low-turnover bone disease. Hypocalcemia in patients with hypoparathyroidism and normal or subnormal glomerular filtration is difficult to treat, because urinary calcium excretion is enhanced in the absence of parathyroid hormone. Corticosteroids may further contribute to hypocalcemia by reducing intestinal calcium absorption. Moreover, patients with hypoparathyroidism may develop low-turnover bone disease due to decreased parathyroid hormone-mediated turnover. Therefore, the indications to parathyroidectomy should be restricted to patients with severe hypercalcemia. Recently, however, the new *calcimimetic cinacalcet* proved to be able to correct hypercalcemia associated with HPTH in many renal transplant recipients (Kruse *et al.*, 2005; Serra *et al.*, 2005), although PTH levels and phosphatemia did not change. Waiting for further studies to give reassurance about the efficacy and tolerability of cinacalcet in the long term, an increasing number of physicians tend to limit more the indications to parathyroidectomy. Nevertheless, patients with symptomatic hypercalcemia not responding to cinacalcet are good candidates for parathyroidectomy. Calciphylaxis and cases with severe hypercalcemic-induced bradycardia may also require urgent parathyroidectomy.

Total or subtotal parathyroidectomy?

The surgical choice between subtotal parathyroidectomy or total parathyroidectomy with subcutaneous autotransplantation largely depends on the experience of the surgeon. From a theoretical point of view, subtotal parathyroidectomy is often preferred, as total parathyroidectomy may expose patients to the risk of hypocalcemia and low-turnover bone disease. Limited resection of a single or double adenoma is indicated in cases with enlargement of only one or two parathyroid glands. Total or subtotal parathyroidectomy should be limited to patients with 3–4-gland hyperplasia (Nichol *et al.*, 2002). However, it is difficult to know whether HPTH is actually caused by a single adenoma, as there is often a concomitant hyperplasia that can be missed by scintigraphy or ultrasonography (Pham *et al.*, 2006). A possible strategy to evaluate whether subtotal parathyroidectomy may be sufficient is based on the intraoperative measurement of serum PTH levels. A decrease in intraoperative PTH levels of >50% at 10 minutes after completion of the operation indicates adequate resection (Haustein *et al.*, 2005). However, if the PTH remains elevated or rises again after an appropriate decrease in levels, then multigland disease or ectopic sources should be considered (Phillips *et al.*, 2005). Subtotal parathyroidectomy with a vascularized parathyroid left *in situ* and tissue cryopreservation (Milas and Weber, 2004), or subcutaneous implantation (Kinnaert *et al.*, 1993), or associated with thymectomy (Triponez *et al.*, 2005) was reported to be effective in treating most renal transplant recipients with tertiary HPTH and could also minimize the recurrence of HPTH in patients with declining renal function.

Osteomalacia

Osteomalacia is a disorder in which mineralization of the organic matrix of the skeleton is defective.

Risk factors

A large number of factors may be responsible for osteomalacia. Some patients may already be affected by *adynamic bone disease* before renal transplantation. In dialyzed patients, aluminum accumulation may be associated with low-turnover osteomalacia, adynamic bone disease, proximal myopathy, microcytic anemia, and progressive dementia and seizures. After successful renal transplantation, the increased urinary excretion may reverse the aluminum accumulation with an improvement of signs and symptoms. Proximal weakness and bone pain may improve quickly. Removal of the bone content of aluminum can take a longer time. However, bone biopsy specimens show markedly improved histologic parameters of bone metabolism (Piraino *et al.*, 1988). Nearly half of cases with pre-transplant adynamic bone disease recover their bone turnover completely, with some improvement observed in the majority of the remaining cases. However, in some patients, osteomalacia may persist after transplantation (Cruz *et al.*, 2004). Treatment with *pamidronate* may significantly improve the bone mineral density after transplantation, but is associated with adynamic bone histology (Coco *et al.*, 2003).

Phosphate depletion can produce osteomalacia. Hypophosphatemia is frequent after renal transplantation due to decreased tubular resorption of phospate. Many factors may concur for post-transplant hypophosphatemia (Table 15.6). When this defect is caused by ischemia–reperfusion injury or rejection, it tends to improve, while it persists or is aggravated in patients with tertiary hyperparathyroidism or with a

Table 15.6   Causes of post-transplant hypophosphatemia

Persistent tertiary hyperparathyroidism
Low levels of 1,25(OH)$_2$ vitamin D$_3$
Corticosteroids
Cyclosporine
Sirolimus
Bisphosphonate?
Bone-derived factor (phosphatonin)?
Tubular dysfunction (ischemia–reperfusion; rejection)

persistent defect of tubular resorption caused by immunosuppressive drugs. Impaired phosphate handling has also been reported in *rapamycine-treated* patients (Schwarz *et al.*, 2001). Hypophosphatemia is associated with an early decrease in osteoblast number and surfaces, as well as an early increase in osteoblast apoptosis. These mechanisms of hypophosphatemia, which are independent of PTH, lead to a reduced bone formation rate and delayed mineralization (Bellorin-Font *et al.*, 2003).

Clinical features

Symptoms include diffuse skeletal pain and bony tenderness. Muscular weakness may be so severe as to confine patients to bed. While adynamic bone disease tends to improve in patients with good allograft function, in the long term many patients show decreased bone formation and prolonged mineralization lag-time associated with persisting bone resorption, and even clear evidence of generalized or focal osteomalacia. Thus, the main alterations in bone remodeling are a decrease in bone formation and mineralization. There are skeletal deformities with radiological features almost indistinguishable from those seen in osteoporosis. A specific finding is the presence of radiolucent bands (Looser's zones) occurring mainly in femoral neck, pelvis, fibula, and metatarsals.

Treatment

Treatment depends on the underlying disorder. Waiting for spontaneous improvement, patients with pre-transplant aluminum intoxication should avoid aluminum-containing compounds. Parathyroidectomy should be considered in patients with tertiary HPTH caused by adenoma, carcinoma, or hyperplasia. In the case of tubular defects, oral inorganic phosphate supplements (1.0–3.6 g/day) and calcitriol (0.5–2.0 μg/day) may be considered. In a small study, a significant improvement in tubular phosphate resorption and hypophosphatemia was seen after short-term treatment with dipyridamole (Balal *et al.*, 2005).

Bone pain

Patients treated with *calcineurin inhibitors* may suffer from a painful leg syndrome characterized by pain over the long bones, localized to the knees and ankles, without joint inflammation. The pain is mostly symmetrical, may interfere with walking, is not relieved by rest, and may wake the patient from sleep. The pain arises between the first and the third month after transplant and usually resolves spontaneously in a few months. The bone pain has been attributed to the intraosseous vasoconstriction caused by cyclosporine or tacrolimus. Bone scans show an increased tracer uptake by the foot bones (Franco *et al.*, 2004). Magnetic resonance imaging demonstrates bone marrow edema in the painful bones (Grotz *et al.*, 2001). An improvement of the syndrome has been reported after the administration of vasodilating calcium-channel blockers (Gauthier and Barbosa, 1994), but in most cases the pain is relieved only with the reduction of withdrawal of calcineurin inhibitors.

Severe bone pain may manifest also in patients treated with *sirolimus*. This can be disabling, and in the most severe cases resolves only after drug withdrawal. Again, it is probably related to changes in the circulation to the bones (Johnson, 2002).

Osteomyelitis

Most cases of osteomyelitis in transplant patients are of bacterial origin. *Staphylococcus aureus* and *S. epidermidis* are the most frequent pathogenic organisms, but Gram-negative bacteria, anaerobic organisms, and *Mycobacterium tuberculosis* may also cause osteomyelitis. Fungi and viruses may also invade and destroy bone.

The *clinical presentation* is characterized by chills, fever, and severe pain of the affected bone. The symptoms are less characteristic for osteomyelitis of the spine, which may present with dull pain, mild fever, and vertebral tenderness, but normal overlying skin.

The location may be identified by labeled leukocyte scanning, gallium scanning, or magnetic resonance. Positron emission tomography seems additionally to have a role (De Winter *et al.*, 2002). Identification of the offending organism may be obtained by blood culture or by deep bone aspiration/biopsy.

Antibiotic *treatment* is based on isolation of the offending organism. Waiting for identification of the microorganism, the intravenous administration of broad-spectrum antibiotics over 4–6 hours is recommended.

β_2-Microglobulin-related amyloidosis

This form of amyloidosis, caused by an accumulation of β_2-microglobulins, typically affects patients undergoing long-term dialysis (Zingraff and Drueke, 1991). It is characterized by cystic bone lesions, destructive arthropathies, and tenosynovitis (Figure 15.4). After transplantation, articular symptoms improve quickly, because of the anti-inflammatory effects of immunosuppressive agents. Unfortunately, since the tissue deposits of the protein cannot be mobilized, cystic bone lesions do not decrease in size, and carpal tunnel syndrome does not ameliorate after transplantation despite the increased renal clearance of β_2-microglobulin (Campistol, 2001).

Joint and muscular complications

Bacterial arthritis

Staphylococci are the most frequent bacteria responsible for septic arthritis, but a number of other Gram-positive and Gram-negative organisms may cause this complication. The *clinical presentation* is characterized by the abrupt onset of pain, swelling, and reddening of a single joint. Chills and fever are frequent. The diagnosis may be confirmed by culture of synovial fluid, which can identify the offending agent. Antibiotic treatment should be given parenterally for 2–4 weeks or more. The choice of antibiotic agent should rely on blood or synovial cultures. They usually attain adequate levels in joint fluid.

Joint pain

Polyarthralgias due to diffuse myalgias and joint effusion may occur after rapid *tapering of corticosteroid* dosage, that is, after the treatment of acute rejection with high intravenous doses of methylprednisolone. The knees are the most symptomatic joints. The synovial fluid is sterile, and tests for rheumatoid factors or antinuclear antibodies are negative. The syndrome is transient, and seems not to be predictive of osteonecrosis. Arthralgias, associated with fatigue, muscular weakness, and other symptoms, can also occur when corticosteroids are withdrawn after long-term administration (Miozzari and Ambuhl, 2004).

Severe *osteoarticular* pain syndrome may occur in the first 6 months after transplantation. Knees and ankles are mainly involved, often bilaterally. The syndrome is probably caused by bone impaction, with consequent inflammation of epiphyseal medulla. Usually the symptoms resolve spontaneously (Goffin *et al.*, 1993).

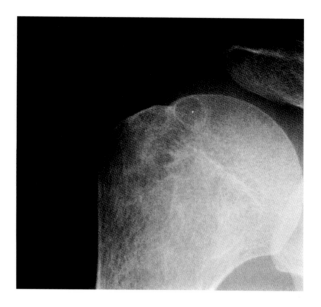

Figure 15.4 Osteoarticular amyloidosis in a patient with a long-term hemodialysis. Osteolysis of the superior epiphysis. This type of lesion does not reverse after successful renal transplantation

Cases of severe arthralgia can also be seen in patients treated with *sirolimus* (Johnson, 2002), with *cyclosporine* (Kart-Koseoglu *et al.*, 2003), and with *mycophenolate mofetil* (Hochegger *et al.*, 2006). The symptoms may improve with a reduction of the dose, but may require withdrawal of the offending drug in some cases.

Tendinitis

Tendinitis and spontaneous *rupture of tendons* may occasionally occur after successful transplantation. Achilles tendons and extensor tendons of quadriceps and of the hand are most commonly affected. The cause remains unknown. As this complication develops more often in patients with a *long history of dialysis*, one may speculate a role for hyperparathyroidism or for deposits of β_2-microglobulin (dialysis amyloidosis). However, in a number of cases, tendinitis also develops in patients with a short period of dialysis. *Pre-transplant hyperphosphatemia* and post-transplant *hypercalcemia* were seen to be associated with tendinitis in a small study (Agarwal and Owen, 1990). It is possible that *corticosteroid*s and *cyclosporine* may play a pathogenetic role (Lucas *et al.*, 1991). *Fluoroquinolones* have been recognized as a possible cause of tendinitis and tendon rupture (Marti *et al.*, 1998). These agents should be used carefully in transplant recipients.

Gout

Gout is frequent in renal transplant patients (Clive, 2000). The cumulative incidence of new-onset gout was 7.6% at 3 years in an analysis of the US Renal Data System (Abbott *et al.*, 2005). *Risk factors* independently associated with post-transplant gout were male sex, older age, higher body mass index, and more recent year of transplant. However, the major cause is represented by *cyclosporine,* which reduces the renal excretion of uric acid. Gout with tacrolimus is less common (Pilmore *et al.*, 2001; Abbott *et al.*, 2005). The use of *diuretics* and *renal dysfunction* can also increase plasma levels of uric acid (Table 15.7).

No therapy is required for asymptomatic hyperuricemia. However, a low-calorie diet with moderate carbohydrate restriction may be suggested. The use of *allopurinol*, which inhibits the xanthine oxidase

Table 15.7	Main factors involved in the pathogenesis of post-transplant gout
Male sex	
Older age	
High body mass index	
Renal dysfunction	
Cylosporine	
Tacrolimus	
Diuretic agents	

enzyme, is usually prescribed to patients with uricemia higher than 10 mg/dl. However, as recent papers have shown that increased serum uric acid is an independent predictor of cerebrovascular or cardiac events (Hayden and Tyagi, 2004; Erdogan et al., 2005), some physicians recommend the use of allopurinol even with lower levels of hyperuricemia. The initial dose of allopurinol should not exceed 100 mg/day in order to avoid exaggerated mobilization of uric acid deposits, which can trigger a gout attack. As *azathioprine* is metabolized to inactive products by xanthine oxidase, the concomitant use of allopurinol and azathioprine causes an accumulation of 6-mercaptopurine that can lead to severe suppression of the bone marrow, with neutropenia, thrombocytopenia, and anemia. Thus, in the case of concomitant administration of allopurinol, the dosage of azathioprine must be reduced by 50–75%, or the patient should be switched to mycophenolic acid salts that do not interfere with azathioprine metabolism. *Uricosuric agents*, such as probenicid or sulfinpyrazone, are not effective when creatinine clearance is lower than 80 ml/min. However, the uricosuric agent benzbromarone may be effective if creatinine clearance is higher than 25 ml/min (Stamp et al., 2005). As uricosuric agents may favor urate stone formation, fluids should be forced, and the urine pH should be kept >6 under uricosuric treatment. In this setting, it should be rememebered that the angiotensin receptor blockers sartans are also uricosuric agents (Dang et al., 2006).

In the case of an acute attack of gout, the agent of choice is *colchicine*, at a dose of 0.6–1 mg, which may be repeated after 1 hour to a maximum of 3–4 mg. Colchicine may cause diarrhea. Often, relief of pain and diarrhea occur simultaneously. Myopathy and neuropathy have been described only occasionally, in spite of the large use of the drug. Renal insufficiency and the concomitant use of statins may favor this rare complication (Alayli et al., 2005). Non-steroidal anti-inflammatory drugs are also effective, but should be used with caution in kidney transplant recipients because they can lead to interstitial nephritis or renal function impairment caused by the inhibition of renal vasodilating prostaglandins.

Myopathy

A number of patients who receive transplantation suffer from weakness, exercise limitation, and rapid-onset tiredness, due to *uremic myopathy*, a condition which may improve, but not resolve completely after transplantation (Campistol, 2002).

A *de novo* myopathy after transplantation may be caused by steroid treatment and/or severe hypophosphatemia. *Steroid-induced* myopathy symmetrically involves proximal muscles, especially of the legs. The first complaint is an inability to climb stairs. Moderate physical training may partially reverse the atrophy and improve exercise capacity. Although the proximal limb muscles are painful, serum enzyme concentrations in the muscles are usually normal.

Hypophosphatemia is frequent, particularly in the first post-transplant months. When the plasma concentration is lower than 1.4 mg/dl, patients complain of muscle weakness. If the phosphate level falls below 0.9 mg/dl, rhabdomyolysis, decreased cardiac contractility, respiratory failure, and hemolytic anemia may occur. Oral supplementation with a neutral phosphate salt may correct hypophosphatemia, increase muscular ATP and phosphodiester content, and improve renal acid excretion (Ambuhl et al., 1999).

Diffuse pain due to rhabdomyolysis, in patients treated with hypolipemic drugs such as *fibrates* and *hydroxy-methylglutaryl coenzyme A* (HMG-CoA). reductase i*nhibitors*, is always accompanied by increased concentrations of muscle enzyme.

Rare cases of acute *quadriplegic myopathy* with myosin-deficient muscle fibers have been reported in organ transplant recipients in the immediate postoperative period. The prognosis is good with early muscle rehabilitation therapy (Miro *et al.*, 1999).

References

Abbott KC, Kimmel PL, Dharnidharka V, et al. New-onset gout after renal transplantation: incidence, risk factors and implications. Transplantation 2005; 80: 1383–91.

Adachi JD, Bensen WG, Brown J, et al. Intermittent etidronate therapy to prevent corticosteroid induced osteoporosis. N Engl J Med 1997b; 337: 382–38.

Agarwal S, Owen R. Tendinitis and tendon ruptures in successful renal transplant recipients. Clin Orthop Relat Res 1990; 252: 270–5.

Alayli G, Cengiz K, Canturk F, et al. Acute myopathy in a patient with concomitant use of pravastatin and colchicine. Ann Pharmacother 2005; 39: 1358–61.

Ambuhl PM, Meier D, Wolf B, et al. Metabolic aspects and phosphate replacement therapy for hypophosphatemia after renal transplantation: impact on muscular phosphate content, mineral metabolism and acid/base homeostasis. Am J Kidney Dis 1999; 34: 875–83.

Apostolou T, Damianou L, Kotsiev V, et al. Treatment of severe hypercalcemia due to refractory hyperparathyroidism in renal transplant patients with the calcimimetic agent cinacalcet. Clin Nephrol 2006; 65: 374–7.

Aroldi A, Tarantino A, Montagnino G, et al. Effects of three immunosuppressive regimens on vertebral bone density in renal transplant recipients. Transplantation 1997; 63: 380–6.

Asano T, Takahashi KA, Fujioka M, et al. Relationship between postrenal transplant osteonecrosis of the femoral head and gene polymorphisms related to the coagulation and fibrinolytic systems in Japanese subjects. Transplantation 2004; 77: 220–5.

Balal M, Paydas S, Seyrek N, et al. Dipyridamole for renal phosphate leak in successfully renal transplanted hypophosphatemic patients. Clin Nephrol 2005; 63: 87–91.

Barreto FC, Barreto DV, Moyses RMA, et al. Osteoporosis in hemodialysis patients revisited by bone histomorphometry: a new insight into an old problem. Kidney Int 2006; 69: 1852–7.

Bellorin-Font E, Rojas E, Carlini RG, et al. Bone remodeling after renal transplantation. Kidney Int 2003; 85 (Suppl): S125–8.

Blake GM, Fogelman I. Bone densitometry, steroids and osteoporosis. Curr Opin Nephrol Hypertens 2002; 11: 641–7.

Body JJ, Gaich GA, Scheele WH. A randomized double-blind trial to compare the efficacy of teriparatide recombinant parathyroid hormone (1–34). with alendronate in postmenopausal women with osteoporosis. J Clin Endocrinol Metab 2002; 87: 4528–35.

Bonarek H, Merville P, Bonarek M, et al. Reduced parathyroid functional mass after successful kidney transplantation. Kidney Int 1999; 56: 642–9.

Bozic KJ, Zurakowski D, Thornill TS. Survivorship analysis of hips treated with core decompression for nontraumatic osteonecrosis of the femoral head. J Bone Joint Surg Am 1999; 81: 200–9.

Brandenburg VM, Ketteler M, Fassbender WJ, et al. Development of lumbar bone mineral density in late course after kidney transplantation. Am J Kidney Dis 2002; 40: 1066–74.

Bryer H, Isserow JA, Armstrong EC, et al. Azathioprine is bone sparing and does not alter cyclosporin A induced bone loss in the rat. J Bone Miner Res 1995; 10: 1191–200.

Campistol JM. Dialysis-related amyloidosis after renal transplantation. Semin Dial 2001; 14: 99–102.

Campistol JM. Uremic myopathy. Kidney Int 2002; 62: 1901–13.

Celik A, Tekis D, Saglam F, et al. Association of corticosteroids and factor V, prothrombin, and MTHFR gene mutations with avascular osteonecrosis in renal allograft recipients. Transplant Proc 2006; 38: 512–16.

Clive DM. Renal transplantation-associated hyperuricemia and gout. J Am Soc Nephrol 2000; 11: 974–9.

Coco M, Glicklich D, Faugere MC, et al. Prevention of bone loss in renal transplant recipients: a prospective, randomized trial of intravenous pamidronate. J Am Soc Nephrol 2003; 14: 2669–76.

Cruz DN, Brickel HM, Wisolmerski JJ, et al. Treatment of osteoporosis and osteopenia in long-term renal transplant patients with alendronate. Am J Transplant 2002; 2: 62–7.

Cruz EA, Lugon JR, Jorgetti V, et al. Histologic evolution of bone disease 6 months after successful kidney transplantation. Am J Kidney Dis 2004; 44: 747–56.

Cueto-Manzano AM, Konel S, Hutchison AJ, et al. Bone loss in long-term renal transplantation: histopathology and densitometry analysis. Kidney Int 1999; 55: 2021–9.

Cueto-Manzano AM, Konel S, Freemont AJ, et al. Effect of 1-25-dihydroxyvitamin D3 and calcium carbonate on bone loss associated with long-term renal transplantation. Am J Kidney Dis 2000; 35: 227–35.

Cvetkovic M, Mann G, Romero D, et al. Deleterious effects of long term cyclosporine A, cyclosporine G, and FK506 on bone mineral metabolism in vivo. Transplantation 1994; 57: 1231–7.

Dang A, Zhang Y, Liu G, et al. Effects of losartan and irbesartan on serum uric acid in hypertensive patients with hyperuricaemia in Chinese population. J Hum Hypertens 2006; 20: 45–50.

De Sevaux RG, Hoitsma AJ, Van Hoof HJ, et al. Abnormal vitamin D metabolism and loss of bone mass after renal transplantation. Nephron 2003; 93: 21–8.

De Winter F, Volegaers D, Gemmel F, Dierckx RA. Promising role of 18-F-fluoro-D-deoxyglucose positron emission tomography in clinical infectious diseases. Eur J Clin Microbiol Infect Dis 2002; 21: 247–57.

Dissanayake I, Goodman C, Bowman A, et al. Mycophenolate mofetil: a promising new immunosuppressant which does not cause bone loss in the rat. Transplantation 1998; 65: 275–8.

Drueke T. The pathogenesis of parathyroid gland hyperplasia in chronic renal failure. Kidney Int 1995; 48: 259–72.

Drueke TB. Therapeutic failure of cinacalcet in a renal transplant patient [Letter]. Nephrol Dial Transplant 2006; 21: 824.

Durieux S, Mercadal L, Orcel P, et al. Bone mineral density and fracture prevalence in long-term kidney graft recipients. Transplantation 2002; 74: 496–500.

Erdogan D, Gullu H, Caliskan M, et al. Relationship of serum uric acid to measures of endothelial function and atherosclerosis in healthy adults. Int J Clin Pract 2005; 59: 1276–82.

Fan S, Kumar S, Cunningham J. Long-term effects on bone mineral density of pamidronate given at the time of renal transplantation. Kidney Int 2003; 63: 2275–9.

Ferrari P, Schroeder V, Anderson S, et al. Association of plasminogen activator inhibitor-1 genotype with avascular osteonecrosis in steroid-treated renal allograft recipients. Transplantation 2002; 74: 1147–52.

First MR. Long-term complications after renal transplantation. Am J Kidney Dis 1993; 22: 477–86.

Franco M, Blaimont A, Albano L, et al. Tacrolimus pain syndrome in renal transplant patients: report of two cases. Joint Bone Spine 2004; 71: 157–9.

Garcia A, Mazuecos A, Garcia T, et al. Effect of parathyroidectomy on renal graft function. Transplant Proc 2005; 37: 1459–61.

Garcia S, Barrios Y, González A, et al. Oral calcitriol prevents early bone loss after renal transplantation. Double-blind placebo controlled study. J Am Soc Nephrol 2000; 11: 575A.

Gauthier V, Barbosa L. Bone pain in transplant recipients responsive to calcium channel blockers. Ann Intern Med 1994; 121: 863–5.

Goffin E, Vande Berg B, Pirson Y, et al. Epiphyseal impaction as a cause of severe osteoarticular pain of lower limbs after renal transplantation. Kidney Int 1993; 44: 98–106.

Greenspan S, Field-Munves E, Tonino R, et al. Tolerability of once-weekly alendronate in patients with osteoporosis: a randomized, double-blind, placebo-controlled study. Mayo Clin Proc 2002; 77: 1044–52.

Grotz WH, Breitenfeldt MK, Braune SW, et al. A calcineurin-inhibitor induced pain syndrome (CIPS): a severe disabling complication after organ transplantation. Transpl Int 2001; 14: 16–23.

Haustein SV, Mack E, Starling JR, Chen H. The role of intraoperative parathyroid hormone testing in patients with tertiary hyperparathyroidism after renal transplantation. Surgery 2005; 138: 1066–71.

Hayden MR, Tyagi SC. Uric acid: a new look at an old risk marker for cardiovascular disease, metabolic syndrome, and type 2 diabetes mellitus: the urate redox shuttle. Nutr Metab 2004; 1: 1–10.

Hirayama T, Athanasou NA. Effects of corticosteroids on human osteoclast formation and activity. J Endocrinol 2002; 175: 155–63.

Hochegger K, Gruber J, Lhotta K. Acute inflammatory syndrome induced by mycophenolate mofetil in a patient following kidney transplantation. Am J Transplant 2006; 6: 852–4.

Inoue S, Horii M, Asano T, et al. Risk factors for nontraumatic osteonecrosis of the femoral head after renal transplantation. J Orthop Sci 2003; 8: 751–6.

Inoue T, Kawamura I, Matsuo M, et al. Lesser reduction in bone mineral density by the immunosuppressant FK 506 compared with cyclosporine in rats. Transplantation 2000; 70: 774–9.

Jeffries CC, Ledgerwood AM, Lucas CE. Life-threatening tertiary hyperparathyroidism in the critically ill. Am J Surg 2005; 189: 369–72.

Joffe I, Katz I, Sehgal S, et al. Lack of change of cancellous bone volume with short term use of the new immunosuppressant rapamycin in rats. Calcif Tissue Int 1993; 53: 45–52.

Johnson RW. Sirolimus (Rapamune) in renal transplantation. Curr Opin Nephrol Hypertens 2002; 11: 603–7.

Julian BA, Laskow DA, Dubovsky J, et al. Rapid loss of vertebral bone density after renal transplantation. N Engl J Med 1991; 325: 544–50.

Julian BA, Qualres LD, Niemann KMW. Musculoskeletal complications after renal transplantation. Am J Kidney Dis 1992; 19: 99–120.

Kart-Koseoglu H, Yucel AE, Isiklar I, et al. Joint pain and arthritis in renal transplant recipients and correlation with cyclosporine therapy. Rheumatol Int 2003; 23: 159–62.

Kifor O, Moore FD, Wang P, et al. Reduced immunostaining for the extracellular Ca^{2+}-sensing receptor in primary uremic hyperparathyroidism. J Clin Endocrinol Metab 1996; 81: 1598–606.

Kinnaert P, Salmon I, Decoster-Gervy C, et al. Total parathyroidectomy and presternal subcutaneous implantation of parathyroid tissue for renal hyperparathyroidism. Surg Gynecol Obstet 1993; 176: 135–8.

Kneissel M, Luong-Nguyen NH, Baptist M, et al. Everolimus suppresses cancellous bone loss, bone resorption, and cathepsin K expression by osteoclasts. Bone 2004; 35: 1144–56.

Kokado Y, Takahara S, Ichimaru N, et al. Factors influencing vertebrate bone density after renal transplantation. Transpl Int 2000; 13 (Suppl 1): S431–5.

Korkor A. Reduced binding of [³H]1,25-dihyroxyvitamin D3 in the parathyroid glands of patients with renal failure. N Engl J Med 1987; 316: 1573–7.

Kruse AE, Eisenberger U, Frey FJ, Mohaupt MG. The calcimimetic cinacalcet normalizes serum calcium in renal transplant patients with persistent hyperparathyroidism. Nephrol Dial Transplant 2005; 20: 1311–14.

Lamy O, Mischler C, Krieg MA. Traitement de l'osteoporose. Rev Med Suisse Romande 2002; 122: 389–93.

Lane NE, Lukert B. The science and therapy of glucocorticoid-induced bone loss. Endocrinol Metab Clin North Am 1998; 27: 465–83.

Leonard MB, Bachrach LK. Assessment of bone mineralization following renal transplantation in children: limitation of DXA and the confounding effects of delayed growth and development. Am J Transplant 2001; 1: 193–6.

Levi M. Post-transplant hypophosphatemia. Kidney Int 2001; 59: 2377–87.

Lewin E, Huan J, Olgaard K. Parathyroid growth and suppression in renal failure. Semin Dial 2006; 19: 238–45.

Lopez-Ben R, Mikuls TR, Moore DS, et al. Incidence of hip osteonecrosis among renal transplantation recipients: a prospective study. Clin Radiol 2004; 59: 431–8.

Lucas VP, Ponge L, Plougastel-Lucas M. Musculoskeletal pain in renal transplant recipients [Letter]. N Engl J Med 1991; 325: 1449.

Marcen R, Caballero C, Pascual J, et al. Lumbar bone mineral density in renal transplant patients on Neoral and tacrolimus: a four-year prospective study. Transplantation 2006; 81: 826–31.

Markowitz GS, Appel GB, Fine PL, et al. Collapsing focal segmental glomerulosclerosis following treatment with high-dose pamidronate. J Am Soc Nephrol 2001; 12: 1164–72.

Marston SB, Gillingham K, Bailey RF, Cheng EY. Osteonecrosis of the femoral head after solid organ transplantation. J Bone Joint Surg Am 2002; 84: 2145–51.

Marti HP, Stoller R, Frey FJ. Fluoroquinolones as a cause of tendon disorders in patients with renal failure/renal transplants. Br J Rheumatol 1998; 37: 343–4.

Martin-Malo A, Rodriguez M, Martinez ME, et al. The interaction of PTH and dietary phosphorus and calcium on serum calcitriol levels in the rat with experimental renal failure. Nephrol Dial Transplant 1996; 11: 1553–8.

McCarron DA, Muther RS, Lentesty B, Brenner WM. Parathyroid function in persistent hyperparathyroidism: relationship to gland size. Kidney Int 1982; 22: 662–70.

Messa PG, Sindici C, Cannella G, et al. Persistent secondary hyperparathyroidism after renal transplantation. Kidney Int 1998; 54: 1704–13.

Meunier PJ, Roux C, Seeman E, et al. The effects of strontium ranelate on the risk of vertebral fracture in women with postmenopausal osteoporosis. N Engl J Med 2004; 350: 459–68.

Mikuls TR, Julian BA, Bartolucci A, Saag KG. Bone mineral density changes within six months of renal transplantation. Transplantation 2003; 75: 49–54.

Milas M, Weber CJ. Near-total parathyroidectomy is beneficial for patients with secondary and tertiary hyperparathyroidism. Surgery 2004; 136: 1252–60.

Miozzari M, Ambuhl PM. Steroid withdrawal after long-term medication for immunosuppressive therapy in renal transplant patients: adrenal response and clinical implications. Nephrol Dial Transplant 2004; 19: 2615–21.

Miro O, Salmeron JM, Masanes F, et al. Acute quadriplegic myopathy with myosin-deficient muscles fibres after liver transplantation: defining the clinical picture and delimiting the risk factors. Transplantation 1999; 67: 1144–51.

Monier-Faugere MC, Mawad H, Qi Q, et al. High prevalence of low bone turnover and ocurrence of osteomalacia after kidney transplantation. J Am Soc Nephrol 2000; 11: 1093–9.

Montalban C, de Francisco ALM, Marinoso ML, et al. Bone disease in long-term adult kidney transplant patients with normal renal function. Kidney Int 2003; 63 (Suppl 85): S129–32.

Morris RE. Rapamycins: antifungal, antitumor, antiproliferative, and immunosuppressive macrolides. Transplant Rev 1992; 6: 39–87.

Movsowitz C, Epstein S, Fallon M, et al. Cyclosporine A in vivo produces severe osteopenia in the rat: effect of dose and duration of administration. Endocrinology 1988; 123: 2571–7.

Movsowitz C, Epstein S, Ismail F, et al. Cyclosporin A in the oophorectomized rat: unexpected severe bone resorption. J Bone Miner Res 1989; 4: 393–8.

Mundy G, Garrett R, Harris S, et al. Stimulation of bone formation in vitro and in rodents by statins. Science 1999; 286: 1946–9.

Nehme D, Rondeau E, Paillard F, et al. Aspectic necrosis of bone following renal transplantation: relation with hyperparathyroidism. Nephrol Dial Transplant 1989; 4: 123–8.

Nichol PF, Starling JR, Mack E, et al. Long-term follow-up of patients with tertiary hyperparathyroidism treated by resection of a single or double adenoma. Ann Surg 2002; 235: 673–8.

Nisbeth U, Lindh E, Liunghall S, et al. Increased fracture rate in diabetes mellitus and females after renal transplantation. Transplantation 1999; 67: 1218–22.

Nizze H, Mihatsch MJ, Zollinger HU, et al. Cyclosporine-associated nephropathy in patients with heart and bone marrow transplants. Clin Nephrol 1985; 30: 248–60.

Parfitt AM. The hyperparathyroidism of chronic renal failure: a disorder of growth. Kidney Int 1997; 52: 3–9.

Pasco JA, Kotowicz MA, Henry MJ, et al. Statin use, bone mineral density, and fracture risk: Geelong Osteoporosis Study. Arch Intern Med 2002; 162: 537–40.

Pham TH, Sterioff S, Mullan BP, et al. Sensitivity and utility of parathyroid scintigraphy in patients with primary versus secondary and tertiary hyperparathyroidism. World J Surg 2006; 30: 327–32.

Phillips IJ, Kurzawinski TR, Honour JW. Potential pitfalls in intraoperative parathyroid hormone measurements during parathyroid surgery. Ann Clin Biochem 2005; 42: 453–8.

Pichette V, Bonnardeaux A, Prudhomme L, et al. Long-term bone loss in kidney transplant recipients: a cross-sectional and longitudinal study. Am J Kidney Dis 1986; 28: 105–14.

Pilmore HL, Faire B, Dittmer L. Tacrolimus for the treatment of gout in renal transplantation: two case reports and review of the literature. Transplantation 2001; 72: 1703–5.

Piraino B, Carpenter BJ, Puschett JB. Resolution of hypercalemia and aluminum bone disease after renal transplantation. Am J Med 1988; 85: 728–30.

Plosker GL, McTavish D. Intranasal salmon calcitonin: a review of its pharmacological properties and in the management of postmenopausal osteoporosis. Drugs Aging 1996; 8: 378–400.

Polak BCP, Baarsma GS, Snyers B. Diffuse retinal pigment epitheliopathy complicating systemic corticosteroid treatment. J Ophthalmol 1995; 79: 922–5.

Ponticelli C, Aroldi A. Osteoporosis after organ transplantation [Letter]. Lancet 2001; 1: 1623.

Raisz LG. Screening for osteoporosis. N Engl J Med 2005; 353: 164–71.

Rejnmark L, Buus NH, Vestergaard P, et al. Statins decrease bone turnover in postmenopausal women: a cross-sectional study. Eur J Clin Invest 2002; 32: 581–9.

Rodan GA, Fleisch HA. Bisphosphonates: mechanism of action. J Clin Invest 1996; 97: 2692–6.

Rojas E, Carlini RG, Clesca P, et al. The pathogenesis of osteodystrophy after renal transplantation as detected by early alterations in bone remodeling. Kidney Int 2003; 63: 1915–23.

Rosen CJ. Postmenopausal osteoporosis. N Engl J Med 2006; 353: 595–603.

Ryu JS, Kim JS, Moon DH, et al. Bone SPECT is more sensitive than MRI in the detection of early osteonecrosis of the femoral head after renal transplantation. J Nucl Med 2002; 43: 1006–11.

Schlosberg M, Movsowitz C, Epstein S, et al. The effect of cyclosporin A administration and its withdrawal on bone mineral metabolism in the rat. Endocrinology 1989; 124: 2179–84.

Schwarz C, Bohmig GA, Steininger R, et al. Impaired phosphate handling of renal allografts is aggravated under rapamycin-based immunosuppression. Nephrol Dial Transplant 2001; 16: 378–82.

Serra AL, Schwarz AA, Wick FH, et al. Successful treatment of hypercalcemia with cinacalcet in renal transplant recipients with persistent hyperparathyroidism. Nephrol Dial Transplant 2005; 20: 1315–19.

Slatopolsky E, Delmez J. Bone disease in chronic renal failure and after transplantation. In Coe FL, Favus MJ, eds. Disorders of Bone and Mineral Metabolism. New York: Raven Press, 1992: 905–17.

Staa TP, Staa TP, Staa TP, et al. The epidemiology of corticosteroid-induced osteoporosis: a meta-analysis. Osteoporosis Int 2002; 13: 777–87.

Stamp L, Searle M, O'Donnell J, Chapman P. Gout in solid organ transplantation: a challenging clinical problem. Drugs 2005; 65: 2593–611.

Sun L, Blair HC, Peng Y, et al. Calcineurin regulates bone formation by the osteoblast. Proc Natl Acad Sci USA 2005; 102: 17130–5.

Taal MW, Masud D, Green D, Cassidy MJ. Risk factors for reduced bone density in haemodialysis patients. Nephrol Dial Transplant 1999; 14: 1922–8.

Takahashi S, Goldring S, Katz M, et al. Down-regulation of calcitonin receptor mRNA expression by calcitonin during human osteoclast-like cell differentiation. J Clin Invest 1995; 95: 167–71.

Tang S, Chan TM, Lui SL, et al. Risk factors for avascular bone necrosis after transplantation. Transplant Proc 2000; 32: 1873–5.

Torregrosa JV, Moreno A, Gutierrez A, et al. Alendronate for treatment of renal transplant patients with osteoporosis. Transplant Proc 2003; 35: 1393–5.

Torres A, Machado M, Concepcion MT, et al. Influence of vitamin D receptor genotype on bone mass after renal transplantation. Kidney Int 1996; 50: 1726–33.

Torres A, Lorenzo V, Salido E. Calcium metabolis and skeletal problems after transplantation. J Am Soc Nephrol 2002; 13: 551–8.

Triponez F, Dosseh D, Hazzan M, et al. Subtotal parathyroidectomy with thymectomy for autonomous hyperparathyroidism after renal transplantation. Br J Surg 2005; 92: 1282–7.

Ulivieri FM, Piodi LP, Aroldi A, Cesana B. Effect of kidney transplantation on bone mass and body composition in males. Transplantation 2002; 73: 612–15.

van den Ham E, Kooman JP, Christiaans MHL, van Hooff JP. The influence of early steroid withdrawal on body composition and bone mineral density in renal transplantation. Transpl Int 2003; 16: 82–7.

Weinstein RS, Jilka RL, Parfitt AM, Manolagas SC. Inhibition of osteoclastogenesis and promotion of apoptosis of osteoblasts and osteoclasts by glucocorticoids: potential mechanisms of their deleterious effects on bone. J Clin Invest 1998; 102: 274–82.

Wells G, Tugwell P, Shea B, et al. Meta-analyses of therapy for postmenopausal osteoporosis. V Meta-analysis of the efficacy of hormone replacement therapy in treating and preventing osteoporosis in postmenopausal women. Endocr Rev 2002; 23: 529–39.

Widler L, Jaeggi KA, Glatt M, et al. Highly potent geminae biphosphonates. From pamidronate disodium (Aredia) to zoledronic acid (Zometa). J Med Chem 2002; 45: 3721–38.

Zeiden B, Shabtal M, Waltzer WC, et al. Improvement in renal transplant function after subtotal parathyroidectomy in a hypercalcemic kidney allograft recipient. Transplant Proc 1991; 23: 2285–8.

Zingraff J, Drueke T. Can the nephrologist prevent dialysis related amyloidosis? Am J Kidney Dis 1991; 18: 1–11.

Zojer N, Keck AV, Pecherstofer M. Comparative tolerability of drug therapies for hypercalcaemia of malignancy. Drug Saf 1999; 21: 389–406.

16 NEUROLOGIC AND OCULAR COMPLICATIONS

Neurologic complications

A number of different neurologic complications may complicate the outcome of renal transplant recipients, leading in the most severe cases to disabling or life-threatening diseases. Some neurologic complications are caused by the inherent disorders that led to transplantation and/or by dialysis. However, the most important role in the genesis of post-transplant neurologic complications is played by immunosuppressive therapy, which may cause direct neurotoxicity or may favor the development of tumors and opportunistic infection. Since the introduction of new immunosuppressive protocols, the nature of post-transplant neurologic complications has changed in the past few years (Ponticelli and Campise, 2005). The prognosis of some neurologic complications in renal transplant recipients has improved substantially, due to progression in diagnostic and therapeutic measures.

Drug-related neurotoxicity

Apart from the non-specific risk of tumor and infection related to the impairment of immune surveillance, some immunosuppressive drugs currently used in renal transplantation may exert direct neurotoxicity (Table 16.1).

Calcineurin inhibitors

Both cyclosporine (CsA) and tacrolimus (TAC) can exert neurotoxic adverse effects, although neurotoxicity seems to occur more frequently in TAC-treated renal transplant recipients (Margreiter, 2002), particularly in children (Flynn et al., 2001). The neurotoxicity of calcineurin inhibitors may be expected, since calcineurin, which accounts for more than 1% of total protein in the brain, plays an important role in the diverse functions of the nervous system and has many and varied roles in both rapid and long-term changes within nerve cells. On the other hand, the neurotoxicity of CsA and TAC may be contrasted by inherent biologic protective mechanisms that limit the access of these drugs to nerve cells, of which the most important is the blood–brain barrier (Tan and Robinson, 2006).

Mild neurologic symptoms are common and include tremor, burning paresthesia, headache, and flushing. *Severe symptoms* include disabling pain syndrome (Grotz et al., 2001), hallucinations, seizures, cerebellar ataxia, and motoric weakness. Delirium and anxiety may occur in transplant patients with high tacrolimus blood concentrations (Corruble et al., 2005).

A reversible *posterior leukoencephalopathy* can develop even at levels of calcineurin inhibitors within the normal range, occipital white matter being particularly vulnerable to the adverse effects of CsA and TAC (Bechstein, 2000). Once again, children are more susceptible to this cerebral complication (Torocsik et al., 1999). Neuroimaging studies show typically low-density white matter lesions involving the posterior areas of cerebral hemispheres. The pathogenesis of CsA- and TAC-related leukoencephalopathy is still unclear. Edema and demyelination have been observed using special magnetic resonance techniques, and probably play a major role (Lacaille et al., 2004). Increased permeability of brain endothelial cells may be responsible for these abnormalities (Dohgu et al., 2000). Recent evidence suggests inhibition of the drug-efflux pump and dysfunction of the blood–brain barrier by enhanced nitric oxide production (Wijdicks et al., 2001). Disruption of the blood–brain barrier could facilitate the passage of calcineurin inhibitors into the cerebral interstitium.

Table 16.1   Neurologic complications caused directly by immunosuppressive agents

Drugs	Mild–moderate	Severe
Calcineurin inhibitors	Ataxia	Posterior leukoencephalopathy
	Weakness	Cerebellar motoric pain
	Tremor	Hallucinations
	Headache	Seizures
	Flushing	
	Paresthesia	Hearing loss
Anti-CD3 monoclonal	Headache	Aseptic meningitis
antibodies	Dizziness	Lethargy
	Blurred vision	Triparesis
		Seizures
Anti-CD52 monoclonal		Myelitis
antibodies		Radiculopathy
Corticosteroids	Emotional lability	Psychiatric reactions
		Myopathy
		Pseudotumor cerebri

A questionnaire completed by 521 liver transplant recipients indicated that 27% developed *hearing impairment* after transplantation. Among them, 52% complained of hearing loss, 38% of tinnitus, and 30% of otalgia. Hearing loss was positively associated with tacrolimus immunosuppression in univariate and multivariate analyses. Patients using a hearing-aid received tacrolimus more frequently than they did cyclosporine. Calcineurin inhibitor-related neurotoxicity could also be responsible for hearing impairment in renal transplant recipients (Rifai *et al.*, 2006).

The symptoms of calcineurin inhibitor neurotoxicity are often reversible with the reduction or withdrawal of the offending drug. However, some patients can have permanent (Esterl *et al.*, 1996; Lacaille *et al.*, 2004) and even fatal complications (Mori *et al.*, 2000), in spite of the withdrawal of calcineurin inhibitors. In view of the lack of neurotoxicity of mTOR (mammalian target of rapamycin) inhibitors (Maramattom and Wijdicks, 2004; Forgacs *et al.*, 2005), either sirolimus or everolimus may be used to replace calcineurin inhibitors in the case of severe neurotoxicity.

Monoclonal antibodies (MAB)

The administration of *anti-CD3 MAB* may cause a *cytokine release syndrome* which may include nuchal rigidity, headache, and blurred vision (Pittock *et al.*, 2003). In the most severe cases, aseptic meningitis, lethargy, seizures, and triparesis can occur (Parizel *et al.*, 1997; Thaisetthawatkul *et al.*, 2001). This *encephalopathy* is often associated with cerebral edema, suggesting a dysfunction of the blood–brain barrier caused by a capillary leak syndrome. Neurologic complications usually reverse after the discontinuation of anti-CD3 MAB. In order to prevent the cytokine release syndrome, the use of lower doses of anti-CD3 MAB (2 mg instead of 5 mg) (Norman *et al.*, 1994), premedication with intravenous high-dose steroids (Ponticelli *et al.*, 1987), and/or anti-human TNF monoclonal antibodies (Charpentier *et al.*, 1992) have been suggested.

In hematologic patients, the use of *anti-CD52 MAB* (Campath®-1H) was associated with severe neurologic disorders in about 9% of cases, the most frequent complications being sensorimotor-radicular neuropathy and/or myelitis (Avivi *et al.*, 2004).

Corticosteroids

Emotional lability or excitability may develop under high-dose steroid administration. Unpredictable *psychiatric* reactions may also occur, particularly in patients with known psychological difficulties. Corticosteroid treatment is frequently associated with transiently impaired attention, concentration, and memory. In rare cases, *cognitive changes* may be prominent and may persist for substantial periods of time after steroid discontinuation (Wolkowitz *et al.*, 2004).

Pseudotumor cerebri, characterized by intracranial hypertension and papilledema, may occur, mainly in children but also in adults, when corticosteroid doses are rapidly decreased. The complication can be managed with lumbar taps or increased doses of corticosteroids. Acetazolamide and furosemide may also be employed. Rarely, permanent *visual loss* occurs in spite of these measures. Optic nerve sheath fenestration or a lumboperitoneal, ventriculoperitoneal, or ventriculoatrial shunting procedure may be considered in patients with deterioration of visual function despite maximum medical treatment.

Corticosteroids have also been implicated in the growth of *lipomas*. A case of intramedullary lipoma of the spinal cord related to corticosteroids has been reported in a renal transplant patient (Agraharkar *et al.*, 2000).

Steroid-induced *myopathy* symmetrically involves proximal muscles, especially of the lower extremities. The first complaint is an inability to climb stairs. Muscle enzymes are normal. Myopathy is not related to the patient's age or to the dosage of therapy. Improvement occurs after steroids are discontinued.

Infection

Infection represents one of the leading causes of neurologic complications in renal transplant recipients (Singh and Husain, 2000). The risk of infection is roughly related to the amount of immunosuppression and to the clinical status of the patient. Central nervous system (CNS) infection usually occurs between 1 and 12 months following transplantation. Rarely, however, the transmission of varicella zoster virus (Fehr *et al.*, 2002) and West Nile virus (Centers for Disease Control, 2002) by the transplanted organ may cause encephalitis within a few days after transplantation.

The *presentation* of CNS infection in transplant patients may be different from that in normal patients. The onset may be subacute and systemic signs may be lacking. The most reliable symptoms that may demonstrate the presence of a CNS infection are headache, alteration in mental status, focal neurologic deficit, and unexplained fever. Patients with such an array of symptoms should undergo magnetic resonance imaging (MRI) with gadolinium. MRI is especially useful for posterior fossa abscesses and in demonstrating cerebritis, surrounding edema, the extent of mass effect, or associated thrombosis. In many cases, lumbar puncture should be performed only after brain imaging excludes the presence of expanded brain abscess or other mass with impending transtentorial herniation. Cerebrospinal fluid examination may allow identification of the etiological agent.

The *etiology* may be variable. *Listeria monocytogenes*, *Cryptococcus neoformans,* and *Aspergillus fumigatus* account for most cases of CNS infections in transplant patients. The *prognosis* of infections of the CNS in renal transplant recipients is severe, and may be negatively influenced by a delay in diagnosis and treatment, since the usual signs of infection are blunted in these immunosuppressed patients and infection with uncommon micro-organisms often occurs.

According to Fishman and Rubin (1998), CNS infection has four distinct patterns: acute meningitis, subacute or chronic meningitis, focal brain infections, and progressive dementia (Table 16.2).

Acute meningitis

This is usually caused by *L. monocytogenes*. *Listeria* meningitis is characterized by fever, altered sensorium, and headache, but some 40% of patients have no meningeal signs on admission. In the cerebrospinal fluid, a high leukocyte count and a high protein concentration may be lacking. One-third of patients have focal neurologic findings and a quarter of patients develop seizures. Meningitis is usually transmitted by an extraneural focus or from a paranasal or paratympanic area (Doganay, 2003). *Haemophilus influenzae*,

Table 16.2   Neurologic infections in renal transplant recipients

Infection	Etiologic agent	Clinical features	Treatment
Acute meningitis	*Listeria monocytogenes*	Altered sensorium Headache	Ampicillin+aminoglycoside
Subacute meningitis	*Cryptococcus neoformans*	Headache Altered consciousness Late occurrence	Amphotericin B + fluconazole or flucytosine
Focal brain infection	*Aspergillus fumigatus*	Seizures Cranial nerve palsies	Amphotericin B+ fluconazole
	Listeria monocytogenes *Nocardia asteroides*		Ampicillin+aminoglycoside Trimethoprim–sulfamethoxazole or aminoglycoside or imipenem
	Varicella zoster		Specific immunoglobulins Acyclovir?
Multifocal leukoencephalopathy	JC virus Herpes virus	Progressive dementia	Cydofovir?

Neisseria meningitides, *Streptococcus pneumoniae*, and other bacteria can also cause acute meningitis in renal transplant recipients. Moreover, meningoencephalitis may also be caused by viruses. The prompt diagnosis of such disorders is critical. It should be noted that drugs such as OKT3 (Pittock *et al.*, 2003) and sulfamethoxazole–trimethoprim (Therrien, 2004) may rarely cause aseptic meningitis, which may make differential diagnosis difficult.

The initial step in the evaluation of CNS infections is usually a MRI study, which may show focal or mass lesions (brain abscess), non-focal lesions or meningoencephalitis, or no lesions, as in the case of meningitis (Singh and Husain, 2000). Cerebrospinal fluid investigation and cultures, latex agglutination tests, countercurrent immunoelectrophoresis, radioimmunoassay, or enzyme-linked immunosorbent assay are helpful in identifying the etiologic agent and the most appropriate treatment.

The *prognosis* of *Listeria* meningitis is severe in transplant patients. Ampicillin for 14–21 days with an aminoglycoside for 7–10 days remains the *treatment* of choice (Mylonakis *et al.*, 1998). A recent meta-analysis showed that the administration of high-dose corticosteroids with the first dose of antibiotic can reduce mortality and neurologic sequelae in patients with acute bacterial meningitis, without detectable adverse effects (Van de Beek *et al.*, 2004).

Subacute or chronic meningitis

Classical meningeal findings may be lacking at the beginning. In a number of cases, patients complain of an unexplained headache in conjunction with a change in the level of consciousness. Other cases may be heralded by seizures, or are characterized by fever, nausea/vomitisng, and headache lasting over several days or weeks, and may be associated with an altered state of consciousness. Subacute meningitis is

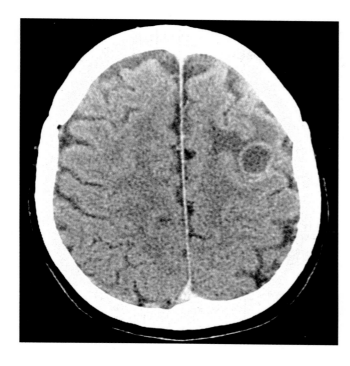

Figure 16.1 Cerebral *Nocardia* infection. Hypodense lesion surrounded by halo in the left parietal area of the brain

usually caused by *C. neoformans,* and tends to be seen relatively late in the transplantation course. The diagnosis is not easy. Based on clinical suspicion and neuroimaging, positive identification of the yeast by using India ink staining and elevated cryptococcal antigen latex agglutination titers in cerebrospinal fluid are needed to confirm the diagnosis (Veerareddy and Vobalaboira, 2004). Elevated intracranial pressure, leading to blindness or hearing loss, may complicate cryptococcal meningitis. Other etiologic microorganisms include *L. monocytogenes, Histoplasma capsulatum, Nocardia asteroides, Strongyloides stercoralis,* and *Mycobacterium tuberculosis.*

Amphotericin B, preferably in its liposomal formulation to reduce nephrotoxicity (Collazos, 2003), is the *therapy* of choice for cryptococcal meningitis. The addition of 5-flucytosine (Vilchez *et al.*, 2002) and/or fluconazole (Larsen *et al.*, 2004) to amphotericin B may be useful.

Focal brain infections

Focal brain infection may present with seizures, alteration in mental status, or focal neurological abnormalities. The most frequent cause is a metastatic *Aspergillus* infection. *Aspergillus* brain abscesses usually occur in the early post-transplant period. The lesions are multifocal, and have a predilection for the gray and white matter junction. The abscesses occur more commonly in the cerebral hemisphere, but the cerebellum or brain system may also be involved. From a practical point of view it must be remembered that almost all brain abscesses in the early post-transplant period are caused by fungi, predominantly by *A. fumigatus.* Brain abscesses in patients with fungal pneumonia are always caused by the same fungus. The mortality rate is virtually 100% (Paterson and Singh, 1999).

L. monocytogenes, Toxoplasma gondii, and *N. asteroides* (Figure 16.1) are other possible causes of brain abscesses. L. *monocytogenes* may occur at any time after transplantation. Although meningitis is the most frequent form of neurologic involvement, *Listeria* may also cause brain-stem encephalitis (also called rhombencephalitis) with cranial nerve palsies or pontomedullary signs. *Toxoplasmosis* usually occurs within 3 months of transplantation, but late-onset disease has been reported. Changes in mental status and seizures are the most frequent clinical manifestations. The lesions are usually multiple, with

Table 16.3 Peripheral neuropathies in renal transplant recipients

Neuropathy	Symptomatology
Mononeuropathy	Carpal tunnel syndrome
	Ischemic monomelic neuropathy
	Acute femoral neuropathy
	Lumbosacral neuropathy
Polyneuropathy	Uremic polyneuropathy
	Guillain–Barré syndrome

periventricular localization. Mortality is elevated, but early diagnosis and treatment may improve the prognosis. *Nocardia* infections usually develop between 1 and 6 months after transplantation. The lesions are usually multiple, with periventricular localization. The primary portal of entry is pulmonary. Cutaneous or soft tissue abscesses may be observed in about 20% of patients with brain abscesses caused by *N. asteroides* (Singh and Husain, 2000).

Infections with the *varicella zoster virus* may cause encephalitis both in pediatric (Lynfield *et al.*, 1992) and in adult transplant recipients (Fehr *et al.*, 2002). Cerebral edema with areas of low attenuation consistent with demyelination can be seen upon CT scan. Lesions involve the gray matter and have contrast enhancement. Because of the severe prognosis of this complication, a pre-transplant vaccination against varicella zoster virus is recommended in children without humoral immunity (Olson *et al.*, 2001). Early treatment with acyclovir and a high-dose specific immunoglobulin should be instituted as early as possible in patients with varicella encephalitis and in patients with relatives affected by active varicella infection. *HHV-6 or JC* virus infection (Koralnik, 2002) may cause progressive multifocal leukoencephalopathy which may be difficult to differentiate from that caused by calcineurin inhibitors.

Apart from the few cases of *West Nile virus* infection transmitted by the donor, other naturally acquired cases of West Nile virus infection have been reported in renal transplant recipients. Most patients developed meningoencephalitis, with flaccid paralysis in about one-third of cases. All patients had cerebrospinal fluid pleocytosis. The prognosis is severe, as 20% of transplanted patients died and 30% had a significant residual deficit (Klinschmidt-De Masters and Marder, 2004).

Peripheral neuropathy (Table 16.3)

Mononeuropathies

Mononeuropathies include *tunnel carpal syndrome* that does not improve after transplantation and the rare ischemic *monomelic neuropathy*. This latter complication requires immediate surgical closure of the arteriovenous fistula to avoid severe and permanent neurologic dysfunction (Pirzada and Morgenlander, 1991).

Acute femoral neuropathy may occur in about 2% of renal transplant patients as the result of perioperative nerve compression and ischemia. As the femoral nerve innervates the iliopsoas (hip flexor) and quadriceps the femoris (knee extensor), the main clinical features may be knee buckling, absent knee jerk, and weak anterior thigh muscles. Symptoms develop between 24 and 48 hours after surgery. Complete recovery of motor function occurs in 4–9 months (Sharma *et al.*, 2002).

Lumbosacral plexopathy has recently been described after dual kidney transplantation. The syndrome consists of pain in the hip with asymmetric weakness of the proximal leg muscles. This complication is uncommon because the plexus has a rich anastomotic blood supply. However, dual kidney transplantation involves a larger and time-consuming dissection requiring more vascular reconstruction. This may predispose the lumbosacral plexus to ischemic injury (Dhillon and Sarac, 2002).

Uremic polyneuropathy

Uremic polyneuropathy is characterized by axonal degeneration with secondary segmental demyelination. Stabilization or improvement almost invariably occurs after successful transplantation. However, *de novo* cases of demyelinating polyneuropathy can occur as a consequence of cytomegalovirus infection (De Maar *et al.*, 1999).

Guillain–Barré syndrome

The Guillain–Barré syndrome is an idiopathic acute inflammatory demyelinating polyradiculoneuropathy, characterized clinically by progressive, symmetric weakness with areflexia. Guillain–Barré syndrome has been reported rarely in renal transplant patients. It is possible, however, that cases of Guillain–Barré syndrome have been underreported. Cytomegalovirus (El Sabrout *et al.*, 2001) and *Campylobacter jejuni* (Maccario *et al.*, 1998) have been found to be associated with the syndrome in renal transplant recipients, but the etiology remains unknown.

The *clinical features* include areflexic motor paralysis with mild sensory disturbance, coupled with an acellular rise of total protein in the cerebrospinal fluid. However, atypical presentations are relatively frequent. Paralysis may spread upwards (ascending paralysis) and may lead to quadriplegia or to acute respiratory failure. Although most patients recover, 5% will die, and more than half suffer residual damage to the peripheral nervous system. Although Guillain–Barré syndrome is thought to be triggered by autoimmune mechanisms that are predominantly T cell-mediated, the syndrome may recover spontaneously in transplant patients even without the return of T-cell function (Bulsara *et al.*, 2001). However, about one-third of patients require ventilatory management. In renal transplant recipients the use of intensive plasmapheresis (daily in the first 5–7 days, then every other day) and/or intravenous high-dose immunoglobulins (0.2–0.4 g/kg) in the first 2 weeks may improve the disability (Mazzoni *et al.*, 2004). However, even if reports concerning intravenous immunoglobulins continue to grow in number, few high-quality randomized controlled trials have been reported (Darabi *et al.*, 2006).

Stroke

By reviewing the files of the Mayo Clinic, Wijdicks *et al.* (1999) reported that intracranial hematomas occurred in nine out of 1573 renal transplant patients and were the cause of death in six of the 530 patients who died. All patients with intracranial hemorrhage had poorly controlled hypertension. The risk of cerebral hemorrhage was ten-fold higher in patients with polycystic kidney disease, due to the frequent presence of aneurysms, particularly in the cerebral anterior circulation, and four-fold in patients with diabetes mellitus compared with other transplant recipients. In an American series, stroke accounted for 8% of deaths in renal transplant recipients (Howard *et al.*, 2002). In a Spanish series the prevalence of stroke was 8% at 10 years. Stroke occurred on average 49 months after kidney transplantation, the main cause being cerebral hemorrhage (Oliveras *et al.*, 2003).

In the general population, arterial hypertension, diabetes, and atherosclerosis are associated with an increased risk of stroke, and the same has been found for renal transplant recipients (Brouns and De Deyn, 2004). Thus, every effort to control these risk factors is warranted to prevent stroke. As occluded internal carotid arteries, stenosis, and/or ulcerative plaque bear a high risk of ischemic complications, hypertensive, diabetic, elderly, and smoking renal transplant patients should be regularly checked using carotid echo color Doppler and receive carotid endarterectomy or surgical treatment when appropriate. Patients with polycystic kidney disease and a family history of strokes should receive angio-MNR to exclude the presence of intracerebral aneurysms.

Tumors

In the past, cadaveric donors with primary brain tumors were accepted because of the rarity of extracerebral spread. Recently, the possibility of metastasis has been demonstrated, particularly in the case of aggressive tumors, a history of craniotomy, and the presence of shunts (Detry *et al.*, 2000). However, with

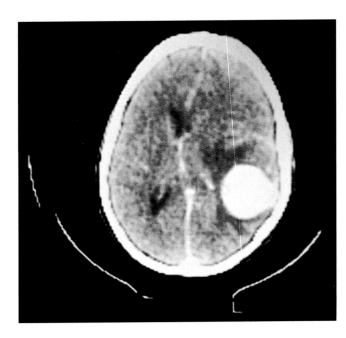

Figure 16.2 Cerebral right parietal lymphoma in a 26-year-old woman transplanted 4 years earlier. The mass, revealed by contrast medium, displaces lateral ventricular

the exception of these few cases, the most frequent neoplasias of the brain in renal transplant patients are lymphomas and metastatic tumors (Martinez, 1998).

B-cell lymphomas

The most frequent primary CNS tumors diagnosed among renal transplant recipients are B-cell lymphomas, while T-cell lymphomas are rare. Patients who receive aggressive immunosuppression with antilymphocyte antibodies are particularly susceptible to lymphomas (Opelz *et al.*, 2006). Central nervous system involvement is uncommon (Figure 16.2) but, when present, occurs in isolation, sparing other organ systems (Brennan *et al.*, 2005). Most B-cell lymphomas are caused by *Epstein–Barr virus* (Penn, 1998). EBV can evade the host responses through restricted gene expression, and can generate a polypeptide analogous in structure and bioactivity to interleukin-10. In immunosuppressed renal transplant recipients, these factors may contribute to impair the ability of the immune system to eliminate EBV, and can lead to the development of polyclonal polymorphic hyperplasia that may evolve into a malignant monoclonal tumor.

In most patients with cerebral lymphoma, the neurologic examination is focally abnormal but not specific. Brain imaging by computed tomography or, even better, by magnetic resonance imaging is indispensable for diagnosis. *Imaging procedures* may show solitary masses or multifocal lesions, of which fewer than half enhance with contrast agent. Differential diagnosis from cerebral abcesses may be difficult, as both disorders may show a ring contrast enhancement (Snanoudj *et al.*, 2003). EBV viral load testing using quantitative DNA amplification of blood samples may help in correct differential diagnosis. However, for definitive diagnosis and adequate treatment planning, a tissue diagnosis should be obtained whenever possible by open or stereotactic biopsy. Unfortunately, however, stereotactic biopsy is often complicated by hemorrhage, which can be fatal (Phan *et al.*, 2000). The prognosis of primary brain lymphomas is severe, with a median survival of 26 months.

Treatment (see also Chapter 11) first consists of the reduction or withdrawal of immunosuppression associated with interferon-α, and chemotherapy and radiation therapy, usually given in small daily fractions to build to a total dose, can significantly improve the patient's survival (Snanoudj *et al.*, 2003).

Patients showing expression of CD20 on neoplastic cells have a good response to treatment with anti-CD20 monoclonal antibodies (Gulley et al., 2003). However, resistance may occur because of either the variable expression of CD20 by neoplastic cells or the elevated apoptotic threshold (Smith, 2003).

Other cancers

Several cases of *glioblastoma* have been reported in kidney transplant patients (Salvati et al., 2003). Because of the putative HIV–glioma association, a pathogenetic link to immunosuppression has been postulated. The prognosis is severe. Cases of *cerebellar hemangioblastoma* (Ozturk et al., 2005), *leiomyosarcoma* (Tahri et al., 2002), intracranial metstasis of *Kaposi's sarcoma* (Bahat et al., 2002), and other tumors (Schwechheimer and Hashemian, 1995) have also been reported.

Progressive dementia

Dementia with or without focal abnormalities may be caused by *JC virus* (Kwak et al., 2002), a polyoma virus belonging to the genus papovavirus, or more rarely by herpes simplex virus, CMV (Salmon-Ceron, 2002), or EBV (Skiest, 2002), which lead to progressive multifocal leukoencephalopathy.

The clinical *signs* and *symptoms* begin insidiously. Blunting of intellectual capacity, aphasia, alteration in personality, and headache may be the first symptoms. The lesions involve the cerebral cortex, are multifocal and asymmetric, and spare the gray matter. The disease is progressive. The efficacy of antiviral treatment is still unclear. As a similar syndrome may be caused by calcineurin inhibitors (see above), differential diagnosis is important, as withdrawal of the offending drug may improve the symptoms in the case of calcineurin inhibitor toxicity.

General recommendations

The transplant physician should be aware of the many neurologic complications that may affect kidney allograft recipients. It should be recalled that the two agents more frequently used for immunosuppression, *calcineurin inhibitors* and *corticosteroids,* may be neurotoxic. When the responsibility of either drug is recognized, its careful reduction may be considered in mild to moderate complications. Withdrawal of the incriminating calcineurin inhibitor is mandatory in the case of posterior leukoencephalopathy. Efforts should be made to control blood pressure, glucose intolerance, and hyperlipemia, and to avoid smoking in order to prevent atherosclerosis and possible stroke.

Even *trivial symptoms* such as headache or mild mental changes should not be underestimated, as they may be the initial clinical expression of a severe underlying disease, such as a brain tumor or a CNS infection. *Evaluation of the mental status* of the patient is of paramount importance. Cognitive deficits, personality changes, and/or memory loss may raise the suspicion of brain tumors, papovavirus JC infection, or cryptococcal infection. The patient should be examined for increased intracranial pressure (papilledema) and for other cranial abnormalities. However, even if the neurologic examination results are normal, the patient should be kept under observation. CT or MRI followed by lumbar puncture should be done in cases of fever (even mild) associated with headache, dysphasia, dyspraxia, or personality change, to rule out meningoencephalitis. A strict collaboration between neurologists and transplant physicians is needed to allow an optimal systematic approach to the many neurologic problems of renal transplant recipients.

Ocular complications

Ocular complications occur frequently in transplant recipients, particularly in the first post-transplant months when immunosuppression is stronger and the doses of corticosteroids are higher (Bradfield et al., 2005). However, in long-term survivors the incidence of sight-threatening complications is relatively low (Jayamanne and Porter, 1998).

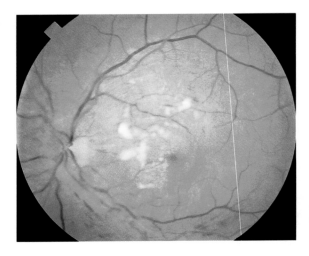

Figure 16.3 Hypertensive retinopathy with exudates, arteriolar narrowing, and tortuosity in a transplant patient. (Courtesy of Professor R Ratiglia, University of Milan.)

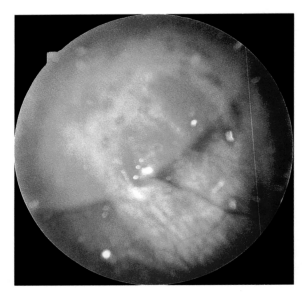

Figure 16.4 Retinal detachment in a transplant patient with severe hypertension and hypercorticism. (Courtesy of Professor R Ratiglia, University of Milan.)

Retinopathy

A number of different causes may lead to retinal lesions in renal transplant recipients. They include arterial hypertension, diabetes, and viral infections. An important contributory role for corticosteroids is also likely in triggering serous retinopathy.

Arterial hypertension

Arterial hypertension may lead to typical retinal lesions characterized by arteriolar narrowing, tortuosity, and arteriovenous nicking (Figure 16.3). In the case of severe hypertension, cotton-wool spots, flame-shaped hemorrhages, and hard exudates may be seen at fundoscopy. Retinal detachment (Figure 16.4), disc edema, and optic atrophy may develop in patients with accelerated, uncontrolled hypertension. In patients with severe and long-standing hypertension, a marked, sudden reduction of blood pressure may

Table 16.4   Classification of viral retinitis

1   Classical acute necrotizing retinitis
2   Slowly progressive necrotizing retinitis
3   Occlusive retinal arteritis
4   Progressive retinal necrosis

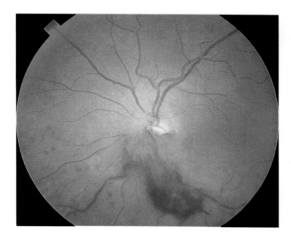

Figure 16.5   Diabetic retinopathy with retinal edema, hemorrhage, and vessel proliferation. (Courtesy of Professor R Ratiglia, University of Milan.)

cause infarction of the optic nerve and visual loss. In other patients, blindness may occur as the result of a cortical infarction.

Viral retinitis

A number of viral infections may lead to severe retinal complications. Various clinical forms may occur (Table 16.4).

Cytomegalovirus retinitis is the most common ocular opportunistic infection in transplant recipients. It is often asympyomatic upon initial examination and bilateral in 60% of cases. It usually involves the posterior pole, and may cause retinal detachment in about half of cases (Wagle *et al.*, 2002). Hemorrhagic and necrotizing retinitis are rapidly progressive in most cases. Intravenous ganciclovir (Lalezari *et al.*, 2002), valganciclovir, foscarnet, and cidofovir (Salmon-Ceron, 2002), are the antivirals most frequently used for CMV retinitis. Leflunomide has also been successfully employed in multidrug-resistant cases (Levi *et al.*, 2006). Each agent has unique advantages and disadvantages that enable the clinician to select a treatment approach tailored to the patient's needs and preferences.

Varicella zoster virus and *herpes simplex virus* may cause acute retinal necrosis. Prolonged antiviral treatment with intravenous acyclovir or oral valacyclovir and reduction of immunosuppression may be tried. However, the visual prognosis is usually poor.

Diabetic retinopathy

Some patients receive renal transplantation because of a previous diabetic nephropathy, and at least 20–25% of renal transplant recipients may develop an overt diabetes *de novo*. The progression of renal and retinal lesions is almost parallel in diabetic patients, and hence the term diabetic renal–retinal syndrome has been introduced. Diabetic retinopathy is characterized by retinal edema, retinal ischemia, and new vessel growth (Figure 16.5). This proliferative retinopathy can be accelerated by arterial hypertension.

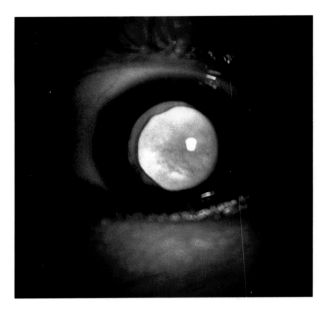

Figure 16.6 Subluxated cataract with dense central opacification. (Courtesy of Professor R Ratiglia, University of Milan.)

Treatment consists of panretinal photocoagulation. Vitrectomy may reduce the progression of proliferative retinopathy, by removing the vitreous hemorrhage and by inducing vitreoretinal traction (Steinmetz et al., 2002).

Serous central retinopathy

This is a disorder in which fluid collects under the central retina (macular area) and disrupts central vision. The cause is unknown. Symptoms include blurred central vision and metamorphopsia. Some patients also develop floaters. Retinal detachment and diffuse retinal pigment epitheliopathy may occur. Renal failure, fluid and electrolyte imbalance, and hypertension may contribute to the pathogenesis of this disorder, but the most important role is probably played by *corticosteroids* (Polak et al., 1995; Fawzi et al., 2006). The reduction of corticosteroids and laser photocoagulation may be tried in order to improve the bad visual prognosis (Kaiserman and Or, 2005).

Cataract

Cataract is the most frequent ocular complication in transplant recipients (Figure 16.6). Posterior subcapsular cataracts have been reported in 20–40% of renal transplant recipients upon slit-lamp examination (First 1993; Pai et al., 2000). Older subjects, diabetics, and patients who have received long-term hemodialysis or pulse corticosteroid therapy are more susceptible to develop cataract. The etiopathogenetic role of *corticosteroids* is well established, and a correlation between the development of cataract and the dose of corticosteroid has been found (Hardie et al., 1992). Today, with the use of small doses of corticosteroids, the risk of cataract is decreased, although some patients show an exquisite sensitivity to these agents. Steroid-free immunosuppression may significantly reduce the risk of cataract in renal transplant recipients (Matas et al., 2005). However, in a randomized prospective trial, a small number of patients given cyclosporine alone developed cataract (Ponticelli et al., 1997). A cataractogen role for *cyclosporine* with broader cataract types and a progressive course has been confirmed by more recent studies (Pai et al., 2000). Regular screening of visual acuity and appropriate surgery for posterior subcapsular or severe cataract are recommended.

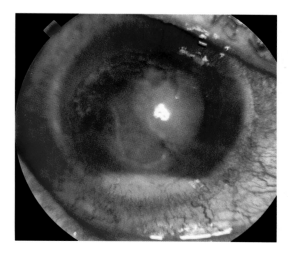

Figure 16.7 Endophthalmitis in a transplant patient with severe sepsis. (Courtesy of Professor R Ratiglia, University of Milan.)

Glaucoma

An increase in intraocular pressure can be found in 1–19% of transplant patients (Jayamanne and Porter, 1998, Asano *et al.*, 1998). The main factor responsible for ocular hypertension and glaucoma is certainly *corticosteroid* therapy (Jones and Rhee, 2006). An unusual sensitivity to corticosteroids in aqueous outflow may lead to an increased resistance to outflow, possibly through an influence on glycosaminoglycans or phagocytic activity in the trabecular network. An association between systemic hypertension and glaucoma has also been found. Common pathogenetic mechanisms in ciliary and renal tubular epithelia may explain the coincidence of glaucoma and systemic hypertension (Langman *et al.*, 2005). Ocular hypertension is usually asymptomatic, and may be detected only on routine eye examination.

Treatment of glaucoma is aimed to reduce the production of intraocular fluid (beta-blockers, carbonic anhydrase inhibitors, cholinesterase α_2-antagonists) or to increase the drainage of intraocular fluid (adrenergic agents, cholinergic drugs, prostaglandin-related drugs). Laser surgery is also used to allow better drainage of intraocular fluid. Eye-lotion treatment with beta-blocker alone or in combination with the above-mentioned drugs may be effective, and allows safe continuation of the administration of corticosteroids. However, a few predisposed patients may develop acute glaucoma.

Drug-induced blurred vision

Blindness is an extremely rare complication of *cyclosporine*. It is completely reversible after drug withdrawal. A single case of permanent blindness after intravenous infusion of cyclosporine has been reported (Esterl *et al.*, 1996). Transient blurred vision may also occur after the first injection of the anti-CD3 monoclonal antibody *OKT3* (Thaisetthawatkul *et al.*, 2001). Blurred vision and headache, due to intracranial hypertension, may occur in children after rapid *tapering of corticosteroids*. The symptoms of intracranial hypertension usually reverse completely, but some children may have permanent visual loss and blindness. All patients receiving high-dose corticosteroids who complain of headache or blurred vision after rapid tapering of steroids should have an ophthalmoscopic examination to exclude this complication. Optic nerve sheath decompression should be considered when medical treatment fails (Patrocinio *et al.*, 2005).

Miscellaneous

Bacterial and fungal infections may be responsible for rare cases of *endophthalmitis* (Figure 16.7). Apart from retinitis, herpes viruses can also cause keratitis. Exceptionally, *ocular neoplasias* may also occur in transplant patients. They include lymphoma of the vitreous, keratoacanthoma, or squamous-cell carcinoma of the eyelids. Persisting hyperparathyroidism and hypercalcemia may cause *corneal calcifications*. A rare case of progressive visual loss to no light perception in the left eye, 20/60 vision in the right eye, and *bilateral papilledema* was reported in a renal transplant patient. Arteriography demonstrated cerebral venous hypertension attributed to the functioning hemoaccess graft. Permanent graft occlusion normalized the papilledema, as well as visual defects in both eyes (Cuadra *et al.*, 2005).

References

Agraharkar A, McGillicuddy G, Ahuja T, Agraharkar M. Growth of intramedullary lipoma in a renal transplant recipient. Transplantation 2000; 69: 1509–11.

Asano T, Tsuji A, Nakajima F, et al. Ocular hypertension in renal transplant recipents. Transplant Proc 1998; 30: 3904–5.

Avivi I, Chakrabarti S, Kottaridis P, et al. Neurological complications following alemtuzumab-based reduced-intensity allogeneic transplantation. Bone Marrow Transplant 2004; 34: 137–42.

Bahat E, Akman S, Karpuzoglu G, et al. Visceral Kaposi's sarcoma with intracranial metastasis: a rare complication of renal transplantation. Pediatr Transplant 2002; 6: 505–8.

Bechstein WO. Neurotoxicity of calcineurin inhibitors: impact and clinical management. Transpl Int 2000; 13: 313–26.

Bradfield YS, Kushner BJ, Gangnon RE. Ocular complications after organ and bone marrow transplantation in children. J AAPOS 2005; 9: 426–32.

Brennan KC, Lowe LH, Yeaney GA. Pediatric central nervous system posttransplant lymphoproliferative disorder. AJNR Am J Neuroradiol 2005; 26: 1695–7.

Brouns R, De Deyn PP. Neurological complications in renal failure: a review. Clin Neurol Neurosurg 2004; 107: 1–16.

Bulsara KR, Baron PW, Tuttle-Nwehall JE, et al. Guillain–Barré syndrome in organ and bone marrow transplant patients. Transplantation 2001; 71: 1169–83.

Centers for Disease Control. West Nile virus infection in organ donor and transplant recipients – Georgia and Florida 2002. JAMA 2002; 288: 1465–6.

Charpentier B, Hiesse C, Lantz O, et al. Evidence that anti-human necrosis factor monoclonal antibody prevents OKT3-induced acute syndrome. Transplantation 1992; 54: 997–1002.

Collazos J. Opportunistic infections of the CNS in patients with AIDS: diagnosis and treatment. Drugs 2003; 17: 869–87.

Corruble E, Buhl C, Esposito D, et al. Psychosis associated with elevated trough tacrolimus blood concentrations after combined kidney–pancreas transplant. Int J Neuropsychopharmacol 2005; 29: 1–2.

Cuadra SA, Padberg FT, Turbin RE, et al. Cerebral venous hypertension and blindness: a reversible complication. J Vasc Surg 2005; 42: 792–5.

Darabi K, Abdel-Wahab O, Dzik WH. Current usage of intravenous immune globulin and the rationale behind it: the Massachusetts General Hospital data and a review of the literature. Transfusion 2006; 46: 741–53.

De Maar EF, Kas-Deelen DM, de Jager AE, et al. Inflammatory demyelinating polyneuropathy in a kidney transplant patient with cytomegalovirus infection. Nephrol Dial Transplant 1999; 14: 2228–30.

Detry O, Honore P, Hans MF. Organ donors with primary central nervous system tumors. Transplantation 2000; 70: 244–8.

Dhillon SS, Sarac E. Lumbosacral plexopathy after dual kidney transplantation. Am J Kidney Dis 2002; 36:1045–8.

Doganay M. Listerosis: clinical presentation. FEMS Immunol Med Microbiol 2003; 35: 173–5.

Dohgu S, Kataoka Y, Ikesue H, et al. Involvement of glial cells in cyclosporine-increased permeability of brain endothelial cells. Cell Mol Neurobiol 2000; 20: 781–6.

El-Sabrout RA, Radovancevis B, Ankoma-Sey V, Van Buren C. Guillain-Barré syndrome after solid organ transplantation. Transplantation 2001; 71: 1311–16.

Esterl RM Jr, Gupta N, Garvin PJ. Permanent blindness after cyclosporine nephrotoxicity in a kidney–pancreas recipient. Clin Neuropharmacol 1996; 19: 259–66.

Fawzi AA, Holland GN, Kreiger AE, et al. Central serous chorioretinopathy after solid organ transplantation. Ophthalmology 2006; 113: 813.e1–5.

Fehr T, Bossart W, Wahe C, Binswanger U. Disseminated varicella infection in adult renal allograft recipients: four cases and a review of the literature. Transplantation 2002; 73: 608–11.

First MR. Long-term complications after transplantation. Am J Kidney Dis 1993; 22: 477–86.

Fishman JA, Rubin RH. Infection in organ-transplant recipients. N Engl J Med 1998; 338: 1741–51.

Flynn JT, Bunchman TE, Sherbotie JR. Indications, results and complications of tacrolimus conversion in pediatric renal transplantation. Pediatr Transplant 2001; 5: 439–46.

Forgacs B, Merhav HJ, Lappin J, Mieles L. Successful conversion to rapamycin for calcineurin inhibitor-related neuro-toxicity following liver transplantation. Transplant Proc 2005; 37: 1912–14.

Grotz WH, Breitenfeldt MK, Braune SW, et al. Calcineurin-inhibitor induced pain syndrome (CIPS): a severe disabling complication after organ transplantation. Transpl Int 2001; 14: 16–23.

Gulley ML, Swinnen LJ, Plaisance KT, et al. Tumor origin and CD20 expression in posttransplant lymphoproliferative disorder occurring in solid organ transplant recipients: implication for immune based therapy. Transplantation 2003; 79: 959–64.

Hardie I, Matsunami C, Hilton A, et al. Ocular complications in renal transplant recipients. Transplant Proc 1992; 24: 177.

Howard RJ, Patton PR, Reed AI. The changing causes of graft loss and death after kidney transplantation. Transplantation 2002; 73: 1923–8.

Jayamanne DG, Porter R. Ocular morbidity following renal transplantation. Nephrol Dial Transplant 1998; 13:2070–3.

Jones R 3rd, Rhee DJ. Corticosteroid-induced ocular hypertension and glaucoma: a brief review and update of the literature. Curr Opin Ophthalmol 2006; 17: 163–7.

Kaiserman I, Or R. Laser photocoagulation for central serous retinopathy associated with graft-versus-host disease. Ocul Immunol Inflamm 2005; 13: 249–56.

Klinschmidt-De Masters BK, Marder BA. Naturally acquired West Nile virus encephalomyelitis in transplant recipients: clinical, laboratory, diagnostic and neuropathological features. Arch Neurol 2004; 61: 1210–20.

Koralnik IJ. Overview of the cellular immunity against JC virus in progressive multifocal leukoencephalopathy. J Neurovirol 2002; 8 (Suppl 2): 59–65.

Kwak EJ, Vilchez RA, Randhawa P, et al. Pathogenesis and management of polyomavirus infection in transplant recipients. Clin Infect Dis 2002; 35: 1081–7.

Lacaille F, Hertz-Pannier L, Nassogne MC. Magnetic resonance imaging for the diagnosis of acute leucoencephalopathy in children treated with tacrolimus. Neuropediatrics 2004; 35: 130–3.

Lalezari JP, Friedberg DN, Bissett J, et al. High-dose oral ganciclovir treatment for cytomegalovirus retinitis. J Clin Virol 2002; 24: 67–77.

Langman MJ, Lancashire RJ, Cheng KK, Stewart PM. Systemic hypertension and glaucoma: mechanisms in common and co-occurrence. Br J Ophthalmol 2005; 89: 960–3.

Larsen CM, Bauer RA, Thomas AM, Graybill JR. Amphotericin B and fluconazole, a potent combination therapy for cryptococcal meningitis. Antimicrob Agents Chemother 2004; 48: 985–91.

Levi ME, Mandava N, Chan LK, et al. Treatment of multidrug-resistant cytomegalovirus retinitis with systemically administered leflunomide. Transpl Infect Dis 2006; 8: 38–43.

Lynfield R, Herrin JT, Rubin RH. Varicella in pediatric renal transplant recipients. Pediatrics 1992; 98: 25–31.

Maccario M, Tarantino A, Nobile-Orazio E, Ponticelli C. *Campylobacter jejumi* bacteremia and Guillain–Barré syndrome in a renal transplant recipient. Transpl Int 1998; 11: 439–42.

Maramattom BV, Wijdicks EF. Sirolimus may not cause neurotoxicity in kidney and liver transplant recipients. Neurology 2004; 65: 337–8.

Margreiter R, European Tacrolimus versus Ciclosporin Renal Transplant Study Group. Efficacy and safety of tacrolimus compared with ciclosporin microemulsion in renal transplantation: a randomised multicentre study. Lancet 2002; 359: 741–6.

Martinez AJ. The neuropathology of organ transplantation: comparison and contrast in 500 patients. Pathol Res Pract 1998; 194: 473–86.

Matas AJ, Kandaswamy R, Gillingham KJ, et al. Prednisone-free maintenance immunosuppression–a 5-year experience. Am J Transplant 2005; 5: 2473–8.

Mazzoni A, Pardi C, Bortoli M. Plasma exchange for polyradiculoneuropathy following kidney transplantation: a case report. Transplant Proc 2004; 36: 716–17.

Mori A, Tanaka J, Kobayashi S, et al. Fatal cerebral hemorrhage associated with cyclosporin A/FK 506–related encephalopathy after allogeneic bone marrow transplantation. Ann Hematol 2000; 79: 588–92.

Mylonakis E, Hohmann EL, Calderwood SB. Central nervous system infection with Listeria monocytogenes: 33 years experience at a general hospital and review of 776 episodes from the literature. Medicine (Baltimore) 1998; 77: 313–36.

Norman DJ, Kimball JA, Bennett WM, et al. A prospective, double-blind, randomized study of high- versus low-dose OKT3 induction immunosuppression in cadaveric renal transplantation. Transpl Int 1994; 5: 356–61.

Oliveras A, Roquer J, Puig JM, et al. Stroke in renal transplant recipients: epidemiology, predictive factors and outcome. Clin Transplant 2003; 17: 1–8.

Olson AD, Shope TC, Flynn JT. Pretransplant varicella vaccination is cost-effective in pediatric renal transplantation. Pediatric Transplant 2001; 5: 44–50.

Opelz G, Naujokat C, Volker D, et al. Disassociation between risk of graft loss and risk of non-Hodgkin lymphoma with induction agents in renal transplant recipients. Transplantation 2006; 81: 1227–33.

Ozturk S, Soyluk O, Gorcin S, et al. A rare post-transplant malignancy, cerebellar hemangioblastoma: a case report. J Nephrol 2005; 18: 781–2.

Pai RP, Mitchell P, Chow VC, et al. Posttransplant cataract: lessons from kidney–pancreas transplantation. Transplantation 2000; 69: 1108–114.

Parizel PM, Snoeck HW, van den Hauwe L, et al. Cerebral complications of murine monoclonal CD3 antibody (OKT3): CT and MR findings. AJNR Am J Neuroradiol 1997; 18: 1935–8.

Paterson DL, Singh N. Invasive aspergillosis in transplant recipients. Medicine 1999; 78: 123–38.

Patrocinio JA, Patrocinio LG, Junior FB, da Cunha AR. Endoscopic decompression of the optic nerve in pseudotumor cerebri. Auris Nasus Larynx 2005; 2: 199–203.

Penn I. The role of immunosuppression in lymphoma formation. Semin Immunopathol 1998; 20: 343–55.

Phan TG, O'Neill BP, Kurtin PJ. Posttransplant primary CNS lymphoma. Neuro-oncol 2000; 2: 229–38.

Pirzada NA, Morgenlander JC. Peripheral neuropathy in patients with chronic renal failure. A treatable source of discomfort and disability. Postgrad Med 1997; 102: 249–50.

Pittock SJ, Rabinstein AA, Edwards BS, Wijdicks FF. OKT3 neurotoxicity presenting as akinetic mutism. Transplantation 2003; 15: 1058–60.

Polak BCP, Baarsma GS, Snyers B. Diffuse retinal pigment epitheliopathy complicating systemic corticosteroid treatment. Br J Ophthalmol 1995; 79: 922–5.

Ponticelli C, Rivolta E, Tarantino A, et al. Rescue of severe steroid-resistant rejection with OKT3PAN. Transplant Proc 1987; 19: 1908–9.

Ponticelli C, Tarantino A, Segoloni GP, et al. A randomized study comparing three cyclosporine-based regimens in cadaveric renal transplantation. Italian Multicentre Study Group for Renal Transplantation (SIMTRe) J Am Soc Nephrol 1997; 8: 638–46.

Ponticelli C, Campise R. Neurological complications in kidney transplant recipients. J Nephrol 2005; 18: 521–8.

Rifai K, Kirchner GI, Bahr MJ, et al. A new side effect of immunosuppression: high incidence of hearing impairment after liver transplantation. Liver Transpl 2006; 12: 411–15.

Salmon-Ceron D. Cytomegalovirus infection: the point in 2001. HIV Med 2002; 2:255–9.

Salvati M, Frati A, Caroli E, et al. Glioblastoma in kidney transplant recipients. Report of five cases. J Neurooncol 2003; 63: 33–7.

Schwechheimer K, Hashemian A. Neuropathologic findings after organ transplantation. An autopsy study. Gen Diagn Pathol 1995; 141:35–9.

Sharma KR, Cross J, Santiago F, et al. Incidence of acute femoral neuropathy following renal transplantation. Arch Neurol 2002; 59:541–5.

Singh N, Husain S. Infections of the central nervous system in transplant recipients. Transpl Infect Dis 2000; 2:101–11.

Skiest DJ. Focal neurological disease in patients with acquired immunodeficiency syndrome. Clin Infect Dis 2002; 34:103–15.

Smith MR. Rituximab (monoclonal anti-CD20 antibody): mechanisms of action and resistance. Oncogene 2003; 22: 7359–68.

Snanoudj R, Durrbach A, Leblond V, et al. Primary brain lymphomas after kidney transplantation: presentation and outcome. Transplantation 2003; 76:930–7.

Steinmetz RL, Grizzard WS, Hammer ME. Vitrectomy for diabetic traction retinal detachment using the multiport illumination system. Ophthalmology 2002; 109: 2303–7.

Tahri A, Noel G, Figuerella-Branger D, et al. Epstein–Barr virus associated central nervous system leiomyosarcoma occurring after renal transplantation: case report and review of the literature. Cancer Radiother 2003; 7: 308–13.

Tan CT, Robinson PJ. Mechanisms of calcineurin inhibitor-induced neurotoxicity. Transplant Rev 2006; 20: 49–60.

Thaisetthawatkul P, Weinstock A, Kerr SL, Cohen ME. Muromonab-DC3-induced neurotoxicity: report of two siblings, one of whom had subsequent cyclosporin-induced neurotoxicity. J Child Neurol 2001; 16: 825–31.

Therrien R. Possible trimethoprim/sulfamethoxazole-induced aseptic meningitis. Ann Pharmacother 2004; 38:1863–7.

Torocsik HV, Curless RG, Post J, et al. FK-506-induced leukoencephalopathy in children with organ transplants. Neurology 1999; 52: 1497–500.

Van de Beek D, de Gans J, McIntyre P, Prasad K. Steroids in adults with acute bacterial meningitis: a systematic review. Lancet Infect Dis 2004; 3: 139–43.

Veerareddy PR, Vobalaboira V. Lipid-based formulations of amphotericin B. Drugs Today 2004; 40: 133–45.

Vilchez RA, Fung J, Kusne S. Cryptococcosis in organ transplant recipients. Am J Transplant 2002; 2: 575–80.

Wagle AM, Biswas J, Gopal L, Madhavan HN. Clinical profile and immunological status of cytomegalovirus retinitis in organ transplant recipients Indian J Ophthalmol 2002; 50: 115–21.

Wijdicks EF. Neurotoxicity of immunosuppressive drugs. Liver Transpl 2001; 7: 937–42.

Wijdicks EF, Torres VE, Schievink WI, Steriof S. Cerebral hemorrhage in recipients of renal transplantation. Mayo Clin Proc 1999; 74: 111–12.

Wolkowitz OM, Lupien SJ, Bigler E, et al. The 'steroid dementia syndrome': an unrecognized complication of gluco-corticoid treatment. Ann NY Acad Sci 2004; 1032: 191–4.

17

HEMATOLOGIC COMPLICATIONS

Hematologic complications are frequent in renal transplant patients. They can involve all types of blood cells and can be triggered by a large number of factors which can cause bone marrow depression or peripheral destruction. Hematologic abnormalities may be mild and reversible or severe and life-threatening. In this chapter the most frequent hematologic abnormalities that may be seen in renal transplant recipients are reviewed, with the exclusion of neoplasias which are treated in Chapter 11.

Anemia

According to the World Health Organization (1968), anemia is defined by hemoglobin levels < 12 g/dl in women and < 13 g/dl in men. Most patients are anemic at the time of transplantation and suffer from a further decrease of hemoglobin levels in the early post-transplant period, which may be caused by blood loss during surgery, frequent blood samples, and/or insufficient erythropoietin production due to delayed graft function. After 1–2 weeks, in most patients with successful renal transplantation hemoglobin gradually increases, reaching normal values within 2–3 months (Beshara et al., 1997; Van Biesen et al., 2005). Little attention has been paid to the problem of anemia in the late post-transplant period. Recent papers, however, have pointed out that anemia is a frequent complication, occuring in between 30 and 40% of renal transplant recipients (Yorgin et al., 2002a; Lorenz et al., 2002; Vanrenterghem et al., 2003). Post-transplant anemia is more frequent in women (Mix et al., 2003), and is particularly frequent in children (Yorgin et al., 2002b; Mitsenef et al., 2005).

Causes of post-transplant anemia

There are several causes of anemia in renal transplant recipients (Table 17.1).

The most frequent cause of post-transplant anemia is *graft dysfunction*, which causes erythropoietin deficiency or resistance. A strong correlation between anemia and serum creatinine has been found both in children (Yorgin et al., 2002b) and in adults (Lorenz et al., 2002; Vanrenterghem et al., 2003). An association between acute rejection and anemia has also been reported in children, probably because a cluster of genes related to hemoglobin synthesis are altered in rejecting patients (Chua et al., 2003).

Iron deficiency is strongly associated with post-transplant anemia (Lorenz et al., 2002; Yorgin et al., 2002b). However, etiological diagnosis may be difficult, as markers of iron deficiency, such as ferritin or transferrin saturation, are frequently inconclusive because of the presence of inflammation and infection (Joist et al., 2006). Anemia associated with iron deficiency may be the first sign of occult gastrointestinal bleeding due to ulcer or malignancy. Persistence of anemia in a patient with normal allograft function should prompt a search for occult sepsis, gastrointestinal bleeding, neoplasia, iron deficiency, or vitamin B_{12} deficiency.

Azathioprine and *mycophenolate salts* can cause bone marrow suppression. Anemia caused by these inhibitors of purine synthesis is usually associated with leukopenia and thrombocytopenia, but rare cases of pure red-cell aplasia have also been reported (Arbeiter et al., 2000). Azathioprine is commonly associated with macrocytosis, but without megaloblastic anemia (Kim et al., 1998). Some studies reported that anemia is more frequent with mycophenolate mofetil (MMF) than with azathioprine (Yorgin et al., 2002a; Vanrenterghem et al., 2003).

The *anti-mTOR (mammalian target of rapamycin) agents* can also cause anemia. In a comparative study in renal transplant recipients, Augustine et al. (2005) found that sirolimus is associated more frequently with anemia than is MMF. Marked erythrocyte microcytosis without persistent anemia has been observed in patients treated with sirolimus and MMF (Kim et al., 2006).

Table 17.1   Main causes of post-transplant anemia
Graft dysfunction
Acute rejection
Malnutrition
Viral infection
Vitamin B_{12} deficiency
Iron deficiency (sepsis, GI bleeding, malignancy)
Nucleotide synthesis inhibitors
mTOR antagonists
ACE inhibitors
Angiotensin receptor blockers
Recurrent hemolytic uremic syndrome
De novo hemolytic uremic syndrome
Hemolytic anemia (anti-A, anti-B donor antibodies)
Hemolytic anemia (passenger lymphocytes)
Autoimmune hemolytic anemia

ACE inhibitors can reduce hematocrit levels by 10% or more in renal transplant patients (Julian *et al.*, 1998). About 43% of patients may develop anemia within 6 weeks after starting treatment with *angiotensin II receptor antagonists* (Ersoy *et al.*, 2005). It has been hypothesized that these agents may function by decreasing insulin-like growth factor-I, which has been demonstrated to promote erythropoiesis (Morrone *et al.*, 1997; Brox *et al.*, 1998).

Cytomegalovirus and *other viral infections* are often associated with anemia. The diagnosis is usually easy because of the accompanying symptoms. More difficult can be the diagnosis of *B19 parvovirus infection*, which can cause chronic anemia and pancytopenia (Yango *et al.*, 2002; Arzouk *et al.*, 2006). In renal transplant patients with recurrent parvovirus B-associated anemia, the administration of intravenous immunoglobulins may obtain positive conversion and long-term remission (Kumar *et al.*, 2005). It should be remembered that *antiviral agents* may cause bone marrow suppression (Danese and Del Tacca, 2004).

Protein energy malnutrition and *chronic inflammation* have also been found to be independently associated with anemia in renal transplant recipients (Molnar *et al.*, 2005).

Symptoms and consequences

The *symptoms* of anemia are mainly represented by fatigability, dizziness, and palpitations. In severe anemia, patients often complain of headache, dizziness, tinnitus, and vertigo. The degree to which symptoms occur depends on several factors. If the anemia develops slowly there is time for compensatory adjustment to the reduced red blood cell mass, and the patient may remain asymptomatic. When there is severe anemia, a hyperdynamic state may develop, and the patient may complain of palpitations and the above-mentioned symptoms. Patients with an underlying cardiovascular disease may have aggravation of angina pectoris or claudicatio intermittens. The main physical signs are pallor, tachycardia, and a systolic ejection murmur.

In the past few years, an increasing number of data suggest that anemia may be responsible for *cardiac complications*. In acute post-hemorrhagic anemia, the drop in hemoglobin dramatically reduces the oxygen transport and delivery to tissues. Tachycardia secondary to anemia leads to a shorter diastolic phase and a reduction in blood pressure, which may result in myocardial damage in patients with coronary disease. As

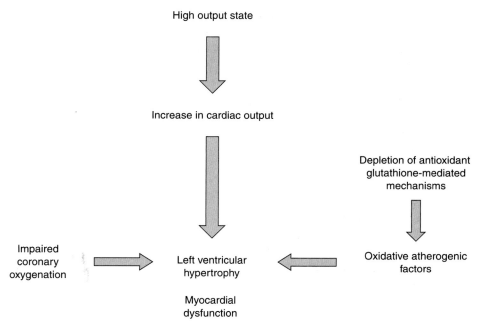

High output state

Increase in cardiac output

Depletion of antioxidant
glutathione-mediated
mechanisms

Impaired
coronary
oxygenation

Left ventricular
hypertrophy

Oxidative atherogenic
factors

Myocardial
dysfunction

Figuer 17.1 Cardiac effects of anemia

a matter of fact, in patients with gastrointestinal bleeding, a value of hemoglobin <8.2 g/dl was an independent variable associated with myocardial injury (Bellotto *et al.*, 2005). Chronic anemia is also a risk factor for cardiac events in the general adult population. In a retrospective study it was found that the percentage of hypochromic cells was an independent risk factor for mortality in kidney transplant recipients (Winkelmayer *et al.*, 2004), and the combination of decreased renal function and anemia is associated with an increasing risk of cardiovascular events and mortality (Astor *et al.*, 2006). Several factors may contribute to the development or aggravation of cardiovascular disease (Figure 17.1). In anemic dialysis patients, tachycardia and high cardiac output increase the ventricular mass index, leading to left ventricular hypertrophy (London, 2003). In transplant patients, the high output state coupled with impaired coronary oxygenation may trigger circulatory congestion and cause myocardial dysfunction (Rigatto *et al.*, 2002; Levin, 2002). On the other hand, as red blood cells represent a paramount antioxidant system, anemia may also lead to the depletion of glutathione-mediated antioxidant mechanisms with consequent prevalence of oxidative atherogenic factors (Campise *et al.*, 2003).

Treatment

As renal transplant patients are particularly susceptible to cardiovascular events, correction of anemia should be recommended. Treatment depends on the precipitating cause. Anemia caused by viral or bacterial infection may respond favorably to treatment of the infection. Corticosteroids may be useful in cases of autoimmune hemolytic anemia (see later). In the case of macrocytic anemia, folate or vitamin B_{12} should be administered. Iron depletion is a frequent cause of post-transplant anemia. In the case of hypochromic, microcytic anemia with additional signs of iron deficiency, an iron supplement should be given while searching for the underlying cause of anemia.

Most cases of post-transplant anemia are related to an insufficient production of erythropoietin. There is little information about the use of *recombinant erythropoietin* (EPO) in the treatment of post-transplant anemia. In a European survey, only 18% of transplant patients with severe anemia were treated with EPO (Vanrenterghem *et al.*, 2003). A number of clinicians are concerned about the risk of hypertension,

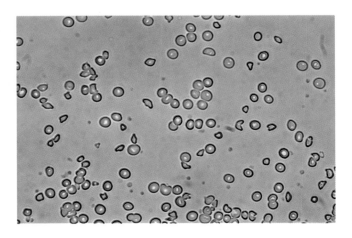

Figure 17.2 Microangiopathic haemolytic anemia in a patient with a de novo posttransplant haemolytic uremic syndrome. Note the fragmented, irregular erthrocytes

thrombotic complications, and/or graft dysfunction with EPO. However, some data suggest that EPO therapy may retard the progression of chronic kidney disease. Becker *et al.* (2002) followed 109 renal transplant patients who received EPO early after transplantation, and 57 given EPO after 10 months or more. The slope of plasma creatinine did not change in patients who received early EPO, while it improved significantly in patients given late EPO. Moreover, the latter group of patients showed a trend toward longer graft survival compared with a group of similar control patients. More recently, McDevitt *et al.* (2005) found no adverse events in 36 renal transplant recipients treated with darbepoetin alfa. The National Kidney Foundation recently provided recommendations for the use of EPO in renal transplant recipients (KDOQI, 2006).

Hemolytic–uremic syndrome

Hemolytic–uremic syndrome (HUS) is a well-recognized complication of renal transplantation. The typical HUS is characterized by acute renal failure, thrombocytopenia, and microangiopathic hemolytic anemia, i.e. severe anemia associated with fragmented red cells (Figure 17.2), unconjugated hyperbilirubinemia, decreased or absent haptoglobin, elevated serum lactate dehydrogenase, and reticulocytosis. It must be pointed out, however, that in transplant recipients not all the hematologic signs and symptoms may be present. Renal lesions are characterized by typical thrombotic microangiopathy, with mucinoid intimal thickening and necrosis of small arteries and arterioles, and glomeruli thrombi.

Recurrent HUS

Most cases of HUS occur in children, and are associated with diarrhea, usually related to exotoxins produced by *Escherichia coli* 0157:H7. These cases do not recur after transplantation (Ferraris *et al.*, 2002). Among the *non-diarrheal forms*, some cases may occur in several members of the same family and may present at any age (Table 17.2). About 30–50% of non-diarrheal HUS (either familial or not) may have a mutation in complement factor I or its cofactors, membrane cofactor protein (MCP) and particularly factor H. Factor I downregulates the activity of both classical and alternative complement pathways. Thus, a deficit in factor I or factor H can cause an overactivity of complement, with consequent endothelial damage and the development of thrombotic microangiopathy. Patients with genetic mutations of factor I or factor H almost regularly show a recurrence of HUS after renal transplantation, while patients with a mutation of MCP only rarely have a recurrence (Atkinson *et al.*, 2005).

Recurrent HUS usually develops in the *early post-transplant period*. Many patients show the typical clinical features and renal failure. However, some cases of recurrence are characterized by rapidly progressive graft dysfunction without the typical signs and symptoms of HUS. The *prognosis* is poor, with a

Table 17.2   Risk of recurrence of the different forms of hemolytic–uremic syndrome after renal transplantation

Forms of hemolytic–uremic syndrome	Risk of recurrence after transplantation
Post-diarrheal (D+)	No recurrence
Non post-diarrheal (D–) or atypical HUS	70%
Mutation in factor H	80%
Mutation in factor I	80–100%
Mutation in MCP	10%
Idiopathic	33–56%
Familial	80–100%

Table 17.3   Possible attempts to avoid HUS recurrence and its consequences

Try to avoid calcineurin inhibitors and anti-mTOR agents
Prolonged plasma infusions or plasma exchange
In failing cases, intravenous immunoglobulins or rituximab

patient survival rate of 50% at 3 years (Reynolds et al., 2003). Particularly ominous is the recurrence of atypical hemolytic–uremic syndrome in adults (Artz et al., 2003) and in patients with a genetic deficit of complement factor H (Ruggenenti, 2002).

Treatment is disappointing (Table 17.3). Plasmapheresis or large plasma infusions may transiently increase the serum levels of factor I and factor H and obtain recovery of thrombocytopenia and microangiopathic hemolytic anemia, but are only rarely effective in preventing renal damage (Gerber et al., 2003). Intravenous immunoglobulins (Banerjee et al., 2003) and rituximab (Yassa et al., 2005) were successfully used as rescue treatment in two patients. A few attempts with simultaneous liver and kidney transplantation failed (Cheong et al., 2004; Remuzzi et al., 2005).

De novo HUS

A *de novo* HUS may be triggered by *cyclosporine* (Franz et al., 1998; Zarifian et al., 1999), *tacrolimus* (Trimarchi et al., 1999; Pham et al., 2000), *sirolimus* (Robson et al., 2003), or *OKT3* (Doutrelepont et al., 1992). More rarely, HUS in allograft recipients is associated with *influenza A* (Asaka et al., 2000) or *cytomegalovirus* infection (Waiser et al., 1999). Cases of HUS have also been reported as a consequence of *E. coli* infection (Chandler et al., 2002), and may be paradoxically worsened by antibiotic therapy directed against *E. coli*. Other risk factors include younger age of the recipient, older age of the donor, and female sex.

The *pathogenesis* of *de novo* HUS is still poorly understood. It is possible that the endothelial lesions caused by ischemia–reperfusion injury, viral infection, and/or rejection may be amplified by the endothelial lesions caused by calcineurin inhibitors. These drugs increase the production of vasoconstrictor agents, such as endothelin, thromboxane A_2, and angiotensin II, while decreasing the vasodilators nitric oxide and prostacyclin. In turn, angiotensin II may enhance the synthesis of plasminogen activator inhibitor. As a result, there is an antifibrinolysis environment that, coupled with the pronecrotic activity of calcineurin

Table 17.4 Different steps of treatment in de novo post-transplant hemolytic–uremic syndrome

Drug-induced	Infection-induced
Stop the offending drug	Treat concomitant viral or bacterial infection aggressively
Plasma infusion or plasma exchange	Plasma infusion or plasma exchange
In refractory cases try intravenous immunoglobulins	In refractory cases try intravenous immunoglobulins

inhibitors, may favor the development of thrombotic microangiopathy. Anti-mTOR agents may act as subsequent aggressors, as they may downregulate the expression of vascular endothelial growth factor, which is required for repairing the endothelial lesions (Schrijvers et al., 2004). A pathogenetic hypothesis is that HUS is linked to deficient production of a metalloprotease called ADAMTS 13, which cleaves the multimers of von Willebrand factor. A deficiency of ADAMTS 13 may be caused either by a congenital defect or by the production of autoantibodies against this cleaving protease (Tsai and Lian, 1998). Although the role of these abnormalities in post-transplant HUS is still unclear, a defective activity of ADAMTS 13 has been reported in a few cases of post-transplant HUS (Pham et al., 2002; Nakazawa et al., 2003).

The *clinical* presentation may be variable. Usually, *de novo* HUS develops in the early post-transplant days (Artz et al., 2003), but may also occur later, even 2 years after transplantation (Katafuchi et al., 1999). Some patients may show the typical clinical and laboratory features of HUS, although milder than those seen in non-transplant patients. Other patients may show progressive graft dysfunction often associated with hypertension and mild anemia. In these cases, the differential diagnosis from vascular rejection may be difficult, even with renal biopsy. Mononuclear and neutrophilic infiltration of the subendothelial layer, and C4d deposits in peritubular capillaries, indicate a diagnosis of vascular rejection. However, overlap of these features has been reported (Mauiyyedi et al., 2002).

The *prognosis* is less severe than with recurrent HUS. It largely depends on the underlying histologic features. Patients with isolated glomerular lesions (Bren et al., 2005), those who have received a kidney from a living donor (Wiener et al., 1997), and those without systemic signs and symptoms of HUS (Schwimmer et al., 2003) usually have a good prognosis if the diagnosis is made early and appropriate therapeutic measures are taken.

Treatment is not well defined (Table 17.4). Withdrawal of the offending drug may resolve the disease, particularly when thrombotic microangiopathy is localized only in the graft (Schwimmer et al., 2003). However, not all cases respond to this maneuver. Some investigators reported reversal of HUS by switching from cyclosporine to tacrolimus (Franz et al., 1998) or from tacrolimus to sirolimus (Yango et al., 2002). However, it should be remembered that all calcineurin inhibitors and anti-mTOR agents may potentially lead to HUS. As a deficiency of a specific plasma protease responsible for the degradation of von Willebrand factor may play a role in the pathogenesis of HUS (Furlan et al., 1998), plasma infusion may be helpful for alleviating severe thrombocytopenia. Also, in transplant patients, plasma exchange in addition to withdrawal of the offending drug resulted in excellent results in several experiences (Trimarchi et al., 1999; Pham et al., 2002; Karthikeyan et al., 2003). In order to remove or neutralize potential autoantibodies directed against ADAMTS 13, plasmapheresis (Karthikeyan et al., 2003) and high-dose intravenous immunoglobulins (Hochstetler et al., 1994; Gatti et al., 2003) have been used with success in renal transplant recipients. In the few cases triggered by cytomegalovirus infection, specific antiviral treatment may obtain recovery of HUS. As a practical recommendation, kidney transplant recipients should have not only baseline but also frequent post-transplant determination of hemoglobin, platelets, lactate dehydrogenase, reticulocytes, and haptoglobin to detect HUS early (Santos *et al.*, 2003). Patients developing post-transplant HUS should first stop calcineurin inhibitors or mTOR inhibitors, which might be replaced by mycophenolic acid. Plasma infusions, plasmapheresis, and/or intravenous imunoglobulins (0.4 g/kg body weight) should be given in patients with microangiopathic anemia and/or severe thrombocytopenia.

Hemolytic anemia

Minor ABO incompatibility

Hemolytic anemia may occur in transplant recipients with minor ABO incompatibility. Patients of group A receiving a kidney of group O or patients of group AB receiving a kidney of group A or B may develop hemolytic anemia, the risk being higher in patients given cyclosporine (Ramsey, 1991). Hemolysis may be triggered by anti-A or anti-B antibodies of the donor or by autoantibodies produced by passenger B lymphocytes (Elhence *et al.*, 1998). In the latter case, a subtype of B cells resistant to cyclosporine would produce anti-A or anti-B antibodies. The hemolysis may be severe enough to require blood transfusions. Spontaneous recovery may occur after 7–10 days. Withdrawal of cyclosporine and the administration of high-dose prednisone is the treatment suggested in the most severe cases. Good results have also been reported by replacing cyclosporine with tacrolimus, which might be more effective for B-cell suppression (Debska-Slizien *et al.*, 2003).

Rhesus D unmatching

Rarely, massive hemolytic anemia with a positive direct antiglobulin test may occur in the early post-transplant period, independent from an ABO incompatibility. Anemia is often associated with thrombocytopenia and requires repeated blood transfusions. In the few cases described, anemia remitted spontaneously within 2 months. This type of anemia is caused by anti-rhesus D antibodies, probably produced by passenger lymphocytes (Frohn *et al.*, 2002; Pomper *et al.*, 2005).

Autoimmune anemia

Autoimmune hemolytic anemia may occur rarely after renal transplantation. The disease may be severe, with poor response to transfusions, pulse steroids, repeat plasma exchange treatments, and intravenous immunoglobulins. Switching from tacrolimus to sirolimus resulted in a prompt response in a recently reported case (Valentini *et al.*, 2006). On the basis of the larger experience in bone marrow transplant recipients, rituximab seems to be the first-line therapy for autoimmune hemolytic anemia refractory to corticosteroids (Endo *et al.*, 2004; Raj *et al.*, 2004).

Hemophagocytic syndrome

Hemophagocytosis is the consumption of hemopoietic cells by phagocytic cells such as activated monocytes/macrophages. The syndrome may be triggered by viruses (HIV, Epstein–Barr, herpes viruses, enteroviruses), bacterial infections causing leukopenia, drugs (phenytoin), lymphoproliferative disorders, solid tumors, systemic lupus erythematosus, ethylene glycol consumption, etc. The syndrome may also occur in renal transplant patients.

The first decription of Risdall *et al.* (1979) reported that 13 of 19 cases with hemophagocytic syndrome were renal transplant recipients. Since then, a number of cases in renal transplant recipients have been described (Calonge *et al.*, 1995; Kursat *et al.*, 1997; Karras *et al.*, 2004). Most of these cases were associated with viral, bacterial, or *Toxoplasma gondii* (Segall *et al.*, 2006) infections. Cases associated with T-cell lymphoma or HHV8-induced primary-effusion lymphoma have also been reported (Peeters *et al.*, 1997; Luppi *et al.*, 2002).

The *pathogenesis* of this syndrome is still unclear. However, the strict link between systemic inflammatory syndrome response and hemophagocytosis coupled with peripheral T cell expansion and deficient

Table 17.5   Possible pathogenesis of hemophagocytic syndrome

1   Failure to overcome infection
2   Overactivity of the immune system
3   Th1 cells activate macrophages
4   Activated macrophages escape NK cell control (genetic factors?) and proliferate
5   Uncontrolled activation and proliferation of macrophages lead to hemophagocytosis

natural killer activity often found in patients with hemophagocytic syndrome (Schmid *et al.*, 2006) strongly supports the hypothesis of a dysregulation in the inflammatory and immune response. Enhanced Th1 cytokine secretion (Chuang *et al.*, 2005), caused by a severe imbalance of IL-18/IL-18BP (Mazodier *et al.*, 2005), has also been documented in patients with hemophagocytic syndrome. The current view (Table 17.5) is that the immune system becomes overactive due to its inability to respond effectively to infections and/or shut down the immune response to such infections. Th1 cytokines would lead to macrophage activation and proliferation with escape of control by natural killer cell cytotoxicity activation (Verbsky and Grossman, 2006). The uncontrolled proliferation of highly activated macrophages eventually leads to hemophagocytosis. The discovery of genetic defects in the secretory pathway of natural killer cells (Villanueva *et al.*, 2005), and of effectors of lymphocyte cytotoxicity such as perforin (Risma *et al.*, 2006), in some patients with hemophagocytosis, further supports this hypothesis.

Clinically, the syndrome is characterized by fever, skin rash, pulmonary infiltrates, hepatosplenomegaly, weight loss, and lymphadenopathy. Neurologic symptoms are frequent in children. Laboratory tests show high serum ferritin levels, liver dysfunction, and a picture of disseminated intravascular coagulation with low factor V and fibrinogen, and severe pancytopenia, which is the most prominent laboratory feature. Bone marrow aspirate shows phagocytosis of hemopoietic cells by histiocytes–macrophages and a decreased number of megakaryocytes. However, the diagnosis is easily missed. If a transplant patient has fever of unknown origin, pancytopenia, and progressive development of multiorgan failure, hemophagocytic syndrome should always be borne in mind.

The *prognosis* is severe. There is a high rate of mortality, and many survivors lose allograft function. The largest series in renal transplant recipients reported that eight of 17 patients died and four of the survivors were submitted to graft nephrectomy (Karras *et al.*, 2004). The *treatment* of etiological factors, such as bacterial or viral infection, can improve the prognosis. High-dose corticosteroids and intravenous γ-globulins may be used to inhibit the release of cytokines by monocytes/macrophages. In non-transplanted patients, success has been obtained in single cases treated with etoposide (Aleem *et al.*, 2005) or infliximab (Henzan *et al.*, 2006).

Erythrocytosis

Erythrocytosis, or polycythemia, is defined as a hematocrit >52% in men and >49% in women. The incidence in renal transplant patients has been reported to vary between 8% (Sumrani *et al.*, 1993) and 22% (Qunibi *et al.*, 1991), being more frequent in males with good graft function (Kessler *et al.*, 1996). In about 30–40% of cases polycythemia may resolve spontaneously, but in the other patients it may persist for years. Many etiologic factors may contribute to post-transplant erythrocytosis (Table 17.6).

Pathogenesis

The pathogenesis of post-transplant erythrocytosis in still to be elucidated. The role of *erythropoietin* has been challenged, as EPO levels have generally been found to be in the normal range. Nevertheless, normal production of EPO in spite of erythrocytosis may be interpreted as an inappropriate secretion of

Table 17.6   Main causes of post-transplant erythrocytosis

Native kidney	Allograft	Patient characteristics
Acquired cystic disease	Graft artery stenosis	Male gender
Polycystic kidney disease	Hydronephrosis	Long-term dialysis
	Rejection-free	Arterial hypertension
	Well-functioning graft	Smoking
		Diabetes mellitus

EPO. In fact, in subjects with normal feedback, the increase in hemoglobin levels is associated with low, not normal, levels of EPO. Other factors may also contribute to post-transplant erythrocytosis. It has been shown that patients with polycythemia vera have elevated levels of *insulin-like growth factor binding protein-I* (IGFBP-1), which stimulates erythroid burst formation (Mirza *et al.*, 1997). Elevated levels of IGFBP-1 have been observed in renal transplant patients with erythrocytosis (Morrone *et al.*, 1997). The role of IGFBP-1 has been confirmed by the demonstration that proliferation of erythroid progenitors could be partially blocked by anti-IGFBP-1 in patients with erythrocytosis and elevated circulating levels of IGFBP-1 (Shih *et al.*, 1999). A role for *angiotensin II* has also be suggested. Angiotensin II can enhance erythro-poietin-stimulated erythroid proliferation through the activation of AT1 receptors present on erythroid progenitors (Mrug *et al.*, 1997). Moreover, angiotensin II might stimulate erythropoiesis as a growth factor (Vlahakos *et al.*, 2003). Erythrocytosis has been found to be more frequent in patients who have *never experienced rejection* and in those with *good graft function* (Einollahi *et al.*, 2005).

Symptoms and clinical outcome

About 60% of patients with post-transplant erythrocytosis experience malaise, headache, plethora, and dizziness. They may also suffer from arterial venous occlusive events associated with thrombocytosis, platelet dysfunction, and hypervolemia. In one study, 11 *thromboembolic* events occurred in 53 poly-cythemic transplant patients in spite of phlebotomies, an incidence significantly higher than in controls (Wickre *et al.*, 1983). Other investigators reported thromboembolic complications in 10–30% of cases (Vlahakos *et al.*, 2003). Moreover, erythrocytosis may increase the risk of *hypertension* and *cardiovascular* complications in renal transplant recipients (Kasiske *et al.*, 2000). It is reasonable to assume that, as in polycythemia vera, the higher is the hematocrit the higher is the risk of life-threatening complications.

Treatment

The goal of treatment of post-transplant erythrocytosis is to reduce the hematocrit to around 45%, a level at which the risk of complications can be minimized. In view of the role of angiotensin II in the pathogenesis of post-transplant erythrocytosis, there is a rationale for the use of *ACE inhibitors*, even because ACE inhibitors may inhibit IGF-I (Jimeno *et al.*, 2005) and induce apoptosis in erythrocyte progenitor cells (Glezerman *et al.*, 2003). As a matter of fact, ACE inhibitors (Beckingam *et al.*, 1995) can significantly reduce the hematocrit in patients with post-transplant erythrocytosis. *Angiotensin receptor blockers* (ARB) have also been used successfully (Julian *et al.*, 1998). Two randomized trials compared the effects of ACE inhibitors and ARB. Yildiz *et al.* (2001) assigned 27 transplant patients with erythrocytosis to receive enalapril 10 mg daily or losartan 50 mg daily for 8 weeks. A greater reduction in hemoglobin but a faster relapse was observed in patients given enalapril. Wang *et al.* (2002) compared the effects of 50 mg of losartan with 5 mg of enalapril in ten transplant patients with erythrocytosis. Enalapril reduced hemoglobin levels more markedly than did losartan. Circulating levels of IGF-I and erythropoietin were reduced with enalapril but not with losartan.

Repeated *phlebotomies* may be used in patients who do not respond to ACE inhibitors. The initial phlebotomy regimen may remove 500 ml of whole blood. The same aliquot may be removed after a few days until the hematocrit falls to 45%. As repeated phlebotomies may lead to iron deficiency, which prevents a rapid increase of hematocrit, some patients may maintain normal hematocrit with only two or three phlebotomies per year.

As ischemic native kidneys may produce erythropoietin, *bilateral nephrectomy* of the native kidney could improve post-transplant erythrocytosis in some cases (Friman et al., 1990).

Theophylline has also been used. This drug is an antagonist of adenosine, which is an important mediator in the biosynthesis of erythropoietin. In one study, the administration of theophylline, at a dose of 8 mg/kg per day for 8 weeks, significantly reduced the levels of hematocrit and erythropoietin in eight patients with post-transplant erythrocytosis (Bakris et al., 1990). However, in another controlled trial, aminophylline proved to be ineffective and inferior to enalapril (Mazzali and Filho, 1998). In a prospective cross-over study, fosinopril proved to be effective in reducing the hemoglobin levels while theophylline was ineffective and poorly tolerated by renal transplant patients (Trivedi and Lal, 2003).

The efficacy and safety of *anti-platelet drugs* in patients with post-transplant erythrocytosis has not been tested. However, as a controlled trial showed that low-dose aspirin (100 mg daily) can safely prevent thombotic complications in polycythemia vera (Landolfi et al., 2004), it is reasonable to administer such a therapy also to transplant patients with erythrocytosis.

Leukopenia

Leukopenia is relatively frequent in renal transplant recipients. A reduction in lymphocyte number is generally caused by immunosuppressive drugs. More worrying may be the development of severe neutropenia, which is an important risk factor for infection. Neutropenia may be considered mild with 1000–2000 cells per μl, moderate when neutrophils range between 500 and 1000 per μl, and severe when neutrophils are less than 500 per μl. In moderate–severe cases it is possible to increase rapidly the number of circulating neutrophils by the administration of granulocyte colony stimulating factor (GCSF) that can stimulate the growth and maturation of neutrophils, eosinophils, and monocytes as well as lymphocytes, platelets, and reticulocytes. The role of GCSF in preventing infection has been debated. However, in cancer patients, GCSF can reduce by 20% the risk of infection in neutropenic patients, being particularly helpful when given in association with prophylactic antibiotics (Pascoe and Cullen, 2006).

Causes of leukopenia

Leukopenia in renal transplant recipients is usually caused by one of two factors, namely toxic effects of drugs and infection.

Drug-induced leukopenia

A number of drugs may cause leukopenia, including several agents used for immunosuppression.

The risk of leukopenia with *azathioprine* is dose-dependent. At the doses currently used with these agents severe leukopenia is rare. However, as azathioprine is transformed into 6-mercaptopurine, which in turn inhibits purine synthesis, standard doses of azathioprine may cause granulocytopenia in patients with a genetic defect of thiopurine methyltransferase, which mediates the *S*-methylation of 6-mercaptopurine (Chocair et al., 1992). The frequency of leukopenia episodes is significantly higher in heterozygous patients, while homozygous patients are more susceptible to severe myelotoxicity (Kurzawski et al., 2005). Severe neutropenia may also occur when azathioprine is given in association with allopurinol, which blocks the enzyme xanthine oxidase, necessary to neutralize the active metabolites of 6-mercaptopurine. Thus, whenever allopurinol is added, the dose of azathioprine should be reduced to a half or a third, or, even better, the drug should be replaced by MMF or sodium mycophenolate, which do not release 6-mercaptopurine.

The risk of leukopenia with mycophenolic acid is increased in patients with high circulating levels of free mycophenolic acid (Weber et al., 2002), and may be further increased by hypoalbuminemia and renal function impairment (Borrows et al., 2006). An interaction between mycophenolic acid and valacyclovir may also lead to neutropenia (Royer et al., 2003).

The anti-mTOR agents *sirolimus* and *everolimus* may also cause leukopenia. Most cases respond to dose reduction. Only exceptionally is temporary suspension required (Hong and Kahan, 2000).

Profound and persistent lymphopenia making the patient more susceptible to infections particularly from viruses can be caused by *antilymphocyte antibodies*, such as antithymocyte globulins, anti-CD3 monoclonal antibodies, anti-CD52 monoclonal antibodies (Campath®-1H), and anti-CD20 monoclonal antibodies (rituximab).

Other drugs used in renal transplantation that may favor leukopenia are ganciclovir, trimethoprim–sulfamethoxazole, penicillins, and α-methyldopa.

Infection

A number of infections, particularly viral infections and overwhelming bacterial infections, may be associated with neutropenia. Severe leukopenia is generally present in hemophagocytic syndrome.

Thrombocytopenia

Thrombocytopenia is defined as a platelet count below 100 000/mm³. In renal transplant recipients, thrombocytopenia may be caused by immunosuppressive drugs such as purine synthesis inhibitors, anti-mTOR agents, antilymphocyte globulins, anti-CD3 monoclonal antibodies, or Campath-1H. CMV and other viral infections as well as antiviral agents are often associated with a low platelet count. Thrombocytopenia is a paramount sign of HUS, and is always present in hemophagocytic syndrome. Although rarely, thrombocytopenia may be caused by the administration of unfractionated heparin (Anderegg *et al.*, 2005).

Rare cases of early and severe *alloimmune thrombocytopenia* have been reported in organ transplant patients. Thrombocytopenia developed as a result of antiplatelet alloantibodies produced by passenger lymphocytes from the donor (West et al., 1999).

Autoimmune thrombocytopenia caused by autoantibodies has been described in a few patients with bone marrow transplantation (Tomonari *et al.*, 2001) or renal transplantation (Orchard *et al.*, 1997). We recently observed a case of severe autoimmune thrombocytopenia (1000 platelets/mm³) that occurred 20 years after renal transplantation in a patient with normal graft function given cyclosporine alone. Treatment with high-dose prednisone and intravenous immunoglobulins obtained a return of platelets to normal values within a few days.

The risk of hemorrhage is inversely proportional to the platelet count. Spontaneous hemorrhage may occur if the platelet count is lower than 20 000/mm³. Fever and anemia render thrombocytopenic patients more susceptible to bleeding. The treatment depends on the etiology. Cases caused by drugs usually respond to withdrawal of the offending agent. Plasma infusion or plasmapheresis may be useful in cases of thrombocytopenia associated with HUS. Splenectomy may be tried in severe cases of alloimmune thrombocytopenia. High-dose prednisone and intravenous immunoglobulins are needed in the case of autoimmune thombocytopenia (Cines and Blanchette, 2002).

References

Aleem A, Al Amoudi S, Al-Mashhadani S, Siddiqui N. Haemophagocytic syndrome associated with hepatitis-B virus infection responding to etoposide. Clin Lab Haematol 2005; 27: 395–8.

Anderegg BA, Baillie GM, Lin A, Lazarchick J. Heparin-induced thrombocytopenia in a renal transplant recipient. Am J Transplant 2005; 5: 1537–40.

Arbeiter K, Greenbaum L, Balzar E, et al. Reproducible erythroid aplasia caused by mycophenolate mofetil. Pediatr Nephrol 2000; 14: 195–7.

Artz MA, Steenbergen EJ, Hojitsma AJ, et al. Renal transplantation in patients with hemolytic uremic syndrome: high rate of recurrence and increased incidence of acute rejection. Transplantation 2003; 76: 821–6.

Arzouk N, Snanoudj R, Beauchamp-Nicoud A, et al. Parvovirus B19-induced anemia in renal transplantation: a role for rHuEPO in resistance to classical treatment. Transpl Int 2006; 19: 166–9.

Asaka M, Ishikawa I, Nakazawa T, et al. Hemolytic uremic syndrome associated with influenza A virus infection in an adult renal allograft recipient: case report and review of the literature. Nephron 2000; 84: 258–66.

Astor BC, Coresh J, Heiss G, et al. Kidney function and anemia as risk factors for coronary heart disease and mortality: the Atherosclerosis Risk in Communities (ARIC) Study. Am Heart J 2006; 151: 492–500.

Atkinson JP, Liszewski MK, Richards A, et al. Hemolytic uremic syndrome: an example of insufficient complement regulation on self-tissue. Ann NY Acad Sci 2005; 1056: 144–52.

Augustine JJ, Knauss TC, Schulak JA, et al. Comparative effects of sirolimus and mycophenolate mofetil on erythropoiesis in kidney transplant patients. Am J Transplant 2005; 4: 2001–6.

Bakris GL, Santer ER, Hussey JL, et al. Effects of theophylline on eythropoietin production in normal subjects and in patients with erythrocytosis after renal transplantation. N Engl J Med 1990; 323: 86–90.

Banerjee D, Kupin W, Roth D Hemolytic uremic syndrome after multivisceral transplantation treated with intravenous immunoglobulin. J Nephrol 2003; 16: 733–5.

Becker BN, Becker YT, Leverson GE, Heisey DM. Erythropoietin therapy may retard progression in chronic renal transplant dysfunction. Nephrol Dial Transplant 2002; 17: 1667–73.

Beckingham IJ, Woodrow G, Hinwood M, et al. A randomized placebo controlled study of enalapril in the treatment of erythrocytosis after renal transplantation. Nephrol Dial Transplant 1995; 10: 2316–20.

Bellotto F, Fagiuoli S, Plebani M, et al. Anemia and ischemia: myocardial injury in patients with gastrointestinal bleeding. Am J Med 2005; 118: 548–51.

Beshara S, Birgegard G, Goch J, et al. Assessment of erythropoiesis following renal transplantation. Eur J Haematol 1997; 58: 167–73.

Borrows R, Chusney G, Loucaidou M, et al. Mycophenolic acid 12-h trough level monitoring in renal transplantation: association with acute rejection and toxicity. Am J Transplant 2006; 6: 121–8.

Bren A, Pajek J, Grego K, et al. Follow-up of kidney graft recipients with cyclosporine-associated haemolytic–uraemic syndrome and thrombotic microangiopathy. Transplant Proc 37: 1889–91.

Brox AG, Mangel J, Hanley JA, et al. Erythrocytosis after transplantation represents an abnormality of insulin-like factor-1 and its binding proteins. Transplantation 1998; 66: 1053–8.

Calonge VM, Glotz D, Bouscary D, et al. Hemophagocytic histiocytosis in renal transplant recipients under cyclosporine therapy: report of two cases. Clin Transplant 1995; 9: 88–91.

Campise M, Bamonti F, Novembrino C, et al. Oxidative stress in kidney transplant patients. Transplantation 2003; 76: 1474–8.

Chandler WL, Jellacic S, Boster DR, et al. Prothrombotic coagulation abnormalities preceding the hemolytic uremic syndrome. N Engl J Med 2002; 346: 23–32.

Cheong HI, Lee BS, Kang HG, et al. Attempted treatment of factor H deficiency by liver transplantation. Pediatr Nephrol 2004; 19: 454–458.

Chocair PM, Duley JA, Simonds HA, Cameron JS. The importance of thiopurine methyltransferase activity for the azathioprine in transplant recipients. Transplantation 1992; 53: 1051–6.

Chua MS, Barry C, Chen X, et al. Molecular profiling of anemia in acute renal allograft rejection using DNA microarrays. Am J Transplant 2003; 3: 17–22.

Chuang HC, Lay JD, Hsieh WC, et al. Epstein–Barr virus LMP1 inhibits the expression of SAP gene and upregulates Th1 cytokines in the pathogenesis of hemophagocytic syndrome. Blood 2005; 106: 3090–6.

Cines DB, Blanchette VS. Immune thrombocytopenia. N Engl J Med 346: 995–1008.

Danesi R, Del Tacca M 2004; Hematologic toxicity of immunosuppressive treatment. Transplant Proc 2003; 36: 703–4.

Debska-Slizien A, Chamiemia A, Krol E. Hemolytic anemia after transplantation: analysis of case reports. Transplant Proc 2003; 35: 2233–7.

Doutrelepont JM, Abramowicz D, Florquin S, et al. Early recurrence of hemolytic uremic syndrome in a renal transplant recipient during prophylactic OKT3 therapy. Transplantation 1992; 53: 1378–83.

Einollahi B, Lessan-Pezeshki M, Nafar M, et al. Erythrocytosis after renal transplantation: review of 101 cases. Transplant Proc 2005; 37: 3101–2.

Elhence P, Sharma RK, Chaudhary RK, Gupta RK. Acquired hemolytic anemia after minor ABO incompatible renal transplantation. J Nephrol 1998; 11: 40–3.

Endo T, Nakao S, Koizumi K, et al. Successful treatment with rituximab for autoimmune hemolytic anemia concomitant with proliferation of Epstein–Barr virus and monoclonal gammopathy in a post-nonmyeloablative stem cell transplant patient. Ann Hematol 2004; 83: 114–16.

Ersoy A, Kahvecioglu S, Ersoy C, et al. Anemia due to losartan in hypertensive renal transplant recipients without posttransplant erythrocytosis. Transplant Proc 2005; 37: 2148–50.

Ferraris JR, Ramirez JA, Ruiz S, et al. Shiga toxin-associated hemolytic uremic syndrome: absence of recurrence after renal transplantation. Pediatr Nephrol 2002; 17: 809–14.

Franz M, Regele H, Schmaldienst S, et al. Posttransplant hemolytic uremic syndrome in adult retransplanted kidney graft recipients: advantage of FK506 therapy? Transplantation 1998; 66: 1258–62.

Friman S, Nyberg G, Blohmel I Erythrocytosis after renal transplantation: treatment by removal of native kidneys. Nephrol Dial Transplant 1990; 5: 969–73.

Frohn C, Jabs WJ, Fricke L, Goerg S Hemolytic anemia after transplantation: case report and differential diagnosis. Ann Hematol 2002; 81: 158–60.

Furlan M, Robles R, Galbusera M, et al. Von Willebrand factor-cleaving protease in thrombotic thrombocytopenic purpura and hemolytic uremic syndrome. N Engl J Med 1998; 339: 1578–84.

Gatti S, Arru M, Reggiani P, et al. Successful treatment of hemolytic uremic syndrome after liver–kidney transplantation. J Nephrol 2003; 16: 586–90.

Gerber A, Kirchhoff-Moradpour AH, Obieglo S, et al. Successful (?) therapy of hemolytic uremic syndrome with factor H abnormality. Pediatr Nephrol 2003; 18: 952–8.

Glezerman I, Patel H, Glicklich D, et al. Angiotensin-converting enzyme inhibition induces death receptor apoptotic pathways in erythroid precursors following renal transplantation. Am J Nephrol 2003; 23: 195–201.

Henzan T, Nagafuji K, Tsukamoto H, et al. Success with infliximab in treating refractory hemophagocytic lymphohistiocytosis. Am J Hematol 2006; 81: 59–61.

Hochstetler LA, Flanigan MJ, Lager DJ. Transplant-associated thrombotic microangiopathy: the role of IgG administration as initial therapy. Am J Kidney Dis 1994; 23: 444–50.

Hong JC, Kahan BD Sirolimus-induced thrombocytopenia and leukopenia in renal transplant recipients: risk factor, incidence, progression and management. Transplantation 2000; 69: 2085–90.

Jimeno L, Rodado R, Barrios Y, et al. Influence of angiotensin-converting enzyme polymorphism gene, IGF-1, and other factors in the response rate of hematocrit to enalapril treatment in patients with posttransplant erythrocytosis. Transplant Proc 2005; 37: 1012–13.

Joist H, Brennan DC, Coyne DW. Anemia in the kidney-transplant patient. Adv Chronic Kidney Dis 2006; 13: 4–10.

Julian BA, Brantley RR Jr, Barker CV, et al. Losartan, an angiotensin II type 1 receptor antagonist, lowers hematocrit in posttransplant erythrocytosis. J Am Soc Nephrol 1998; 6: 1104–8.

Karras A, Thervet E, Legendre C; for the Group Coopératif de Transplantation de l'Ile de France. Hemophagocytic syndrome in renal transplant recipients: report of 17 cases and review of the literature. Transplantation 2004; 77: 238–43.

Karthikeyan V, Parasuraman R, Shah V, et al. Outcome of plasma exchange therapy in thrombotic microangiopathy after renal transplantation. Am J Transplant 2003; 3: 1289–94.

Kasiske BL, Vazquez MA, Harmon WE, et al. Recommendations for the outpatient surveillance of renal transplant recipients. J Am Soc Nephrol 2000; 11: S1–6.

Katafuchi R, Saito S, Ikeda K, et al. A case of late-onset cyclosporine-induced hemolytic uremic syndrome resulting in renal graft loss. Clin Transplant 1999; 13 (Suppl 1): 54–8.

KDOQI; National Kidney Foundation IV. Clinical practice recommendations for anemia in chronic kidney disease in transplant recipients. Am J Kidney Dis 2006; 47 (Suppl 3): S109–16.

Kessler M, Heistin D, Mayeux D, et al. Factors predisposing to post-renal transplant erythrocytosis. A prospective matched-pair control study. Clin Nephrol 1996; 45: 83–9.

Kim CJ, Park KI, Inoue K, et al. Azathioprine-induced megaloblastic anemia with pancytopenia 22 years after living-related renal transplantation. Int J Urol 1998; 5: 100–2.

Kim MJ, Mayr M, Pechula M, et al. Marked erythrocyte microcytosis under primary immunosuppression with sirolimus. Transplant Int 2006; 19: 12–18.

Kumar J, Shaver MJ, Abul-Ezz S. Long-term remission of recurrent parvovirus-B associated anemia in a renal transplant recipient induced by treatment with immunoglobulin and positive conversion. Transpl Infect Dis 2005; 7: 30–3.

Kursat S, Cagirgan S, Ok E, et al. Haemophagocytic–histiocytic syndrome in renal transplantation. Nephrol Dial Transplant 1997; 12: 1058–60.

Kurzawski M, Dziewanowski K, Gawronska-Szklarz B, et al. The impact of thiopurine S-methyltransferase polymorphism on azathioprine-induced myelotoxicity in renal transplant recipients. Ther Drug Monit 2005; 27: 435–41.

Landolfi R, Marchioli R, Kutti J, et al. Efficacy and safety of low-dose aspirin in polycythemia vera. N Engl J Med 2004; 350: 114–24.

Levin A. Anemia and left ventricular hypertrophy in chronic kidney disease populations: a review of the current state of the knowledge. Kidney Int 2002; 64 (Suppl 80): S35–8.

London GM. Left ventricular hypertrophy: why does it happen? Nephrol Dial Transplant 18 2003; (Suppl 8): 2–6.

Lorenz M, Kletzmayr J, Perschl A, et al. Anemia and iron deficiency among long-term renal transplant recipients. J Am Soc Nephrol 2002; 13: 794–7.

Luppi M, Barozzi P, Rasini V, et al. Severe pancytopenia and hemophagocytosis after HHV8 primary infection in a renal transplant patient successfully treated with foscarnet. Transplantation 2002; 74: 131–2.

Mauiyyedi S, Crespo M, Collins AB, et al. Acute humoral rejection in kidney transplantation: II Morphology, immunopathology, and pathologic classification. J Am Soc Nephrol 2002; 13: 779–87.

Mazodier K, Marin V, Novick D, et al. Severe imbalance of IL18/IL18BP in patients with secondary hemophagocyticsyndrome. Blood 2005; 106: 3483–9.

Mazzali M, Filho GA. Use of aminophylline and enalapril in posttransplant polycythemia. Transplantation 1998; 65: 1461–4.

McDevitt LM, Smith LD, Somerville KT, et al. A retrospective assessment of pre-treatment variables on the response to darbepoetin alfa after renal transplantation. Am J Transplant 2005; 8: 1948–56.

Mirza AM, Ezzat S, Axelrad AA. Insulin-like growth factor binding protein-1 is elevated in patients with polycythemia vera and stimulates erythroid bust formation in vitro. Blood 1997; 89: 1862–9.

Mitsenef MM, Subat-Dezulovic M, Khoury PR, et al. Increasing incidence of post-kidney transplant anemia in children. Am J Transplant 2005; 7: 1713–18.

Mix T, Kazmi W, Khan S, et al. Anemia: a continuing problem following kidney transplantation. Am J Transplant 2003; 3: 1426–33.

Molnar MZ, Novak M, Ambrus C, et al. Anemia in kidney transplanted patients. Clin Transplant 2005; 19: 825–33.

Morrone LF, Di Paolo S, Logoluso F. Interference of angiotensin-converting enzyme inhibitors in erythropoiesis in kidney transplant recipients. Transplantation 1997; 64: 913–18.

Mrug M, Stopka T, Julian BA, et al. Angiotensin II stimulates proliferation of normal early eythroid progenitors. J Clin Invest 1997; 100: 2310–14.

Nakazawa Y, Hashikura Y, Urata K, et al. Von Willebrand factor-cleaving protease activity in thrombotic microangiopathy after living donor liver transplantation: a case report. Liver Transpl 2003; 9: 1328–33.

Orchard TR, Neild GH. Immune thrombocytopenic purpura presenting in an immunosuppressed patient after renal transplantation. Nephrol Dial Transplant 1997; 12: 2436–8.

Pascoe J, Cullen M. The prevention of febrile neutropenia. Curr Opin Oncol 2006; 18: 325–9.

Peeters R, Sennesael J, De Raeve H, et al. Hemophagocytic syndrome and T-cell lymphoma after kidney transplantation: a case report. Transpl Int 1997; 10: 471–4.

Pham PT, Peng A, Wilkinson A, et al. Cyclosporine- and tacrolimus-associated thrombotic microangiopathy. Am J Kidney Dis 2000; 36: 844–50.

Pomper GJ, Joseph RA, Hartmann EL, et al. Massive immune hemolysis caused by anti-D after dual kidney transplantation. Am J Transplant 2005; 5: 2586–9.

Qunibi WY, Barri Y, Devol E, et al. Factors predictive of post-transplant erythrocytosis. Kidney Int 1991; 40: 1153–9.

Raj A, Bertolone S, Cheerva A. Successful treatment of refractory autoimmune hemolytic anemia with monthly rituximab following nonmyeloablative stem cell transplantation for sickle cell disease. J Pediatr Hematol Oncol 2004; 26: 312–24.

Ramsey G. Red cell antibodies arising from solid organ transplants. Transfusion 1991; 31: 76–86.

Remuzzi G, Riggenenti P, Colledan M, et al. Hemolytic uremic syndrome: a fatal outcome after kidney and liver transplantation performed to correct factor H gene mutation. Am J Transplant 2005; 5: 1146–50.

Reynolds JC, Agodoa LY, Yuan CM, Abbott KC. Thrombotic microangiopathy after renal transplantation in the United States. Am J Kidney Dis 2003; 5: 1058–68.

Rigatto C, Parfrey P, Foley R, et al. Congestive heart failure in renal transplant recipients: risk factors, outcomes, and relationship with ischemic heart diseases. J Am Soc Nephrol 2002; 13: 1084–90.

Risdall RJ, McKenn RW, Nesbit ME, Krivit W. Virus-associated hemophagocytic syndrome. A benign histiocytic proliferation distinct from malignant histiocytosis. Cancer 1979; 44: 993–1002.

Risma KA, Frayer RW, Filipovich AH, Sumegi J. Aberrant maturation of mutant perforin underlies the clinical diversity of hemophagocytic lymphohistiocytosis. J Clin Invest 2006; 116: 182–92.

Robson M, Cote I, Abbs I, et al. Thrombotic microangiopathy with sirolimus-based immunosuppression: potentiation of calcineurin-inhibitor-induced endothelial damage? Am J Transplant 2003; 3: 324–7.

Royer B, Zanetta G, Berard M, et al. A neutropenia suggesting an interaction between valacyclovir and mycophenolate mofetil. Clin Transplant 2003; 17: 158–61.

Ruggenenti P. Post-transplant hemolytic–uremic syndrome. Kidney Int 2002; 62: 1093–26.

Santos ES, Raez LE, Kharfan-Dabaja MA, et al. Survival of renal allograft following de novo hemolytic uremic syndrome after kidney transplantation. Transplant Proc 2003; 35: 1370–4.

Schmid JM, Junge SA, Hossle JP, et al. Transient hemophagocytosis with deficient cellular cytotoxicity, monoclonal immunoglobulin M gammopathy, increased T-cell numbers, and hypomorphic NEMO mutation. Pediatrics 2006; 117: 1049–56.

Schrijvers BF, Flyvbjerg A, De Vries AS. The role of vascular endothelial growth factor (VEGF) in renal pathophysiology. Kidney Int 2004; 65: 2003–17.

Schwimmer J, Nadasdy TA, Kaplan KL, Zand MS. De novo thrombotic microangiopathy in renal transplant recipients: a comparison of hemolytic uremic ssyndrome with localized renal thrombotic microangiopathy. Am J Kidney Dis 2003; 41: 471–9.

Segall L, Moal M-C, Doucet L, et al. Toxoplasmosis-associated hemophagocytic syndrome in renal transplantation. Transpl Int 2006; 19: 76–80.

Shih LY, Huang JY, Lee CT. Insulin-like growth factor I plays a role in regulating erythropoiesis in patients with end-stage renal disease and erythrocytosis. J Am Soc Nephrol 1999; 10: 315–22.

Sumrani NB, Daskalakis P, Miles AM, et al. Erythrocytosis after renal transplantation: a prospective analysis. ASAIO J 1993; 39: 51–5.

Tomonari A, Tojo A, Lseki T, et al. Severe autoimmune thrombocytopenia after allogeneic bone marrow transplantation for aplastic anemia. Int J Hematol 2001; 74: 228–32.

Trimarchi HM, Troung LD, Brennans S, et al. FK 506-associated thrombotic microangiopathy: report of two cases and review of the literature. Transplantation 1999; 67: 539–43.

Trivedi H, Lal SM. A prospective, randomized, open labeled crossover trial of fosinopril and theophylline in post renal transplant erythrocytosis. Ren Fail 2003; 25: 77–86.

Tsai HM, Lian E. Antibodies to Von Willebrand factor-cleaving protease in acute thrombotic thrombocytopenic purpura. N Engl J Med 1998; 339: 1585–94.

Valentini RP, Imam A, Warrier I, et al. Sirolimus rescue for tacrolimus-associated post-transplant autoimmune hemolytic anemia. Pediatr Transplant 2006; 10: 358–61.

Van Biesen W, Vanholder R, Veys N, et al. Efficacy of erythropoietin administration in the treatment of anemia immediately after renal transplantation. Transplantation 2005; 79: 367–8.

Vanrenterghem Y, Ponticelli C, Morales J, et al. Prevalence and management of anemia in renal transplant recipients: a European Survey. Am J Transplant 2003; 3: 835–45.

Verbsky JW, Grossman WJ. Hemophagocytic lymphohistiocytosis: diagnosis, pathophysiology, treatment, and future perspectives. Ann Med 2006; 38: 20–31.

Villanueva J, Lee S, Giannini EH, et al. Natural killer cell dysfunction is a distinguishing feature of systemic onset juvenile rheumatoid arthritis and macrophage activation syndrome. Arthritis Res Ther 2005; 7: R30–7.

Vlahakos DV, Marathias KP, Agroyannis B, Madias NE. Posttransplant erythrocytosis. Kidney Int 2003; 63: 1187–94.

Waiser J, Budde K, Rudolph B, et al. De novo hemolytic uremic syndrome postrenal transplant after cytomegalovirus infection. Am J Kidney Dis 1999; 34: 556–9.

Wang AYM, Yu AWY, Lam CWK, et al. Effects of losartan and enalapril on hemoglobin, circulating erythropoietin, and insulin-like growth factor-1 in patients with and without posttransplant erythrocytosis. Am J Kidney Dis 2002; 39: 600–8.

Weber LT, Shipkava M, Armstrong VW, et al. The pharmacokinetic–pharmacodynamic relationship for total and free mycophenolate mofetil therapy. A report of the German study group on mycophenolate mofetil therapy. J Am Soc Nephrol 2002; 13: 759–68.

West KA, Anderson DR, McAlister VC, et al. Alloimmune thrombocytopenia after organ transplantation. N Engl J Med 1999; 341: 1504–7.

Wickre CG, Norman DJ, Bennison A, et al. Postrenal transplantation erythrocytosis: a review of 53 patients. Kidney Int 1983; 23: 731–7.

Wiener Y, Nakhle RE, Lee MW, et al. Prognostic factors and early resumption of cyclosporine A in renal allograft recipients with thrombotic microangiopathy and hemolytic uremic syndrome. Clin Transplant 1997; 11: 157–62.

Winkelmayer WC, Lorenz M, Kramar P, et al. Percentage of hypochromic cells is an independent risk factor for mortality in kidney transplant recipients. Am J Transplant 2004; 12: 2075–81.

World Health Organization. Nutritional anamias. Report of a WHO scientific group. WHO Tech Rep Ser 1968; 405: 3–37.

Yango AJR, Morrissey P, Gohh R, Wahbeh A. Donor-transmitted parvovirus infection in a kidney transplant recipient presenting as pancytopenia and allograft dysfunction. Transpl Infect Dis 2002; 4: 163–6.

Yassa SK, Blessios G, Marinides G, Venuto RC. Anti-CD20 monoclonal antibody (rituximab) for life-threatening hemolytic–uremic syndrome. Clin Transplant 2005; 19: 423–6.

Yildiz A, Cine N, Akkayo V, et al. Comparison of the effects of enalapril and losartan on posttransplantation erythrocytosis in renal transplant recipients: prospective randomized study. Transplantation 2001; 72: 542–4.

Yorgin PD, Scandling JD, Belson A, et al. Late post-transplant anemia in adult renal transplant recipients. An underrecognized problem? Am J Transplant 2002a; 2: 429–35.

Yorgin PD, Belson A, Sanchez J, et al. Unexpectedly high prevalence of posttransplant anemia in pediatric and young adult renal transplant recipients Am J Kidney Dis 2002b; 40: 1306–18.

Zarifian A, Meleg-Smith S, O'Donovan R, et al. Cyclosporine-associated thrombotic microangiopathy in renal allografts. Kidney Int 1999; 55: 2457–66.

18 THROMBOTIC COMPLICATIONS

Renal allograft thrombosis

Renal allograft thrombosis is responsible for 2–7% of early allograft losses (Irish, 1999). Graft thrombosis is characterized by anuria, and generally causes irreversible loss of function. Venous thrombosis in the transplanted kidney is more common than arterial thrombosis.

Causes of graft thrombosis

Apart from *technical errors,* a number of factors may contribute to graft thrombosis. It is likely that in most cases of renal allograft thrombosis there is an interaction between acquired hypercoagulability as a result of the renal disease, genetic risk of thrombosis, technical problems, characteristics of the kidney, and environmental stress, such as surgery (Table 18.1).

Vascular abnormalities in the donor kidney are often responsible for graft thrombosis. In allografts with multiple renal arteries, up to 36% graft thrombosis has been reported (Dodhia *et al.*, 1991).

Atherosclerosis of the donor or recipient may predispose to graft thrombosis. The donor kidney endothelium may also suffer from reperfusion injury and activation of a procoagulant surface due to cytokines and the recipient immune response (Irish, 1999).

Donor age is also a risk factor. In pediatric transplant patients, recipients of kidneys from cadaver donors less than 5 years of age had a significantly higher thrombosis rate than did recipients from older donor groups (Singh *et al.*, 1997). On the other hand, an increased risk of graft thrombosis has also been reported in kidney transplants from elderly donors (Englesbe *et al.*, 2004).

Cold ischemia time: a retrospective analysis in pediatric renal transplant recipients showed that the duration of cold ischemia was significantly longer in children with graft thrombosis (Singh *et al.*, 1997). In adult transplant recipients, some reports found an association between cold ischemia time and graft thrombosis (Penny *et al.*, 1994), while other studies did not (Bakir *et al.*, 1996).

Age of the recipient: small children are particularly susceptible to graft thrombosis, probably because of the discrepancy in the size of vessels compared with the donor. A review of the North American Pediatric Renal Transplant Cooperative Study reported a graft loss caused by thrombosis in 51 of 2750 renal transplants in children. This represented the main cause of graft failure, 35%, in the first year (Smith *et al.*, 2006).

Genetic coagulation abnormalities: a number of transplant recipients may have an autosomal dominant inherited antithrombin deficiency (Hara and Naito, 2005), factor V Leiden mutation (G1691A), or prothrombin (PT G20210A) and methylenetetrahydrofolate reductase (MTHFR T677T) variants (Heidenreich *et al.*, 2003). In the immediate postoperative period, these abnormalities may concur with dehydration, hypovolemia, and postoperative hypercoagulability in favoring thrombosis. A hypercoagulable state was demonstrated in most episodes of graft thrombosis (Friedman *et al.*, 2001).

Hypovolemia may be a contributing factor to graft thrombosis. Some patients who receive hemodialysis-immediately before transplantation may be submitted to excessive dehydration. In other instances, massive post-transplant polyuria may lead to hypovolemia if water and salt losses are not adequately replaced.

Type of dialysis: hypofibrinolysis is present in patients treated both by long-term hemodialysis and by peritoneal dialysis (Opatrny *et al.*, 2002). Some reports pointed out that arterial allograft thrombosis was more frequent in peritoneal dialysis (7.1%) than in hemodialysis (1.8%) patients (Murphy *et al.*, 1994). However, other studies have reported either no difference in the incidence of renal graft thrombosis between peritoneal dialysis and hemodialysis patients (Penny *et al.*, 1994; Bakir *et al.*, 1996) or an increased risk in hemodialysis patients (Snyder *et al.*, 2002).

Table 18.1   Main causes of renal graft thrombosis

Kidney	Recipient	Drugs
Vascular abnormalities	Small children	OKT3
Donor age	Coagulation abnormalities	Methylprednisolone pulses
Atherosclerosis	Hypovolemia	Calcineurin inhibitors?
Cold ischemia time	Type of dialysis	
Ischemia–reperfusion	Antiphospholipid antibodies	

Delayed graft function: allograft thrombosis is particularly frequent in patients with acute tubular necrosis and delayed graft function (Bakir *et al.*, 1996; Singh *et al.*, 1997).

Antiphospholipid (aPL) syndrome: in a multicenter study, all four patients with antiphospholipid antibodies who did not receive anticoagulation after transplantation lost their allograft within 1 week as a consequence of thrombosis, while only one of the seven patients given anticoagulants had a graft thrombosis (Vaidya *et al.*, 2000).

Immunosuppressive drugs may be responsible for hypercoagulability. Renal graft thrombosis may be triggered by the administration of OKT3, which can exert a procoagulant activity (Lozano *et al.*, 2001; Shankar *et al.*, 2001). The risk is increased in patients pretreated with high-dose intravenous methylprednisolone. Thus, it is recommended that the dose of methylprednisolone, for premedication, should not exceed 8 mg/kg (Abramowicz *et al.*, 1996). Calcineurin inhibitors may cause hypofibrinolysis by enhancing the expression of plasminogen activator inhibitor (Verpooten *et al.*, 1996), but there is no good evidence that they may be responsible for an increased risk of graft thrombosis.

Diagnosis

The peak incidence of vascular thrombosis is around 48 hours after transplantation; exceptionally, graft thrombosis may occur after 7 days of initially good function (Balachandra and Tejani, 1997). A sudden onset of anuria is the main sign of allograft thrombosis. The suspicion of graft thrombosis merits urgent investigation, as it may be potentially correctable, while a delay in the diagnosis or management of this complication can result in graft loss (Humar and Matas, 2005). Echo color Doppler is a simple and reliable technique, and is generally used to evaluate the perfusion of transplanted kidneys, and detect renal artery stenosis or renal vein thrombosis. Contrast-enhanced magnetic resonance angiography is also a valuable non-invasive technique (Jain and Sawhney, 2005).

Prevention and treatment

It is still under discussion whether it is worth giving anticoagulation to transplant recipients at a low risk of thrombosis. Nevertheless, in spite of the hemorrhagic risks of anticoagulation, the prevention of thrombosis with low molecular-weight heparin is considered to be effective and safe (Alkhunaizi *et al.*, 1998). More prolonged heparin administration is recommended in patients at high risk of arterial thrombosis (Irish, 2004). In patients with aPL or congenital coagulation abnormalities, heparin treatment has been recommended in the first postoperative period (McIntyre and Wagenknecht, 2003). Whether long-term anticoagulation is also needed to prevent cardiovascular complications is still unknown. Patients who have lost a first kidney transplant because of graft thrombosis not related to technical errors should receive a thrombophilic work-up before retransplantation. Patients with an identified disorder should undergo adequate prophylaxis before retransplantation. With these cautions, the results of retransplantation may be equivalent to those obtained in primary transplant recipients (Humar *et al.*, 2001).

Treatment of vascular thrombosis is generally disappointing. However, a few cases of renal graft vein thrombosis have been successfully rescued by intra-arterial injections of antifibrinolytic agents, such as

Table 18.2   Risk factors for deep vein thrombosis

General	Transplant-related
Fractures of legs or pelvis	Surgery
Immobilization	Tacrolimus
Heterozygosity for factor V Leiden	Antithymocyte globulins
Antiphospholipid positivity	Proteinuria
Diabetes mellitus	CMV infection
Oral contraception	Left or right ventricular failure
Deficiency of antithrombin III, protein C, protein S	

recombinant tissue plasminogen activator or urokinase (Rouviere et al., 2002), or by percutaneous endoluminal thromboaspiration carried out with full heparinization (Rerolle et al., 2000).

Deep venous thrombosis

The risk for deep vein thrombosis (DVT) in renal transplant patients ranges between 4 and 9% (Humar et al., 1998; Poli et al., 2006). DVT may be asymptomatic in about 39% of cases. It usually occurs in the first 12 months after transplantation, but recurrence may occur in about half of patients (Poli et al., 2005). Rare cases of late renal vein thrombosis have also been reported (Kim et al., 2002).

Risk factors (Table 18.2)

The three main factors that promote DVT are stasis, abnormalities of the vessel wall, and coagulation abnormalities. *Surgery, fractures of the legs or pelvis*, and *immobilization* are major risk factors for deep venous thrombosis. The presence of *heterozygosity for factor V Leiden* (Wutrich et al., 2001) and/or of *antiphospholipid antibodies* (Wagenknecht et al., 1999) may be associated with venous thrombosis and related complications. *Erythrocytosis* may also favor thromboembolic events in transplant patients. An incidence of 10–30% of cases of thrombosis in polycythemic transplant recipients has been reported (Vlahakos et al., 2003). Other subjects at risk are those with a family or personal *history* of venous thrombosis, women taking *oral contraceptives*, and patients with *diabetes mellitus* (Kessler et al., 1998) or *atherosclerosis*.

Following a *transplant operation*, fibrinolysis may be impaired, and coagulation remains activated as a consequence of tissue trauma, inflammation, and the expression of tissue factor. *Cyclosporine* has a procoagulant activity, and may theoretically predispose to vein thrombosis (Dodhia et al., 1991; Verpooten et al., 1996). However, some studies failed to find any difference between transplant patients who took cyclosporine and those who did not (Penny et al., 1994). Although the addition of sirolimus may increase the area-under-the-curve for cyclosporine, it did not result in an increased risk of postoperative DVT in renal transplant recipients (Langer and Kahan, 2003). In a randomized study comparing tacrolimus with cyclosporine, patients assigned to *tacrolimus* had a significantly higher risk of deep vein thrombosis (5%) than those assigned to cyclosporine (0.5%), suggesting a potential thrombogenic effect of tacrolimus (Pirsch et al., 1997). Cases of vein thrombosis caused by *rabbit antithymocyte* globulins have also been desctibed (Mathis and Rao, 2004). Vein thrombosis may also be favored by the occurrence of severe *proteinuria,* which causes urinary loss of antithrombin III and other anticoagulant proteins while causing increased production of fibrinogen and von Willebrand factor in response to hypoalbuminemia. Patients with left or right *ventricular failure* are also at high risk for DVT. *Cytomegalovirus* (CMV) infection can modify the endothelial phenotype from anticoagulant to procoagulant. A frequent association between CMV infection and DVT has been reported in a series (Kazory et al., 2004).

In transplant candidates with an increased risk for DVT, it may be of particular importance to search for thrombophilic factors to prevent thrombotic complications. Investigations should include *factor V Leiden mutation*, *lupus anticoagulant*, and/or *antiphospholipid antibodies*. As the risk of antithrombin III deficiency (0.02–0.2%) and protein S or protein C deficiency (0.1–0.5%) is quite low in the general population, the measurement of these parameters is usually omitted. However, although rarely, inherited antithrombin deficiency may lead to renal failure (Hara and Naito, 2005) and increase the risk for thrombotic complications after transplantation. Screening for a hypercoagulable state is particularly important in transplant patients with previous episodes of DVT (Morrissey *et al.*, 2002).

Complications

Apart from the risks of venous claudication and chronic venous insufficiency, asymptomatic deep vein thrombosis in the popliteal and femoral vein may also precipitate *renal allograft thrombosis* (Ramirez *et al.*, 2002; Giustacchini *et al.*, 2002). However, the most important consequence is *pulmonary embolism*. Available data indicate that more than 95% of pulmonary emboli derive from thrombi in the deep venous system. In renal transplant recipients, about 25% of patients with DVT develop pulmonary embolism (Andrassy *et al.*, 2004). The immediate result of thromboembolism is the complete or partial obstruction of pulmonary arterial blood flow to the lung, with consequent hypoperfusion, alveolar collapse, and often arterial hypoxemia. The extent of embolic obstruction is the key prognostic factor. Most deaths caused by embolism occur within 1 or 2 hours.

Prevention and treatment

General measures to reduce the risk of deep vein thrombosis include subcutaneous heparin, early mobilization, calf stimulators, and graduated compression stockings. Although controlled studies evaluating the role of anticoagulation for the prevention of venous thrombosis are lacking, *low-dose heparin prophylaxis* for 3–4 weeks can be used as standard therapy to prevent the occurrence of DVT after kidney transplantation (Alkhunaizi *et al.*, 1998). Short-term anticoagulation may not be sufficient for concurrent disorders of blood homeostasis, such as elevated levels of antiphospholipid antibodies, lupus anticoagulant, prothrombin gene G20210A polymorphism, or a combined inherited thrombophilia. These patients may need prophylactic anticoagulation with coumarins, starting prior to transplantation and being continued for at least 1 year or even lifelong (Andrassy *et al.*, 2004). Only randomized trials can answer the question concerning the optimal duration and safety of coumarins in this setting. A significant reduction in the incidence of DVT but not its abolition has been reported with the addition of low-dose aspirin (Robertson *et al.*, 2000).

Besides heparin therapy, in the case of ileofemoral venous thrombosis, thrombolytic therapy with urokinase (Tamim and Arous, 1999) or thrombectomy (Sundberg *et al.*, 2004) may be tried in order to rescue the transplanted kidney.

Complications of anticoagulant treatment

Treatment with low-dose heparin is not devoid of complications. A *major hemorrhage* may occur in 2.6% of patients, and injection-site hemorrhage in 10% of patients. A major hemorrhage may be more likely in older patients, in patients with chronic liver disease and impaired renal function, in patients receiving prolonged enoxaparin therapy, and in patients receiving warfarin or a proton pump inhibitor (Ellis *et al.*, 2006).

Type II *heparin-induced thrombocytopenia* (HIT) is a rare but life-threatening event. HIT type II is an immunologically mediated platelet reduction caused by platelet-activating antibodies that increase the risk of *arterial* or *venous thrombosis*. It has been reported in up to 5% of patients receiving unfractionated heparin. Unlike other thrombocytopenic coagulopathies, HIT is associated with a high risk of thromboembolic events if not treated with an appropriate anticoagulant alternative. Diagnosis is dependent on the assessment of platelet reduction, identification of previous heparin exposure, detection of thrombotic complications, and evaluation of laboratory assays. HIT has been well described in surgical patient populations; however, the abdominal organ transplant population is an exception.

HIT should be included in the differential diagnosis of patients presenting with thrombocytopenia after transplantation, in order to prevent or treat thrombotic complications that can pose a risk to patient or graft survival (Anderegg et al., 2005). Nevertheless, platelet count determination must be systematic during heparin therapy (Sturtevant et al., 2006). Treatment consists of alternative thrombin inhibitors such as danaparoid and lepirudin. The platelet count usually requires fewer than 10 days to recover normal values after heparin withdrawal.

Thrombophilic state and graft function

In a prospective study in 165 renal allograft recipients, heterozygous factor V Leiden mutation (G1691A) and PT G20210A and MTHFR T677T variants were significantly associated with rejection rates of 68%, 67%, and 71%, respectively, compared with 35% in patients not carrying these genotypes. Many rejections were vascular. Patients with the genotype PT G20210A had the highest prothrombotic activity pre-transplant and the lowest 1–year graft survival, around 50% (Heidenreich et al., 2003). The presence of antiphospholipid antibodies has also been found to be associated with a higher incidence of acute vascular rejection (Ekberg et al., 2000) and delayed graft function (Wagenknecht et al., 1999).

Other studies found that in transplant recipients with a mutation of factor V Leiden (GA genotype), not only the occurrence of delayed graft function and acute rejection episodes were increased but also the slope of the reciprocal of serum creatinine was significantly worse and the annual increase in daily proteinuria significantly higher than in patients with the normal GG genotype (Hocher et al., 2002). In one study, transplant recipients heterozygous for the G20210A mutation in the prothrombin gene showed a median graft survival significantly lower (65.9 vs. 149 months) than in patients homozygous for the normal PT G20210G allele (Fischereder et al., 2001). On the other hand, another single-center study reported that the 30-day and 1-year graft survivals in recipients with thrombophilic mutations were similar to those in patients without mutations (Pherwani et al., 2003).

References

Abramowicz D, De Pauw L, Le Moine, et al. Prevention of OKT3 nephrotoxicity after kidney transplantation. Kidney Int 1996; 49: S39–43.

Alkhunaizi AM, Olyaei AJ, Barry JM, et al. Efficacy and safety of low molecular weight heparin in renal transplantation. Transplantation 1998; 66: 533–4.

Anderegg BA, Baillie GM, Lin A, Lazarchick J. Heparin-induced thrombocytopenia in a renal transplant recipient. Am J Transplant 2005; 5: 1537–40.

Andrassy J, Zeier M, Andrassy K. Do we need screening for thrombophilia prior to kidney transplantation? Nephrol Dial Transplant 2004; 19 (Suppl 4): 64–8.

Balachandra S, Tejani A. Recurrent vascular thrombosis in an adolescent transplant recipient. J Am Soc Nephrol 1997; 8: 1477–81.

Bakir N, Sluiter WJ, Ploeg RJ, van Son Tegzess AM. Primary renal graft thrombosis. Nephrol Dial Transplant 1996; 11: 140–7.

Dodhia N, Rodby RA, Jensik SC, Korbet SM. Renal transplant arterial thrombosis association with cyclosporine. Am J Kidney Dis 1991; 17: 532–6.

Ekberg H, Svensson PJ, Simanatis M, Dahlbäck B. Factor VR506Q mutation (activated protein C resistance) is an additional risk factor for early renal graft loss associated with acute vascular rejection. Transplantation 2000; 69: 1–5.

Ellis MH, Hadari R, Tchuvrero N, et al. Hemorrhagic complications in patients treated with anticoagulant doses of a low molecular weight heparin (enoxaparin) in routine hospital practice. Clin Appl Thromb Hemost 2006; 12: 199–204.

Englesbe MJ, Punch JD, Armstrong DR, et al. Single-center study of technical graft loss in 714 consecutive renal transplants. Transplantation 2004; 78: 623–6.

Fischereder M, Schneeberger H, Lohse P, et al. Increased rate of renal transplant failure in patients with the G20210A mutation of the prothrombin gene. Am J Kidney Dis 2001; 38: 1061–4.

Friedman GS, Meier-Kriesche HU, Kaplan B, et al. Hypercoagulable states in renal transplant candidates: impact of anticoagulation upon incidence of renal allograft thrombosis. Transplantation 2001; 72: 1073–8.

Giustacchini P, Pisanti F, Citterio F, et al. Renal vein thrombosis after renal transplantation: an important cause of graft loss. Transplant Proc 2002; 34: 2126–7.

Hara T, Naito K. Inherited antithrombin deficiency and end stage renal disease. Med Sci Monit 2005; 11: RA346–54.

Heidenreich S, Juncker K, Wolters H, et al. Outcome of kidney transplantation in patients with inherited thrombophilia: data of a prospective study. J Am Soc Nephrol 2003; 14: 234–9.

Hocher B, Slowinski T, Hauser I, et al. Association of factor V Leiden mutation with delayed graft function, acute rejection episodes and long-term graft dysfunction in kidney transplant recipients. Thromb Haemost 2002; 87: 194–8.

Humar A, Johnson EM, Gillingham KJ, et al. Venous thromboembolic complications after kidney and kidney–pancreas transplantation. Transplantation 1998; 65: 229–34.

Humar A, Key N, Ramcharan T, et al. Kidney retransplants after initial graft loss to vascular thrombosis. Clin Transplant 2001; 15: 6–10.

Humar A, Matas AJ. Surgical complications after kidney transplantation. Semin Dial 2005; 18: 505–10.

Irish A. Renal allograft thrombosis: can thrombophilia explain the inexplicable? Nephrol Dial Transplant 1999; 14: 2297–303.

Irish A. Hypercoagulability in renal transplant recipients. Identifying patients at risk of renal allograft thrombosis and evaluating strategies for prevention. Am J Cardiovasc Drugs 2004; 4: 139–49.

Jain R, Sawhney S. Contrast-enhanced MR angiography (CE-MRA) in the evaluation of vascular complications of renal transplantation. Clin Radiol 2005; 60: 1171–81.

Kazory A, Ducloux D, Coaquette A, et al. Cytomegalovirus-associated venous thromboembolism in renal transplant recipients: a report of 7 cases. Transplantation 2004; 77: 597–9.

Kessler L, Wiesel ML, Attali P, et al. Von Willebrand factor in diabetic angiopathy. Diabetes Metab 1998; 24: 327–36.

Kim JK, Han DJ, Cho KS. Post-infectious diffuse venous stenosis after renal transplantation: duplex ultrasonography and CT angiography. Eur Radiol 2002; 12 (Suppl 3): S118–20.

Langer RM, Kahan BD. Sirolimus does not increase the risk for postoperative thromboembolic events among renal transplant recipients. Transplantation 2003; 76: 318–23.

Lozano M, Oppenheimer F, Cofan F, et al. Platelet procoagulant activity induced in vivo by muromonab-CD3 infusion in uremic patients. Thromb Res 2001; 104: 405–11.

Mathis AS, Rao V. Deep vein thrombosis during rabbit antithymocyte globulin administration. Transplant Proc 2004; 36: 3250–51.

McIntyre JA, Wagenknecht DR. Antiphospholipid antibodies and renal transplantation: a risk assessment. Lupus 2003; 12: 555–9.

Morrissey P, Ramirez PJ, Gohh RY, et al. Management of thrombophilia in renal transplant patients. Am J Transplant 2002; 2872–6.

Murphy BG, Hill CM, Middleton D, et al. Increased renal allograft thrombosis in CAPD patients. Nephrol Dial Transplant 1994; 9: 1165–9.

Opatrny K Jr, Zemanova P, Opatrna S, Vit L. Fibrinolysis in chronic renal failure, dialysis and renal transplantation. Ann Transplant 2002; 7: 34–43.

Penny MJ, Nankivell BJ, Disney APS, et al. Renal graft thrombosis. Transplantation 1994; 58: 565–9.

Pherwani AD, Winter PC, McNamee PT, et al. Is screening for factor V Leiden and prothrombin G20210A mutations in renal transplantation worthwhile? Results of a large single-center UK study. Transplantation 2003; 73: 603–18.

Pirsch JD, Miller J, Deierhoi MH, et al. A comparison of tacrolimus (FK506) and cyclosporine for immunosuppression after cadaveric renal transplantation. FK506 Kidney Transplant Study Group. Transplantation 1997; 63: 977–83.

Poli D, Zanazzi M, Antonucci E, et al. High rate of recurrence in renal transplant recipients after a first episode of venous thromboembolism. Transplantation 2005; 80: 789–93.

Poli D, Zanazzi M, Antonucci E, et al. Renal transplant recipients are at high risk for both symptomatic and asymptomatic deep vein thrombosis. J Thromb Haemost 2006; 4: 988–92.

Ramirez PJ, Gohn RY, Kestin A, et al. Renal allograft loss due to proximal extension of ileofemoral deep venous thrombosis. Clin Transplant 2002; 16: 310–13.

Rerolle JP, Antoine C, Raynaud A, et al. Successful endoluminal thrombo-aspiration of renal graft venous thrombosis. Transpl Int 2000; 13: 82–6.

Robertson AJ, Nargund V, Gray DW, Morris PJ. Low dose aspirin as prophylaxis against renal-vein thrombosis in renal-transplant recipients. Nephrol Dial Transplant 2000; 15: 1865–8.

Rouviere O, Berger P, Beziat C, et al. Acute thrombosis of renal transplant artery: graft salvage by means of intra-arterial fibrinolysis. Transplantation 2002; 73: 403–9.

Shankar R, Bastani B, Salinas-Madrigal L, Sudarshan B. Acute thrombosis of the renal transplant artery after a single dose of OKT3. Am J Nephrol 2001; 21: 141–4.

Singh A, Stablein D, Tejani A. Risk factors for vascular thrombosis in pediatric renal transplantation. Transplantation 1997; 63: 1263–7.

Smith JM, Stablein D, Singh A, et al. Decreased risk of renal allograft thrombosis associated with interleukin-2 receptor antagonists: a report of the NAPRTCS. Am J Transplant 2006; 6: 585–8.

Snyder JJ, Kasiske BL, Gilbertson T, Collins AJ. A comparison of transplant outcomes in peritoneal and hemodialysis patients. Kidney Int 2002; 62: 1423–30.

Sturtevant JM, Pillans PI, Mackenzie F, Gibbs HH. Heparin-induced thrombocytopenia: recent experience in a large teaching hospital. Intern Med J 2006; 36: 431–6.

Sundberg AK, Rohr MS, Hartmann EL, et al. Conversion to sirolimus-based maintenance immunosuppression using daclizumab bridge therapy in renal transplant recipients. Clin Transplant 2004; 18 (Suppl 12): 61–6.

Tamim W, Arous E. Thrombolytic therapy: the treatment of choice for iliac vein thrombosis in the presence of kidney transplant. Ann Vasc Surg 1999; 13: 436–8.

Vaidya S, Sellers R, Kimball P, et al. Frequency, potential risk and therapeutic intervention in end-stage renal disease patients with antiphospholipid antibody syndrome: a multicenter study. Transplantation 2000; 69: 1348–52.

Verpooten GA, Cools FJ, Van der Planken MG, et al. Elevated plasminogen activator inhibitor levels in cyclosporin-treated renal allograft recipients. Nephrol Dial Transplant 1996; 11: 347–51.

Vlahakos DV, Marathias KP, Agroyannis B, Madias NE. Posttransplant erythrocytosis. Kidney Int 2003; 63: 1187–94.

Wagenknecht DR, Becker DG, LeFor WM, McIntyre JA. Antiphospholipid antibodies are a risk factor for early renal allograft failure. Transplantation 1999; 68: 241–6.

Wutrich RP, Cicvara-Muzar S, Booy C, et al. Heterozygosity for the factor V Leiden (G1691A) mutation predisposes renal transplant recipients to thrombotic complications and graft loss. Transplantation 2001; 72: 549–50.

INDEX